Communications in Computer and Information Science 374

Constantine Stephanidis (Ed.)

HCI International 2013 – Posters' Extended Abstracts

International Conference, HCI International 2013
Las Vegas, NV, USA, July 21-26, 2013
Proceedings, Part II

Springer

Volume Editor

Constantine Stephanidis
Foundation for Research and Technology - Hellas (FORTH)
Institute of Computer Science (ICS)
N. Plastira 100, Vassilika Vouton
70013 Heraklion, Crete, Greece
and
University of Crete
Department of Computer Science, Crete, Greece
E-mail: cs@ics.forth.gr

ISSN 1865-0929 e-ISSN 1865-0937
ISBN 978-3-642-39475-1 e-ISBN 978-3-642-39476-8
DOI 10.1007/978-3-642-39476-8
Springer Heidelberg Dordrecht London New York

Library of Congress Control Number: 2013942203

CR Subject Classification (1998): H.5, K.3, J.3, J.5, H.3, K.4, I.2.7, K.6.5

Typesetting: Camera-ready by author, data conversion by Scientific Publishing Services, Chennai, India

Printed on acid-free paper

Springer is part of Springer Science+Business Media (www.springer.com)

Foreword

The 15th International Conference on Human–Computer Interaction, HCI International 2013, was held in Las Vegas, Nevada, USA, 21–26 July 2013, incorporating 12 conferences / thematic areas:

Thematic areas:

- Human–Computer Interaction
- Human Interface and the Management of Information

Affiliated conferences:

- 10th International Conference on Engineering Psychology and Cognitive Ergonomics
- 7th International Conference on Universal Access in Human–Computer Interaction
- 5th International Conference on Virtual, Augmented and Mixed Reality
- 5th International Conference on Cross-Cultural Design
- 5th International Conference on Online Communities and Social Computing
- 7th International Conference on Augmented Cognition
- 4th International Conference on Digital Human Modeling and Applications in Health, Safety, Ergonomics and Risk Management
- 2nd International Conference on Design, User Experience and Usability
- 1st International Conference on Distributed, Ambient and Pervasive Interactions
- 1st International Conference on Human Aspects of Information Security, Privacy and Trust

A total of 5210 individuals from academia, research institutes, industry and governmental agencies from 70 countries submitted contributions, and 1666 papers and 303 posters were included in the program. These papers address the latest research and development efforts and highlight the human aspects of design and use of computing systems. The papers accepted for presentation thoroughly cover the entire field of Human–Computer Interaction, addressing major advances in knowledge and effective use of computers in a variety of application areas.

This volume, edited by Constantine Stephanidis, contains extended abstracts of posters addressing the following major topics:

- Learning and Education
- Health and Medicine
- Media, Art and Culture
- Transport
- Web and Social Media

- Information Search and Retrieval
- Work, Collaboration and Creativity
- Text and Storytelling
- Agents, Avatars and Robots
- Smart Environments
- Virtual and Mixed Environments
- Security and Privacy

The remaining volumes of the HCI International 2013 proceedings are:

- Volume 1, LNCS 8004, Human–Computer Interaction: Human-Centred Design Approaches, Methods, Tools and Environments (Part I), edited by Masaaki Kurosu
- Volume 2, LNCS 8005, Human–Computer Interaction: Applications and Services (Part II), edited by Masaaki Kurosu
- Volume 3, LNCS 8006, Human–Computer Interaction: Users and Contexts of Use (Part III), edited by Masaaki Kurosu
- Volume 4, LNCS 8007, Human–Computer Interaction: Interaction Modalities and Techniques (Part IV), edited by Masaaki Kurosu
- Volume 5, LNCS 8008, Human–Computer Interaction: Towards Intelligent and Implicit Interaction (Part V), edited by Masaaki Kurosu
- Volume 6, LNCS 8009, Universal Access in Human–Computer Interaction: Design Methods, Tools and Interaction Techniques for eInclusion (Part I), edited by Constantine Stephanidis and Margherita Antona
- Volume 7, LNCS 8010, Universal Access in Human–Computer Interaction: User and Context Diversity (Part II), edited by Constantine Stephanidis and Margherita Antona
- Volume 8, LNCS 8011, Universal Access in Human–Computer Interaction: Applications and Services for Quality of Life (Part III), edited by Constantine Stephanidis and Margherita Antona
- Volume 9, LNCS 8012, Design, User Experience, and Usability: Design Philosophy, Methods and Tools (Part I), edited by Aaron Marcus
- Volume 10, LNCS 8013, Design, User Experience, and Usability: Health, Learning, Playing, Cultural, and Cross-Cultural User Experience (Part II), edited by Aaron Marcus
- Volume 11, LNCS 8014, Design, User Experience, and Usability: User Experience in Novel Technological Environments (Part III), edited by Aaron Marcus
- Volume 12, LNCS 8015, Design, User Experience, and Usability: Web, Mobile and Product Design (Part IV), edited by Aaron Marcus
- Volume 13, LNCS 8016, Human Interface and the Management of Information: Information and Interaction Design (Part I), edited by Sakae Yamamoto

- Volume 14, LNCS 8017, Human Interface and the Management of Information: Information and Interaction for Health, Safety, Mobility and Complex Environments (Part II), edited by Sakae Yamamoto
- Volume 15, LNCS 8018, Human Interface and the Management of Information: Information and Interaction for Learning, Culture, Collaboration and Business (Part III), edited by Sakae Yamamoto
- Volume 16, LNAI 8019, Engineering Psychology and Cognitive Ergonomics: Understanding Human Cognition (Part I), edited by Don Harris
- Volume 17, LNAI 8020, Engineering Psychology and Cognitive Ergonomics: Applications and Services (Part II), edited by Don Harris
- Volume 18, LNCS 8021, Virtual, Augmented and Mixed Reality: Designing and Developing Augmented and Virtual Environments (Part I), edited by Randall Shumaker
- Volume 19, LNCS 8022, Virtual, Augmented and Mixed Reality: Systems and Applications (Part II), edited by Randall Shumaker
- Volume 20, LNCS 8023, Cross-Cultural Design: Methods, Practice and Case Studies (Part I), edited by P.L. Patrick Rau
- Volume 21, LNCS 8024, Cross-Cultural Design: Cultural Differences in Everyday Life (Part II), edited by P.L. Patrick Rau
- Volume 22, LNCS 8025, Digital Human Modeling and Applications in Health, Safety, Ergonomics and Risk Management: Healthcare and Safety of the Environment and Transport (Part I), edited by Vincent G. Duffy
- Volume 23, LNCS 8026, Digital Human Modeling and Applications in Health, Safety, Ergonomics and Risk Management: Human Body Modeling and Ergonomics (Part II), edited by Vincent G. Duffy
- Volume 24, LNAI 8027, Foundations of Augmented Cognition, edited by Dylan D. Schmorrow and Cali M. Fidopiastis
- Volume 25, LNCS 8028, Distributed, Ambient and Pervasive Interactions, edited by Norbert Streitz and Constantine Stephanidis
- Volume 26, LNCS 8029, Online Communities and Social Computing, edited by A. Ant Ozok and Panayiotis Zaphiris
- Volume 27, LNCS 8030, Human Aspects of Information Security, Privacy and Trust, edited by Louis Marinos and Ioannis Askoxylakis
- Volume 28, CCIS 373, HCI International 2013 Posters Proceedings (Part I), edited by Constantine Stephanidis

I would like to thank the Program Chairs and the members of the Program Boards of all affiliated conferences and thematic areas, listed below, for their contribution to the highest scientific quality and the overall success of the HCI International 2013 conference.

This conference could not have been possible without the continuous support and advice of the Founding Chair and Conference Scientific Advisor, Prof. Gavriel Salvendy, as well as the dedicated work and outstanding efforts of the Communications Chair and Editor of HCI International News, Abbas Moallem.

I would also like to thank for their contribution towards the smooth organization of the HCI International 2013 Conference the members of the Human–Computer Interaction Laboratory of ICS-FORTH, and in particular George Paparoulis, Maria Pitsoulaki, Stavroula Ntoa, Maria Bouhli and George Kapnas.

May 2013

Constantine Stephanidis
General Chair, HCI International 2013

Organization

Human–Computer Interaction

Program Chair: Masaaki Kurosu, Japan

Jose Abdelnour-Nocera, UK
Sebastiano Bagnara, Italy
Simone Barbosa, Brazil
Tomas Berns, Sweden
Nigel Bevan, UK
Simone Borsci, UK
Apala Lahiri Chavan, India
Sherry Chen, Taiwan
Kevin Clark, USA
Torkil Clemmensen, Denmark
Xiaowen Fang, USA
Shin'ichi Fukuzumi, Japan
Vicki Hanson, UK
Ayako Hashizume, Japan
Anzai Hiroyuki, Italy
Sheue-Ling Hwang, Taiwan
Wonil Hwang, South Korea
Minna Isomursu, Finland
Yong Gu Ji, South Korea
Esther Jun, USA
Mitsuhiko Karashima, Japan
Kyungdoh Kim, South Korea
Heidi Krömker, Germany
Chen Ling, USA
Yan Liu, USA
Zhengjie Liu, P.R. China
Loïc Martínez Normand, Spain
Chang S. Nam, USA
Naoko Okuizumi, Japan
Noriko Osaka, Japan
Philippe Palanque, France
Hans Persson, Sweden
Ling Rothrock, USA
Naoki Sakakibara, Japan
Dominique Scapin, France
Guangfeng Song, USA
Sanjay Tripathi, India
Chui Yin Wong, Malaysia
Toshiki Yamaoka, Japan
Kazuhiko Yamazaki, Japan
Ryoji Yoshitake, Japan
Silvia Zimmermann, Switzerland

Human Interface and the Management of Information

Program Chair: Sakae Yamamoto, Japan

Hans-Jorg Bullinger, Germany
Alan Chan, Hong Kong
Gilsoo Cho, South Korea
Jon R. Gunderson, USA
Shin'ichi Fukuzumi, Japan
Michitaka Hirose, Japan
Jhilmil Jain, USA
Yasufumi Kume, Japan
Mark Lehto, USA
Hiroyuki Miki, Japan
Hirohiko Mori, Japan
Fiona Fui-Hoon Nah, USA
Shogo Nishida, Japan
Robert Proctor, USA
Youngho Rhee, South Korea
Katsunori Shimohara, Japan

Engineering Psychology and Cognitive Ergonomics

Program Chair: Don Harris, UK

Universal Access in Human–Computer Interaction

Program Chairs: Constantine Stephanidis, Greece, and Margherita Antona, Greece

Virtual, Augmented and Mixed Reality

Program Chair: Randall Shumaker, USA

Waymon Armstrong, USA
Juan Cendan, USA
Rudy Darken, USA
Cali M. Fidopiastis, USA
Charles Hughes, USA
David Kaber, USA
Hirokazu Kato, Japan
Denis Laurendeau, Canada
Fotis Liarokapis, UK
Mark Livingston, USA
Michael Macedonia, USA
Gordon Mair, UK
Jose San Martin, Spain
Jacquelyn Morie, USA
Albert "Skip" Rizzo, USA
Kay Stanney, USA
Christopher Stapleton, USA
Gregory Welch, USA

Cross-Cultural Design

Program Chair: P.L. Patrick Rau, P.R. China

Pilsung Choe, P.R. China
Henry Been-Lirn Duh, Singapore
Vanessa Evers, The Netherlands
Paul Fu, USA
Zhiyong Fu, P.R. China
Fu Guo, P.R. China
Sung H. Han, Korea
Toshikazu Kato, Japan
Dyi-Yih Michael Lin, Taiwan
Rungtai Lin, Taiwan
Sheau-Farn Max Liang, Taiwan
Liang Ma, P.R. China
Alexander Mädche, Germany
Katsuhiko Ogawa, Japan
Tom Plocher, USA
Kerstin Röse, Germany
Supriya Singh, Australia
Hsiu-Ping Yueh, Taiwan
Liang (Leon) Zeng, USA
Chen Zhao, USA

Online Communities and Social Computing

Program Chairs: A. Ant Ozok, USA, and Panayiotis Zaphiris, Cyprus

Areej Al-Wabil, Saudi Arabia
Leonelo Almeida, Brazil
Bjørn Andersen, Norway
Chee Siang Ang, UK
Aneesha Bakharia, Australia
Ania Bobrowicz, UK
Paul Cairns, UK
Farzin Deravi, UK
Andri Ioannou, Cyprus
Slava Kisilevich, Germany
Niki Lambropoulos, Greece
Effie Law, Switzerland
Soo Ling Lim, UK
Fernando Loizides, Cyprus
Gabriele Meiselwitz, USA
Anthony Norcio, USA
Elaine Raybourn, USA
Panote Siriaraya, UK
David Stuart, UK
June Wei, USA

Augmented Cognition

Program Chairs: Dylan D. Schmorrow, USA, and Cali M. Fidopiastis, USA

Robert Arrabito, Canada
Richard Backs, USA
Chris Berka, USA
Joseph Cohn, USA
Martha E. Crosby, USA
Julie Drexler, USA
Ivy Estabrooke, USA
Chris Forsythe, USA
Wai Tat Fu, USA
Rodolphe Gentili, USA
Marc Grootjen, The Netherlands
Jefferson Grubb, USA
Ming Hou, Canada
Santosh Mathan, USA
Rob Matthews, Australia
Dennis McBride, USA
Jeff Morrison, USA
Mark A. Neerincx, The Netherlands
Denise Nicholson, USA
Banu Onaral, USA
Lee Sciarini, USA
Kay Stanney, USA
Roy Stripling, USA
Rob Taylor, UK
Karl van Orden, USA

Digital Human Modeling and Applications in Health, Safety, Ergonomics and Risk Management

Program Chair: Vincent G. Duffy, USA and Russia

Karim Abdel-Malek, USA
Giuseppe Andreoni, Italy
Daniel Carruth, USA
Eliza Yingzi Du, USA
Enda Fallon, Ireland
Afzal Godil, USA
Ravindra Goonetilleke, Hong Kong
Bo Hoege, Germany
Waldemar Karwowski, USA
Zhizhong Li, P.R. China
Kang Li, USA
Tim Marler, USA
Michelle Robertson, USA
Matthias Rötting, Germany
Peter Vink, The Netherlands
Mao-Jiun Wang, Taiwan
Xuguang Wang, France
Jingzhou (James) Yang, USA
Xiugan Yuan, P.R. China
Gülcin Yücel Hoge, Germany

Design, User Experience, and Usability

Program Chair: Aaron Marcus, USA

Sisira Adikari, Australia
Ronald Baecker, Canada
Arne Berger, Germany
Jamie Blustein, Canada
Ana Boa-Ventura, USA
Jan Brejcha, Czech Republic
Lorenzo Cantoni, Switzerland
Maximilian Eibl, Germany

Anthony Faiola, USA
Emilie Gould, USA
Zelda Harrison, USA
Rüdiger Heimgärtner, Germany
Brigitte Herrmann, Germany
Steffen Hess, Germany
Kaleem Khan, Canada
Jennifer McGinn, USA
Francisco Rebelo, Portugal
Michael Renner, Switzerland
Kerem Rızvanoğlu, Turkey
Marcelo Soares, Brazil
Christian Sturm, Germany
Michele Visciola, Italy

Distributed, Ambient and Pervasive Interactions

Program Chairs: Norbert Streitz, Germany, and Constantine Stephanidis, Greece

Emile Aarts, The Netherlands
Adnan Abu-Dayya, Qatar
Juan Carlos Augusto, UK
Boris de Ruyter, The Netherlands
Anind Dey, USA
Dimitris Grammenos, Greece
Nuno M. Guimaraes, Portugal
Shin'ichi Konomi, Japan
Carsten Magerkurth, Switzerland
Christian Müller-Tomfelde, Australia
Fabio Paternó, Italy
Gilles Privat, France
Harald Reiterer, Germany
Carsten Röcker, Germany
Reiner Wichert, Germany
Woontack Woo, South Korea
Xenophon Zabulis, Greece

Human Aspects of Information Security, Privacy and Trust

Program Chairs: Louis Marinos, ENISA EU, and Ioannis Askoxylakis, Greece

Claudio Agostino Ardagna, Italy
Zinaida Benenson, Germany
Daniele Catteddu, Italy
Raoul Chiesa, Italy
Bryan Cline, USA
Sadie Creese, UK
Jorge Cuellar, Germany
Marc Dacier, USA
Dieter Gollmann, Germany
Kirstie Hawkey, Canada
Jaap-Henk Hoepman, The Netherlands
Cagatay Karabat, Turkey
Angelos Keromytis, USA
Ayako Komatsu, Japan
Ronald Leenes, The Netherlands
Javier Lopez, Spain
Steve Marsh, Canada
Gregorio Martinez, Spain
Emilio Mordini, Italy
Yuko Murayama, Japan
Masakatsu Nishigaki, Japan
Aljosa Pasic, Spain
Milan Petković, The Netherlands
Joachim Posegga, Germany
Jean-Jacques Quisquater, Belgium
Damien Sauveron, France
George Spanoudakis, UK
Kerry-Lynn Thomson, South Africa

Julien Touzeau, France
Theo Tryfonas, UK
João Vilela, Portugal
Claire Vishik, UK
Melanie Volkamer, Germany

External Reviewers

Maysoon Abulkhair, Saudi Arabia
Ilia Adami, Greece
Vishal Barot, UK
Stephan Böhm, Germany
Vassilis Charissis, UK
Francisco Cipolla-Ficarra, Spain
Maria De Marsico, Italy
Marc Fabri, UK
David Fonseca, Spain
Linda Harley, USA
Yasushi Ikei, Japan
Wei Ji, USA
Nouf Khashman, Canada
John Killilea, USA
Iosif Klironomos, Greece
Ute Klotz, Switzerland
Maria Korozi, Greece
Kentaro Kotani, Japan
Vassilis Kouroumalis, Greece
Stephanie Lackey, USA
Janelle LaMarche, USA
Asterios Leonidis, Greece
Nickolas Macchiarella, USA
George Margetis, Greece
Matthew Marraffino, USA
Joseph Mercado, USA
Claudia Mont'Alvão, Brazil
Yoichi Motomura, Japan
Karsten Nebe, Germany
Stavroula Ntoa, Greece
Martin Osen, Austria
Stephen Prior, UK
Farid Shirazi, Canada
Jan Stelovsky, USA
Sarah Swierenga, USA

HCI International 2014

The 16th International Conference on Human–Computer Interaction, HCI International 2014, will be held jointly with the affiliated conferences in the summer of 2014. It will cover a broad spectrum of themes related to Human–Computer Interaction, including theoretical issues, methods, tools, processes and case studies in HCI design, as well as novel interaction techniques, interfaces and applications. The proceedings will be published by Springer. More information about the topics, as well as the venue and dates of the conference, will be announced through the HCI International Conference series website: http://www.hci-international.org/

General Chair
Professor Constantine Stephanidis
University of Crete and ICS-FORTH
Heraklion, Crete, Greece
Email: cs@ics.forth.gr

Table of Contents – Part II

Learning and Education

Health and Medicine

Media, Art and Culture

Transport

Web and Social Media

Information Search and Retrieval

Work, Collaboration and Creativity

Text and Storytelling

Agents, Avatars and Robots

Smart Environments

Virtual and Mixed Environments

Security and Privacy

Table of Contents – Part I

HCI Design Approaches, Methods and Techniques

Usability Methods, Techniques and Studies

Universal Access and eInclusion

Multimodal and Ambient Interaction

Cognitive and Psychological Aspects of Interaction

Ergonomic and Human Modelling Issues

Capturing Gaze, Biosignals and Brainwaves

Development Environments

Part I
Learning and Education

Interactive Screening for Learning Difficulties: Analyzing Visual Patterns of Reading Arabic Scripts with Eye Tracking

Arwa Al-Edaily[1], Areej Al-Wabil[2], and Yousef Al-Ohali[3]

[1] Information Technology Dept,
[2] Software Engineering Dept,
[3] Computer Science Dept
College of Computer and Information Sciences, King Saud University, Saudi Arabia
{aedaily,aalwabil,yousef}@ksu.edu.sa

Abstract. Dyslexia Explorer is a screening program for dyslexia that focuses on mapping visual patterns of reading Arabic scripts to reading difficulties. Dyslexia Explorer is designed to process the eye gaze patterns exhibited by readers with Specific Learning Difficulties (SpLDs) in screening sessions with Arabic stimuli. The screening is based on gaze measures of eye fixation duration for the Area Of Interest (AOI), mean fixation duration, fixation count for the AOI, total fixations count, backward patterns (within words, lines and paragraph). The system is a novel contribution in screening for reading difficulties in the Arabic language. It helps in diagnosing dyslexia by specifying reading deficits, providing objective gaze metrics and linking them to phonological processing difficulties of readers.

Keywords: Dyslexia, Learning Difficulties, Specific Learning Difficulty, Reading Difficulties, Eye tracking, SpLD.

1 Introduction

Specific Learning Difficulties (SpLDs) such as Dyslexia are persistent problems in reading and information processing affecting an estimated 5 to 10% of the Arabic-speaking population [1-3]. Over the past 30 years, abundant evidence has accumulated to indicate that erratic eye movements of people with SpLDs are a reflection of a language processing deficit [5]. In this paper, we describe the design and development of an interactive screening system, called Dyslexia Explorer, for examining visual attention and reading patterns of individuals in their processing of Arabic scripts.

Eye tracking is used to capture visual attention which was otherwise unattainable to specialists dealing with diagnosing this 'invisible disability' [4]. In this system, several near-infrared illuminators, invisible to the reader's eye, create reflection patterns on the cornea. At a high sampling rate of 120Hz, image sensors register the image of the reader's eyes. Image processing is utilized to create a 3D model of the reader's eyes, accurately detect the pupil's position, and identify the correct reflections from the illuminators and their exact positions. A mathematical model of the eye is

C. Stephanidis (Ed.): Posters, Part II, HCII 2013, CCIS 374, pp. 3–7, 2013.

used to calculate the eyes' position in the space allocated for displaying the Arabic script stimuli and the reader's point of gaze. Freedom of head movement was 30x22x30 cm. Head movement compensation algorithms ensured accuracy of gaze detection and precision when subjects, especially children with co-morbid attention deficit and hyperactivity disorders, moved during recordings in relation to the eye tracker. This system is the first Arabic language screening tool, based on visual attention analysis, in the domain of assistive technologies for SpLDs.

2 Dyslexia Explorer

Dyslexia Explorer is a screening program based on visual attention patterns in reading Arabic scripts. It is designed to capture eye gaze of readers in their processing of Arabic script and to decode visual patterns of reading in Arabic and classify them into phonological difficulties in order to help specialists in the SpLDs area to identify problems that individuals with SpLDs experience and design effective remedial programs. The context of use for this interactive screening program and its conceptual design were reported in [11]; and is illustrated in Fig. 1 in which an unobtrusive eye tracking device is placed within range of computer monitor viewing for readers.

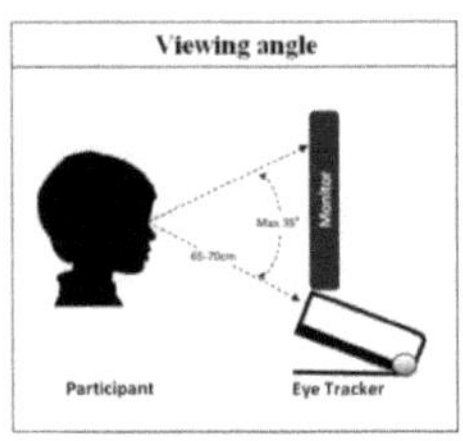

Fig. 1. Setup for the Dyslexia Explorer system

A structured system analysis and design approach was adopted to effectively develop the algorithmic eye gaze analysis screening program. This automated processing depends on some measurements, gathered by eye tracking, to analyze the patterns and produce analytical reports of patterns for special-education practitioners to assist then in identifying the specific reading difficulties of subjects and develop effective remedial programs. The measures are chosen based on the eye gaze metrics and patterns examined in an exploratory study described in [1]. Analysis is based on what is called Area Of Interest (AOI) for each stimuli. The AOIs are for individual words and lines within a segment of Arabic script as depicted in Fig. 2.

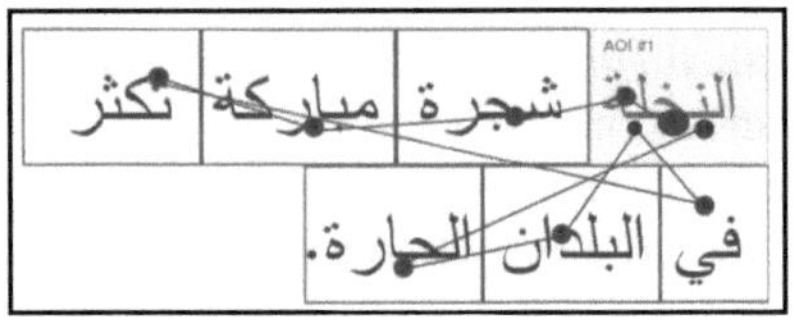

Fig. 2. Areas of Interest for Analyzing Visual Reading Patterns in Arabic Scripts

The system is comprised five key components as illustrated in the architecture in Fig. 3. The first component is "Manage participants" this component manages participants' information either add new participant's info or edit it. This component is comprised of demographic data and cognitive profile of subjects, which can be used in the exploratory component of the system when eye gaze metrics are used to explore the measures that can differentiate between struggling readers and normal readers. The next two components are calculation processes that depend on the eye gaze measurements. The eye gaze raw data are files generated from the eye tracker and contain all information related to each participant's recorded session. The information include: eye fixation coordinates, time stamp for each fixation, and index for each fixation. The component "Filter raw gaze data" filters eye gazes into fixations and saccades based on the Filtering Fixation Algorithm and then the component "Analyze fixations" analyzes and processes fixations to calculate measurements mentioned before. The component "Format and produce report" produces the main output in this system which is an analytical report of aggregate data from all subjects (i.e. 'profile') that is aimed at aiding specialists in their exploration of the dataset. Although normative screening data does not exists for Arabic readers, the specialist can examine the percentile of where the subject exists with regards to different eye gaze measures. This report contains participant information and his/her reading analysis measurements (Mean fixation duration, total fixation count, backward patterns, etc). Finally, "Explore thresholds" component helps specialists to have general overview about results in comparison to the scores recorded previously. Also, shows the degrees of differences between participants. This component plays an important role to design remedial plans for dyslexic children.

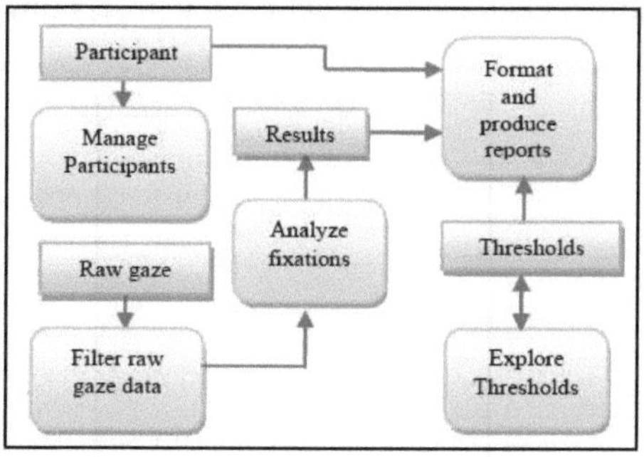

Fig. 3. Architecture of the Dyslexia Explorer system

3 Visual Attention Analysis with Eye Tracking

The Dyslexia Explorer system mainly consists of two processes: Fixation Filtering, and Reading Analysis. The system filters raw gaze data (contains eyes' x/y coordinates, timestamps, and validity code of each gaze), captured by the eye tracker, to fixations and saccades using Fixation Filtering Algorithm. Filtering fixations is the process of grouping raw gaze data collected from the eye tracker to fixation points and saccades lines. This process is important because the tracking process generates fixation points that are close in positions and time stamps. In addition, raw fixations are related to fine-course analysis which hinder the process of synchronizing or mapping them to human cognitive processes [7,4]. The filtering process starts with mapping the gaze data points to the scene coordinates (i.e. viewing plane) [7]. Following that, it classifies gaze points to fixations or saccades depending on separation thresholds related to the algorithm specification [8]. The Dyslexia Explorer system uses Fixation Filtering Algorithm; a velocity algorithm with two thresholds: velocity and distance [9,10]. This algorithm is chosen because it is suitable for the off-line processing mode as in this system [8].

The system analyzes the fixations under number of measurements (baseline measures were described in [1]): total fixation duration for all Areas of Interest (AOI) in the stimuli, mean fixation duration, fixations' count for all AOI in stimulus and backwards saccades (regressive saccades). The backward saccade may pass on one word, many words or cross lines in the stimulus. An example of this analysis is depicted in Fig. 4. Part-1 of the Reading Analysis component is comprised of visual attention overlaid on the stimulus that has been read. This is illustrated with fixations on the AOI (the green boundaries in Fig. 4). This image shows the raw gaze data of recorded reading after filtered to eye fixations. The circles in the image are the fixations while the lines are saccades. The size of the fixations links directly to the duration of this fixation during the reading process. It helps SpLD practitioners in understanding the flow of the reading and the difficult words that the child spent more time in reading them (this is often depicted in visual scan-paths with several fixations on an AOI or fixations with a relatively large radius). These visual patterns facilitate mapping reading abilities of the individuals to the phonological processing difficulties exhibited in the reading of the stimuli. Part-2 presents quantitative measurements of visual attention distribution in reading; each measure depicted in a separate tab.

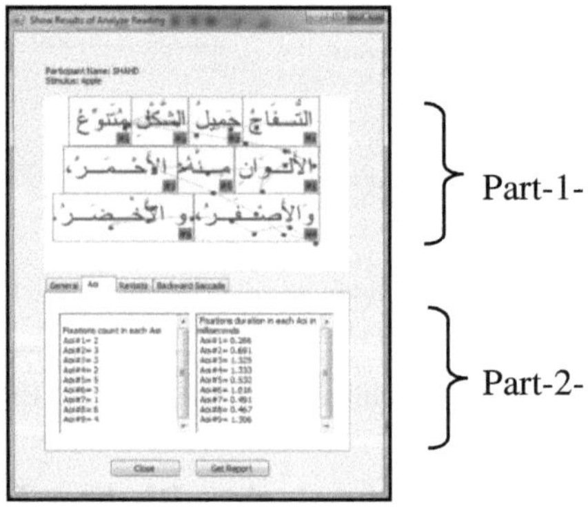

Fig. 4. Reading Analysis in Dyslexia Explorer

4 Conclusion

In this paper, we described the design and development of an interactive screening system for dyslexia in Arabic. The system's key contribution is providing SpLD practitioners with objective screening tools for dyslexia in Arabic by specifying reading deficits, and linking gaze metrics to phonological processing difficulties. Experimental evaluations comparing visual reading patterns of controls and participants with SpLDs revealed marked differences in the intensity and visual scan-patterns of gaze between the two groups. Evaluations provided evidence of accuracy in capturing visual patterns, and efficiency in screening for irregular visual exploration patterns, particularly regression reading patterns and abnormal intensity on words for struggling readers.

Acknowledgment. This project was supported in part by Research Group Grant RGP-VPP-157 from the Deanship of Scientific Research in King Saud University. Authors would like to thank the staff at the 186' elementary school for their help in our experimental evaluations. Our thanks also to Mrs. Areej Al-Salamah, an SpLD specialist from King Saud University, for her contribution in test phases of this project's development cycle.

References

1. Al-Wabil, A., Al-Sheaha, M.: Towards an Interactive Screening Program for Developmental Dyslexia: Eye Movement Analysis in Reading Arabic Texts. In: Miesenberger, K., Klaus, J., Zagler, W., Karshmer, A. (eds.) ICCHP 2010, Part II. LNCS, vol. 6180, pp. 25–32. Springer, Heidelberg (2010)
2. Abu-Rabia, S.: Reading Arabic Texts: Effects of Text type, Reader Type, and Vowelization. Reading and Writing: An Interdisciplinary Journal 10, 106–119 (1998)
3. Abu-Rabia, S.: Dyslexia in Arabic. In: Smyth, I., Everatt, J., Salter, R. (eds.) International Book of Dyslexia: A Cross-Language Comparison and Practice Guide, pp. 31–38. John Wiley & Sons, West Sussex (2004)
4. Duchowski, A.: Eye Tracking Methodology: Theory and Practice, 2nd edn. Springer, London (2007)
5. Rayner, K.: Eye Movements in Reading and Information Processing: 20 Years of Research. Psychological Bulletin 124, 372–422 (1998)
6. Savage, R., Stuart, M., Hill, V.: The role of scaffolding errors in reading development: Evidence from a longitudinal and a correlation study. British Journal of Educational Psychology 71, 1–13 (2001)
7. obii Team, Tobii Studio 2.X User Manual, Tobii Technology (2010)
8. Salvucci, D., Goldberg, J.: Identifying fixations and saccades in eye-tracking protocols. In: Proc. Symposium on Eye Tracking Research & Applications (ETRA 2000), Palm Beach Gardens, pp. 71–78 (2000)
9. obii Team, Tobii Studio 2.3 Release Notes, Tobii Technology (2011)
10. Ollson, P.: Real-time and Offline Filters for Eye Tracking: Master's degree Project, KTH Electrical Engineering (2007)
11. Al-Edaily, A., et al.: Dyslexia Explorer: A Screening System for Learning Difficulties in the Arabic Language Using Eye Tracking. In: Proc. SouthCHI: International Conference on Human Factors in Computing and Informatics, Maribor, Slovenia (2013)

Android vs. iOS Interaction Design Study for a Student Multiplatform App

Abimael Barea, Xavier Ferre, and Lorenzo Villarroel

Universidad Politécnica de Madrid
Campus de Montegancedo
28660 - Boadilla del Monte (Madrid), Spain
{abimaelbarea,villarroel.lorenzo}@gmail.com,
xavier.ferre@upm.es

Abstract. When aiming to develop a multiplatform mobile application or app there is a dichotomy between following each platform interaction philosophy and creating a common cross-platform interaction design. iOS and Android are the two most common mobile platforms used by university students, and they are the obvious choice when planning to develop a mobile app for students in just two platforms. We have compared the particularities of the interaction philosophy of both, and we have studied how four popular apps have addressed the contradiction between following each platform interaction philosophy and having a common interaction design between iOS and Android versions. The results show that there are three possible approaches for multiplatform interaction design, with different pros and cons.

Keywords: Interaction design for mobile platforms, cross-platform consistency.

1 Introduction

User experience has a big effect in mobile application development [1]. Smartphone users enjoy a user experience that is particular to their device mobile platform. According to Wasserman, mobile apps must share common elements of the user interface with other apps in the same platform, and must adhere to platform-dependent user interface guidelines [2]. Mobile application developers need to consider both constraints when creating the interaction design: formal norms in the form of platform-specific user interface guidelines (like [3] and [4]), and 'de facto' norms comprising the common strategies used in the interaction design of the most popular apps. While the former are readily available, it is difficult for developers to get to know the second ones, unless they are highly specialized in a given platform. When an app is designed following both official and 'de facto' norms, users will be able to build on their previous app usage experience, therefore improving their learning curve and their overall satisfaction.

For various market or organizational reasons, most teams must support apps on multiple platforms [1]; therefore maximizing the user base an app may reach. Multiplatform developers hold a dilemma between cross-platform consistency for the

C. Stephanidis (Ed.): Posters, Part II, HCII 2013, CCIS 374, pp. 8–12, 2013.

interaction design and offering interaction designs unique to each platform that follow its specific norms. Cross-platform consistency keeps the user experience coherent across multiple platforms [5], but when going against platform conventions it contributes negatively to novice user learnability. Existing generic design guidelines for mobile development, like [6], do not consider these issues, since they address more abstract interaction design concerns to consider when designing for mobility. For the development of a multiplatform app addressed to university students, we have carried out a survey between freshmen, with two aims: First, to choose the two most used mobile platforms as development platforms for the app; and, second, to identify the most popular apps. We have studied popular apps in terms of cross-platform interaction design consistency, to help in the decision of cross-platform consistency vs. platform-specific interaction design.

2 Students Survey about Mobile Platforms and Popular Apps

The survey was delivered to freshmen Computer Science students at UPM, during orientation week in September 2012. 188 responses were received, showing that platform distribution among respondents is as follows: Android (54.25%), iOS (19.68%), BlackBerry (7.98%), Symbian (7.44%), Windows Phone (1.06%) and other (9.57%). Android and iOS cover 74% of the students, so they are the best choice when choosing to develop for just two platforms in this context of use. Given that Android and iOS account together to 85% of the smartphone market [7], this choice may be also adequate for other more generic contexts of use. Participating students were also asked about the three apps they used most. This question received 180 responses, with the following apps mentioned: WhatsApp (67.2%), Twitter (40.56%), Tuenti (30%), Facebook (15.56%), Youtube (6.67%), Safari (5.56%), Gmail (5%), Spotify (3.33%), Shazam (2.22%), and Skype (1.667%).We chose the top three apps (Whatsapp, Twitter, and Facebook) for our study, discarding Tuenti because it is a local Spain-based social network, which would be less representative from a global point of view. Additionally, we considered Skype as well because mobility students typically use this app to communicate with their families, and any app offering information about the campus would consider mobility students as a relevant profile.

3 Comparison of iOS - Android Interaction Design Philosophy

We carried out a study of the iOS and Android versions of the four apps mentioned in the previous section, and the platform stores (iOS App Store and Android Google Play) to understand the main interaction design solutions that users of each platform find in their apps, interpreted according with the advice present in the corresponding platform guidelines ([3] and [4]). It is necessary to look at the interaction design of specific apps in order to fully understand the possibilities offered in platform guidelines. Additionally, we have identified for each app the differences and similarities between iOS and Android versions in terms of interaction design. Table 1 shows the results of the study. The Look column reflects how close the appearance of the user interface in both platforms is; the Feel column reflects how different the dynamic part of the interaction in both versions is; and the Compliance column reflects the fidelity to each platform user interface guidelines.

Table 1. Comparison of Android and iOS versions of four popular apps

Apps version considered: (iOS; Android)	**Look**	**Feel**	**Compliance with guidelines**	
			iOS	**Android**
Facebook (v5.0.1; v1.9.10)	The same	The same	Low	High
Skype (v4.1.1310; v2.9.0.315)	Different	Different	Very high	High
Twitter (v5.0.3; v3.4.0)	Similar	Similar	Very high	Very high
WhatsApp (v2.8.4; v2.8.5310)	Different	Different	Very high	Very high

3.1 Main Interaction Design Differences between iOS and Android

After studying the interaction design of these four apps and the platform stores, we have distilled the main interaction design elements that stand out as different between Android and iOS:

- Navigation: Whereas iOS navigation relies on the top-positioned navigation bar, Android offers the action bar on the same position and the (physical or virtual) back button in the bottom part of the screen. iOS navigation bar contains the back button, a title for the current screen and, optionally, buttons in its right part. Android action bar contains the app icon (doubling as the "up" button), a control to alternate views, and action buttons like the search.
- Screen logical regions: Both platforms have a status bar in the top position of the screen, but each one considers different regions in the rest of the screen. iOS divides the rest of the screen in three regions from top to bottom: the navigation bar, the content area, and a tool area that may hold a toolbar, a segmented bar or a tab bar. Android only considers the main action bar on top and the rest is dedicated to a content area, but this content area may be further divided into an optional upper bar, the main content and a lower split action bar to optionally hold additional controls. Android also offers the possibility of a sliding drawer to show a menu hidden under the current view.
- Settings: The overall approach to setting up options strongly differs between both platforms, and it affects to where users expect to find the functionality to change app settings. iOS distinguishes between app settings and app preferences: App settings are accessed through the system settings part of the operating system, and they are expected not to change very often; while app preferences refer to options changed regularly, which are configured from inside the app. Alternatively, Android only considers one kind of setting: app settings located inside the app, and

they must be situated inside the action overflow with the name "Settings".We have also observed that iOS offers a narrower variety of options and elements for interaction design than Android. Therefore, it is easier to adapt an iOS design to Android than the other way round.

4 Multiplatform Interaction Design Approaches

We have observed three possible approaches to cross-platform interaction design consistency: Platform-Dependent, Own Cross-Platform and Adapted Cross-Platform. A description of each approach, along with their main advantages and disadvantages follows.

4.1 Platform-Dependent

The Platform-dependent approach consists on creating a different interaction design for each platform, closer to each platform interaction philosophy. This is the approach followed by WhatsApp and Skype.

- Pros: The user experience is better adapted to each platform philosophy. There is a higher ease of learning for users, since the delivered experience of use matches their previous experience
- Cons: It is required a higher effort from the development team, since multiple designs need to be created and maintained. Regarding team expertise, more specialized skills in the interaction design for each platform are required.

4.2 Own Cross-Platform

In this approach the interaction design is the same in both platforms, not necessarily following platform norms and conventions. The Facebook app follows this approach.

- Pros: The user experience is coherent between both platforms, so users in one platform may help users in the other one, and users changing from one platform to the other one may directly apply their previous knowledge. There is a lower maintenance effort for the development team, and brand image is reinforced.
- Cons: The app defines its own way of doing things, departing from conventions typically used in other apps. Novel users experience a higher difficulty in learning to use the app, with possible decreased satisfaction.

4.3 Adapted Cross-Platform

This approach is a compromise between the two previous approaches, delivering an app with a similar appearance in both platforms, but with an interaction design that follows platform conventions to a high extent. Twitter follows this approach.

– Pros: The user experience is better adapted to each platform, favoring a positive reaction from the user while still offering some coherence between platforms. With regard to the development team, there is a slightly lower maintenance effort compared to the platform-dependent approach due to both designs sharing the same basic interaction design scheme.
– Cons: The compromise between platforms may leave out some interesting interaction design functionalities present in just one platform. A high level of expertise in each platform interaction design skills is required from (possibly part of) the development team.

5 Discussion

We have carried out a study on the multiplatform interaction design decisions taken in four popular apps in iOS and Android, observing three possible approaches for addressing cross-platform consistency. The choice of a specific approach in a particular multiplatform app development project will depend on business and marketing objectives, available resources and skills in the development team, and usability requirements. When the chosen approach is Platform-Dependent or Adapted Cross-Platform, due to the more constrained variety of options in iOS, it is advisable to conceive first the iOS interaction design than the Android one. Then the resulting iOS-oriented interaction design can be further extended or modified with the increased options offered in the Android platform. We expect to carry out usability studies with users to test how adherence to platform conventions is perceived and the effect it has on app acceptance and user satisfaction.

References

1. Charland, A., Leroux, B.: Mobile application development: web vs. native. Communications of the ACM 54(5), 49–53 (2011)
2. Anthony, I.: Wasserman. Software engineering issues for mobile application development. In: Proc. of the FSE/SDP Workshop on Future of Software Engineering Research (FoSER 2010), pp. 397–400. ACM, New York (2010)
3. Apple. iOS Human Interface Guidelines (2012), `http://developer.apple.com/library/ios/documentation/UserExperience/Conceptual/MobileHIG/`
4. Google Inc. and the Open Handset Alliance. Android User Interface Guidelines (2012), `http://developer.android.com/design/`
5. Antila, V., Lui, A.: Challenges in Designing Inter-usable Systems. In: Campos, P., Graham, N., Jorge, J., Nunes, N., Palanque, P., Winckler, M. (eds.) INTERACT 2011, Part I. LNCS, vol. 6946, pp. 396–403. Springer, Heidelberg (2011)
6. Hoober, S., Berkman, E.: Designing Mobile Interfaces. O'Reilly, Beijing (2011)
7. IDC. Android and iOS Surge to New Smartphone OS Record in Second Quarter (2012), `http://www.idc.com/getdoc.jsp?containerId=prUS23638712`

Designing Educational Interfaces for Saudi Students

Abeer A. Boreqqah[1], Amandeep Dhir[2], and Khalid Buragga[3]

[1] College of Education, King Faisal University, Saudi Arabia
[2] Department of Computer Science and Engineering, Aalto University, Finland
[3] Department of Information Systems, CCSIT, King Faisal University, Saudi Arabia
{aboregeh,kburagga}@kfu.edu.sa, amandeep.dhir@aalto.fi

Abstract. Traditional forms of educational instruction have witnessed a sharp inclination towards the use of educational technology and various e-learning tools and platforms. Educational technology is seen as a facilitator for learning, it motivates students and tends to increase their confidence. Up to the present day, the majority of the available research on this subject has been dominated by a Western perspective, while the needs and expectations of Arabic speaking students in context to educational technology has been ignored in the past. The focus of our on-going research is to understand the potential needs, requirements and expectations of the Saudi students (including college level, undergraduate, graduate and postgraduate students) in regards to educational interfaces and technology. In this work in progress paper, we have presented our on-going research by discussing its motivation, the methodology (including detailed information on the underlying questions characterising the research), methods and study participants, and finally research process practiced in the on-going research is presented.

Keywords: Educational technology, information technology, e-learning tools, students, instruction.

1 Introduction

The last decade has witnessed a growing interest among educational researchers, information technology specialists and educational psychology researchers regarding the design and development of educational technology (Culén, 2011). In the context of the recent emergence of educational technology, it could even argue that this technology has revolutionized our traditional forms of instruction, which more or less revolve around chalks and blackboards (Albirini, 2007). Some of the notable forms of educational technology are interactive tablets such as iPad, the surface table, and learning management systems such as the blackboard (Timmermann, 2010). Educational technology is seen as a facilitator for the learning and educational process, motivating students towards learning and course work (Plowman and Stephen, 2005), tending to increase their confidence (Chester & Gwynne, 1998; Earle, 2002) and has positive impact on the academic performance and learning outcomes (Dunlap, 2009; Churchill, 2012). Educational technology and related research has attracted some

C. Stephanidis (Ed.): Posters, Part II, HCII 2013, CCIS 374, pp. 13–17, 2013.

much-needed attention from various multidisciplinary researchers, including technology specialists, educational researchers and information system experts. This is based on the recent availability of an abundant amount of literature on educational technology development, covering different topics under the umbrella term of "development of e-learning platforms and tools". Interestingly, the majority of the present research on the development of educational technology or e-learning platforms and tools is dominated by the viewpoint of western countries or developed nations (Al-Wabil et. al., 2012). This means previous as well as on-going research on this subject has been mostly designed and organized in western countries and other developed nations. Subsequently, the needs and expectations of other specific communities (forexample Arabic speaking students) have been ignored in the past. In 2013 Dhir and Alsumait performed an up-to-date systematic literature review on the educational user interface, technology and related pedagogy needs of Arabic speaking community. Some of the prominent achievements of this systematic literature review were:

1. Presenting an educational technology research agenda underpinned by extensive research and studies.
2. Noting various missing interconnections between the empirical findings of published studies and the various educational theories.
3. Presenting various open challenges in the design and development of educational technology and related instructional strategies.
4. Finally, the study proposed various guidelines and recommendations for future research so as to overcome some of the existing challenges in the design and development of educational technology platforms.

The focus of our on-going research is to understand the potential needs, requirements and expectations of the Saudi students (i.e. college level, undergraduate, graduate and postgraduate students) in regards to educational interfaces and technology. We argue that by understanding the needs and expectations of the students, we can deliver a positive user-experience in the context of e-learning platforms. This argument is based on the user-experience literature that has scientifically proven that the user's needs later transform into user experience (Roto et. al., 2009; Heikkinen et. al., 2009). Based on the investigated needs and requirements of students, we aim to provide insightful design considerations, frameworks, both low and high level prototypes for other researchers and practitioners involved in the development of educational technology platforms particularly e-learning tools.

The primary focus of this research is centered on the development of various e-learning platforms and other relevant educational tools that can support learning and engagement of students. This kind of research is important as it satisfies the growing present need of development of educational technology for Arabic speaking students, which has been mostly ignored and until the present date has received little attention from other educational technology researchers and practitioners. Additionally, we believe that our on-going work will serve as a reference for developing better educational technology for Arabic speaking students in other parts of the world.

2 Research Methodology

In this section, we have briefly presented the methodology for our ongoing research. The discussion includes questions used in our ongoing research, to-be practiced methods employed, a profile of the study participants and of the process followed by us.

Research Questions. The four main questions of this ongoing research are:

1. To examine the existing literature on developing educational technology frameworks and platforms in the context of Arabic speaking users
2. To understand the various needs, expectations and requirements of Arabic speaking students in Saudi Arabia in the context of educational technology, particularly e-learning platforms
3. To utilise the various collected needs and expectations of Saudi young people to prepare insightful design considerations, frameworks and platforms governing the development of e-learning platforms for the Arabic speaking community.
4. To provide essential design guidelines, frameworks and prototypes for policy makers, educationalists, government officials, product developers and designers in terms of "developing suitable and appropriate educational technologies and tools for Arabic speaking students in Saudi Arabia."

Research Methods. This ongoing study consists of a combination of various qualitative and quantitative research methods. Our research philosophy has been influenced by the social science principle referred to as triangulation (Jick, 1979). The principle of triangulation argues that one should employ a combination of different qualitative and quantitative questionnaires in order to examine any given problem and/or behaviour. For this reason, the present study consists of systematic literature review of existing work (qualitative method), large-scale questionnaire surveys (quantitative study involving students), open-ended questionnaires and sentence completion forms (qualitative study involving students), prototype development, usability evaluation and finally framework preparation. The combination of qualitative and quantitative methods will ensure that the underlying theme (the needs and requirements of Saudi students related to educational technology) is examined scientifically and systematically.

Study Participants. Since the main research questions of this study are focused on the different needs, requirements and expectations of Arabic speaking students in Saudi Arabia in the context to educational technology platforms and tools, the primary study participants are undergraduate and graduate level students in the King Faisal University (KFU) of Saudi Arabia. However, considering the role of other educational stakeholders (namely educators, teachers, instructors, curriculum designers, educational policy makers), we aim to involve all of them as secondary participants in the research process. The aforementioned stakeholders will be involved in brainstorming sessions, focus discussions and one to one interviews, so as to understand their opinions and receive their feedback based on the development of frameworks, tools and models governing development of futuristic educational technology platforms aimed at Arabic speaking students in Saudi Arabia.

Research Process. The research process of our ongoing study is divided into four phases and each of them are explained below (see Figure 1):

1. First Phase: In the first phase, systematic literature review of earlier literature governing development of educational technology for Arabic speaking community will be carried out. This kind of rigorous examination will include all three types of literature (theoretical, conceptual and empirical studies).
2. Second Phase: In the second phase, based on the literature review of existing work, we aim to design questionnaire surveys, sentence completion tasks and open ended forms so that a combination of qualitative and quantitative data is gathered. The target participants will be undergraduate and graduate students at King Faisal University, Saudi Arabia.
3. Third Phase: In the third phase, collected empirical data (both qualitative and quantitative) will be analysed and results will be interpreted in the light of research questions behind our present study. Based on the study results, potential design considerations and frameworks will be defined which will govern the development of futuristic educational technology platforms aimed at Arabic speaking community in Saudi educational spaces.
4. Fourth Phase: In the fourth phase, we aim to develop low fidelity and high fidelity prototypes representing some of the potential uses of educational technology platforms. These potential scenarios will be developed based on the needs and expectations of the students in Saudi Arabia (as the collected empirical datasets). These prototypes and their evaluation by students will certainly bring newer insights into the design and development of educational technology platforms, especially e-learning platforms aimed at the Arabic speaking population in Saudi Arabia.

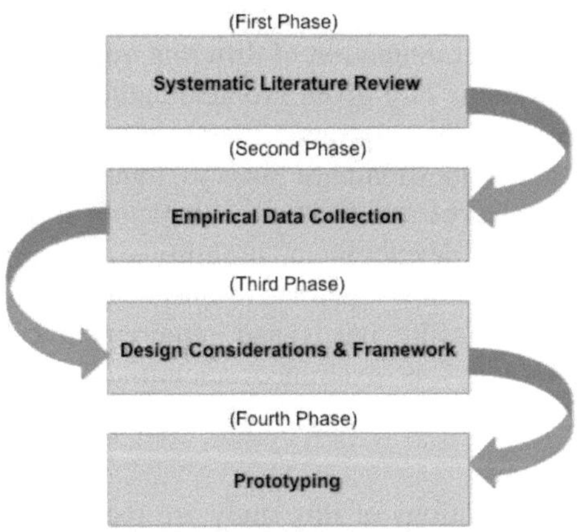

Fig. 1. Research process for the study

3 Conclusions and Future Work

In this paper, we have presented an outline of our ongoing study at King Faisal University (KFU) that is aimed at understanding the various needs, expectations and requirements of Arabic speaking Saudi students in regard to different e-learning platforms and tools and educational technology in general. In this work in progress, we have presented our ongoing research by discussing its motivation, the methodology (including detailed information on underlying research questions), information about methods and study participants and finally the process of our ongoing research.

Acknowledgements. The Deanship of Scientific Research (DSR), King Faisal University (KFU), Saudi Arabia, funds this ongoing research.

References

1. Albirini, A.: The Crisis in Educational Technology, and the Prospect of Reinventing Education. Educational Technology & Society 10(1), 227–236 (2007)
2. Timmermann, P.: Is my iPad in my backpack? Journal of Digital Research & Publishing, University of Sydney
3. Churchill, D., Fox, B., King, M.: Study of Affordances of iPads and Teachers' Private Theories. Int. J. of Information and Education Technology 2(3) (June 2012)
4. Culén, C.A.L., Gasparini, A.: iPad: a new classroom technology? A report from two pilot studies. In: INFuture Proceedings, 2011, pp. 199–208 (2011)
5. Dunlap, J.C., Lowenthal, P.R.: Tweeting the night away: Using Twitter to enhance social presence. Journal of Information Systems Education 20(2) (2009)
6. Al-Wabil, A., Dhir, A., Al-Musaaed, H., Al-Sheaha, A.: Screening Program for Learning Difficulties in Arabic Speaking Students: Design Considerations for Educational Interfaces. In: Workshop on Interaction Design in Educational Environments (IDEE) 15th International Conference on Enterprise Information Systems (ICEIS), June 28 (2012)
7. Dhir, A., Alsumait, A.: Examining Educational User Interface, Technology and Pedagogy for Arabic Speaking Children in Kuwait, J. of Universal Computer Science (JUCS) special issue Interaction Design in Educational Environments (2013) (currently in press)
8. Roto, V., Rantavuo, H., Väänänen-Vainio-Mattila, K.: Evaluating User Experience of Early Product Concepts. In: Proceedings of International Conference on Designing Pleasurable Products and Interfaces, DPPI 2009, Compiegne (October 2009)
9. Heikkinen, J., Olsson, T., Väänänen-Vainio-Mattila, K.: Expectations for User Experience in Haptic Communication with Mobile Devices. In: Proc. Of MobileHCI 2009, Bonn, Germany, September 15-18. ACM Press (2009)
10. Plowman, L., Stephen, C.: Children, play, and computers in pre-school education. British Journal of Educational Technology 36(2), 145–157 (2005)
11. Chester, A., Gwynne, G.: Online teaching: encouraging collaboration through anonymity. Journal of Computer Mediated Communication 4, 2 (1998), `http://jcmc.indiana.edu/vol4/issue2/chester.html`
12. Earle, R.S.: The integration of instructional technology into public education: Promises and challenges. Educational Technology 42(1), 5–13
13. Jick, T.D.: Mixing qualitative and quantitative methods: Triangulation in action. Administrative Science Quarterly, 24 (4), pp. 602-611 (December 1979); Qualitative Methodology

Facebook an Open Education Platform: Exploring Its Educational Uses*

Khalid Buragga[1], Amandeep Dhir[2], and Abeer A. Boreqqah[3]

[1] Northern Border University, Saudi Arabia
[2] Institute of Behavioral Sciences, University of Helsinki, Finland
[3] College of Education, King Faisal University, Saudi Arabia
nbu10@hotmail.com, amandeep.dhir@helsinki.fi, aboregeh@kfu.edu.sa

Abstract. Past few years have witnessed the growing popularity of Facebook among young people particularly school and college going students. Due to the ever-growing user community of Facebook educational researchers and practitioners believe that Facebook could be used for delivering educational content and act as a learning tool. In this work in progress submission, we aim at exploring if and how Facebook could be used as an open education platform and explore its educational uses. Facebook for educational users has received some attentions from educational researchers but majority of this research is focused on University and college going students. In contrast to previous research, we have organized a questionnaire survey with 424 high school students in India. This questionnaire survey investigates different aspects addressed the bigger issue i.e. how Facebook can be used for educational purposes. This study addresses if and how Facebook could be used as a medium for open education, different affordances (such as technical, social, communication) offered by Facebook for educational purposes, various benefits and limitations of Facebook in context to educational spaces and finally various policy level implications of Facebook use on education institutions and its stakeholders.

Keywords: Educational technology, Facebook, information technology, information systems, open education, quantitative survey.

1 Introduction

Past decade has witnessed the emergence of online social networks such as Facebook, Orkut and LinkedIn. However, among these different social media platforms, the role and usage of Facebook has always been dominant since its emersion. Over past few years, Facebook has emerged as the preferred social media platform for expression and communication among young people. The popularity of Facebook can be seen

* Statistics 1, 2013, http://newsroom.fb.com/Key-Facts
Statistics 2, 2013, http://news.yahoo.com/number-active-users-facebook-over-230449748.html
Statistics 3, 2013, http://www.socialbakers.com/facebook-statistics/ (India statistics)

C. Stephanidis (Ed.): Posters, Part II, HCII 2013, CCIS 374, pp. 18–22, 2013.

from the statistics published by Facebook (Statistics 1, 2013), as of December 2012, it has around a billion of users who are active on monthly basis (Statistics 2, 2013). Furthermore, there are around 1.06 billion Facebook users around the world as of December 2012 out of which 62.6 million users from India (Statistics 3, 2013). Due to this overwhelming popularity of Facebook among young people particularly students from all three educational levels i.e. primary, secondary and tertiary, educational technology practitioners and researchers are optimistic about using Facebook for educational purposes [1]. This claim gets more strength after looking at the ever-growing user community of Facebook, which has recently crossed 1 billion. Educational technology practitioners see this large community of Facebook users as a lucrative market while educational technology researchers believe that Facebook can be used as a communication channel for hosting learning related content and reach the masses [2]. This becomes more realistic considering the recent emergence of newer concepts of "openness in education" in the educational instruction. The last few years have witnessed the emergence of a newer phenomena referred to as "openness in education" that calls for an unrestricted access to any educational content or material so that different stakeholders of any educational system namely students, teachers, parents, and even institutions can access them anytime and anywhere [3]. The success of the concept of educational technology is extending its roots by significantly contributing to the emergence of new concepts such as Massive Open Online Courses (MOOCs). Existing studies on "open education" have coined MOOCs and Open educational resources (OER), which are commonly referred as new high profile development in the field of education and instruction [3]. The seeds of such educational learning concepts was sown by MIT in 2001 by introducing their first Open-CourseWare (OCW) based courses for their undergraduate and graduate level students [3]. Such new initiatives can be perceived as: 1) promising tools for enhancing the learning experience. 2) These account for shaping the future of the educational sector. 3) They might have profound impact in shaping the future of any economy by providing easy access to educational material to its youth [3]. In this regard, [3] also extend their support to emergence such concepts for facilitating future learning considering the changes occurring in the existing lifestyles of the users and economical issues being faced by the governments owing to increasing population loads especially in the developing countries such as India and Africa. Previous research on this topic has predicted several policy level implications of "open education" on our social, political, and educational system [4]. These implications are: 1) "open education" has led to the reduction of geographic and economic barriers to education. 2) Loosening of the institutional grip over access to knowledge. 3) Massification of educational opportunities for the learners from low-income groups [4]. Despite its growing popularity and value-added advantages for traditional forms of educational instruction, research pertaining to open education is still in its early phases, which is under-theorized and under-researched.

Considering various added advantages provided by "openness in education" supported by newer concepts namely OER and MOOC, our present study tends to examine: 1) if and how Facebook could be used as a medium for open education 2) investigating different affordances (such as technical, social, communication) offered by Facebook for educational purposes 3) understanding various benefits and limitations of Facebook in context to educational spaces 4) determining various policy level implications of using Facebook on education institutions and its stakeholders. Furthermore the essence of our ongoing study is to "How Facebook can be used as an open education tool therefore open access to various learning and educational material". Additionally this study examines whether Facebook can be successfully used as a learning tool in high schools, understanding various perceptions of high school students towards using Facebook for learning purposes, benefits and limitations of using Facebook for educational purposes and finally examining various implications of study on educational instruction and policy making in regard to using Facebook in schools. Our study brings a new perspective to the existing research agenda on "open education" i.e. if and how Facebook, a popular social networking site (SNS) especially among Indian teenagers, can serve as a cost effective medium for open education in Indian schools. Developing countries like India requires cost-effective and economical open-education tools that can serve the masses, especially in schools with lower computing infrastructure. This study has examined the perception of students towards the use of Facebook for learning and other educational reasons through a questionnaire survey with 424 respondents from grade 8 to grade 12. In this work in progress submission, we have outlined the background literature on this subject and presented research methodology behind this study covering research questions, study design, sample size and other details related to its implementation.

2 Background Research

Existing Facebook related statistics have clearly shown the ever-growing popularity of Facebook. However despite this popularity, little research has examined Facebook's role for learning and various other educational purposes. Facebook could potentially offer various affordances related to its environment, technology, connectivity and presence of huge user community [1]. Considering this need, we argue that it will be useful to investigate different ways in which Facebook can be used utilized for enhancing the learning experience in different educational settings. Learning is an active and social process [5] so Facebook might support the learning experience of students in various ways. The usage of Facebook for learning can add fun element in the process, which will also attract students towards its use. Due to this reason, Facebook has the capability to promote concentration and engagement among young people. Furthermore, the presence of possibility of indulging in informal communications around the clock also enhances the learning experience and learning curve of the students. It also enables the students to engage in communications regarding the problems that they encounter while they are not in the class or in close proximity with peers ([3], [6]. Even though Facebook has been popular among school, college and University level students however little has studied Facebook usage for educational purposes. Existing studies on this subject have mainly examined Facebook role in the tertiary levels of our education system i.e. for University level students. This earlier work mostly focused on following aspects namely examining usage of Facebook as a Learning-management system (LMS), teacher-student relationship in context to Facebook use, exploring students' educational related uses of Facebook and modeling its various educational usages ([7], [8], [9], [10], [11], [12]). In contrast to these earlier studies, our present study is focused on examining the usage of Facebook for educational purposes in high schools in India. This examination includes understanding perception of high school students on using Facebook as a learning tool and examining various gratifications of Facebook use among high school students. To our best of knowledge, no previous study has examined educational uses of Facebook for high schools and that too in India. Almost all of the existing studies are organized in western countries or in China and other East Asian countries.

3 Research Methodology

Research Questions. The study consists of following research questions: To examine whether Facebook can be successfully used for learning and other educational purposes in high schools; To understand the perception of school students towards using Facebook for educational purposes; To examine various limitations and benefits of using Facebook for educational purposes in schools? To outline various implications and design considerations on various aspects related to educational set up, policy making and classroom instruction.

Research Method and Study Design. A comprehensive questionnaire survey was prepared for collecting quantitative data on various underlying themes directly supporting the main research questions behind this study. This questionnaire survey consists of three parts namely: Part A consists of 23 items designed for collecting demographics information about the participating students which includes information on their age, class, academic performance, economic condition and various other statements related to Facebook use. Part B consists of 93 items designed for examining various gratifications and affordances (namely technological, learning, social, connectivity, educational and pedagogical, school performance, and economical) related to Facebook use. Part B consists of 15 items examining impact of Facebook on learning, teaching and students skill improvement in subjects namely science, mathematics and English language.

Study Process. This questionnaire study was organized in November-December 2012 and 424 participants mainly students (age 12 to 19 years) studying in different English speaking high schools in India answered it. The respondents were either already using Facebook or those who have recent joined Facebook. Before the actual study, a pilot study was performed where 20 participants (10 males and 10 female students) of same age group participated and answer this questionnaire. After the pilot study, the survey questionnaire was updated based on the feedback and study results as participants were instructed to point out difficult, complex and confusing statements and words. Afterwards, the updated questionnaire study was advertised in 5 local schools in Northwestern India where all students from grade 8 to grade 12 were informed about the study objective, purpose and background information. It was informed that this study is purely voluntary in nature and no negative consequences will occur to those students who will withdraw their participant at anytime before and during the study questionnaire survey. However, there was no possibility to withdraw their participation once survey is answered and returned since we did not keep any identification or coding of the answer sheets so it was impossible for us to find the returned answer sheet from the pile of respondents. The study was organized during the school hours and inside the normal classrooms in the presence of their class-teachers. Interested students received the questionnaire survey inside the classroom and it took 30 minutes on average to complete this study. No monetary or other kind of incentive was given to the participating students.

4 Conclusion and Future Work

In this work in progress submission, we have addressed the growing concern among educational technology researchers on how Facebook could be used for delivering open educational content and act as a learning tool. Towards this direction, we have organized a questionnaire survey with 424 high school students in India. This questionnaire survey investigates different aspects addressed the bigger issue i.e. how Facebook can be used for educational purposes. This study addresses if and how Facebook could be used as a medium for open education, different affordances offered by Facebook for educational purposes, various benefits and limitations of Facebook in context to educational spaces and finally various policy level implications of Facebook use on education institutions and its stakeholders.

In our future work, we aim to organize the same questionnaire survey in other countries namely Pakistan, Saudi Arabia and Finland. This kind of data collection in other parts of the world would enable us to perform cross-cultural analysis, which would in way help us in understanding the underlying subjects from different point of view. Additionally, we aim to generalize the findings of the study by comparing the results received from India with other countries.

References

1. Wang, Q., Woo, H.L., Quek, C.L., Yang, Y., Liu, M.: Using the Facebook group as a learning management system: An exploratory study. British Journal of Educational Technology 43(3), 428–438 (2012)
2. Shiu, H., Fong, J., Lam, J.: Facebook – Education with Social Networking Websites for Teaching and Learning. In: Tsang, P., Cheung, S.K.S., Lee, V.S.K., Huang, R. (eds.) ICHL 2010. LNCS, vol. 6248, pp. 59–70. Springer, Heidelberg (2010)
3. Brown, S., Adler, R.P.: Minds on fire. Open Education, the Long Trail, and Learning 2.0. Educause 43, 17–32 (2008)
4. McAuly, A., Bonnie, S., Siemens, G., Cormier, D.: The MOOC Modelfor Digital Practice, Knowledg Synthesis Grants on the Digital Economy. University of Prince Edward Island (2010), `http://www.edukwest.com/wp-content/uploads/2011/07/MOOC_Final.pdf`
5. Motschnig-Pitrik, R., Holzinger, A.: Student-Centered Teaching Meets New Media: Concept and Case Study. IEEE J. of Educ. Tech. & Society 5(4), 160–172 (2002)
6. Siemens, G.: Connectivism: A Learning Theory for the Digital Age. International Journal of Instructional Technology and Distance Learning 2(1) (January 2005)
7. Grossecka, G., Bran, R., Tiru, L.: Dear teacher, what should I write on my wall? A case study on academic uses of Facebook. Procedia Social and Behavioral Sciences 15, 1425–1430 (2011)
8. Hew, K.F.: Review: Students' and teachers' use of Facebook. Computers in Human Behavior 27, 662–676 (2011)
9. Munoz, C.L., Towner, T.L.: Opening Facebook: How To Use Facebook In The College Classroom. Paper presented at the Proceedings of Society for Information Technology and Teacher Education Conference, Charleston, South Carolina (2009)
10. Ellison, N.B., Steinfield, C., Lampe, C.: The Benefits of Facebook "Friends:" Social Capital and College Students' Use of Online Social Network Sites. Journal of Computer-Mediated Communication 12, 1143–1168 (2007)
11. Wilson, R.E., Gosling, S.D., Graham, L.T.: A Review of Facebook Research in the Social Sciences. Perspectives on Psychological Science 7, 203 (2012)
12. Ross, C., Orr, E.S., Sisic, M., Arseneault, J.M., Simmering, M.G., Orr, R.R.: Personality and motivations associated with facebook use. Computers in Human Behavior 25(2), 578–586 (2009)

Constructing an Embodied Interaction for Concept Mapping

Andreea Danielescu[1], Caroline Savio-Ramos[2], and John Sadauskas[2]

[1] School of Computing, Informatics, and Decision Systems Engineering Arizona State University Tempe, Arizona, USA
[2] Mary Lou Fulton Teachers College. Arizona State University Tempe, Arizona, USA
{lavinia.danielescu,caroline.savio,john.sadauskas}@asu.edu

Abstract. Creating learning experiences that are meaningful and motivational is crucial in learning. Research demonstrates that effectively organizing ideas via concept maps allows students to view prior knowledge with new perspectives. Recently, embodied computation has emerged as an effective means of meeting educational objectives due to its intuitive, gesture-based control and to its promotion of associating knowledge with physical events. Unfortunately, a majority of systems tailored for such interaction are expensive prototypes. However, the release of depth cameras has brought embodied interaction into the commercial realm, allowing users' bodies to "become" controllers. This research presents a novel, low cost system that provides embodied interaction with a computer and depth camera, through which learners can create concept maps with gestures. Current work involves defining intuitive gestural controls. Future work will involve evaluating the system for use in a classroom with the aim to create opportunities to easily incorporate embodiment into collaborative learning.

Keywords: embodied learning, computer supported collaborative learning, concept mapping, gestural interaction.

1 Introduction

A discontinuity exists between technological tools and our ability to interact with them in natural, beneficial, and, most importantly, creative ways [1]. Embodied computation has emerged as an effective means of meeting educational objectives due in part to its natural, intuitive, gesture-based control and to its promotion of associating knowledge and concepts with physical events, collaborative interaction, and movement. Embodied interactions provide immersive, novel and memorable educational opportunities, but a majority of systems tailored for such interaction are expensive prototypes and thus not widely employed in classrooms due to both cost and scarcity. However, electronic gaming has brought embodied interaction into the commercial realm with the release of the Microsoft Kinect, a depth-camera controller that allows users' bodies to "become" controllers.

We present a novel, low cost system that allows for embodied interaction with a computer via a depth camera. Through this system learners create and organize

C. Stephanidis (Ed.): Posters, Part II, HCII 2013, CCIS 374, pp. 23–27, 2013.

concept maps with gestures. Concept maps have been shown to encourage meaningful learning by helping students depict a set of relationships between known and new concepts [2], [3], [4]. Additional research demonstrates that effectively organizing ideas via concept maps allows students to view prior knowledge with new perspectives [5], [6]. In constructing a concept map, learners must explicitly define relationships between concepts, considering how to link them in meaningful ways. The skill "requires learners to think harder about the subject matter domain being studied while generating thoughts that would be impossible without the tool" [7].

Our goal is to foster collaboration, creativity, and retention in students through an embodied concept mapping system. In this paper, we discuss our gestural interaction development process for this system, as well as challenges we faced while designing the system. We will introduce our plans for user studies to refine the GUI and future work aimed at evaluating the system for use in a classroom setting. Our ultimate goal is to create opportunities to more easily incorporate embodiment into daily collaborative learning in both educational and professional settings.

2 Related Work

Ishii & Ulmer's interactive physical desktops and ambient office workspace alerts [8], and the RoBallet digitally augmented theatrical performance system [9] provided inspiration for the embodied interaction presented in our system. Several recent efforts in embodied collaborative tools particularly informed our design, including: a touch-table system for creating affinity diagrams in group settings, controlled by tangible tokens and paper Post-It notes [10]; Wilensky's HubNet design allowing participants to "become" interactive nodes of organizational systems via handheld devices [11]; and TRACES, a floor-based system utilizing Kinect for embodied organization of digitized concepts in brainstorming sessions [12]. Additionally, our system was greatly inspired by SMALLab, an interactive digital environment for K-12 educational applications [13].

3 Theoretical Framework: Embodied Cognition

Embodied interactions can offer fun and motivational learning environments. Additionally, research has demonstrated that optimal learning and retention occurs when learning is embodied [14], and gestures influence strategy choices in problem solving [15]. Embodied cognition states that cognitive processes are rooted and derived from the body's interactions with its physical environment [16]. Understanding guides literal action and is closely related to bodily abilities [17]. Lakoff and Johnson have argued that human cognition is inherently embodied, from the metaphors we construct [18] to the way we perceive color, objects, and other concepts in the world. Our perceptions are influenced by our language and by our physical relationship to the world. Furthermore, Glenberg has demonstrated that even abstract concepts are represented in the physical body, through activation of motor circuits [17], [5]. Therefore, students will have a more meaningful and memorable experience if they are able to physically act out activities. Beach's work [19] also validates embodied cognition's role in learning. Experienced thinkers use embodied and tangible tools to aid in memory recall, which allows them to recover from interruptions. Related research affirms that gestures can be used as memory aids as well – for instance, when children learn to count, they may gesture to different points in space as a mnemonic device [20].

4 Embodied Concept Mapping

Our embodied concept mapping system consists of a depth camera, a projection screen, and a computer with an attached webcam. Users can create both image and text concepts. Mouse interaction is currently provided for concept creation. Once the concepts are created, users use the gestural interface to move the newly created concepts, create relationships between concepts, and group concepts.

The Kinect is a motion sensing input device originally intended for the Xbox 360 video game console. It allows users to move around and interact with a computer or console through gestural movements. Our system maps the user's hand positions to cursors, and uses z-depth to trigger click events. Two hand silhouettes mirror the tracked position of the user's hands and serve as pointers (See Figure 1). The current supported actions are: selecting, deselecting, dragging, linking, deleting, and grouping. The gestures used are similar to those used on multi-touch devices (for example, pushing towards the screen to select), but on a larger scale. Large buttons replace right-click contextual menus, which are unwieldy in a gestural interface.

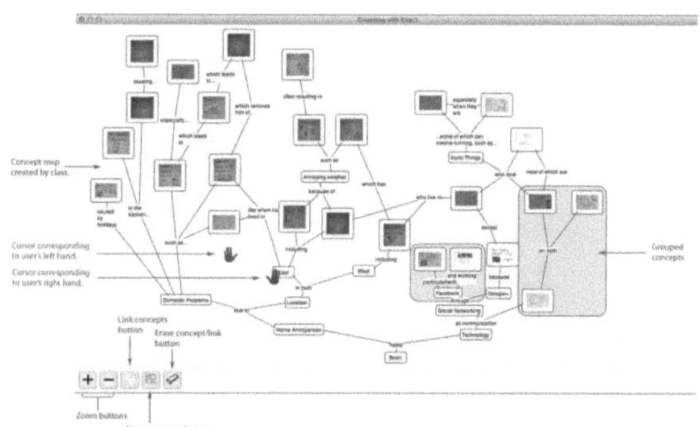

Fig. 1. Annotated screenshot of the concept mapping application

We envision the system to be used in the following way in a classroom: The activity begins with a focus question posed for the students. Students then brainstorm concepts and ideas related to that question. These ideas can be written, drawn, or photographed and become the "nodes" for the concept map. The brainstormed concepts are input into the computer system by scanning them, taking pictures of them, or importing digital images. The images will automatically appear in a concept-mapping workspace, as seen in Figure 2. This, in turn, is projected onto a whiteboard or screen. Using the embodied concept-mapping workspace, the images are organized and links are created defining their relationships to each other.

Although the system only supports one user at a time, this design is still conducive to collaboration due to its enlarged scale. Another user can use the computer keyboard to enter text labels, since the Kinect system affords node manipulation and linking. Ultimately users will be able to create a complete concept map through embodied interaction, as shown in Figure 1.

5 Conclusion and Future Work

We have described a novel concept mapping system for encouraging collaborative embodied learning. We have collected survey results from the larger university student population on user expectations when using a Kinect to interact with a computer. We have also distributed the survey as Mechanical Turk task. 267 responses have been collected and we are currently analyzing the results. We will further refine our gestural interaction based on these results before beginning pilot studies. We hope to integrate our embodied concept mapping application into a classroom and evaluate its effectiveness in motivating students to learn, as well as measuring learning gains using embodied concept mapping compared to traditional concept mapping techniques (paper and pencil, and standard desktop based concept mapping). It is our aim that by further development of this system will create opportunities to more easily incorporate embodiment into daily collaborative learning in both educational and professional settings.

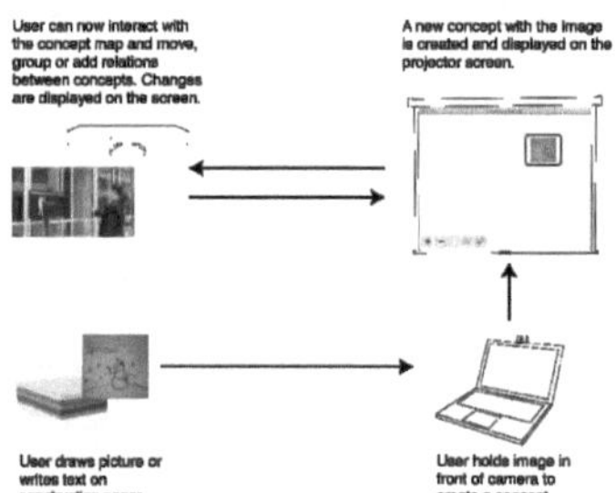

Fig. 2. System diagram showing the process a user would take to create a concept map in the embodied concept mapping application

References

1. Burleson, W., Selker, T.: Creativity and Interface. Communications of the ACM 45(10), 89 (2002)
2. Barenholz, H., Tamir, P.: A comprehensive use of concept mapping in design instruction and assessment. Research in Science & Technological Education 10(1), 37–53 (1992)
3. Leake, D., Maguitman, A., Reichherzer, T.: Understanding knowledge models: Modeling importance of concept importance in concept maps. In: Proc. 26th Annual Meeting of the Cognitive Science Society (2004)
4. Novak, J., Cañas, A. (The Theory Underlying Concept Maps and How to Construct and Use Them. Technical Report IHMC Cmap Tools 2006-01 Rev 01 (2008)

5. Glenberg, A.M.: How reading comprehension is embodied and why that matters. International Electronic Journal of Elementary Education 4(1), 5–18 (2011)
6. Martínez-Cañas, R., Ruíz-Palomino, P.: Concept Mapping As a Learning Tool For The Employment Relations Degree. Journal of International Educational Research 7(5), 23–28 (2011)
7. Jonassen, D.H., Carr, C., Yueh, H.: Computers as Mindtools for engaging learners in critical thinking. TechTrends 43(2), 24–32 (1998)
8. Ishii, H., Ulmer, B.: Tangible Bits: Towards seamless interfaces between people, bits and atoms. In: Proc. CHI (1997)
9. Cavallo, D., Sipitakiat, A., Basu, A., Bryant, S., Welti-Santos, L., Maloney, J., Chen, S., Amussen, E., Solomon, C., Ackerman, E.: RoBallet: Exploring learning through expression in the arts through constructing in a technologically immersive environment. In: Proc. International Conference of the Learning Sciences, pp. 105–112 (2004)
10. Geyer, F., Pfeil, U., Hochtl, A., Budzinski, J., Reiterer, H.: Designing reality-based interfaces for creative group work. In: Proc. ACM Creativity & Cognition (2011)
11. Wilensky, U.: Embodied Learning: Students enacting complex dynamic phenomena with the HubNet Architecture. In: Proc. Annual Conference of the American Educational Research Association (2001)
12. Van Dijk, J., Vos, G.W.: Traces in creative spaces. In: Proc. ACM Creativity & Cognition (2011)
13. Birchfield, D., Johnson-Glenberg, M.C.: A next gen interface for embodied learning: SMALLab and the geological layer cake. International Journal of Gaming and Computer-mediated Simulation 2(1), 49–58 (2010)
14. Johnson-Glenberg, M., Birchfield, D., Savvides, P., Megowan-Romanowicz, C.: Semi-Virtual Embodied Learning – Real World STEM Assessment. Serious Educational Game Assessment: Practical Methods and Models for Educational Games, Simulations and Virtual Worlds. pp. 225-241 (2010)
15. Alibali, M., Spencer, R., Knox, L., Kita, S.: Spontaneous Gestures Influence Strategy Choices in Problem Solving. Psychological Science 22(9), 1138–1144 (2011)
16. Wilson, M.: Perceiving Imitatible Stimuli: Consequences of isomorphism between input and output. Psychological Bulletin 127 (2001)
17. Glenberg, A.M.: Embodiment as a unifying perspective for psychology. Wiley Interdisciplinary Reviews: Cognitive Science 1 (2010)
18. Lakoff, G., Johnson, M.: Metaphors We Live By. University Of Chicago Press (2003)
19. Beach, K.: Becoming a Bartender: The Role of External Memory Cues in a Work-directed Educational Activity. Applied Cognitive Psychology 7(3), 191–204 (1993)
20. Cook, S.W., Mitchell, Z., Goldin-Meadow, S.: Gesturing makes learning last. Cognition 106, 1047–1058 (2008)

My iPad: A New Learning Tool for Classrooms

Amandeep Dhir[1] and Mohammed Al-kahtani[2]

[1] Department of Computer Science and Engineering, Aalto University, Finland
[2] Computer Engineering Department, Salman Bin Abdulaziz University, Saudi Arabia
amandeep.dhir@aalto.fi, alkahtani@sau.edu.sa

Abstract. The iPad is a well-known handheld interactive multimedia tool that has been quite popular lately among educators and students. Previous research investigating the iPad's role as a learning device indicated that the iPad encourages young children to feel engaged with learning and related activities, helps to bridge the communication gap between educators and students, supports educational literacy, collaborative work practices and helps the leaner connect with his or her peers. However, empirical and conceptual studies focused on the iPad are still in short supply at the moment. There is a growing need to examine the use of the iPad in educational arenas, such as classrooms and laboratories. Additionally, a thorough examination of the instructional and pedagogical advantages and disadvantages of using iPad for educational reasons is also required. Finally, longitudinal user studies with students (ipad users and potential ipad users) will bring a newer perspective to the body of research, which examines the use of iPad as a learning tool. With this aim in mind, an e-learning research project was launched at Salman Bin Abdulaziz University in Saudi Arabia. The aim of this research was to examine new forms of digital technology (namely the iPad) and ascertain if and how this device might act as a learning tool for Saudi students. This submission (a work in progress) will present the aims and objectives of this study, research methodology, research questions, and ultimately outline some research objectives based upon our recent extensive literature review on the use of iPad for educational reasons.

Keywords: Classrooms, iPad, instruction, learning, pedagogy, technology integration and technology acceptance.

1 Introduction

The past few years have witnessed the emergence of newer forms of interactive technology aids that have revolutionised the educational sector as a whole. Some of these highly-used interactive technologies include electronic teaching-boards, interactive markers, multi-touch interfaces and augmented reality based learning tools which are known for providing newer means of presenting concepts, ideas and opinions in educational settings [1, 2, 4, 6]. In this work in progress, we present a quick summary of our ongoing research, which is focused on evaluating the use of the iPad tablet as a learning tool in classrooms in Saudi Arabia. This evaluation requires careful examination of various internal and external factors: for example, the effect of iPad use on

C. Stephanidis (Ed.): Posters, Part II, HCII 2013, CCIS 374, pp. 28–32, 2013.

academic performance of students, learning and academic responsibilities. Furthermore, the potential effect of the iPad on various educational stakeholders should be discussed on both a short and long-term scale. Earlier research about developing educational technology for Arabic speaking students is scarce at the moment e.g. [1, 2, 3], and subsequently the current research topic becomes more appealing and necessary at the present time. Most countries are now making efforts to implement large-scale reforms in their traditional educational systems, so as to experience the potential benefits of educational technology [7]. Saudi Arabia has emerged as one of the top spenders in the field of education, spending 55 billion USD during the financial year of 2013: 10% of country's total GDP (especially relevant as more than 50% of its total population is below 25 years old) [9]. Part of this educational spending was an e-learning research project launched at Salman Bin Abdulaziz University. The aim of this research is to examine new forms of digital technology, namely the iPad, and ascertain if and how this device can act as a learning tool for Saudi students. This on-going research is very relevant for the Saudi educational community and society, considering the fact that lately Saudi Arabia has emerged as one of the top spenders in education related budget. The aforementioned reasons make the Saudi educational scenario very lucrative for the iPad and other digital handheld devices capable of providing learning aid to students. The iPad is now considered a preferred tool for learning and performing various educational instructions due to its smaller screen size, multimedia support, longer battery life and light-weight [8, 10]. In 2012 Churchill noted that the iPad came to commercial market only in 2010 but within two and half years had successfully made an impact in the educational sector [10]. Due to the relatively new use of the iPad in education, instances of its use and integration of iPad as a learning aid are still scarce and they are considered as relatively unexplored learning and educational tools [10, 11]. This work in progress submission will present the aims and objectives of this study, research methodology, and research questions and finally outline some research objectives determined based on our recent extensive literature review on use of iPad for educational reasons.

2 Our Study and Research Methodology

The research methodology of this long-term and multidisciplinary study (which involves technology specialists, e-learning experts and educational researchers) has been influenced by the social science principle of triangulation that aims to combine qualitative and quantitative data to offer rich insight about any underlying problems and challenges [12]. The research methodology behind this study consists of various qualitative and quantitative methods. Our on-going research involves qualitative methods namely sentence completion, interviews, an open-ended questionnaire, focus groups and brainstorming, while the quantitative part mainly includes survey questionnaires. The primary study participants are students (mainly at university level, which includes undergraduate, graduate and post-graduates), teachers (both junior and senior) and other people involved in the education policy and decision-making procedures at University level. Based on our literature review, four emerging and open research questions have been outlined in the context of the use of an iPad as a learning tool in classrooms and educational environment. The open research questions are:

Study Research Questions:

1. How can we effectively examine and evaluate various instructional benefits of iPad use in context to educational domain?
2. What are the long-term effects of iPad use on students' literacy skills, academic performance, learning outcomes, educational policies, and pedagogical and instructional skills of the educators and responsibilities of different educational stakeholders in this regard?
3. What are the different tools, techniques, methods and strategies that educators can adopt for making use of the iPad in order to have a positive impact on students' learning and their various academic responsibilities?
4. Finally, what are the potential challenges, constraints and hurdles in the successful integration of the iPad or similar interactive digital technology into educational settings?

Research Objectives:

1. **Effect of iPad**: In order to properly capture the effect of iPad use on various attributes (for example learning, academic performance, classroom instruction and pedagogy), well-designed and controlled experiments that are long enough to assess the impact of iPad before and after the adoption of it as a learning mechanism.
2. **iPad and Educational Stakeholders**: Proper examination of various implications of using the iPad on different stakeholders of our education system including students (learners), teachers (educators) and education policy makers.
3. **iPad and Learning**: Experiment-based analysis of the possible impact of iPad use on the learning process, which includes reading, comprehension, and problem-solving skills in science, mathematics and other related subjects.
4. **Innovative ways of utilizing iPad in day-to-day classroom instruction**: Integrating the iPad with already existing devices and technologies such as smart boards, creating an orchestrated environment using iPad so that educational stakeholders can interact and collaborate throughout the learning process, and finding other similar mechanisms of preparing iPad based instruction, which are more engaging.
5. **Guidelines and recommendations**: Developing various guidelines and recommendations governing new curricula, instruction and pedagogy so that iPad-based instruction becomes smooth and easy for educators. Similarly, providing guidelines for application developers so that due focus can be given on developing education-oriented iPad based applications
6. **Developing Frameworks**: Preparing technology-independent analysis and design frameworks for education, as they are needed. These frameworks should be based on a solid educational, collaborative, and psychological learning ground, so that smooth implementation of the best educational technology and easy transition from one form of educational technology to another can takes place. If this vision is not practically realised then we might experience negative consequences in economical technological, and motivational terms, as a result of out-dated and constraining technologies at our educational institutions.

3 Challenges of iPad Integration into Classrooms

Existing studies on the subject have informed us that the iPad shares the workload of teachers, helping them in various classroom activities by enabling easy and quick content production [13]. Earlier literature on the teachers' attitude towards the adoption of educational technology has reflected that teachers have a high impact on whether or not technology is adopted in the educational space, as teachers influence their students' habits and behaviour [14, 15]. For this reason, Dhir et. al., argued that teachers might also influence the successful integration of newer technologies into the classroom environment e.g. iPad [4] and Twitter [5]. There are many challenges in this regard, namely teachers' limited IT backgrounds, their lack of troubleshooting skills required for regular iPad use [15], unfavourable school infrastructure, pedagogical and administrative obstacles as schools might want to stick with old traditional curriculum [11]. In this regard, Dhir et. al., [4] gave recommendations and guidelines that might ensure the successful integration of iPad use into an educational context. They included: (i) Customization of the iPad (such as screen size, language and images) so as to comply with the needs of students and teachers; (ii) Determining newer, innovative ways of organising and evaluating students' assignments; (iii) Proper IT training for teachers, so that they can address troubleshooting if and when needed; (iv) Understanding the needs and expectations of different stakeholders in our education system regarding iPad use; (v) Schools should calibrate their existing instructional strategies and curriculum so as to integrate iPad into the existing settings in a smooth fashion; (vi) Introducing iPad supported teaching strategies that can inculcate playful interaction, feedback and engaging learning among students in classroom environment.

4 Conclusions and Future Work

The iPad tablet offers tempting technological features for both learners and educators, due to its inbuilt support for advanced usability and ease of use. Lately, educators have emphasized the incorporation and integration of iPad into mainstream educational instruction and learning. However, research governing iPad use in an educational context is relatively new and scientific studies are scarce. At present, there is a pressing need to answer questions related to the potential impact of iPad use on students' literacy skills, academic performance and learning. Similarly what is the impact of iPad use on educational policies, pedagogical and instructional skills of the educators? Furthermore, the long-term effects of iPad use on learning outcomes, instruction, academic performance, learning and responsibilities of different educational stakeholders is worth investigation. This work in progress submission will present the aims and objectives of this study, research methodology, and research questions and finally outline some research objectives determined based on our recent extensive literature review on use of iPad for educational reasons.

References

1. Dhir, A., Alsumait, A.: Examining Educational UI, Technology and Pedagogy for Arabic Speaking Children in Kuwait. In: 2012. Workshop on Interaction Design in Educational Environments (IDEE), 15th Int. Conf on Enterprise Information Systems, ICEIS (2012)
2. Al-Wabil, A., Dhir, A., Al-Musaaed, H., Al-Sheaha, A.: Screening Program for Learning Difficulties in Arabic Speaking Students: Design Considerations for Educational Interfaces. In: 2012. Workshop on Interaction Design in Educational Environments (IDEE), 15th Int. Conf. on Enterprise Information Systems, ICEIS (2012)
3. Dhir, A., Alsumait, A.: Examining Educational User Interface, Technology and Pedagogy for Arabic Speaking Children in Kuwait, J. of Universal Computer Science (JUCS) Special Issue Interaction Design in Educational Environments (2013) (currently in press)
4. Dhir, A., Gahwaji, M.N., Nyman, G.: The Role of the iPad in the Hands of the Learner. J. of Universal Computer Science (JUCS) Special Issue Innovative Instructional Technologies, 2013(currently in press)
5. Dhir, A., Buragga, K., Boreqqah, A.A.: Tweeters on Campus: Twitter a Learning Tool in Classroom? J. of Universal Computer Science (JUCS) Special Issue Innovative Instructional Technologies, 2013 (currently in press)
6. Dhir, A., Olsson, T., Elnaffar, S.: Developing Mobile Mixed Reality Application Based on User Needs and Expectations. In: Proc. of 2012 IEEE Int. Conf. on Innovations in Information Technology (IIT), United Arab Emirates, March 18-21, pp. 83–88 (2012)
7. Timmermann, P.: Is my iPad in my backpack? Journal of Digital Research & Publishing, University of Sydney (2010)
8. Ostashewski, N., Reid, D., Ostashewski, M.: Mobile Teaching and Learning Technologies: Ukrainian Dance Instruction in Canada. Paper presented at IADIS Mobile Learning 2009, Barcelona, Spain (February 27, 2009)
9. Kingdom tops world in education spending (January 2, 2013), `http://www.arabnews.com/saudi-arabia/kingdom-tops-world-education-spending`
10. Churchill, D., Fox, B., King, M.: Study of Affordances of iPads and Teachers' Private Theories. Int. J. of Information and Education Technology 2(3) (June 2012)
11. Hutchison, A., Beschorner, B., Schmidt-Crawford, D.: Exploring the Use of the iPad for Literacy Learning. The Reading Teacher 66(1), 15–23 (2012)
12. Jick, T.D.: Mixing qualitative and quantitative methods: Triangulation in action. Administrative Science Quarterly 24(4), 602–611 (1979); Qualitative Methodology
13. Walters, E.A.: Will the iPad revolutionize education? (2011), `http://www.iste.org/learn/publications/learning-leading/issues/may-2011/point-counterpoint-will-the-ipad-revolutionize-education-`
14. Baylor, A.L., Ritchie, D.: What factors facilitate teacher skill, teacher morale, and perceived student learning in technology-using classrooms? Comp. & Education 39, 395–414
15. Culén, C.A.L., Gasparini, A.: IPad: a new classroom technology? A report from two pilot studies. In: INFuture Proceedings, pp. 199–208 (2011), `http://infoz.ffzg.hr/INFuture/papers/3-02%20Culen,%20Gasparini,%20iPad%20-%20A%20New%20Classroom%20Technology.pdf`

Use of Assistive Technology Resources for Low Vision Students

Maria Elisabete R. Freire Gasparetto[1] and Marília C.C. Ferroni[2]

[1] Campinas State University, Campinas, Brazil
gasparetto@fcm.unicamp.br
[2] Colégio Tema Objetivo, Jardinópolis, Brasil
marilia_ferroni@hotmail.com

Abstract. Background: Access of low vision students to school should also be secured through the use of assistive technology resources. Assistive resources are any devices used to enhance visual functioning. Objective: The aim of this study was to check and analyze the use of assistive technology by low vision students. Material and Methods: A descriptive study was conducted and interviews were applied. The sample comprised 19 low vision students. Results: Of the low vision students 52.6% declared to use far optical resources. Information Technology was the better-accepted resource in use as 73.7% declared to work with software's like DosVox, Virtual Vision, Jaws and Windows Magnifier. Conclusion: It is preoccupant to see that those low vision students are using Information Technology only at the specialized institution while computer labs are available in regular schools and could be used for the introduction to the use of this important resource.

Keywords: Low Vision, Rehabilitation, Assistive Technology, Information Technology, Educational Technology, Visually Impaired Persons.

1 Introduction

Vision is the sense that supplies information about the environment, and it is capable of organizing other sensorial information. The visual deficiency can dramatically affect life experiences, limiting routine duties in the every day life thus compromising life quality [1].According to the 2010's Demographic Census, the IBGE (Instituto Brasileiro de Geografia e Estatística) data bank shows 45.6 million people having some kind of disability in Brazil. This figure corresponds to 23.91% of the Brazilian population. From those, 12.7 millions (6.7% of total population) have at least one serious disability with prevalence of visual disability on 3.5% of the population [2].Service restriction for low vision results in a detection difficulty of visually impaired children and consequent lack of ophthalmologic assessment to investigate the need for assistive technology and orientation for efficient use of vision either in or off school [3].Low vision is visual acuity less than 6/18 and equal to or better than 3/60 in the better eye with best correction (WHO, 2003). Vision of 20/70 to 20/200 is considered moderate visual impairment, or moderate low vision. Vision of 20/200 to

C. Stephanidis (Ed.): Posters, Part II, HCII 2013, CCIS 374, pp. 33–37, 2013.

20/400 is considered severe visual impairment, or severe low vision and 20/500 to 20/1000 is considered profound visual impairment, or profound low vision [4]. People with low vision need to know strategies, resources and equipment to facilitate daily activities and learning to read and write [5]. The role of interdisciplinary team habilitation and rehabilitation foster this knowledge. Assistive technology is an interdisciplinary field of knowledge comprising products, resources, methodologies, strategies practices and services that aims to promote functionality for low vision people with regard autonomy and independence [6].Information technology applied to students with disabilities can be defined as computers with programs that allow accessing the digital environment, promoting individual life and educational and social inclusion [7].Low vision students may have difficulties with their daily activities, even when they use both optical resources, to magnify the image, and no optical resources which can be material adaptation and changes in the environment [10]. These students can benefit from the combined use of classical and Information Technology resources, such as screen magnification software and speech synthesis systems [11]. The aim of this study was check and analyze assistive technology, with a special focus on the Information Technology, used by low vision students in their daily activities.

2 Material and Methods

A transversal descriptive study [12] has been conducted and data collection instrument used was a questionnaire applied to low vision students during a personal interview. Questionnaire was made up with discursive and multiple choice questions, elaborated from an exploratory study specifically developed. This methodology was justified because aimed to obtain frequency and values for the variables under focus also providing knowledge on the ensemble of low vision students engaged into Vision Rehabilitation Services. Data were collected from March to August of 2010, part by the Visual Habilitation and Rehabilitation services at Ribeirão Preto's Association of Visual Disability (ADEVIRP) and part by the Center of Studies and Research in Rehabilitation Prof. Dr. Gabriel Porto of Medical Sciences Faculty of Campinas State University (CEPRE/FCM/UNICAMP).This study was approved by the Research Ethics Committee of the Medical Sciences Faculty of Campinas State University: process number 1077/2009.

3 Results

The population was composed of 19 low vision students at ages between 12 and 17 years old, average of 14.7 years, with 52.6% female and 47.4% male. Far vision acuity in the better eye ranged within 20/60 to 20/1000 and near acuity ranged from 0.8M to 3.2M. Most of the students (94.7%) reported having congenital low vision and only 5.3% had acquired low vision. The main causes for low vision included: Congenital Cataract, Leber Congenital Amaurosis, Retinopathy of Prematurity, Optic Atrophy, Macular Retinochoroiditis due to Congenital Toxoplasmosis and Coloboma. As indicated in Figure 1, most of the students, 78.9%, present a moderate low vision,

15.8% profound and only one (5.3%) was classified as severe. Considering the best eye, far visual acuity ranged from 20/60 to 20/1000 and near visual acuity from 0.8M to 3.2M. About resources, 52.6% declared to use far and near optical aids classified as glasses, telescopes and hand magnifiers. About non optical-aids, 57,9% declared to use large print items and contrast. Information Technology was the best-accepted resource in use as 73.7% declared to work with softwares like DosVox, Virtual Vision, Jaws and the tools available in Windows. Students declared to be introduced and trained in the use of Information Technology resources only at the Habilitation Services but not at the regular school.

*FC= far correction for the acuity of the best eye. / *NC= near correction for the acuity of the best eye.

Subject	**Visual Acuity**		**Low vision degree**	**Use of optical resources**		**Use of non optical resources**	**Use of IT resource**
	FC*	NC*		FC*	NC*		
1.	20/100	1.0M	Moderate	No	No	Large print	Dosvox Windows magnifier
2.	20/700	1.2M	Profound	Glasses	Glasses	Large print	Dosvox
3.	20/100	2.0M	Moderate	Glasses	Glasses	Large print	No
4.	20/1000	1.6M	Profound	Glasses	Glasses	No	Dosvox
5.	20/100	1.0M	Moderate	No	No	Large print	Windows magnifier
6.	20/70	0.8M	Moderate	No	No	No	No
7.	20/200	2.0M	Moderate	No	No	Large print	Virtual Vision
8.	20/70	0.8M	Moderate	Glasses	Glasses	Large print	No
9.	20/100	1.2M	Moderate	Glasses	Glasses	Large print	Dosvox
10.	20/400	3.2M	Severe	No	Hand magnifier	No	Jaws
11.	20/70	0.8M	Moderate	Glasses	No	No	No
12.	20/200	1.2M	Moderate	Telescope	Hand magnifier	Large print High contrast	Virtual Vision
13.	20/70	0.8M	Moderate	Glasses	Glasses	No	Virtual Vision
14.	20/100	0.8M	Moderate	No	No	Large print	Virtual Vision

Fig. 1. Characterization of the student population considered in this study

Subject	**Visual Acuity**		**Low vision degree**	**Use of optical resources**		**Use of non optical resources**	**Use of IT resource**
15.	20/100	0.8M	Moderate	Glasses	Glasses Hand magnifier	Large print High contrast	Virtual Vision
16.	20/70	0.8M	Moderate	No	No	No	Windows magnifier
17.	20/70	1.0M	Moderate	No	No	No	Virtual Vision
18.	20/640	1.0M	Profound	No	No	Large print	No
19.	20/70	1.6M	Moderate	Glasses	Glasses Hand magnifier	No	Dosvox Windows magnifier

Fig. 4. (*Continued*)

It is possible to assume that 47.4% of the low vision students reporting as not using far correcting optical resources might be avoiding this use due to typical teens psychological factors. It is known that, especially in adolescence, group acceptance is a determinant factor in the behavior therefore the use of goggles or aesthetically weird resources that differs from conventional might cause discomfort on self-esteem and self-acceptance resulting from the condition of individual with special needs [13].Regarding the use of IT resources, the majority (76.7%) makes use of specific software for the visually impaired as Dosvox, tools of Windows, Virtual Vision and Jaws. About these resources,[8] states that since the creation of the Braille System in 1825, probably no technological advance overcame the impact of computers in the quality of life of people with visual impairments.

4 Conclusion

This study showed that a large number of low vision students do not use optical resources either for near or far but they do have those resources available and this is because the resources do not provide adequate amplification of images present in their activities. Although optical resources are portable and liable to be used in any kind of environment, psychological factors might be associate to the resistance on their use, mainly by the teenagers because of this may affect the acceptance within the group.Information Technology resources, on the contrary, is something present in daily life in computers, automatic bank cashiers, games and represent a method of fast and confidential access. It is preoccupant to see those low vision students using Information Technology only at the specialized institution while at regular schools Information Technology labs are available and could be used for the introduction to its use. Information Technology is a valuable resource for the teaching-learning process that could bring the low vision student to a status of comparable level with sighted students and also access to daily activities.

References

1. Montilha, R.C.I., Arruda, S.M.C.P.: Habilitação e Reabilitação de adultos e idosos com deficiência visual. In: Masini, E.F.S. (ed.) A pessoa com deficiência visual: um livro para educadores. São Paulo. Vetor, pp. 113–118 (2007)
2. IBGE.: Instituto Brasileiro de Geografia e Estatística. Censo demográfico. Disponível em, http://www.ibge.gov.br (accessed April 05, 2012)
3. Sampaio, M.W., Haddad, M.A.O., Costa Filho, H.A., Siaulys, M.O.C.: Baixa visão e cegueira: os caminhos para a reabilitação, a educação e à inclusão. Rio de Janeiro, Cultura Médica: Guanabara Koogan. Rio de Janeiro. Cultura Médica: Guanabara Koogan (2010)
4. World Health Organization.: Prevention of Blindness & Deafness. Consultation on Development of Standards for Characterization of Visual Loss and Visual Functioning. WHO, Geneva (2003)
5. Ferroni, M.C.C., Gasparetto, M.E.R.F.: Students with low vision: perception about visual difficulties, opinions on relations with the school community and use of assistive technology resources in daily activities. Rev. Bras. Educ. Espec. 18(2) (2012); Marília
6. Cook, A., Hussey, S.M.: Assistive Technologies: principles and practice, 2nd edn. Mosby, St. Louis (2002)
7. Mortimer, R.: Recurso de informática para pessoa com deficiência visual. In: Sampaio, M.W., Haddad, M.A.O., Costa Filho, H.A., Siaulys, M.O.C (eds.) Baixa visão e cegueira: os caminhos para a reabilitação, a educação e à inclusão. Rio de Janeiro. Cultura Médica: Guanabara Koogan; pp. 221- 234 (2010)
8. Gasparetto, M.E.R.F., Montilha, R.C.I., Arruda, S.M.C.P., Sperque, J., Azevedo, T.L., Nobre, M.I.R.S.: Utilização de recursos de tecnologia assistiva por escolares com deficiência visual. Informática na Educação: teoria e prática. Porto Alegre 15(2), 113–130 (2012)
9. Gil, A.C.: Como elaborar Projetos de Pesquisa. 4 edn. 10. reimpr. Atlas, São Paulo (2007)
10. Montilha, R.C.I., Temporini, E.R., Nobre, M.I.R.S., Gasparetto, M.E.R.F., Kara-Jose, N.: Utilização de recursos ópticos e equipamentos por escolares com deficiência visual. Arq. Brás. Oftalmol. 69(2), 207–211 (2006)

Intelligent Student-Bot for an Interactive Question and Answer User Interface

Emmanuel Günther and Bettina Harriehausen-Mühlbauer

University of Applied Science, Department of Computer Science, Darmstadt, Germany
Emmanuel-Maurice.Guenther@stud.h-da.de,
Bettina.Harriehausen@h-da.de

Abstract. We face the task to minimize hours of email-answering for similar questions that were being asked by so-called incoming students, i.e. foreign students that would like to spend some time in our department. We wanted to create an information system that was more intelligent than previous BOTs working on the level of ELIZA, i.e. on the basis of a simple pattern-matching algorithm. Our paper describes the use and implementation of technologies for these steps and discusses pros and cons of our implementation in comparison to alternative solutions, including the vector-space-model, the cosine similarity and web search with n-grams.

Keywords: Intelligent Bot, vector-space-model, cosine similarity, web search, n-grams.

1 Introduction

In most international offices the staff receives a lot of e-mails from incoming students and potential students who want to study abroad with questions regarding university related issues. Some of these staff members are using pre-defined text blocks to answer the questions they have in many e-mails and send them as a response. But it takes the staff many hours to answer all the e-mails. We are seeking ways to minimize this time of email-answering for similar frequently asked questions. For handling this problem we created an information system to answer the questions directly therefore eliminating the need for incoming students to write an e-mail to the staff of an international office.

In order to be able to provide answers to questions from incoming students, several goals were defined. The first goal was to provide an easily integrated and usable system for different universities worldwide. In order to achieve this goal, the system should be implemented in a generalized way to easily provide the necessary data and configuration parameters. The second goal was to get a wider range of available information. In order to achieve this, the system should not only have a static database, rather a second source should be available to search for information – the internet.

C. Stephanidis (Ed.): Posters, Part II, HCII 2013, CCIS 374, pp. 38–42, 2013.

2 Background

One other system, the Jabberwacky AI[1], is using contextual pattern matching techniques to find an answer or a response text to a given text. Jabberwacky stores all questions and responses in a self-learning database, which stores everything everyone has given as an input. From this information, Jabberwacky finds the most appropriate response text. In order to have a sufficient database and intelligent answers to a given input can be computed, the self-learning database takes a very long time to be called "intelligent". Another system called "Alice"[2] is using the Artificial Intelligence Markup Language (short AIML)[3]. "Alice" has a self-learning database as well.

In order to build an information system for incoming students, a self-learning database is not usable because we need a static database which already has enough information stored to answer questions of incoming students.

A group project of the natural language processing course at the University of Applied Science in Darmstadt developed a program to answer questions. This program tokenizes a given question, checking the spelling of these tokens and is filtering out unnecessary tokens with a so-called "stop word" list to get a list of keywords, which are lemmatized and synonyms created. This list of keywords and synonyms is ranked against keywords of questions in the database using the vector space model. The resulting rank value is compared against a threshold value and if the rank value is higher and also the highest rank value of all rank values, the defined answer of this rank value is returned. If there is no higher rank value, the program starts a web search using the web service of SearchBlox [4].

The use of a third party web service includes the problem to achieve the goal of a generalized system which can easily be integrated and usable in university environments. Our design is based on these features.

3 Design

Our design includes the extraction of keywords, building synonyms and ranking them against the keywords of questions in the database. In order to accomplish a better keyword extraction we are using a part-of-speech tagger to tag all word tokens and delete unnecessary tags from this list. This is a preferred, more generalized approach to the stopword list, as it is not limited to one language only. We chose the part-of-speech tagger from the Natural Language Processing Group of Stanford University[5]. Our design is programmed as a Java Servlet.

For a generalized system an external web service for performing a web search is not optimally performant, as an internal API. That is why we integrated the index and search function directly into the system, using the Apache Lucene API to index and

---

[1] `http://www.jabberwacky.com/`

[2] `http://www.alicebot.org/`

[3] A derivative of XML (Extensible Markup Language).

[4] `http://www.searchblox.com/`

[5] `http://nlp.stanford.edu/software/tagger.shtml`

search web pages on the internet. We are also including the Apache PDFBox API into Lucene to search specifically for pdf files on web pages. In addition, a Web Crawler is included which searches a web site for all its pages. To easily update the web data, a second servlet is integrated into the design which calls the update mechanism of the system architecture.

Avoiding hardcoded parameters, we add a single configuration file for setting up all the necessary parameters. For example, the web page URL, the file endings searched for (e.g. html, pdf) and predefined replies. This system design approach enables easy integrating options within a wider range of different environments.

4 Architecture

The following flowchart shows the system architecture.

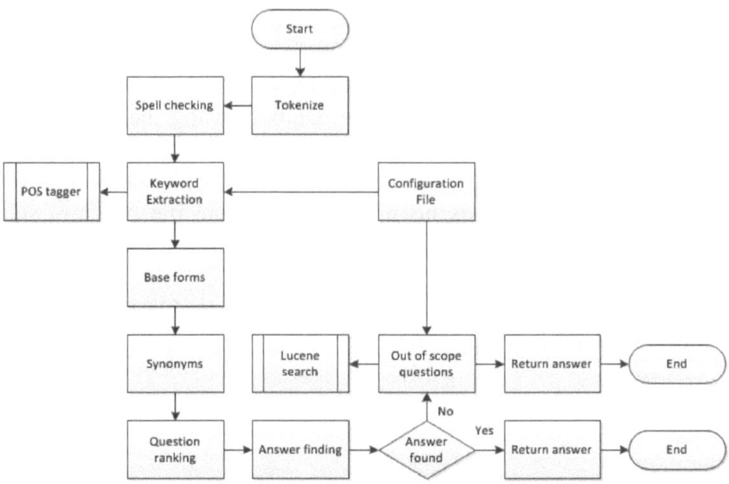

Fig. 1. System Architecture Flowchart

The working process of the system starts with the tokenization of the question. The Tokenizer splits plain text into logical sequences, which are called tokens, and removes punctuation marks. The word tokens are listed in a Java ArrayList and transformed into lowercase to avoid token repetitions because of case differences. This word token list is then forwarded to the spell checker.

The spell checker uses a list of all words of the database containing questions and answers. The complete list is searched for the most similar word using the Levenshtein distance [6] and Keyboard Proximity [7]. The original word token and the found word token are then compared against each other. If they are equal nothing is done,

[6] Minimal number of character changes to transform one word into another.

[7] Hitting wrong key on the keyboard.

otherwise the original word token is replaced by the found word token. The corrected word token list is now forwarded to the keyword extraction with the POS tagger.

The keyword extraction is using a POS tagger, which is using the Penn Treebank POS tag set for tagging the word tokens. All word tokens having a tag of the removable tags are removed from the list and the remaining word tokens are then used as keywords. Removable word tags are: CC, IN, DT, RB, VBP, VB, MD, VBZ, VBD, PRP, PRP$, WRB, LS, these are the tags of conjunctions, determiner, adverbs, verbs in various tenses, modals, pronouns, wh-adverbs and a list item marker.

In the next step the Lemmatizer is generating a lemma for every word, which is called lexical root or the base form. The system is using the English Lemmatizer of the "MorphAdorner" project [8], which is using a combination of irregular forms and grammar rules to determine the lemma of a word token. The remaining lemmatized word tokens are then forwarded to the synonym resolution.

The Synonym resolution in our system is done by using the Java API for WordNet Searching [9] which uses the WordNet [10] database to retrieve synonyms. The synonym resolution process returns a HashMap with the word as key and a weighting value as value, which is for obtaining a different weighting for synonyms then for previous keywords. The HashMap is then forwarded to the question ranking.

The question ranking process in our system is using the vector space model to represent the question and answer documents as a vector. The similarity between the vector of keywords and synonyms of the given question and the vector of keywords from the questions for one answer are calculated with the cosine similarity. The inverse document frequency is also included into the cosine similarity formula. In (1) A and B are two vectors, representing the query (A) and one document (B).

$$similarity = \frac{\sum_{i=1}^{n} A_i * B_i * idf_i^{\,2}}{\sqrt{\sum_{i=1}^{n}(A_i * idf_i)^2} * \sqrt{(B_i * idf_i)^2}} \qquad (1)$$

The similarity of the vectors is the probability for one answer to be related to the query. The result is a list of answer and probability pairs which is forwarded to the find answer process.

The list of answer and probability pairs is now processed to find the best matching answer and the probability of all answers is analyzed for these pairs. The probability has to be higher than a threshold value which is defined as 0.5 [11] and the highest value of all probabilities. The answer with the highest probability value above the threshold is returned to the user. If there is no probability value higher than the threshold value, the given question is forwarded to the web search.

The web search is performed on the basis of the previously extracted keywords of the given question. These keywords are concatenated in one list of single keywords n-grames, where n is the maximum number of keywords. This results in a list of search

---

[8] `http://morphadorner.northwestern.edu/morphadorner/lemmatizer/`

[9] `http://lyle.smu.edu/~tspell/jaws/index.html`

[10] `http://wordnet.princeton.edu`

[11] This value is set as a result of testing because most non matching answers are below this value and matching answers above.

tokens. All web pages identified are saved in a list with their weighting value, which is the percentage matched. If the weighting is higher than the previously stored weighting value for a specific URL, it is updated with every search performed on one search token. A number of web links, specified in the configuration file, is then returned to the user or if no web link is found, the last answer is returned. For indexing the web pages the system has a second servlet to create or update the web search data.

The configuration file includes: the possibility for setting up the database filename, the web site URL, the link endings of pages and documents, the maximum number of displayed link results, the possibility to enable or disable the robot.txt file, the name of the tag model for the POS tagger, the predefined answers displayed before the web links and the last answer if no result is found.

5 User Evaluation

Our program was evaluated at the University of Applied Science in Darmstadt, Germany and at the Reykjavík University in Iceland. The target user group was made up of incoming exchange students. We used a very small database with only a few frequently asked questions. The outcome of the evaluation was that 20 % of the test users would trust information of a BOT and 30 % would not. The program answered 87 questions in total of which 14 % were correctly answered, 46 % wrong and 40 % were unknown questions.

6 Conclusion

After analyzing the results of the user evaluation, our BOT can be used, but its answers are not totally reliable, which is mainly caused by the limited data in our database. To prevent the program from answering so many questions incorrectly, the database should have at least 2 to 3 related questions for a single answer and the dataset should be as large as possible. During the evaluation the test user asked many questions which were not part of the database, that led to a majority of the incorrect answers. However, the main problem is that not all of the test users actually trusted the answers returned by the BOT. We believe that this problem will be resolved by enhancing the database with more current data.

References

1. Jurafsky, D., Martin, J.H.: Speech and language processing (2008)
2. McCandless, M., Hatcher, E., and Gospodnetic, O.: Lucene in Action. Manning Pubs. Co. Series. Manning. (2010) ISBN 9781933988177
3. Toutanova, K., Klein, D., Manning, C., Singer, Y.: Feature-rich part-of-speech tagging with a cyclic dependency network (2003), `http://nlp.stanford.edu/~manning/papers/tagging.pdf`

The Site-Specific Learning Model on Mobile Phones Using Zeigarnik Effect

Designing Collaboration Tool for Outdoor Studying

Yuko Hiramatsu[1], Atsushi Ito[2], and Fumihiro Sato[1]

[1] Chuo University, 742-1 Higashinakano, Hachioji, Tokyo 192-0393, Japan
susana_y@tamacc.chuo-u.ac.jp, fsato@tamacc.chuo-u.ac.jp
[2] KDDI Research and Development Laboratories, 3-10-10 Iidabashi, Chiyoda-ku, Tokyo, 102-8460, Japan
at-itou@kddi.com

Abstract. What is the best way to feel the spirit of the location? In Japan, junior high school students go to several day school trip with classmates. This differs from ordinary sightseeing tours, as its purpose is to encourage students to learn about history and nature in a proactive way. After studying about the area in the school, students walk around there by themselves in small groups. Such on-site outdoor activities are very precious, however, they cannot recognize the artistic points and understand that meaning and value if they just look at the objects or scenery. To solve this problem, we have developed a new learning model for outdoor studies using Zeigarnik effects.

1 Introduction

In Japan, students go to several day school trips with classmates to visit famous places to learn histories. For that purpose, 87.3 % of junior high schools allow students to walk around the area by themselves in small groups [1]. Such site-specific outdoor studies are very precious [2], however, they cannot recognize the artistic points and understand that meaning and value if they just look at the objects or scenery. To solve this problem, we developed a new learning model for outdoor studies using Zeigarnik effects [3]; human beings feel some interesting in object unfinished. This paper examines our learning model for outdoor study and our original application. In addition we will mention the results of the research using our application on September, 2013.

2 Our Methods for Students to Be Interested in Objects

2.1 Using Cognitive Model for Out Door Study

We, human beings do not recognize what we are looking at. For example some like a game named photo hunt. If we can recognize all the things our eyes catch, photo hunt would not be a game. We sometimes do not find the differences between

C. Stephanidis (Ed.): Posters, Part II, HCII 2013, CCIS 374, pp. 43–47, 2013.

two resemble photos. However, once we have caught the object, we cannot help looking at that particular one.If students walk around the area without any marks, their memory would become ambiguous. We utilize this special quality of human beings and use a quiz as the trigger to focus on the object from whole scenery in front of them. Then they would feel the special point of the object deeply. The quizzes are triggers to accept objects positively.

In addition we treat the class in which student prepare to outdoor study as an incomplete experience. Before the trip students have learned history and specific arts in the area and they made some quizzes for other classmates by making use of the preparation. They do not know what kinds of quizzes are preparing for them each other. Such an incomplete experience rouses human beings interest in the object. On the basis of a version of the Zeigarnik tasks that have been completed are recalled less well than tasks that have not been completed. Nowadays some engineers have created detailed navigation systems for trips, however, we create the incomplete experience by design based on the Zeigarnik effects for students.

2.2 Related Works

For the Zeigarnik effects, a study done by Greist-Bousquet and Schiffman 1992 [4] provided evidence. There are several related works about Environmental psychology and tourism. Pearce and Stringer 1991 [5] studied from the view point of physiology, cognition and individual variation etc. Fridgen 1984[6], van Raaij 1996 [7], Toshiji Sasaki also studied about this field. T.Sasaki told that we can part into 3 scenes in a trip: before the trip, during the trip and after the trip. And it is important for travelers to be impressed in each part [8]. As we will mention on chapter 4, we focus this three points and have made our application.

3 Designing Quizzes for Site-Specific Learning

3.1 Using Zeigarnik Effects

The tendency of leaning evaluation is changing from input knowledge to Learning outcomes recently. On our methods students learn about the area (input the knowledge).Then they make Quizzes by preparation of the trip (Learning outcomes). Students learned new knowledge about the area: famous persons, arts, architecture etc. They make quizzes about the objects they are interested in and then they study more. For, if they want to win the game, they should remember many kinds of things about the area. They do not know the quizzes they will answer and they do not know their course to walk exactly till the trip. Teachers make the courses and choose quizzes. In such an incomplete situation students go to the trip and then they will complete their study on the trip.

3.2 Site-Specific Learning

We also consider the trip as a site-specific learning. Using the quizzes, we make some special points to keep students eyes on. This is an example.

Quiz :Do all dragons have wings on their back?

1. Yes, all dragons have wings
2. No, dragons dont have wings.
3. Though eastern dragons have wings, Japanese dragons dont have wings.
4. There are several kinds of dragons in Japan. Some have wings and some dont have wings.

Right answer is 4.

Explanation:There are several kinds of dragons in Japanese legend. Some belong to water and some belong to sky. A dragon of the sky, called TENRYU, has wings. Lets go to the temple and look at the sculpture of a flying dragon. After answering this quiz, students looked at the sculpture with more interest.

4 Outline of Our System

In our model, students walk around the assigned area with smart phone. On the screen, quizzes relating to that area are displayed by using GPS. The quizzes are triggers to accept objects positively. Figure 1 shows the outline of implementation of our learning model. The behavior of this system is as follows.

Scene 1. Preparation: Students make quizzes and set up walking routes before going to outdoor studying. Teachers check routes and quizzes. ((1) and (2) in Figure 1)Students use PC at this step.

Scene 2. During the outdoor study: When a group of students visit the places, they should answer a quiz and find the next place of visiting as orienteering game. They also can see the status, such as points and location, of other

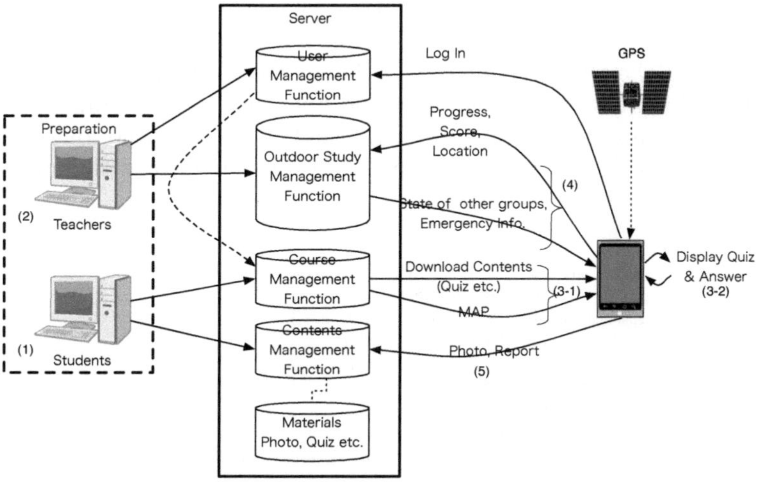

Fig. 1. Outline of implementation of our site-specific learning model

groups. Teachers can get the same information. They may upload photos and comments. ((3)(4)(5) in Figure 1) Students use mobile phones

Scene 3. After the trip:After the trip, the first prize becomes open to everybody at the goal. In addition students have a file of photos that they have taken each point of quiz on the way to the goal. It will be a memorial album for them. Students can look at the file both at PC s and at mobile phones.

5 The Results of a Trial

5.1 Outline of the Trial

We had a trail on September, 2012 around Tokyo Sky Tree. Tokyo Sky Tree is the tallest tower in the world is the new symbol of Tokyo, but also that area was a downtown of Edo. Traditional culture is remaining and there are many historical Japanese temples, gardens and architecture in that area. Summary of the trial is as follows. 30 persons, inclosing high school students, university students and adults, made 8 groups (3 or 4 persons per group). Each group has a smart phone with our site-specific learning application, named Stasta Eye. They walked using this application. 10 quizzes ware prepared for one group. We assigned different route to each group and we set average trip time about 2 hours. After they answered one quiz, then the next point was shown. They could look at the map around the point on smart phone. In addition they could telephone to the curator any time from the application at the emergency situation. Also, the curator used PC in which the places, telephone numbers and the records of the quizzes of all groups were indicated.

5.2 Evaluation Based on Questionnaires

The results of questionnaires show us that people were strongly interested in objects and nature they saw by answering quizzes (Figure 2). We had high valuation about the planning and our methods of learning. In Figure 3, we would like to show the evaluation of planning and operation. The average point of the planning was 4.50 and that of operation was 3.65. People who joined this trial were interested in this kind of study (planning), but the evaluation of operation

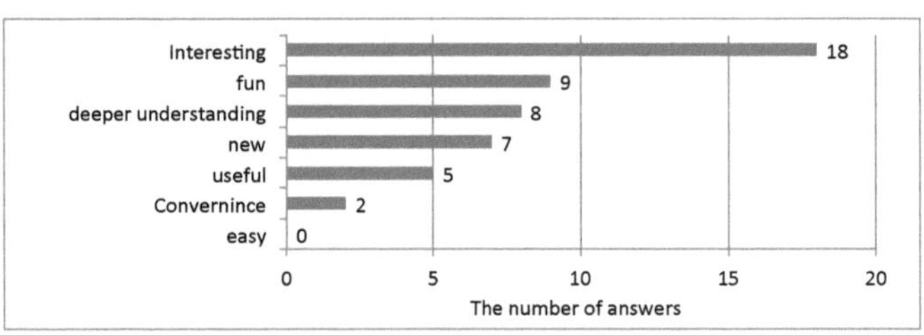

Fig. 2. Impresion of using Stasta Eye (multiple answer)

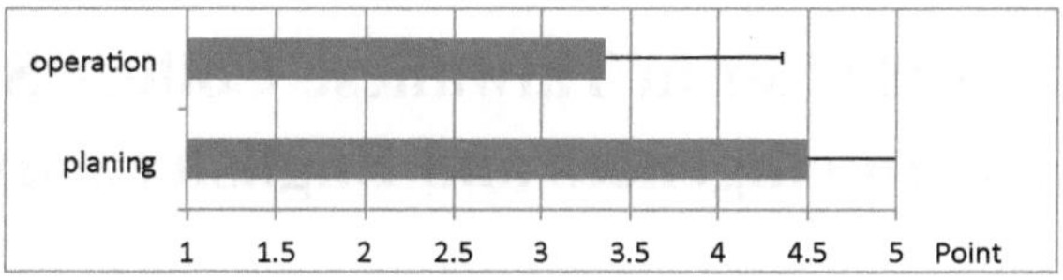

Fig. 3. Evaluation about the planning and the operation Likert scale

was lower than planning. In this trial, who joined this research was high school students, professors of universities and engineers. So that, We think that the evaluation of UI might be divorced and the average score was not so good.

6 Conclusion

We proposed a new idea of site-specific learning using Zeigarnik effect to make school trip more valuable and developed a trial system for evaluation. Smart phone is a useful devise that connects classroom study and outdoor study. It is small and light to bring with. Of course it is not the main object. Smart phone is a subordinating tool to know about the area, in another word, spirit of the place. The site-specific learning could make chances for students to feel and know about the objects in the location. We will continue this research based on experiment, making quizzes and enjoy sightseeing, as educational activities.

Acknowledgment. We would like to thank Prof. Watanabe, Prof. Fujii and Mr.Ogawara of Utsunomiya University who implemented this system. We also thank all volunteer who joined the evaluation and member of Study Group on School Trips [9].

References

1. http://www.travelnews.co.jp/news/kankou/1007301042.html
2. Hatta, N.: The Commitment of Placeto the Birth and the Appreciation of Art Workse. Shimane Journal of Policy Studies 8 (December 2004)
3. Zeigarnik, B.V.: On finished and unfinished tasks. In: Ellis, W.D. (ed.) A Sourcebook of Gestalt Psychology, Humanities Press, New York (1967)
4. Schiffman, N., Greist-Bousquet, S.: Psychology and toursim. Bulletin of the Psychonomic Society 30(1), 9–11 (1992)
5. Pearce, P.L., Stringer, P.F.: The effect of task interruption and closure on perceived duration. Annals of Tourism Research 18, 136–154 (1991)
6. Fridgen, J.D.: Environmental psychology and tourism. Annals of Tourism Research 11(1), 19–39 (1984)
7. Van Raaij, W.E.: Consumer Research on tourism:Mental and behavioral consructs. Annals of Tourism Research 13, 1–9 (1986)
8. Sasaki, T.: Kankoo-Ryoko no Sinrigaku, Kitaoji Shobo, p. 38 (2007)
9. http://joyful-shu-gaku.com/

How Genders Differ in Taiwanese College Students' Multiple Intelligences and English Learning

Yi-an Hou

Kaomei Junior College of Healthcare and Management, Taiwan
hynhyn.tw@yahoo.com.tw

Abstract. The study aims to explore how genders differ in multiple intelligences and English learning. Subjects are 254 Taiwanese EFL college freshmen in a private university in Taiwan, including 113 males and 141 females. They were arranged to take an English proficiency test and fill out questionnaires dealing with their intelligences (MI) (Gardner, 1993) and foreign language learning anxiety (Horwitz, Horwitz, and Cope, 1986). It's suggested that teachers take students' individual differences of intelligences and anxiety into consideration for more effective foreign language teaching and learning.

Keywords: gender difference, multiple intelligences, anxiety.

1 Introduction

Many research findings have revealed the gender differences in language learning performance and behaviors. Since the early 2000s, there have been a growing number of studies about language learning anxiety of Asian learners of Japan, China, Taiwan, Korea, Vietnam, the Philippines, and many others. In addition, many teachers and educators have recognized the important role of Multiple Intelligences (MI). To put the two crucial factors together, the study intends to investigate how multiple intelligences and anxiety predict students' English learning, in particular, how genders differ in multiple intelligences, learning anxiety, and English performance in a Taiwanese EFL setting.

2 Literature Review

Ellis (2003) pointed out that "Sex (or gender) is, of course, likely to interact with other variable in determining L2 proficiency' (p.204). Other research studies have indicated that the learning style preferences by gender make a significant difference in language learning. Girls like to work in groups and used "take-part" methods when reading books together. They also did not want to stop when the reading time had finished. Based on the research findings mentioned above, female students tend to be more positive in learning behaviors and perform better in foreign language learning.

C. Stephanidis (Ed.): Posters, Part II, HCII 2013, CCIS 374, pp. 48–51, 2013.

Learning anxiety is "a distinct complex of self-perceptions, beliefs, feelings, and behaviors related to classroom language learning" (Horwitz, Horwitz, & Cope, 1986, p.128), and affect language learners' performance to some extent. Not until 1978 when Scovel reviewed the sparse literature concerning anxiety's role in language learning, did researchers become interested in investigating the role of anxiety in foreign/second language learning. Nevertheless, many findings are inconsistent and unable to establish a clearcut relationship between anxiety and overall foreign language achievement (Horwitz, Horwitz & Cope, 1986), nor establish a clear picture of how anxiety affects language learning and performance.

The Multiple Intelligence theory (MI), proposed by Gardner (1983) offers teachers a way to examine and adopt the best teaching techniques and strategies in light of student's individual differences. It also encourages educators to view learners as equals regardless of quotient produced from a traditional intelligence exam. Without doubt that Gardner deserves everyone's gratitude, in particular, language teachers appreciate how well the theory applies in the language-learning process. With the help of the theory, language teachers can create activities flexible, reflective, logical, and creative for diverse students' individual differences.

3 Methodology

The study intends to answer the following research questions:

1. Are multiple intelligences and foreign language learning anxiety predictive to Taiwanese EFL college students' English proficiency?
2. How genders differ in students' multiple intelligences, anxiety, and English performance?

The purposes of the study are to investigate gender differences in Taiwanese EFL college students' multiple intelligences and English learning anxiety, as well as the prediction of multiple intelligences and foreign language learning anxiety to their English proficiency.

A case study and convenience sampling were used for the research methodology. It is the study of a bounded system, which is in a particular circumstance and with a particular problem, and also gives readers 'space" for their own opinions (Stake, 1988). In addition, the subjects included in the sample were "whoever happen to be available at that time" (Gay & Airasian, 2003, p.112).

Subjects are 254 Taiwanese EFL college freshmen in a private university in Taiwan, including 113 males and 141 females. In addition to their English scores of College Entrance Exam adopted, they were arranged to take an English proficiency test and fill out questionnaires dealing with their intelligences (MI) (Gardner, 1993) and foreign language learning anxiety (Horwitz, Horwitz, and Cope, 1986).

The research instruments include questionnaires of Multiple Intelligences (MI) (Gardner, 1985), Foreign Language Classroom Anxiety Scale (FLCAS) (Horwits, Horwitz, and Cope ,1986), as well as English scores of College Entrance Exam (CEE) and National English Test of Proficiency All on Web (NETPAW). Along with descriptive statistics of mean, standard deviation, and percentages, Regression Analysis and T-test analysis were used to answer the research questions. All available data were processed by SPSS 16 (Statistical Package of Social Science). In this study, the significance level was set at $p<.05$.

4 Findings and Discussions

The reliability of the questionnaire of MI and Foreign Language Classroom Anxiety Scale (FLCAS) is Cronach Alpha =.732 and Cronach Alpha =.930. The results indicate that the research instruments of the study are acceptable and reliable.

The results reveal that students' English proficiency is not satisfactory and their anxiety level is above average (M=3.08/5.00). Furthermore, they are with strong Musical Intelligences (M=3.94), followed by Interpersonal Intelligences (M=3.53), but weak with Visual/Spatial Intelligences (M=3.13) and Logical/Mathematical Intelligences (M=2.70). As for Foreign Language Classroom Anxiety Scale (FLCAS), the top sources of their anxiety come from worrying about the consequences of failing the English class, having to speak without preparation, feeling that the other students speak better, having not prepared in advance when English teacher asks questions, finding themselves thinking about things that have nothing to do with the course, and keeping thinking that other students are better than they are.

By Regression Analysis, it's found that score of NETPAW is predictive of CEE ($p<.01$). But for the scores of NETPAW, the best predictors are students' scores CEE ($p<.01$), Anxiety (FLCAS) ($p<.01$) and Verbal/Linguistic intelligence ($p<.05$). In other words, students with higher scores of CEE, higher level of anxiety, and stronger Verbal/Linguistic intelligences, tend to have better scores of NETPAW.

The findings show that significant differences exist in English scores of CEE ($p<.01$), **Logical**/Mathematical intelligence ($p<.01$), and **Bodily**/Kinesthetic intelligence ($p<.05$) between male students and female students. Female students have better English scores of CEE than males, but male students are with stronger **Logical**/Mathematical intelligence and **Bodily**/Kinesthetic intelligence than females. As for anxiety, female students tend to have higher level of anxiety than male students, in particular, when they don't understand what the teacher is saying in English class ($p<.01$), worry about the consequences of failing English class ($p<.05$), and get nervous when English teachers asks questions which they haven't prepared in advance ($p<.05$).

5 Conclusion and Implication

5.1 Conclusion

1. The reliability of the research instrument is Cronbach's Alpha=.93 and .73 for the Foreign Language Classroom Anxiety Scale (FLCAS) and Multiple Intelligences (MI), respectively. The results reveal the acceptability and reliability of the research instruments.

2. Students are with stronger Musical intelligence, but with weaker Logical/ Mathematical intelligence (especially females), and their anxiety level is above average.
3. Factors predictive to students' English scores of NETPAW are Verbal/Linguistic intelligence ($p<.05$) and anxiety ($p<.01$), positively.
4. Male students are stronger with Logical/Mathematical intelligence ($p<.01$) and Bodily/ Kinesthetic intelligence ($p<.05$), but female students have better English scores of NETPAW. In addition, female students tend to have higher level of anxiety and genders do differ in anxiety to some extent.

5.2 Implication

1. Students' English performance is predictive by Verbal/linguistic intelligences ($p<.05$) and Anxiety ($p<.01$), positively. However, students are weak in Verbal/linguistic intelligences. So teachers should help students strengthen their Verbal/Linguistic intelligences (especially male students) by "teaching strategies for Verbal/Linguistic Intelligence", including "storytelling, brainstorming, tape recording, journal writing, and publishing" (Armstrong, 2000, pp.51-53).
2. Anxiety is also predictive to students' English performance ($p<.01$), positively. It proves that some kind of anxiety is essential. So, teachers should let the students know that anxiety is normal and likely to arouse in every language learning stage, and encourage students to try to make the best use of anxiety's positive effects on learning.

References

1. Gardner, H.: Multiple Intelligences: The Theory in Practice. Basic Books, New York (1993)
2. Horwitz, E.K., Horwitz, M.B., Cope, J.: Foreign language classroom anxiety. The Modern Language Journal 70, 125–132 (1986)
3. Hu, G.: Recent important developments in secondary English-language teaching in the People's Republic of China. Language, Culture, Curriculum 15, 30–49 (2002)
4. Kim, J.H.: Foreign language listening anxiety: A study of Korean students' learning English. Unpublished doctoral dissertationl. the University of Texas, Austin (2000)
5. Nguyen-thuy, L.: Foreign language learning anxiety among 1st-year students at FELTE. Thesis of Bachelor degree. Vietnam National University, Hanoi (2011)
6. Lucas, R.I.: English language learning anxiety among foreign language learners in the Philippines. Philippine ESL Journal 7, 3–27 (2011)
7. Scovel, T.: The effect of affect on foreign language learning: A review of the anxiety research. Language Learning 28, 129–142 (1978)
8. Stake, R.E.: Case study methods in educational research: Seeking sweet water. In: Jaeger, R.M. (ed.) Complementary Methods for Research in Education, pp. 253–300. American Educational Research Association, Washington, DC (1988)

Mapping Peace Ideas around the Table

Andri Ioannou, Panayiotis Zaphiris, Fernando Loizides, and Christina Vasiliou

Cyprus University of Technology, Department of Multimedia and Graphic Arts, Limassol, Cyprus
{andri.i.ioannou,panayiotis.zaphiris,fernando.loizides, c.vasiliou}@cut.ac.cy

Abstract. This work is concerned with the exploration of an educational tabletop application designed to facilitate dialog and collaborative decision making. The application was enacted in the context of two sensitive scenarios related to Peace and Immigration. Results showed that despite the sensitivity of the scenarios, the interactions observed were rich in cognitive and physical elements and typical to small group collaboration around problem-based activities. Moreover, the taxonomies of ideas constructed by the groups highlight a number of areas where research could focus in terms of using technology for peace making.

Keywords: collaborative decision making, surface computing, interactive tables, tabletops, peace, immigration.

1 Introduction

Multi-touch interactive tables (or tabletops) have recently attracted the attention of the human computer interaction (HCI) and Learning Technology communities. As discussed by [2], multi-touch tabletops afford cooperative gestures which can enhance users' sense of teamwork. In this work, an educational tabletop application designed to facilitate dialog and collaborative decision making was enacted in the context of two sensitive scenarios related to Peace and Immigration. These are topics of interest to the HCI and Learning Technology communities, but for which empirical research is currently lacking. The study sought to explore two research questions (RQs): (1) What kinds of interactions occur amongst the participants and the tabletop; (2) What themes and ideas relevant to Peace and Immigration are demonstrated during the collaborative activity. We briefly report on the functionality of the tabletop application. We then report empirical findings from two studies.

2 The Tabletop Application

Ideas Mapping is a tabletop application designed to support collaborative decision making by allowing the participants to analyze a problem and brainstorm around possible solutions, while they actively construct a consensus artifact -- namely, a taxonomy of their ideas. A user-centered design approach was followed for the design

C. Stephanidis (Ed.): Posters, Part II, HCII 2013, CCIS 374, pp. 52–56, 2013.

of the application. The detailed functionality of the application, design methodology and user experience evaluation are reported elsewhere [3]. Below we briefly report the three stages of the application:

Stage 1: With a problem at hand, each collaborator generates new ideas. Ideas are typed into a web application through the use of a mobile device such as a laptop or tablet (brainstorming).

Stage 2: The ideas are presented one-by-one, as digital post-it notes in the middle of the tabletop and become subject to discussion amongst the collaborators. For each idea, collaborators make an effort to categorize it in a thematic unit - thematic units can be created by any participant (collaborative decision making).

Stage 3: Participants can finalize their taxonomy by editing ideas or generating new ones, deleting ideas or thematic units that are less promising, and relocating ideas into thematic units for a better fit (collaborative decision making).

3 Methodology

Participants. For study 1, we recruited 17 MA/PhD students at a public university in Cyprus, aged between 22-45 years old (M=30). The participants formed five groups: 3 groups of 3 students and 2 groups of 4 students, suitable for the four-sided tabletop. For study 2, we recruited 20 new students (forming 4-member groups), aged between 22-35 years old (M=25) from the same school. Three groups were composed of 4-year undergraduate students and another two groups were composed of MA/PhD students.

Procedures. In study 1, the following scenario was presented to the students: "Your team works at a non-governmental organization dealing with global peace. Your project is to create a taxonomy of ideas regarding how we can promote global peace using technology." Students were given a week to think creatively and record their ideas into the Ideas Mapping web application (brainstorming). Then, each group met face-to-face around the table and engaged in collaborative work as required by Stages 2 and 3 of Ideas Mapping. Briefly, the group categorized the different views and ideas of the participants into thematic units (collaborative decision making, see Fig. 1), aiming to create a taxonomy of how global peace can be promoted through technology (collaborative decision making, see Fig. 2). In Study 2, the procedures were identical to those of Study 1, but with the new scenario focused on immigration: "Your team works at a non-governmental organization dealing with immigration issues. Your project is to create a taxonomy of ideas regarding how we can promote the integration of immigrants in Cyprus using technology."

Data Collection and Analysis. The sessions of all five groups were video recorded; more than four hours of video data were collected across groups (approximately 50 minutes for each group). Detailed video analysis was conducted guided by the RQs of the study. In particular, all utterances in the video were first transcribed to assist with subsequent analysis. A coding scheme was then developed to describe the cognitive and physical interactions present during the activity (RQ1). Finally, the taxonomies constructed by the groups were explored for consistent themes and ideas (RQ2).

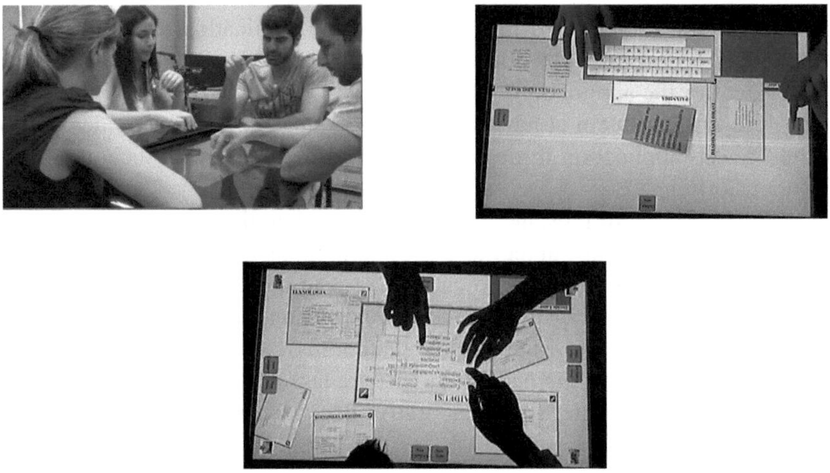

Fig. 1. Categorization of ideas in thematic units (up); Consensus on group artifact (down)

4 Results

The resulting coding scheme (see Table 1) showed that, despite the sensitivity of the scenarios, the cognitive interaction patterns observed were typical to small group collaboration on problem-based activities as described in previous research (e.g., [1]). Additionally, there was focused physical interaction with the application with the participants maintaining joint attention on the content of the notes and categories.

Table 1. Coding Scheme - Cognitive and Physical Contributions around the Tabletop

Cognitive Contributions
1.Knowledge Sharing –Description of views and ideas on the problem
2.Proposing – Proposing a thematic unit or a new idea
3.Elaborating – Building on previous statements, Clarifications
4.Negotiating meaning – Evaluation of proposal, Questioning/ answering, Expressing agreement/disagreement, Providing arguments for/against
5.Stating consensus – Summary of ideas, Metacognitive reflections
6.Other talk – Tool-related talk, Social talk, Laughter
Physical Contributions
7.Communicative Gestures – Show on the table without touching, Dominating/blocking gestures
8.Touch Gestures – Resize, Rotate, Type, Move something across, Random touching or touching to explore

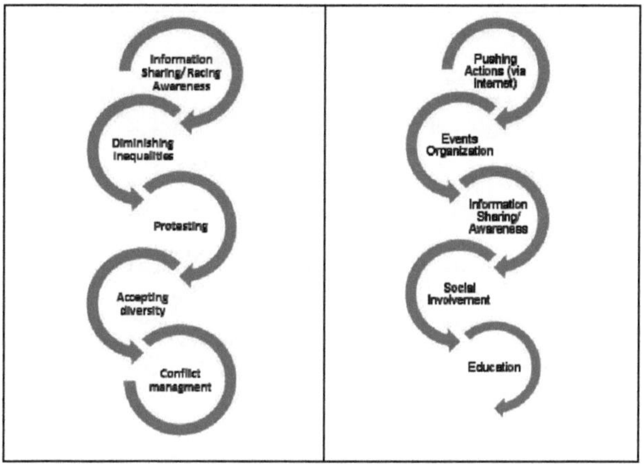

Fig. 2. Sample taxonomies of using technology to promote peace

With regards to taxonomies created, there was some overlap in the general thematic categories formulated across groups. Yet, there was less overlap in the ideas included in the categories. In fact, each group had a few unique and creative ideas within each category. On the other hand, some similar ideas were categorized differently by different groups as a result of the negotiation process and the views of the participants. The taxonomies of two participating groups from each study are illustrated in Fig. 2 and 3 for a sample (read as "Using Technology for…").

Overall and across both investigations, we found that the ideas contributed revolved around (and can be consolidated into) three themes: (1) the use of specific technologies to promote peace-related outcomes (e.g., the use of YouTube to broadcast favorable images of the "other"/"enemy"/"immigrant" and to promote awareness of their culture, (2) the use of technology to promote empowerment (e.g., allowing "access" to technology seeking to "include" the children of the developing world/the immigrant and enable a means for learning), and (3) the use of technology for understanding conflict (e.g., discussions and collaboration on conflict resolution among the conflicting parties using weblogs and wikis etc.). All of these provide insights and directions relevant for future research in the area of using technology for peace making.

5 Discussion

In the HCI and Learning Technology research communities there is not much work reporting empirical findings from using technology to facilitate co-located collaboration around sensitive topics such as Peace and Immigration. We now have some evidence on how educational tabletop applications can be tailored toward this direction; our investigation of Ideas Mapping showed that participants were actively engaged in the group activity, both cognitively and physically.

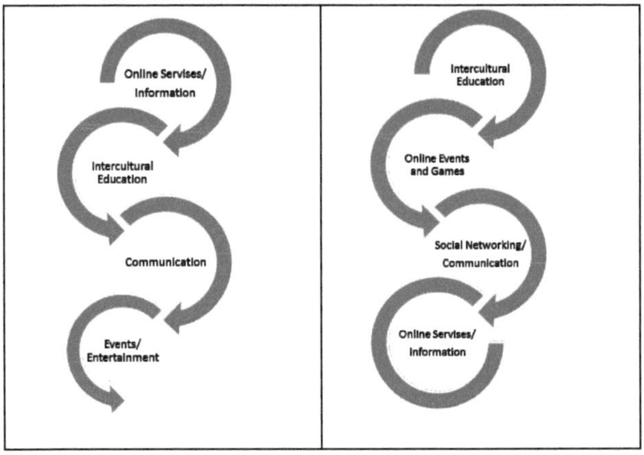

Fig. 3. Sample taxonomies of using technology to promote the integration of immigrants

Additionally, the study showed that, despite the sensitivity of the scenarios, the cognitive interactions observed during the activity were typical to small group collaboration around problem-based activities. This finding enforces the use of Peace and Immigration -related problem-based scenarios as fruitful collaborative activities that also serve an important purpose.

Last but not least, groups in both investigations produced interesting taxonomies of their ideas which reflected the result of their consensus decision making. These taxonomies highlight a number of areas where research could focus in terms of using technology to promote peace and immigrants' integration in the society.

References

1. Hmelo-Silver, C.E.: Analyzing collaborative knowledge construction: Multiple methods for integrated understanding. Computers and Education 41(4), 397–420 (2003)
2. Morris, M.R., Huang, A., Paepcke, A., Winograd, T.: Cooperative gestures: Multi-user gestural interactions for co-located groupware. In: Proc. CHI, pp. 1201–1210. ACM (2006)
3. Zaphiris, P., Ioannou, A., Loizides, F., Vasiliou, C.: User Expreicne in Using Surface Computing for Collaborative Decision Making. Interactive Technology and Smart Education (in press)

Exploring the Impact of School Culture on School's Internet Safety Policy Development

Birgy Lorenz[1], Kaido Kikkas[1,2], and Mart Laanpere[1]

[1] Institute of Informatics, Tallinn University, Narva Road 25, 10120 Tallinn, Estonia
[2] Estonian Information Technology College, Raja St 4C, 12616 Tallinn, Estonia
{Birgy.Lorenz,Kaido.Kikkas,Mart.Laanpere}@tlu.ee

Abstract. This paper describes an exploratory study on school-level e-safety policy development. The research was based on the participatory design-based methodology, involving various stakeholders in a school-level policy development exercise. Our aim was to find out whether the schools with open and participatory culture would choose more flexible, emancipatory and participatory approach to e-safety policy development, while schools with rational-managerial organizational culture tend to rely on prescriptive approaches and technology-driven solutions in their e-safety policies. Regarding future research, we plan to continue the work to construct a new design and development platform to be used in a more flexible and bottom-up manner instead of strict prescriptive rule sets provided on the national level.

Keywords: policy development, internet safety, participatory design-based methodology, school culture, privacy issues.

1 Background

Since the Children's Internet Protection Act ("CIPA") in 2000, USA requires recipients of federal technology funds to comply with Internet filtering and policy requirements[1] and Internet Safety Act from 2009 gave responsibility to log to the police. In Europe, the Safer Internet Programme[2] and the European Network of Awareness Centres have developed an award system for schools called 'E-Safety label'[3] since 2012. The weakness here is that decision-making about e-safety policies on the global level takes time and compromises, while the world is changing more rapidly than legislation. In order to increase the sense of ownership towards e-safety policies at schools, we propose a new, bottom-up approach to e-safety policy development [6].

The process of policy development usually involves steps like issue identification, analysis, generating solutions, involving experts for prediction and performance

---

[1] CIPA: http://www.e-ratecentral.com/CIPA/

[2] InSafe Programme: http://www.saferinternet.org/web/guest/about-us

[3] Esafety Label: http://www.esafetylabel.eu/web/guest/about

C. Stephanidis (Ed.): Posters, Part II, HCII 2013, CCIS 374, pp. 57–60, 2013.

measurement [3]. Stakeholders should always be involved. The timeframe depends on the situation: the pace is hastened if the policy development is initiated as a reaction to recent e-safety incidents. In most cases policies are developed with proactive approach – with application research and input from interested parties [2]. The context of our study is framed by the lack of national-level e-safety policies in Estonia and an increasing demand for school-level policies, guidelines and intervention schemes which could help the schools to counter potential e-safety related threats and manage incidents. As the schools in Estonia enjoy large degree of freedom in policy development and examples from other countries are widely available, our schools are sometimes taking very different perspectives on e-safety policy development as well content [4]. The current study explores to what extent these differences could be attributed to the school culture and how can we support (on the national level) a set of alternative approaches to e-safety policy development, which should be sensitive to the school culture.

Our general approach to the development is following the tradition of scenario-based design by Carroll (1999). The main advantages of this method are enhanced ownership and relevance for the target group, but also flexibility and agility. In addition, this method allows describing the policy goals and measures in the target group's own language [1]. We also include in our methodology ideas from the field of school culture research [5]. Eventually, our aim is to demonstrate that local development of e-safety rules and regulations works better in case the process is adapted in accordance with the organisational culture in a given school. The current paper addresses only the first phase of this research.

2 Methods

The first stage of our study involved interviews with representatives of 5 stakeholder groups in one school: school board (4 persons), teaching staff (15), students (2) and parents (4). Semi-structured interviews focused on perceived needs and problems regarding e-safety policy, the policy development process and its participants. In the second stage, we developed and validated through online survey an original 8-step model for bottom-up e-safety policy development and pilot-tested it in one school, in order to find out how our model could be improved. Our model consisted of eight steps (an extended description is available online[4]): (1) collecting accounts on e-safety incidents and fictional stories; (2) specifying the policy-related needs of the school; (3) participatory design of e-safety rules and recommendations; (4) voting for the important and disputable topics; (5) evaluating findings; (6) getting feedback to initial policy from stakeholders; (7) developing final set of regulations or repeat some steps; (8) rolling out, promoting and enforcing the final policy document. In the third stage, we plan to carry out a design experiment in 20 schools, which go through the e-safety policy development process in line with our 8-step model. Prior to the pilot test, the school culture survey will be carried out in all participating schools, based on

[4] http://goo.gl/0eyrE

Maslowski (2001). In the fourth stage, we will modify our 8-step policy development model so that it could be dynamically adapted to the school culture in selected organization. This paper reflects on the model design and validation survey carried out in the second phase in 20 schools selected for participation in design experiment to be carried out in the third phase.

3 Results and Discussion

Estonian schools reported students' good understanding of the concept of internet safety (76%), existence of e-safety policies in 48% of schools, school e-safety trainings (64%) and blind trust in technical restrictions (84%). 50% of the schools are interested to deal with e-safety policy-making more deeply. All groups mentioned mobile phones, WiFi and BYOD (bring your own device) being the issue of disagreement. Both teachers and students mentioned there are a lot of oral guidelines and it differs by class and school. While teachers felt that filtering or other technological restrictions would make the school safer, ICT managers disagreed: "Blocking and filtering can only restrict beginners, not advanced users. Only teachers are affected by technical restrictions, students just override them". Almost all teachers and 72% of students agreed that schools need e-safety policy. Yet it was unclear how this policy should be developed: some respondents see it a responsibility for ICT staff and administration. Students stated that when they are not active in the development of school rules, they are not eager to follow them. About 85% of school IT-specialists expected to take initiative over their e-safety policy development and to involve in this process teachers (in 32% of schools), administration (31%), students (23%), and parents (15%).

We introduced our 8-step model for e-safety policy development to 20 schools and conducted an online survey among IT-specialists of these schools to validate our model. 16 out of 20 respondents agreed that explicit e-safety policy is needed in their school. Two schools reported that they do not have currently any rules about e-safety, nor do not they provide WiFi for their students. Seven schools had a policy only for behavior in computer labs; ten schools have addressed e-safety issues in their general house rules document.

4 Conclusion

The participatory design of e-safety policy development model requires flexibility to meet the needs of schools with highly heterogeneous school culture. Yet, the schools would also appreciate if the efforts related with participatory policy development could be reduced through providing clear guidelines, templates, survey instruments, examples on data collecting, sorting and voting process. We found that decision making works better in a small committee that includes members of school board, the school's ICT specialist and a teacher. Developing rules and regulations should not be automated in a uniform manner or let some small expert group handle it, as through participatory design the ownership, awareness and commitment to the new policy could be achieved significantly more effectively.

The next step in our research is to involve 20 schools in pilot study where they go through the full-scale process of participatory development of their local e-safety policy, based on our 8-step model. As the participating schools will be selected so that they represent four different school culture types, this allows us to explore the needs for modifying our model according to the school culture.

Acknowledgements. This research was supported by European Social Fund's Doctoral Studies and Internationalization Programme DoRa, which is carried out by Foundation Archimedes and also by Estonian Information Technology Foundation.

References

1. Carroll, J.: Five Reasons for Scenario-Based Design. In: Proceedings of the 32nd Hawaii International Conference on System Sciences (1999), http://testingeducation.org/BBST/testdesign/CarrollScenarios.pdf (retrieved)
2. Dukeshire, S., Thurlow, J.: A Brief Guide to Understanding Policy Development, Rural Communities Impacting Policy (2002), http://www.ruralnovascotia.ca/documents ISBN 0-9780913-0-2 (retrived)
3. Frag, M.: A Guide To Policy Development, Office of the Auditor General Manitoba Technology (2003), http://www.oag.mb.ca/wp-content/uploads/2011/06/ (retrieved)
4. Marandi, T., et al.: IKT ja Eesti koolikultuur, Tiigrihüppe SA (2003), http://www.tiigrihype.ee/sites/default/files/tekstifailid/IKT_ja_Eesti%20koolikultuur_2003.pdf (retrieved)
5. Maslowski, R.: School Culture and School Performance. Ph. D. thesis Twente University Press (2001), http://doc.utwente.nl/36122/1/t0000012.pdf (retrieved)
6. Niemi, H., Kynäslahti, H., Vahtivuori-Hänninen, S.: Towards ICT in everyday life in Finnish schools: seeking conditions for good practices. Learning, Media and Technology 38(1), 57–71 (2013)

Choosing and Using a Common Book in an Undergraduate Research Experience

D. Scott McCrickard[1], Woodrow Winchester[2], Marlow Lemons[3], and Robert Beaton[1]

[1] Department of Computer Science,
[2] Grado Department of Industrial and Systems Engineering,
[3] Department of Statistics,
Virginia Tech, Blacksburg VA 24061, USA
{mccricks,wwwinche,lemons,rbeaton}@vt.edu

Abstract. This paper describes efforts in using a common book in an undergraduate research experience, including choosing a book, crafting activities (both inside and outside the classroom) around book readings, and evidence of the effectiveness of the methods in selection and use. The experiences highlight the value to educators seeking to include a common book as part of a research course or experience—but also value for anyone seeking to use a common book as an integral part of teaching efforts.

Keywords: computer science education, human factors, common book.

1 Introduction

Introduction of a *common book*, a short and appealing manuscript to be provided to all students within a certain demographic, has been adopted by universities and colleges as a way to encourage a sense of community and togetherness among members of the student population. Selection of the common book generally takes place at a high level within the university by a large and diverse committee—with the mandate to use the book passed on to the professors teaching the students. Suggested methods for utilizing a common book include creation of discussion groups around book topics, in-class reference to select sections or quotations, and an invitation of relevant speakers on the book to class—generally methods that are not graded but have potential to broaden student understanding through shared experience. In a survey of 130 administrators of common book programs, the top three goals in adopting common books were developing community outside of the classroom, fostering intellectual engagement, and encouraging a breadth of reading toward understanding diverse perspectives [14]—goals that seem relevant for our research-centered experience.

This paper describes our efforts in using a common book in multi-university undergraduate research experiences. We describe the methods used to choose a book, activities (both inside and outside the classroom) designed around book readings, and empirical and anecdotal evidence of the effectiveness of our methods. We expect that

C. Stephanidis (Ed.): Posters, Part II, HCII 2013, CCIS 374, pp. 61–65, 2013.

our experiences will be of the most value to educators seeking to include a common book as part of a research course or experience—but we see value for anyone seeking to use a common book as a central part of teaching and research efforts. Primarily, our data come from experiences with undergraduate students at an alliance of universities, funded by a National Science Foundation (NSF) Broadening Participation in Computing (BPC) alliance and an NSF Research Experience for Undergraduates (REU) grant. The alliance focused on building research skills and desires among undergraduate students. We administered this program for six years and, in each instance, made reading integral to their weekly activities.

2 Choosing a Common Book and Crafting Activities

Guidelines for choosing a common book generally center on issues like readability, low cost, potential for student engagement, relevance and appeal to target student populations, richness of content, and connection to college initiatives [6]. These guidelines, and others like them, have relevance to our more focused target group—but the guidelines we found typically focus on university-wide common book programs for incoming freshmen. We seek to establish four categories for these themes that are particularly relevant to computing and HCI disciplines—current events, group demographic, task, and topic—and to provide examples of books in each category. This does not represent a complete list of themes, or a mutually exclusive list, but rather ones relevant in the selection of books for our program.

A *current events* theme leverages highly-visible books, authors, and events, toward increasing relevance and appeal for the student readers. Examples include Randy Pausch's *The Last Lecture* [10], authored by a computing researcher after receiving a diagnosis of terminal pancreatic cancer, and Casey's *Atomic Chef* and Petroski's *To Engineer is Human*, both aggregates of news stories that highlight how technological innovations can have tragic results when designers fail to consider the possibility for human error [3,11]. The *group demographic* theme focuses on books that are appealing or relevant to certain characteristics of the target demographic. Examples include Quart's *Branded* [13], examining how advertisers target teenagers toward maximizing profits, and Lightman's *Einstein's Dreams* thought experiment a young Einstein's thoughts and dreams [7]. A *task* theme informs the readers about a common task all will be seeking to accomplish; for example, undertaking a research effort, pursuing a college degree, or writing a professional paper. Examples of common books with a task theme are Booth's *The Craft of Research* and Peters' *Getting What You Came For* [1,10]. A *topical* theme focuses on the topic that will engage the students—in our case, human-computer interaction (HCI) that was the focus of our program. Examples of common books with a topical theme include Norman's *Design of Everyday Things* and Vicente's *The Human Factor* [9,15].

A common book is often intended to establish informal common talking points among students, creating opportunities for dialog and raising issues for deep thought. However, it has proven important to engage students—both in formal classroom settings and through external activities—through highly interactive activities related to the common book. Generally, we provide a brief recap of the readings for the day—but with lots of embedded questions to highlight the need to do the reading. Perhaps most inspiring to students is the connection of concepts in the book to personal anecdotes—both from the discussion leader and from the students. This begins to foster creative and interactive thought that is essential in the next component of our weekly classroom activities.

Vital in encouraging engagement from students is the inclusion of interactive activities that exercise their creative energies. An effective technique for inspiring this engagement is to turn around the arguments and techniques from readings and have them apply it creatively to a common situation—or to another reading. The importance of creativity is evidenced by the successes of such innovators as Apple and IDEO. Activities crafted from book themes often have a creative component of sketching, sculpting, or cooking, with connections to computing and research that can exercise creativity, connect design with engineering, and lead to richer learning experiences [2,4,5,8,14].

3 Assessing the Importance of a Common Book

Assessment of educational approaches is vital in creating a foundation that others can leverage. Much of the evaluation for common books relies on opinions of organizers based on their observations—and often it is only mildly positive [15]. As described previously in this paper, research exemplifies the value that can be obtained through a common reading for freshmen students [6, 15]. This section presents our evaluation approach for benefits from common readings undertaken by more senior students—focusing on empirical evidence, anecdotal evidence, and post-program reflection from the first three years of our program.

In an effort to understand the value that students place on a common book experience—particularly in comparison with other factors like the year of study and an annual research symposium—we administered several surveys and analyzed them for relevant influential factors: a Demographics survey, a Post Orientation survey, a Progress survey, and a Post Summer survey. We applied an item response theory (IRT) model to measure how the summer experience gave our students an intellectually value-added experience. Variables such as the year of the summer program (which we will call YEAR), students' responses to participating in an end-of-summer research symposium (SYMP), and students' responses to the book-centered courses taken each summer (i.e. COURSES) were used to measure their likelihood of enhancing their interest in HCI (which we will name this response variable HCI_INT). We used a backward regression modeling technique, logit, removing insignificant variables and reproducing a smaller model, toward categorizing explanatory and response variables. Phase 1 of the logit regression model included all three explanatory variables, concluding that all of the explanatory variable, with the exception of YEAR, were significant in measuring HCI. After Phase 2, the SYMP variable was not significant and was, thus, removed from the model. Finally, Phase 3 concluded that only the COURSES variables remained significant.

We found that students that reacted very positive (or very negative) toward taking the Monday meetings and participating in the research symposium have a higher (or lower) odds ratio of being classified as one who has a 'Very Strong' level of interest in HCI research versus an 'At Most Neutral' interest. We infer from this finding that these students understood the value of a research symposium where key personnel from the Center, the university, and local technology companies attended. Following up on this result, we used a logit regression model once more to estimate the likelihood of our student participants pursuing graduate studies in HCI at Virginia Tech based on the YEAR, SYMP, and COURSES variables. The response variable, which we will call GRAD_STUD, was categorized where '2' represents those that are "Strongly" encouraged to pursue graduate studies in HCI, '1' represents those that are "Slightly to Moderately" encouraged, and '0' represents those students that are 'At Most Neutral'. We found the COURSES variable to be the only significant variable in predicting GRAD_STUD—students who had a positive experience in the weekly meetings were more likely to strongly desire to pursue research further. This suggests a need to focus even more on providing positive, inclusive, and interactive experiences during our Monday sessions, with close repetition and integration of the lessons related to creativity, technology, computing, and human-computer interaction.

Anecdotal qualitative evidence suggests that using a common book (1) encourages peer-to-peer debate on what our key program focus (research) really means to the students, (2) helps participants experience different viewpoints of research and processes in conducting it, and (3) encourages participants to gain more knowledge to network with other researchers. In return, the common book gives students a panoramic view of what it means to be called a "researcher".

Online discussions with students who took part in the common book initiative revealed how the books shaped their careers. Three students took part in the discussions, all of whom are part of Ph.D. programs. All three recognized value in the books during the course of the program, and two still own the books. One acknowledged recommending it to others. Learning sessions that were more active (e.g., videos with discussions, relating to metaphors) stood out to the students. However, none have re-read the book since the initiative ended (though one noted an occasional desire to do so). It seems that the book was useful during the program and still sparks discussion, but none became favorites of the program participants.

4 Conclusions and Future Work

This paper describes our efforts in using a common book in undergraduate research experiences, providing four themes for common books—current events, group demographic, task, and topic. We describe how activities inside and outside of the classroom can assist in the use of a common book, with examples and support from empirical and anecdotal evidence. We expect that our experiences will be of the most value to educators seeking to include a common book as part of a research course or experience—but we see value for anyone seeking to use a common book.

Acknowledgements. Thanks to all of the student participants, grad facilitators, and faculty for taking part in our common book program and for providing great feedback about the common reading. Thanks to the NSF for providing relevant funding through grants IIS-0552732, CNS-0540509, IIS-0851774, and IIS-1134960.

References

1. Booth, W.C., Colomb, G.G., Williams, J.M.: The craft of research. The University of Chicago Press, Chicago (2003)
2. Buxton, B.: Sketching User Experiences. Morgan Kaufmann Publishers, San Francisco (2007)
3. Casey, S.: The atomic chef and other true talks of design, technology, and human error. Aegean Publishing Company, Santa Barbara (2006)
4. Fallman, D.: Design-oriented Human-Computer Interaction. In: Proceedings of ACM SIGCH, pp. 225–232 (2003)
5. Gelb, M.: How to Think like Leonardo da Vinci. Dell Publishing, New York (1998)
6. Laufgraben, J.L.: Common reading programs: Going beyond the book. Columbia, SC: National Resource Center for the First-Year Experience & Students in Transition. University of South Carolina (2006)
7. Lightman, A.: Einstein's Dreams. Warner Books, New York (1992)
8. McCrickard, D.S., Chewar, C.M., Somervell, J.P.: Design, science, and engineering topics: Teaching HCI with a unified method. In: Proceedings of SIGCSE, pp. 31–35 (2003)
9. Norman, D.: The Design of Everyday Things. Doubleday, New York (1990)
10. Pausch, R., Zaslow, J.: The last lecture. Hyperion Press, New York (2008)
11. Peters, R.L.: Getting what you came for: The smart student's guide to earning a Master's or Ph.D. The Noonday Press, New York (1997)
12. Petroski, H.: To engineer is human: The role of failure in successful design. Vintage Books, New York (1992)
13. Quart, A.: Branded: The buying and selling of teenagers. Basic Books, Cambridge (2003)
14. Stouffer, W.B., Russell, J.S., Oliva, M.G.: Making the strange familiar: Creativity and the future of engineering education. In: Proceedings of the 2004 American Society for Engineering Educational Annual Conference & Exposition (2004)
15. Twiton, A.: Common reading programs in higher education. Technical paper, Gustavus College (2007), `http://gustavus.edu/academics/library/Pubs/Lindell2007.html`
16. Vicente, K.: The human factor: Revolutionizing the way people live with technology. Routledge, New York (2004)

Impression Management Support System for Teachers in Computer-Mediated Communication

Tamotsu Mukaiyachi[1] and Toshikazu Kato[2]

[1] Industrial and Systems Engineering, Graduate School of Science and Engineering, Chuo University, 1-13-27 Kasuga, Bunkyo-ku, Tokyo, 112-8551, Japan
a12.5jwc@g.chuo-u.ac.jp
[2] Chuo University, 1-13-27 Kasuga, Bunkyo-ku, Tokyo, 112-8551, Japan
kato@indsys.chuo-u.ac.jp

Abstract. Recently, due to development of Internet technology, online teaching has become very popular. Building good interpersonal relationships between teachers and students is important for the students' performance in online teaching. In this study, we propose an impression management support system for teachers in Computer-Mediated Communication instruction. The system suggests improvements in instruction to teachers to give good impressions and to develop interpersonal relationships with students. As the first step to realize the system, we performed an experiment to investigate impression factors in email instruction. From the experiment, we found that seven e-mail elements which become the factors of the impressions.

Keywords: Teacher support system, Impression management, Computer-Mediated Communication.

1 Introduction

Recently, due to development of Internet technology, online teaching such as distance tutoring has become very popular. Building good interpersonal relationships between teachers and students is important for the students' outcome and satisfaction in online teaching as well as in face-to-face (FtF) teaching [1]. Liu has proposed instructional strategy for achieving positive impression in Computer-Mediated Communication (CMC) instruction to develop interpersonal relationships with students [2]. Walther has indicated that CMC has rich enough cues to form interpersonal impressions [3]. Many studies have also investigated the cues of the impressions such as the emoticons [4], the frequency and duration [5]. Such process by which people control impressions others form of them is called "impression management" [6]. Conventional impression studies have considered that an attitude gives the same impressions to people (Fig 1). On the other hand, we consider that an attitude of a teacher gives the different impressions to students (Fig 2).

In this study, we propose an impression management support system for teachers which adapts to each student in CMC instruction. The system suggests improvements

C. Stephanidis (Ed.): Posters, Part II, HCII 2013, CCIS 374, pp. 66–70, 2013.

in instruction to teachers to give good impressions. Following the system, teachers can control their attitudes to give good impression to each student easily.

In this study, we will consider situation where teachers feedback to students via e-mail to focus on text-based interaction.

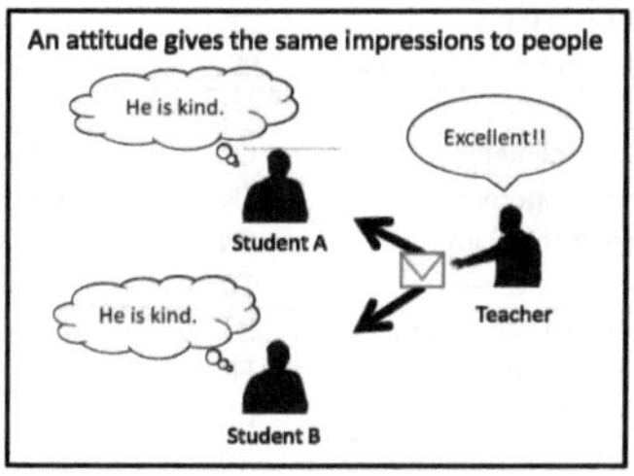

Fig. 1. Conventional framework of interpersonal impressions

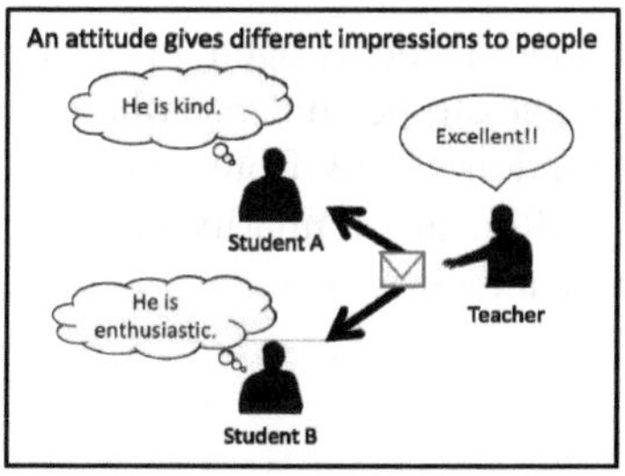

Fig. 2. Our framework of interpersonal impressions

2 Experiment: Investigation of Impression Factors in E-Mail

First of all, we performed an experiment to investigate impression factors in email instruction. We chose fourteen email elements shown in Table 1 as candidates of impression factors, expressed them quantitatively as feature values. We referred to five elements used by Kato[7]: EM, EX, NL, TO, RT, and two elements used by Liu[5]: FR, DU(not used in this experiment because of impression modeling for one email). We added three feature values as the indexes of a Japanese readability: SLA, KR, PIA. We also added four feature values as email instruction elements from the result of the free description questionnaire: PO, CO, EN, CN. We divided these elements into three types: Syntax, Content, and Temporal elements. The appropriateness of the feature values is judged by prediction accuracy of the impression models, not by exploratory data analysis.We produced thirty-six emails following orthogonal array testing method on email feature values. Using the orthogonal array, we can expect that the set of email are balanced samples of the minimum number.

Table 1. Email feature values and the levels

Element Type	Element	Acronym	Level		
Syntax Elements	Emoticon	EM	presence		absence
	Exclamation	EX	presence		absence
	The Number of the Letters	NL	~99	100~249	250~
	Sentence Length Average	SLA	~19	20~31	32~
	Kanji Rate	KR	~29	30~39	40~
	Punctuation Interval Avarage	PIA	~9	10~14	15~
Content Elements	Point Out	PO	presence		absence
	Compliment	CO	presence		absence
	Encouragement	EN	presence		absence
	Calling the Name	CN	presence		absence
	Tone	TO	polite		colloquial
Temporal Elements	Responce Time (days)	RT	2	6	10
	Frequency	FR		NA	
	Duration	DU		NA	

2.1 Procedure

We experimented on 20 graduate students aged 21-24 at a university in Tokyo. The subjects were assumed themselves to be students who had solved an arithmetic problem, and read thirty-six instruction emails from teachers. Then, they classified these emails into some groups based on the similarity of the impressions of the teachers. The number of the groups was at their will.

2.2 Data Analysis

The result of grouping was analyzed by decision tree analysis that is a method to detect the rules of the classification. The procedures of analysis were as follows.

i. Made the decision trees for each subject.
ii. Examined the number of people using each feature value for the email classification (Table 2).
iii. Evaluated classification accuracy for each subject with all feature values.
iv. Reevaluated the classification accuracy while excluding feature values which seemed little influence.
v. Repeated this evaluation until the classification accuracy of all subjects became over 75.0% with as few feature values as possible.

3 Results

Table 2 shows that 19 of 20 subjects used NL (the number of letters) for classification. The order from the second to the fifth is RT (used by 14 subjects), EM (used by 10 subjects), EX (used by six subjects), and TO (used by six subjects). These are the top 5 elements which are used for classification by subjects. The average classification accuracy with the top 5 elements is 84.6%, while the accuracy with all elements is 88.7% (Table 3). With the top 5 elements, classification accuracy of five subjects are under 75.0%. When we add PIA which is the sixth place to the top 5, the average classification accuracy is 86.1%. When we add PO which is the seventh place to the top 5, the accuracy is 87.2% which is higher than when PIA is added. When we add PO and EN to the top 5, the accuracy is 88.6% which is the highest with as few elements as possible, and classification accuracy of all subjects are more than 75.0%.

Table 2. Email feature values used for classification by each subject

Subject	EM	EX	NL	SLA	KR	PIA	PO	CO	EN	CN	TO	RT
A	O	O	O									
B	O	O	O	O	O				O			
C	O		O								O	
D		O	O				O		O			O
E			O						O		O	O
F			O									O
G	O		O			O			O			O
H			O									O
I	O		O			O					O	O
J			O			O	O					O
K	O	O	O								O	O
L			O									O
M	O		O				O					
N	O	O	O									O
O	O	O			O	O	O				O	
P			O									O
Q	O		O			O						O
R			O									
S			O									O
T			O	O							O	O
The Number of Users	10	6	19	2	2	5	4	0	4	0	6	14

Table 3. Classification Accuracy

	All Elements	EM+EX+NL +TO+RT (Top 5)	Top 5+PO	**Top 5 +PO+EN**	Top 5+PIA
Average Classification Accuracy	88.7%	84.6%	87.2%	**88.6%**	86.1%
The Number of Subjects Less than 75.0% Classification Accuracy	0	5	2	**0**	3
The Number of Elements Used for Classification	12	5	6	**7**	6

4 Discussion

From the results, it appears that these seven elements (EM, EX, NL, TO, RT, PO, EN) become the factors of the impressions in e-mail instruction. Thus, teachers may control their impressions on students by paying attention to these e-mail elements.

Table 2 shows that important elements for classification are different among individuals. For example, Subject A classified the e-mails from the viewpoint of EM, EX, and NL. On the other hand, subject L classified them from the viewpoint of NL and RT. Thus, we must make impression model for each subject.

The average classification accuracy when we add PO is higher than when we add PIA. We think PIA has little influence to impressions, though many subjects used it for classification.

5 Conclusion

In this study, we propose an impression management support system for teachers which adapts to each student in CMC instruction. To realize the system, we performed an experiment to investigate impression factors in email instruction. From the results, we found that seven elements (EM, EX, NL, TO, RT, PO, EN) become the factors of the impressions in e-mail instruction. Now, we investigated image words suitable to evaluate impressions of teachers in e-mail. If we find out the image words, we will analyze the relations between the e-mail elements which are the factor of impressions and impression evaluation. Then we will make impression model and predict the impressions of teachers.

Acknowledgements. This work was partially supported by JSPS KAKENHI grants, "Effective Modeling of Multimodal KANSEI Perception Processes and its Application to Environment Management" (No. 24650110), "Robotics modeling of diversity of multiple KANSEI and situation understanding in real space" (No. 19100004) and TISE Research Grant of Chuo University, "KANSEI Robotics Environment".

References

1. Liu, Y., Ginther, D.: Managing Impression Formation in Computer-Mediated Communication. Educause Quarterly 24(3), 50–54 (2001)
2. Walther, J.B.: Interpersonal Effects in Computer-Mediated Interaction: A Relational Perspective. Communication Research 19(1), 52–90 (1992)
3. Walther, J.B., D'Addario, K.P.: The Impacts of Emoticons on Message Interpretation in Computer-Mediated Communication. Social Science Computer Review 19(3), 324–347 (2001)
4. Liu, Y., Ginther, D., Zelhart, P.: How Do Frequency and Duration of Messaging Affect Impression Development in Computer-Mediated Communication? Journal of Universal Computer Science 7(10) (2001)
5. Liu, Y., Ginther, D.: Instructional Strategies for Achieving a Positive Impression in Computer-Mediated Communication (CMC) Distance Education Courses. In: Sixth Annual Mid-South Instructional Technology Conference Proceedings, Murfreesboro, Tennessee (April 10, 2001)
6. Leary, M.R., Kowalski, R.M.: Impression management literature review and two-component model. Psychological Bulletin 107(1), 34–47 (1990)
7. Kato, Y., Sugimura, K., Akahori, K.: Influence of Contents of E-mail Messages on Occurrences of Emotions in Communications by E-mail. Japan Journal of Educational Technology 29(2), 93–105 (2005)

Terminal Tablet as Electric Textbooks for Nursing Practicum

Yumiko Nakamura[1,*], Yukie Majima[2], and Kaori Fukayama[1]

[1] School of Nursing, Osaka Prefecture University, Japan
naka-yu@nursing.osakafu-u.ac.jp
[2] College of Sustainable System Sciences, Osaka Prefecture University, Japan
majima@kis.osakafu-u.ac.jp

Abstract. Based on the Nursing Learning Support System, which was developed and tested by this university, this study developed the "Digital Nursing Dictionary (ver. 2)," a terminal tablet with a new function of an electronic books, by taking advantage of the developed ICT. This report describes development of the "Digital Nursing Dictionary (ver. 2)" by a terminal tablet and presents an interim report of the results of those assessments.

Keywords: mobile learning, terminal tablet, nursing education, nursing practicum.

1 Introduction

System development and the operational model construction of e-learning have advanced in the educational engineering field. However, even given high needs for e-learning, the nursing field is confronting important problems of the deficiency of educational materials and wide gaps in informational technological literacy.

In 2007, O University's nursing department adopted the "e-learning support for nursing practice ability" according to a support program responding to current educational needs by the Ministry of Education, Culture, Sports, Science and Technology. As learning support of nursing practicum, "Digital Nursing Dictionaries (ver. 1)," portable game consoles (PSP; Sony Corp.) with skill images (video images) of educational material contents and knowledge cards (slides) were lent to students.

Now, the Digital Nursing Dictionary (ver. 2), with educational material contents and electric textbooks loaded on a terminal tablet, has been developed. This report describes the development of the terminal tablet and presents an interim report of the results of performance assessments.

2 Purposes

This study was undertaken as a performance assessment using the terminal tablet in nursing practicum to verify its effectiveness and utility.

---

* Corresponding author.

C. Stephanidis (Ed.): Posters, Part II, HCII 2013, CCIS 374, pp. 71–75, 2013.

3 Research Methods

3.1 Research Methods

1. We examined 92 of 137 juniors of O University's nursing department, who consented to participation in this research.
2. Period of performance assessment: October 2012 – July 2013 (Questionnaires were and will be circulated and gathered at the end of November 2012, and in February and July 2013)
3. Main research contents of Self-completed questionnaire survey: The status, time, and place of terminal tablet's use, the status of the internet connection, the usefulness of the contents, and the evaluation of functions, etc.
4. Data analysis: Data were analyzed using statistical methods with basic descriptive statistics and analysis of free description response contents.
5. Intervention contents: To juniors of the nursing department, a terminal tablet was lent during 2–3 months in nursing practicum, during October 2012 to July 2013, which period was divided into three sub-periods. Research participants had free access to the tablet for learning.

3.2 Ethical Considerations

We explained the following orally and in writing to participants and gained consent to participation in writing from each: the research intent; use and disposal of data; data are to be used for research purposes only; data are unrelated to a participant's academic results. We obtained permission to conduct the study from this university's ethical commission.

4 Regarding the Terminal Tablet Development

4.1 Contents

1. Electronic textbooks

Of the books purchased by students, we computerized 17 which the publishers had permitted us to use for this study. We created electronic books using PDF data of the text and index provided by the publishers.

2. Educational material contents for the nursing support system

Web contents for the nursing support system, which had been developed by this university, were changed for the terminal tablet. They include 132 scenes of nursing simulated examples (sound and video, analytical points, and text input and capture), nursing skill video images with 100 titles (video), 1,000 pages of knowledge cards (slide images), and 180 questions from the national examination (questions and answers).

4.2 Specifications of the Terminal Tablet

The terminal tablet we used (RW-T110; Sharp Corp.), which weighed about 640 g. had a 10.1 inch TFT liquid crystal screen. The platform was AndroidTM 2.3. Wireless LAN communication was used. Functions of the terminal tablet is

3. Handwriting (marker), bookmark function: Users were able to mark points they learned by filling them in with a marker, underlining, and bookmarks on any page of electric books.
4. Text input: Users were able to input into text the answers of analytical points for simulated examples and their own notes while reading the textbooks.
5. Dictionary search function: Users were able to cross-search the index of the electrical textbooks and the text information of example materials. Furthermore, they were able to web search by accessing the internet.

5 Results

5.1 Basic Information of Participants

In this report, we describe data of 63 participants in the first and second periods, of whom 56 used the terminal tablet and 54 of whom answered the questions.

Of the participants, 52 (96.3%) were female and 46 (85.2%) were 20–22 years old. Also, 50 (92.6%) used a smart phone, 26 (48.1%) used WiFi by wireless LAN, and 34 (63.0%) used wireless LAN at home.

5.2 Status of the Terminal Tablet Use

Regarding the use frequency by practicum subjects, the percentage of answers "often used it" and "used it" were the highest in child Care nursing (60.8%), followed by maternity nursing, Critical nursing, and chronic nursing (Fig.1.). Regarding places of use, the devices were most frequently used at home and in dormitories, but less at college and practicum facilities. Regarding times of use, they were most frequently used during 21:00–24:00 and 16:00–21:00, but less during practicum.

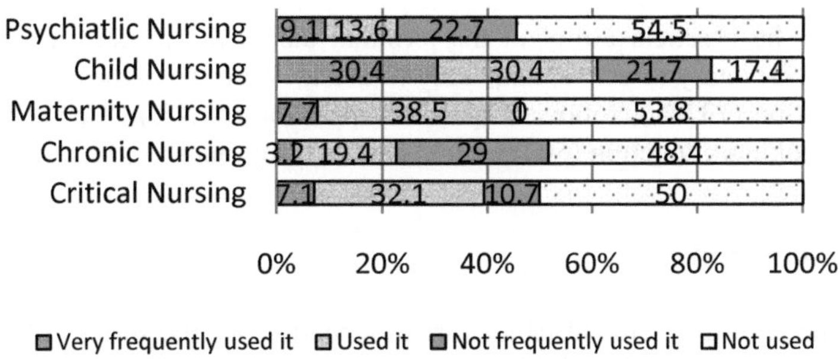

Fig. 1. Use frequency for using the terminal tablet by practicum subjects

The use frequency of educational material contents on the terminal tablet shows that the percentage responding that they "often used it" and "used it" were the highest (66.7%) for the electronic textbook, followed by nursing skill videos (31.5%), knowledge cards, and example educational materials. Regarding the use frequency of the terminal tablet's functions, the percentage of those who answered "often used it" and "used it" were the highest (51.9%) in the dictionary search function, followed by bookmark (31.5%) and web search functions (27.8%)(Fig. 2.).

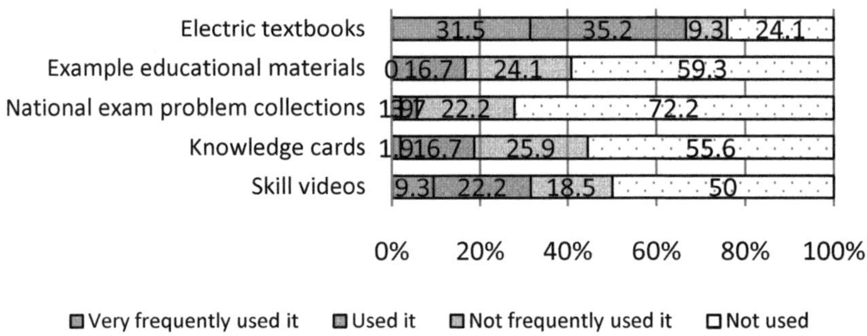

Fig. 2. Use frequency of contents for using the terminal tablet

5.3 Usefulness of the Terminal Tablet

Regarding the usefulness of the terminal tablet's educational material contents, the percentage of those who answered "very useful" and "useful" were the highest for electronic textbooks (59.2%), followed by skill videos (40.0%), knowledge cards, and example educational materials. As to the usefulness of the terminal tablet's functions, the percentage of those who answered "very useful" and "useful" were the highest in the dictionary search function (62.0%), followed by the Web search function (39.6%), bookmark function (37.5%) and hand writing (marker) function (31.9%).

5.4 Practical Utility of the Terminal Tablet

In terms of the practical utility of the terminal tablet, the percentage of those who responded "very easy to use it" and "easy to use it" were the highest in the dictionary search function (73.9%), followed by basic operation (69.4%), Web search function (57.1%), bookmark function (50.0%), and hand writing (marker) function (50.0%).

6 Discussion

The use status of the terminal tablet varied depending on the subject of practicum. It was more frequently used in child nursing and maternity nursing; it was less commonly used in chronic nursing and psychiatric nursing. As to frequently used contents, the electric textbooks were frequently used. Furthermore, the high use frequency of utilization of the search function and bookmark function shows that participants often used the electronic textbooks.

Among the electronic contents, nursing skill videos were frequently used. Because nursing students need to confirm the nursing skills in advance before helping nurse patients in nursing practicum, it is very useful to see the videos of nursing skills anytime, which are expected to contribute to achieving their learning effects.

In addition, the terminal tablet, even if mobile, was used more frequently at home. It was necessary to encourage the participants to use practicum facilities and ask the staff of the practicum facilities for their cooperation. Furthermore, although the web search function was often used, because the penetration of wireless LAN at home is about 50%, if penetration expands, the web search function's use rate can be expected to grow.

In terms of practical utility, the size and weight of the terminal tablet were evaluated as appropriate. Therefore, it is suggested that the device used this time should present no problems. However, even given the tablet's basic operation, dictionary search, and web search functions were evaluated to be easy to use, note-making functions were not frequently used and availability was also not good, which suggest room for improvement.

7 Conclusion

The "Digital Nursing Dictionary (ver. 2)" with the terminal tablet developed this time had electronic contents and electronic textbooks provided by a web system. Because it allows the users to use electric educational material contents and electronic textbooks in a unified manner, it is expected that these books will contribute to achieving the users' learning effects. Among them, the utilization rate of the electronic textbooks was high. Their availability would be improved if users became accustomed to using them, making them an effective educational material for use in future studies.

The use frequencies of the terminal tablet's functions vary. Therefore, we must make improvements by narrowing down the necessary functions and by making actions easily accessible for anyone to use it.

Acknowledgements. We are deeply grateful to the students of the nursing department for participating in the survey and to Sharp Corp. for collaborating in development of the terminal tablet.

References

1. Majima, Y., Sou, Y.: Development of E-learning for Problem solving Approach of Nursing Students. Studies in Health Technology and Informatics 122, 919 (2006)
2. Majima, Y., Nakamura, Y., Maekawa, Y., So, Y.: Development of ubiquitous on demand study support environment for nursing students. In: Jacko, J.A. (ed.) HCI International 2009, Part IV. LNCS, vol. 5613, pp. 149–155. Springer, Heidelberg (2009)

Interaction in Distance Education: Student, Teaching Material, Information Technology and Communication

Sônia Regina Gouvêa Rezende, Valter Gomes Campos, Pollyana dos Reis Pereira Fantone, and Melca Moura Brasil

State University of Goiás-UEG
soniarez2@yahoo.com.br, {valtergc1,pollyana_reis}@hotmail.com, melacabrasil@gmail.com

Abstract. Distance education requires the development and production of teaching materials with their own peculiarities, on which stand out the clarity, objectivity, the interactivity and the reference to the dialogue. These characteristics imply the qualification of teachers for the development of differentiated skills and competencies for their manufacture. This article presents the methodology of the course "Development and Production of Teaching Materials for Distance Education", in the State University of Goiás - UEG. At first it is presented the demanded qualifications of the content teacher that needs to master the covered content and be able to promote student motivation, prompting him to search for knowledge. Still, in this context, it discusses the specifics of teaching materials for distance education. In the second phase, it presents the historical background of the university, its work in this area and its future challenges. As a last step, it describes the methodology used in the course of the University Unit of Distance Education (UnUEAD) UEG to train its teachers to act as content teachers of teaching material for this type of education. This methodology consists of the following phases: planning, structure and organization of the course. The design is characterized by the construction of the conceptual map, a tool that assists in defining the theoretical and practical approaches to be worked. From these fundamentals, the course is structured and its modules are organized. In the final evaluation of the course the content teacher consolidates his learning through the development of the Subject Production Plan and a production of a text, according to the characteristics of materials for distance education. It stands out, as a final consideration of this article, that the development and production of teaching material at UnUEAD is guided by the same methodology used in training its contents teachers.

Keywords: Methodology, Distance Education, Instructional Materials, Training, Information Technology and Communication.

1 Introduction

The Information and Communication Technologies - ICT and implementation of flexible learning models and intelligent educational activities based on Web, provided a rapid growth of Distance Education (DE), and made it an educational modality even

C. Stephanidis (Ed.): Posters, Part II, HCII 2013, CCIS 374, pp. 76–79, 2013.

more challenging. Information Technologies and Communication alone are not able to promote student learning, so it is necessary that communication can be the focus of the case and planned in a way that is efficient in promoting the interaction among the student, the teacher and knowledge. In this process the didactic material is the key role and requires its own methodology for its preparation, as it has different characteristics and should be well planned and produced and has appropriate language and formatting.

Thus, it is evident the need and importance of the content teacher training to the development of teaching specific materials, appropriate and qualified to distance education requirement. With this vision, the State University of Goiás (UEG), through the Crew Pedagogical University Unit of Distance Education (UnUEAD) developed the course "Training Development and Production of Teaching Materials for Distance Education." To be offered at a distance, gives opportunity to apply the knowledge built as the course develops.

2 Training Teachers to Work in DE

Teaching is a complex activity that includes technical and pedagogical questions, knowledge and subjectivities, which requires consistent training. Hence the importance of training institutions, which according to Nóvoa (1995), occupy a central place in the production and reproduction of knowledge and system of standards of the teaching profession and play a fundamental role in the assertion of professional identity. In turn, the teacher must take his professional identity, being a researcher, dealing with everyday school life, with new knowledge and new educational methods.

With the rapid development of knowledge and education in the face of current reality, it is observed that for proper training of educators is not enough just the technical approach and educational content. It is increasingly evident the need for a solid education, which includes the binomial theory and practice and the quest for the development of skills and competencies, especially, learning to learn, research and the use of innovative teaching practices. Learning is essential to the challenges that present itself in the educational context (POZO, 1998).

The use of Information and Communication Technologies - ICT in education has increased in recent years, especially with the expansion of Internet access. This added to the network usage by students has become a major challenge for professionals working in and with education. Thus, it is necessary a comprehensive teacher training, both initial and continuing, that, beyond the mastery of the content covered, teachers are able to use ICT, and select teaching materials and work to promote student motivation in order that it cannot position itself as being passive receiver of information, but as one who instigates the whole time to seek the necessary knowledge for his/her formation.

For this to happen we need to understand education as a practice of social construction of meaning by the individuals who participate and, in this context, understanding the importance of student autonomy, which is accentuated in Distance Education (PRETI, 2000).

It is therefore important to use methodological strategies that provide autonomy and at the same time, cooperation among students around a didactic purpose, for which ICT has proven very useful. It should be noted, however, that technology should not be seen as an end but as a means to assist in the construction of knowledge, because it itself does not guarantee success in education. Belloni (2009) discusses the use of Information Technologies and Communication becomes the process of teaching and learning more complex, requiring a segmentation of the act of teaching in different and multiple tasks. Therefore, one must understand its pedagogical value, how, and why to use ICT in education.

In this scenario, it is necessary training for the job as content teacher, who is the one responsible for designing and producing educational material in a particular discipline to DE. To act as a content teacher, the teacher must first of all overcome the barriers and rejections of the modality. Secondly, the teacher should have an appropriate profile, manifest by aligning with the Information and Communication Technologies. And, thirdly, he/ she must know the peculiarities and characteristics of teaching materials for distance education, as well as the drafting and production of this material.

3 Teaching Materials for DL

In Distance Education the process of teaching and learning takes place primarily through the courseware, because communication happens through interaction with texts and hypertexts, with the authors' interpretation of thinking through writing. In Distance Education, the teaching material is the basis on which sets the methodologies of teaching and interactions. It is one of the main elements of mediation among the subjects of this educational modality, thus it requires different characteristics as to be able to promote communication and dialogical.

The teaching materials for Distance Education must have appropriate language and formatting. In it is important to use teaching resources and methodological strategies that provide autonomy in the context of various forms of cooperation among students around a didactic purpose. It must be carefully planned and presented, taking into account the student's profile and establishing relationships with his/her everyday issues, so that the teaching material is an instrument of permanent dialogue.In this sense, context, clarity, objectivity, and interactivity dialogicity are essential peculiarities and characteristics to the quality of educational material. As Oliveira and Nogueira (2005), to address these specificities, courseware must be prepared by multidisciplinary or transdisciplinary, incorporation and adaptation of technology tools that will be used, the collaboration of tutors and the student as the center of the teaching process learning.

Given this, it is evident the necessity and importance of this training for the professional development of teaching materials specific, appropriate and quality that distance education requires. With this vision, the State University of Goiás (UEG), through the Pedagogical Crew of the University Unit of Distance Education (UnUEAD) developed the course "Training Development and Production of Teaching

Materials for Distance Education." To be offered at a distance, this course gives opportunity to apply the knowledge built as the course develops. This article aims to describe the methodology used by the State University of Goiás, through the Unit University of Distance Education (UnUEAD), to train its staff in the development and production of teaching material for distance education. It is presented in the first part of this article the need for training of teachers to act as content teacher in distance education. The second part describes the peculiarities of teaching materials for this educational modality and presents techniques for interactivity as the foundation of its development. The last section presents the methodology of the course "Training Development and Production of Teaching Materials for Distance Education." The planning is characterized by the construction of the concept map, a tool that assists in defining the theoretical and practical approaches to be worked. From this foundation, the course is structured and its modules are organized. In the final evaluation of the course content teacher consolidates their learning through the development of the Production Plan of Discipline and production of a text, according to the specificities and characteristics of materials for Distance Education. It stands out as a final consideration of this article, the development and production of teaching materials in the UnUEAD is guided by the same methodology used in the training of its content teachers.

References

1. Belloni, M.L.: Educação a Distância. São Paulo: Autores associados (2009)
2. Landim, C.M., Das, M.P.F.: Educação a Distância: algumas considerações. Edição do Autor, Rio de Janeiro (1997)
3. Oliveira, E., da, S.G.: e Nogueira, M. L de L. Educação a Distância e Formação Continuada de Professores: novas perspectivas. A revista digital da CVA-RICESU. v. 3 – n.10, nov, Universidade do Estado do Rio de Janeiro (UERJ), Faculdade de Educação – Brasil (2005)
4. Preti, O.: Autonomia do Aprendiz na Educação a Distância: significados e dimensões Disponível, http://www.nead.ufmt.br/documentos/autonomia_-ooreste_I07.doc. (Acesso March 20, 2011)
5. UnUEAD. Pesquisa realizada nas Unidades Universitárias da Universidade Estadual de Goiás (2010)

English for Specific Purposes via Distance Learning: Opportunities for Academic and Professional Qualification

Sônia Regina Gouvêa Rezende[1], Francisco Alberto Severo de Almeida[2], and Carla Conti de Freitas[1]

[1] State University of Goiás-UEG, Brazil
[2] State University of Goiás-UEG, and University of Porto, Portugal
soniarez2@yahoo.com.br, serevo@ueg.br, carlacontif@gmail.com

Abstract. The objective of the course "English for Specific Purposes" (E.S.P), focusing on textual genres developed in a virtual environment, is to enable course participants in understanding and interpreting texts in the English language as well as involving the students of the Linguistics Course at UEG in mentoring activities. This paper discusses an extension project of E.S.P via Distance Learning in the State University of Goiás-UEG that presents in its capillary a multicampi structure of 42 units. UEG aims at the integral formation of the human being to a socio-professional solidarity performance and the concern for the exercise of citizenship. This project reveals the UEG policy of engagement and participation in integrated development of the state of Goiás besides aligning the purpose the university to prepare its students to participate in the Science Without Borders program.

Keywords: Project extension, Distance Learning, English for Specific Purposes via Distance Learning, Academic and professional qualifications.

1 English for Specific Purposes" (E.S.P)

This paper discusses the extension project of "English for Specific Purposes" (E.S.P) via Distance Learning in the State University of Goiás-UEG that presents in its capillary a multicampi structure of 42 units. In its policy of engagement and participation in integrated development of the state of Goiás, UEG aims at the integral formation of the human being to a socio-professional solidarity performance and the concern for the exercise of citizenship.

This project proposes to enhance socio-economic and cultural life of the academic community (students and teachers), thus enhancing their chances for integration and / or consolidation in the labor market, as well as integrate the university community to society in a joint action with full citizenship construction.

Distance Learning, part of a broader educational process of innovations, which includes the integration of Information and Communication Technologies (ICT) in the educational processes (BELLONI, 2002) is the link between the University and the community in Goiás.

C. Stephanidis (Ed.): Posters, Part II, HCII 2013, CCIS 374, pp. 80–83, 2013.

In view of Aranha (2002) the interaction of individuals in a formal and even informal organization is associated with their acquired knowledge, developed skills and attitudes in converting their skills in the most essential function of human life: work. The adaptability of the human being to the most vital social activities, work, allows the use of their potential to provide for their own needs. Participants' difficulties in continuing their professional development goals by factors such as time availability, locomotion troubles and objectivity of the course failed attempts at resolving the teachers' problem. As for the students of Linguistics obstacles in practice the knowledge acquired in their graduation.

Thus, given the limitations encountered by the target audience that sometimes are overcome by its competitors due to lack of training, this English for Specific Purposes pilot project in the form of distance learning aims to expand the opportunities for integration into the labor market to the Linguistics students in the UEG offering a consistent and skilled preparation. The Linguistics students will be able to effectively work out in their area.

In another aspect the project directs to UEG teachers as a grant proposal to hone their skills in understanding and interpreting English texts in order to facilitate the insertion in different knowledge areas in post-graduation courses. This duality strategic process for the project concerns to guide both participants as Linguistics students in the use of English for reading and interpreting texts and offers an opportunity for Linguistics students to work in the area of tutoring in an English for Specific Purposes Course in the UEG. These students will receive ongoing training to perform their activities.

This project is founded on methodological aspect focuses on the development of students' ability to extract the message that contains the text. Thus, the English for Specific Purposes Course focusing on instrumental textual genres will be developed in virtual environment, involving Linguistics students of UEG in tutoring activities. Tutoring has become a constitutive part of the distance learning mode, which occupies a key place in the development of courses in this way to make education (PRETI, 2001). So it is up to tutoring, mediation and guidance between students and the resources needed for the realization of "didactic conversation".

In its instrumental approach this course demands that students need to take control over their learning process, learning to overcome the difficulties they will face when reading a text in a foreign language, developing strategies that allow them to solve understanding problems at both the content of the text as the linguistic level. The teaching material prepared exposes the student tasks that take them to reflect on the meaning of the text, and also to focus and analyze the English language in concrete use situations by reading in a variety of textual genre, leveraging the practical opportunities of interpretation and understanding of various communication styles.

In his work, Swales (1990) focuses attention on the analysis of textual genres, emphasizing its use for both academic situations and for professional contexts. The methodology of distance learning, as well as the techniques and reading strategies, among them scanning and skimming, inference, flexibility and basic structure of English will be used in the process of teaching and learning (MUNHOZ, 2000). The operation of the project for 2013 was approved by the referees of the Pro-Dean for Extension and Culture of UEG therefore future research could be conducted to analyze the results of the project.

For the development of Distant Learning actions that is proposed in this project, we believe that it is necessary to maintain a communication network that enables the connection of multiple units where the course is offered. Therefore, it is imperative to organize physical structure, pedagogical and academic to guarantee:

- Maintenance of a multidisciplinary team to guide the course participant; Appointment of coordination that will be responsible for monitoring the course both administrative and pedagogical;
- Maintenance of laboratories in the units that support the communication required for current arrangements of the course;
- Organization of a system of communication between units of UEG and UNUEAD.

Through the Virtual Learning Environment Moodle, students will receive feedback on their performance, guidelines and exchange of information with respect to the content covered in developed exercises especially those that have been answered incorrectly, leading to new elaborations and referrals reassessment.

The English course will be taught instrumental in two modules, developed in distance mode, with a total duration of 200 hours, spread over eight months. From action at a distance in a virtual environment, the following topics will be covered with their workload:

- Module 1 - Getting Started - 100 hours
- Module 2 - Citizen of the global environment - 100 hours

The course participants reach 75% (seventy five percent) of frequency and perform the activities required during the course and present a conclusive work will be certified. As well as for students of the Linguistics Course that act with tutors and report performance of their students. Certificates will be issued by this entity, signed by the director of the University Unit of Distance Education and the Course Coordinator. The certification will show support from Extension, Culture and Student Affairs Pro – Deanship, as its delegated power.

References

1. Aranha, M.S.F.: Formando educadores para a escola inclusiva.MEC. Secretaria de Educação a Distância. Programa TV Escola – Salto para o futuro (November 2002)
2. Belloni, M.L.: Ensaio sobre educação a distância no Brasil. IN: Educação e Sociedade, ano XXIII, (78), p. 124, abr (2002)

3. Munhoz, R.: Inglês Instrumental: estratégias de leitura. Módulo I. Texto novo, SãO Paulo (2000)
4. Preti, O.: A formação do professor na modalidade a distância (des)construindo metanarrativas e metáforas. R. bras. Est. pedag., BrasÌlia, v. 82, n. 200/201/202, p. 26-39, jan./dez (2001)
5. Swales, J.: Genre Analysis: English In Academic And Research Settings. Cambridge University Press, Cambridge (1990)

Digital Badges: Signposts and Claims of Achievement

Răzvan Rughiniş[1] and Stefania Matei[2]

[1] University Politehnica of Bucharest, Splaiul Independenţei 313, Bucharest, Romania
razvan.rughinis@cs.pub.ro
[2] University of Bucharest, Faculty of Sociology and Social Work, Bucharest, Romania
stefania.matei@sas.unibuc.ro

Abstract. We discuss digital badges in education, focusing on two functions of badge architectures: mapping a learning system and offering a vocabulary to present one's achievements. We have designed, implemented and evaluated two badge architectures; our research findings support the conclusion that students see these medals less as extrinsic motivations than as signposts that point out relevant learning targets. Also, because trainers and students define badges mainly as fun, locally relevant prizes, there is little concern for how they can be used to communicate merits outside the learning community. Badge architectures can be designed to support local or public reputations; if public visibility is desired, the system should assist holders' work of claiming merit.

1 Introduction

Digital badges are increasingly considered an alternative to grades and degrees (Casilli, 2012; Davidson, 2011, 2012; Hickey, 2012a, 2012b). Large-scale initiatives such as Mozilla Open Badges (The Mozilla Foundation, 2012) and the DML Competition (HASTAC Initiative, 2012) have brought them to public debate. We examine two prominent claims based on our research, and we discuss implications for design[1]:

- Badges are extrinsic incentives (Hickey, 2012a; Resnick, 2012) that run the risk of crowding out intrinsic motivation;
- Badges are evidence-based credentials (Casilli, 2012; Davidson, 2012) easily communicated and understood by observers.

Our discussion is based on an evaluation research concerning two badge architectures that we designed and implemented in University Politehnica of Bucharest: the Cisco Networking Academy CCNA.ro medals, and the Local Networks Course (RL) Hit List[2]. The evaluation relies on semi-structured interviews with 12 students and 4 instructors for the CCNA.ro system, and with 14 students and 4 teaching assistants for the RL course.

The CCNA.ro medal system (see Fig.1) awards medals for a variety of student involvements and achievements. For each CCNA training track, 'Bronze', 'Silver' and

[1] This research has been supported by the program EXCEL, grant POSDRU/89/1.5/S/62557.
[2] https://systems.cs.pub.ro/teaching/courses/rl/hit-list/

C. Stephanidis (Ed.): Posters, Part II, HCII 2013, CCIS 374, pp. 84–88, 2013.

'Gold' medals reward final GPAs greater than 75%, 85% and 95%, respectively; 'Inquisitive mind' rewards student involvement in class discussions; 'Technical stamina' is awarded to students who complete all laboratories; 'Perfectionist' acknowledges students with all scores above 90%, and 'Community catalyst' is granted to participants with 3 or more forum contributions. Each medal is available to any student who fits the criteria, and can be displayed on students' profile as a credential (for potential recruiters, employers, peers, and other interested observers).

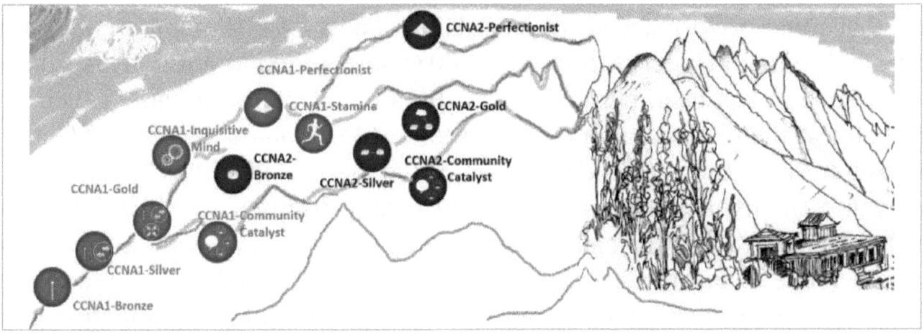

Fig. 1. The CCNA.ro Medal Architecture: Signposts for Exploration

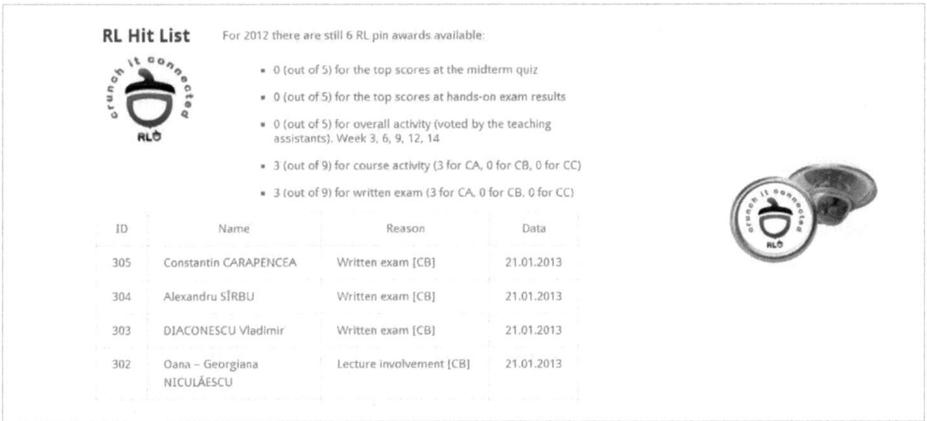

Fig. 2. The RL Hit List: Design for Reputation across Generations

The RL Hit List[3] has a different mission and design (see Fig. 2): it awards a limited number of medals to top 10% student performers on selected activities. Each medal consists of a digital mention on the online 'Hit List', and a metallic pin badge conferred publicly, in a special section of the lecture. The Hit List is designed as a chronologically numbered list that spans multiple generations, aiming to assemble a community of recipients sharing a memorable course-related experience.

[3] https://systems.cs.pub.ro/teaching/courses/rl/hit-list/

2 The "Motivation" vs. "Attention" Issue

Badges are often discussed as extrinsic motivators (Hickey, 2012a; Resnick, 2012) – pointing to their potentially corrosive role on the development of an intrinsic, authentic learning involvement. We argue that focusing on badges as incentives obscures their cognitive role as 'signposts': badge architectures chart learning routes, through their conditionalities and entitlements (Rughiniş, 2013a, 2013b).

This cartographic function is visible for designers, who face the challenge of selecting relevant points of recognition throughout the learning system. By making explicit that some performances are remarkable, badges *focus attention*, *map* the curriculum, and *nudge* (Thaler & Sunstein, 2008) student exploration. This function of drawing attention has been particularly visible in students' accounts of their evaluation of badges: the distinction between a score of 90% and a score of 95% becomes visible as a meaningful difference because of the associated 'Silver' / 'Gold' medals; the relevance of involvement in course and forum discussion is highlighted by the associated medals. CCNA.ro badges are seen by students as having a function of visualizing achievement, of translating numbers or unarticulated merits into a language of praise, for themselves and for others; it is because of their attention-grabbing power that medals acquire positive valence.

3 The "Evidence" vs. "Interpretation" Issue

Badges create 'bragging rights' for peer conversations, but also become boundary objects (Akkerman & Bakker, 2011) – that is, credentials for employers, recruiters, and significant others in various domains of practice. Badges can acknowledge in/formal instruction, personal experience and peer evaluation, complete and partial achievements. Because of their flexibility, badges are clues that invite interpretation (Rughiniş, 2013a): What does a medal or collection of medals *actually say* about its holder?

Badges are 'evidence-based' insofar the conditions for their award are publicly available, together with other information about the issuing authority and the recipient. In a strict sense, badges are explicit descriptions of merit – but they are easy to make sense of especially if the interlocutor is familiar with the activity and the community in which the badge was awarded. On the contrary, a problem of interpretation arises for interlocutors that are distant, professionally and/or socially – as it may be the case for recruiters in Human Resource departments. Even self-presentation of one's medals may not be straightforward, in contexts with an unfamiliar public.

Holders (in our case, students) are directly interested in invoking their medals, to highlight their merits. At the same time, students themselves may not be aware of the potential of badges to 'say something' meaningful about their skills and achievements. This is especially the case for badges that are introduced as secondary, playful achievements, accompanying traditional, 'hard' credentials such as grades and points – as it is the case in our two architectures.

We have observed, in interviews, that some students define badges as minor in public significance – being rather 'for fun', or for self-motivation. Even students who see their badges as an indication of special merit are unsure of how to practically introduce them in a CV, a personal online profile, or in discussions with employers. This uncertainty was stronger for the RL Hit List: the very innovations that make this architecture attractive also render it difficult to interpret for outsiders. The medal, in RL Hit List, is a number that is awarded chronologically; although there is a brief description of the related merit (see Fig.2), the RL Hit List falls short of being self-explanatory.

Therefore, our evaluation of the badge architectures employed for CCNA.ro and the Local Networks RL course indicates that designers should explicitly take into account holders' interpretive work in communicating for other observers, such as recruiters, what their badges say about them. There are two main possibilities of using badges for building holders' reputations:

1. Badges for *local community use*: in this case, badges appear on participants profiles in the system, with little concern for their outside relevance. Stack Overflow badges offer such an example (Stack Exchange, 2012a). Stack Overflow encourages users to create professional CV's that are distinctive from their user profiles, and which do not refer to badges at all, including instead a variety of other information about their activity on the platform (Stack Exchange, 2012b);
2. Badges for *public use*: in this case, holders are encouraged to include their medals on various public profiles. Mozilla Open Badge infrastructure is designed to support such public display; the Khan Academy, for example, encourages learners to publish their badges on Facebook (Khan Academy, 2012).

Badge designers that aim for public visibility can take a series of steps to encourage holders' interpretive work in presenting their achievements:

a) Create a public, online description of the badge architecture, that would offer holders and other interested persons a vocabulary in which to make sense of the significance of each achievement;
b) Provide technical means for publishing badges as digital awards on various public profiles; for example, badg.us[4] offers a quick and easy platform for badge generation compatible with Mozilla Open Badges;
c) Present samples of public profiles (CVs, Facebook, LinkedIn) in which badges are included, with examples of how to classify them (as learning outcomes, distinctions, community recognition etc.) and how to describe them.

4 Conclusions

There is a gap between public debates on digital badges, and learners' views and practices. While badges are much discussed as incentives, they also have an attention-focusing role, as signposts that map learning systems and make visible

[4] http://badg.us/en-US/

significant learning outcomes. Badges are also discussed as clear, evidence-based credentials; still, if badges are to support public reputations, holders must make them visible and 'translate' them for external observers. This requires a publication and interpretation work, which should be supported through the design of badge architectures, and through vivid examples and communication between instructors and learners.

References

1. Akkerman, S.F., Bakker, A.: Boundary Crossing and Boundary Objects. Review of Educational Research 81(2), 132–169 (2011)
2. Casilli, C.: Mozilla Open Badges: The Ecosystem Begins to Take Shape, `http://carlacasilli.wordpress.com/2012/07/31/mozilla-open-badges-the-ecosystem-begins-to-take-shape/` (retrieved December 19, 2012)
3. Davidson, C.: Why Badges Work Better Than Grades. In: HASTAC (2011), `http://hastac.org/blogs/cathy-davidson/why-badges-work-better-grades` (retrieved November 20, 2012)
4. Davidson, C.: Can Badging Be the Zipcar of Testing and Assessment (2012), `http://dmlcentral.net/blog/cathy-davidson/can-badging-be-zipcar-testing-and-assessment` (retrieved October 13, 2012)
5. HASTAC Initiative. Digital Media Learning Competition, `http://dmlcompetition.net` (retrieved November 20, 2012)
6. Hickey, D.T.: Intended Purposes Versus Actual Functions of Digital Badges. In: Re-Mediating Assessment (2012a), `http://remediatingassessment.blogspot.ro/2012/09/intended-purposes-versus-actual.html` (retrieved October 13, 2012)
7. Hickey, D.T.: Open Badges and the Future of Assessment. In: Re-Mediating Assessment (2012b), `http://remediatingassessment.blogspot.ro/2012/03/open-badges-and-future-of-assessment.html` (retrieved November 20, 2012)
8. Khan Academy, Share your Khan Academy badges on Facebook in style (2012), `http://www.khanacademy.org/about/blog/post/23071271279/facebook-opengraph` (retrieved April 2, 2013)
9. Resnick, M.: Still a Badge Skeptic. In: HASTAC, `http://hastac.org/blogs/mres/2012/02/27/still-badge-skeptic` (retrieved October 13, 2012)
10. Rughiniș, R.: Talkative Objects in Need of Interpretation. Re-Thinking Digital Badges in Education. In: ACM SIGCHI Conference on Human Factors in Computing Systems, Alt-CHI 2013, pp. 1–10. ACM, Paris (2013a)
11. Rughiniș, R.: Badge Architectures in Engineering Education. Blueprints and Challenges. In: The 5th International Conference on Computer Supported Education CSEDU 2013. INSTICC, Aachen (2013b)
12. Stack Exchange, Stack Overflow Badges (2012a), `http://stackoverflow.com/badges` (retrieved November 20, 2012)
13. Stack Exchange, Stack Overflow Sample Profile (2012b), `http://careers.stackoverflow.com/spolsky` (retrieved April 2, 2013)
14. Thaler, R.H., Sunstein, C.R.: Nudge: Improving Decisions About Health, Wealth, and Happiness. Yale University Press, New Haven (2008)
15. The Mozilla Foundation, Mozilla Open Badges, `http://openbadges.org` (retrieved November 20, 2012)

Preliminary Design of a Network Protocol Learning Tool Based on the Comprehension of High School Students: Design by an Empirical Study Using a Simple Mind Map

Makoto Satoh[1], Ryo Muramatsu[2], Mizue Kayama[3], Kazunori Itoh[3], Masami Hashimoto[3], Makoto Otani[3], Michio Shimizu[4], and Masahiko Sugimoto[5]

[1] Division of Science & Technology Master's Program, Shinshu University, Nagano, Japan
[2] Graduate School of Science & Technology, Shinshu University, Nagano, Japan
[3] Shinshu University, Nagano, Japan
[4] Nagano Prefectural College, Nagano, Japan
[5] Takushoku University Hokkaido Junior College, Hokkaido, Japan
{12tm524h,11ta549f}@shinshu-u.ac.jp,
{kayama,itoh,hasimoto,otani}@cs.shinshu-u.ac.jp,
michio@nagano-kentan.ac.jp, sugimoto@takushoku-hc.ac.jp

Abstract. The purpose of this study is to develop a learning tool for high school students studying the scientific aspects of information and communication networks. More specifically, we focus on the basic principles of network protocols as the aim to develop our learning tool. Our tool gives students hands-on experience to help understand the basic principles of network protocols.

Keywords: Learning Tool, High School Student, Empirical Comprehension, Mind Map, Network Protocol.

1 Introduction

In her proposal statement on Computational Thinking (CT), Wing pointed out the importance of educational opportunities for college/university freshmen and pre-college students [1,2]. Based on her paper, Phillips described the CT concepts as follows [3] : Algorithms, Data (variables, data bases, queue), Abstraction (conceptualizing, modularizing), Queries (search, conditionals, boolean), Sensing & Feedback(robotics), Iterations (loops, recursion) and Systems. CATA and ISTE have discussed bringing CT to K-12 [4]. Some schools / universities also have started new lectures on CT education [5].

In Japan, CT related education starts in elementary school [6-8]. Especially at high school, "information study" has been one of the compulsory subjects for all students from 2003. The core curricula for information study can be divided into three parts, "using information in practice", "scientific understanding of information study", and "proper attitudes for participating in an information society". To design an appropriate learning tool related to these topics, we examined the comprehension of high school students and university freshmen about information and communication

C. Stephanidis (Ed.): Posters, Part II, HCII 2013, CCIS 374, pp. 89–93, 2013.

networks through a simple mind map. A Simple mind map consists of nothing but nodes with a word and edges between nodes. These objects do not have any colors or graphical parts like the original mind map [9].

2 Comprehension of High School Students for Informatics

2.1 Methods

The subjects were 270 high school students (1st, 2nd and 3rd grade students) and 96 university freshmen. We asked them to draw a simple mind map about "information and communication network" from three aspects of core topics in information study. These maps were called student maps. On the other hand, we made a "text map" based on some textbooks authorized by the Japanese government for information study at high school. This text map had 91 words. From all student maps, we (1) counted the number of words in each map, (2) separated all words in two groups: formal (in the text map) and informal (not in the text map), and (3) counted the use frequency of all words.

2.2 Results

Based on (1) and (2), there was no significant change in number of formal words for only "the scientific understanding of information" related to the school grades of the subjects. Therefore, the comprehension level of this domain does not change or avoids increasing at those developmental stages (from 1st grade in high school to freshmen in university). Based on (2) and (3), the number of formal words which 10% or more of the subjects used was 6 for high school students and 7 for university freshmen. We called these words typical words. Of these words, 50% or more students used only 3 words: e-mail, mobile phone and internet. Two typical student maps were made based on these frequently used words (see Fig. 1 (a) and (b)). The words in double circles are typical words. The words in single circles are "related words", which are connected by edges with each typical word in all student maps. From these maps, the concept hierarchy of our subjects is unarranged and unsuitable. Any words related to scientific fundamental rule, architecture or mechanism do not appear in those maps.

Meanwhile, based on the text map, (2) and (3), we showed comprehension maps of our subjects (see Fig2 (a) and (b)). The text map had 8 divisions: internet, packet switching, network protocol, file transfer, security, e-mail, data transmission speed and network services. In those divisions, whole words of 10% or more of the high school students described in their maps are matched to only 3 divisions. In the case of university freshmen, 5 divisions were matched to our subjects' words. The number of divisions which were not matched was 3. They were protocol, file transfer and data transmission speed.

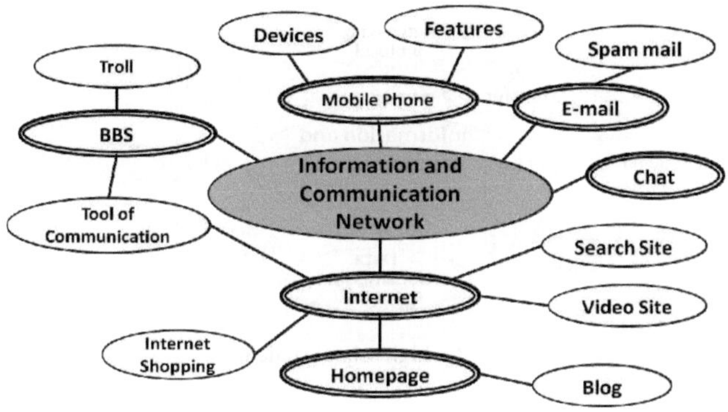

(a) high school student

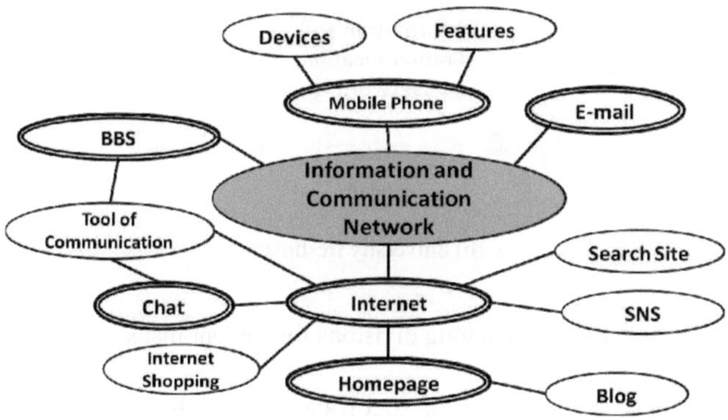

(b) university freshman

Fig. 1. Typical maps

More specifically, we focused on the basic principles of network protocols as the aim to develop our learning tool. Our tool gives students hands-on experience to help understand the basic principles of network protocols.

3 Preliminary Design of a Network Protocol Learning Tool

Referring to previous research, we ordered the basic principles of network protocols and summarized them into the four following points:

1. the start of the data to be communicated,
2. the end of the data to be communicated,
3. the format of the data to be communicated,
4. how to recover when a communication error occurs.

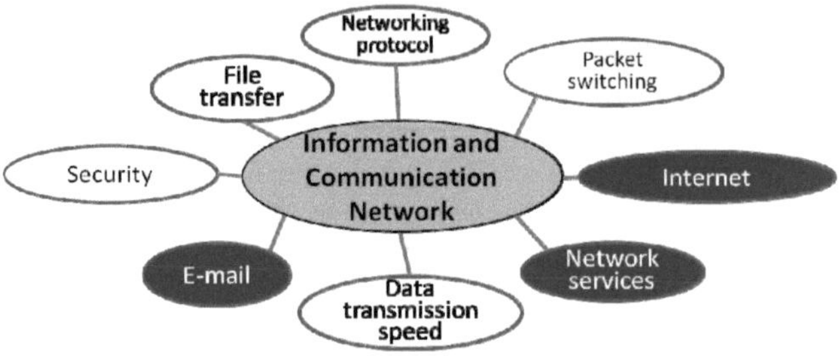

(a) high school student

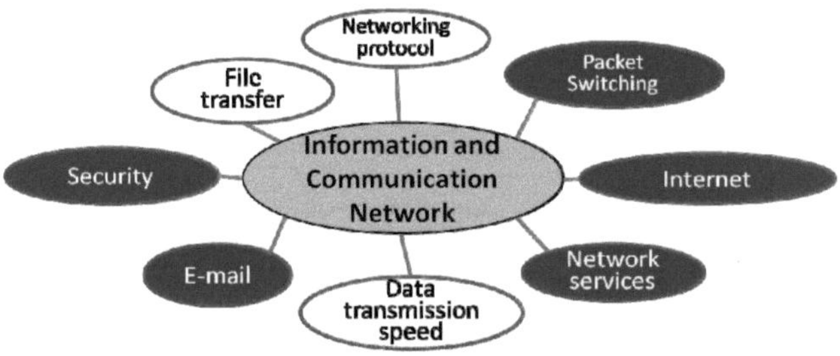

(b) university freshman

Fig. 2. Matching divisions for student maps

We embodied these points into the specifications of the learning tool. Also, we made our hands-on size learning tool experimentally on an electronic circuit using Arduino [10]. We defined the data to be sent and received as the start code, message, and stop code. This learning tool allows learners to set up the start code and stop code, and assemble outgoing messages. These functions correspond to points 1. and 2. above (see Fig.3 (a)). To show the message body, the user can make a choice between two formats: ASCII code(8 bits / 1 ASCII character) or ASCII character. This function corresponds to point 3. above (see Fig.3 (b)). Daily objects such as "distance" and "fall" are easily presented credible threats to wireless communication. By using IT technology, we can recover from these communication errors. Our tool helps the user to be aware of the existence of these technologies. This function corresponds to point 4. above (see Fig.3 (c)).

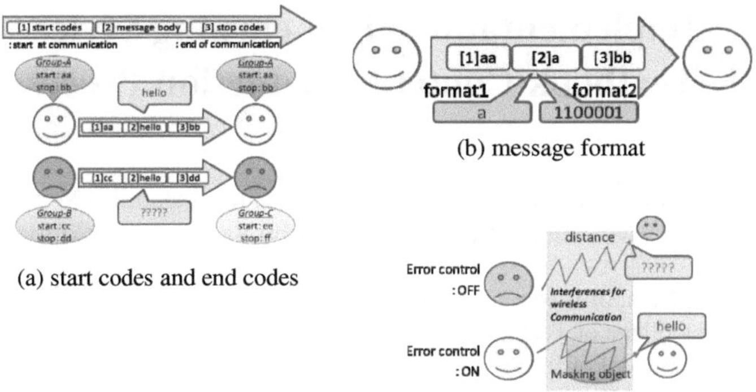

(a) start codes and end codes

(b) message format

(c) error control

Fig. 3. Features of our proposed tool

References

1. Wing, J.M.: Computational Thinking. CACM 49(3), 33–35 (2006)
2. Wing, J.M.: Computational Thinking: What and Why? Link Magazine, http://www.cs.cmu.edu/~CompThink/papers/TheLinkWing.pdf (accessed April 09, 2013)
3. Phillips, P.: Computational Thinking. A Problem-Solving Tool for Every Classroom, http://www.cs.cmu.edu/~CompThink/resources/ct_pat_phillips.ppt (accessed April 09, 2013)
4. Barr, V., Stephenson, C.: Bringing computational thinking to K-12: what is Involved and what is the role of the computer science education community? ACM Inroads 2(1), 48–54 (2011)
5. Yadav, A., Zhou, M., Mayfield, C., Hambrusch, S., Korb, J.T.: Introducing computational thinking in education courses. In: Proc. of the 42nd ACM Technical Symposium on Computer Science Education, pp. 465–470 (2011)
6. Japanese Ministry of Education, Culture, Sports, Science and Technology (MEXT): Government guidelines for elementary school education, ch. 1, General Provisions, http://www.mext.go.jp/component/a_menu/education/micro_detail/__icsFiles/afieldfile/2011/04/11/1261037_1.pdf (accessed April 09, 2013)
7. MEXT: Government guidelines for junior high school education, Section 8 Technology and Home Economics, http://www.mext.go.jp/component/a_menu/education/micro_detail/__icsFiles/afieldfile/2011/04/11/1298356_9.pdf (accessed April 09, 2013)
8. MEXT: High School Subject names in government guidelines for high school education, http://www.mext.go.jp/a_menu/shotou/new-cs/youryou/eiyaku/__icsFiles/afieldfile/2011/04/11/1298353_0.pdf (accessed April 09, 2013)
9. Buzan, T., Buzan, B.: The Mind Map Book: Radiant Thinking - Major Evolution in Human Thought. BBC Books (1993)
10. Arduino, http://www.arduino.cc/ (accessed April 09, 2013)

Implementation of a Learning Style by E-Textbook Contents Reduction Processing

Haruya Shiba[1], Kousei Ueta[1], Yoshino Ohishi[1], Takahiko Mendori[2], Yusuke Nishiuchi[1], Masanobu Yoshida[1], Hironobu Satoh, and Takumi Yamatuchi[1]

[1] Dept. of Electrical Engineering and Information Science, Kochi National College of Technology, 200-1 Monobe-Otsu, Nankoku-city, Kochi, Japan

[2] School of Information, Kochi University of Technology, 185 Miyanokuchi, Tosayamda, Kami-city, Kochi, Japan

{shiba,nishiuchi,myoshida,satoh,yama}@ee.kochi-ct.ac.jp, {e4702,e4707}@gm.kochi-ct.jp, mendori.takahiko@kochi-tech.ac.jp

Abstract. The majority of Japanese classrooms are teacher-centered. Teachers lecture one-sidedly and write explanatory notes on blackboard matching the content of the textbook. The students just listen and copy the content that the teacher wrote on the blackboard.

We have begun using an electronic textbook (e-textbook) that students can edit. When the student understands the teacher's explanation, leaving out an important term, or obscuring the part where it is explained allows students to remake the textbook into their personal notebook. Because copying the blackboard becomes unnecessary, the students can better focus on the teacher's explanation while becoming more engaged in the learning process. We have developed a WEB application that changes a textbook into a personalized notebook which better engages students in a teacher-centered environment.

Keywords: ICT-based learning, e-textbook, reduction edit, learning style.

1 Introduction

In recent years, portable information devices have become ubiquitous. Numerous projects introduce electronic equipment and computer based texts into school lessons [1] and evaluate the educational effect [2], [3]. However, it is difficult to dramatically improve effectiveness by only learning environment computerization. New education and learning methods to improve instructional effectiveness are needed.

The majority of Japanese classrooms are teacher-centered. Teachers lecture one-sidedly and write explanatory notes on blackboard matching the content of the textbook. The students just listen and copy the content that the teacher wrote on the blackboard. Students spend too much time only copying from the blackboard. This amount of time can be reduced and used in a more interactive and engaging manner.

C. Stephanidis (Ed.): Posters, Part II, HCII 2013, CCIS 374, pp. 94–97, 2013.

We have begun using an electronic textbook (e-textbook) that students can edit. When the student understands the teacher's explanation, leaving out an important term, or obscuring the part where it is explained allows students to remake the textbook into their personal notebook. Because work to copy the content of the blackboard is no longer necessary, students can concentrate fully on the teacher's explanation, students can be expected to acquire knowledge in a short time. The e-textbook is rewritten by an electronic operation. The parts students understand and become unnecessary are obscured, but not deleted. Therefore, a number of degrees of cancellation and editing are possible.

In the class, an important word or equation will noted electronically. This can be easily achieved to make a wordbook by extracting the marked-up words, and for making problem-solving exercises. These functions might be useful so that the student may review or complete homework. When this kind of electronic textbook is used, taking notes will be simplified, and study and problem solving made more transparent. As a result, student learning might be improved.

The WEB application that remakes the e-textbook into the notebook has been developed. We call this framework the "Gakuzai system". "Gakuzai" is a compound word of two Japanese words. The word of “gaku” means the learning processes until knowledge is acquired and the word of "zai" is the material. The Gakuzai system offers an environment to support all processes of study from a class by teacher to homework by student. This paper proposes a suitable next generation learning method in the e-textbook generation, and aims at a system preparation that doesn't depend on an operating system or browser.

2 Gakuzai System Overview

The Gakuzai system should have the following functions.

1. The e- textbook should be able to be edited quickly during the lesson.
   (a) Unnecessary parts are hidden or replaced a short word.
   (b) Important words can be marked up (text color, under line, bold-faced type, highlight).
2. The content of 1) must be reproduced in the next class.
3. Two or more learners are able to edit jointly.
4. Collaborative learning via sharing editing results among learners.

All processes from individual study to group study can be supported by these functions. EPUB and PDF are formats for general computerised books, which don't adapt, and are dependent on software/hardware for specific usage. Freedom to customize is low. Using HTLM enables flexibility and freedom from software dependencies.

The server computer was prepared to distribute the e-textbooks and to keep the edited data. The Gakuzai system was constructed by using the PHP language and JavaScript on this server computer. Currently implemented functions are the 1st and 2nd function of the Gakuzai system in above.

2.1 Classroom Phase

Sentences that could be understood enough are hidden on the e-textbook or replaced by a short key word. The e-textbook makes a change to the formulary or the wordbook by this function. To explain study that uses the Gkuzai system, Kirchhoff's current law is an example. [Text from Wikipedia: Kirchhoff's current law, (2013)]

> This law is also called Kirchhoff's first law, Kirchhoff's point rule, or Kirchhoff's junction rule (or nodal rule).
>
> The principle of conservation of electric charge implies that:
>
> At any node (junction) in an electrical circuit, the sum of currents flowing into that node is equal to the sum of currents flowing out of that node, or:
>
> The algebraic sum of currents in a network of conductors meeting at a point is zero.
>
> Recalling that current is a signed (positive or negative) quantity reflecting direction towards or away from a node, this principle can be stated as:
>
> $$\sum_{k=1}^{n} I_k = 0$$
>
> n is the total number of branches with currents flowing towards or away from the node.

Only a formula summation of I is left because the chapter of the explanation will only have to record the name and the expression of the law that becomes not necessary for the student who understood this content, and the rest will be concealed.

2.2 Home Study Phase

If an underline is pulled during the lesson importantly, - in the example above, the under line has already been pulled -, the exercise that removes this term from the explanation can be made from an automatic operation. The automatically generated exercise can help self-learning. Therefore, retention can be expected to increase.

The system responds to the fact of adding words because the replacement of the characters only doesn't shorten the long one. Moreover, images can be added the same as words and though the Gakuzai system students can use take notes with traditionally.

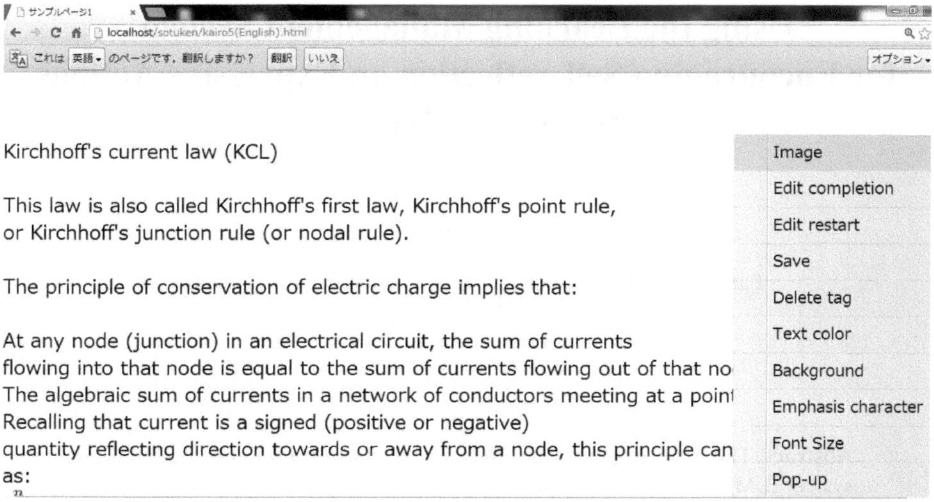

Fig. 1. The e-textbook editing form in the Gakuzai sytem. The content of the textbook is displayed on the left side. User selects the strings for editing on this screen and edits with the right side menu.

3 Conclusions and Future Work

We proposed a new education / learning method with the e-textbook. The WEB application software to practice this method was developed. Currently we are using this system in the classroom, and the educational effect will be evaluated in the future.

Acknowledgments. This study was supported by JSPS KAKENHI Grant Number 25330431 and 24501236.

References

1. Japan Ministry of Internal Affairs and Communications: Future School Promotion Research Society
2. http://www.soumu.go.jp/main_sosiki/joho_tsusin/eng/Releases/Telecommunications/110720_a.html
3. Rockinson-Szapkiw, A.J., Courduff, J., et al.: Electronic versus traditional print textbooks: A comparison study on the influence of university student's learning. Computers & Education 63, 259–266 (2013)
4. Matsuuchi, N., Nishiuchi, Y., et al.: TERAKOYA Learning System Linking Multipoint Remote Users for Supplementary Lessons. The Journal of Information and Systems in Education 9, 35–44 (2011)

Using the Learning Management System for Encouraging Self-reflection on Expressive Actions in Higher Education

Shoko Shiroma

Faculty of School Education, Joetsu University of Education,
1, Yamayashiki-machi, Joetsu, Niigata 943-8512, Japan
shoko@juen.ac.jp

Abstract. This study examines the effectiveness of using a learning management system (LMS) for learning expressive actions in higher education. The author intended to use the LMS as a tool for students' self-reflection on their class experiences. Students in the course "Seminar on expression" were given writing assignments with the LMS. An analysis of the student essays showed that the students were able to reflect on their class experiences and improve their understanding of expressive actions. Specifically, through their essay writing using the LMS, they related changes in their way of thinking with regard to expressive actions with their class learning experiences.

Keywords: learning management system, self-reflection, conceptual change, expressive education, teacher-training course.

1 Introduction

This study examines the effectiveness of using a learning management system (LMS) for learning about expressive actions in higher education.

LMSs are an application for e-learning. LMSs such as Moodle, Blackboard, and WebCT are widely used for effective learning in higher education. They allow teachers to handle students' learning outside the classroom, as they can both create and deliver course materials and track student progress. Students can access the provided materials, submit their homework, and exchange their opinions on lesson topics. However, in only a few universities in Japan students can complete an entire course online. About half of Japan's higher education institutions use a LMS to complement the face-to-face classes [1].

This study focuses on self-reflection in expressive education. Experience-based learning is prevalent as the method of education in this field, with students typically engaging in performance and appreciation activities. However this learning style has been criticized for failing to ensure that students acquire conceptual knowledge. Therefore, reflecting on their learning experiences is essential for students to gain a better understanding of course contents [2]. The author intended to use the LMS as a tool for students to reflect on their classroom experiences. The purpose of this study is to demonstrate the effect of self-reflection with the LMS.

C. Stephanidis (Ed.): Posters, Part II, HCII 2013, CCIS 374, pp. 98–102, 2013.

2 Method

2.1 Outline of the Course

The course "Seminar on expression" was offered for college students who aim to become teachers. One hundred sixty-six freshmen took the course held in 2012. The purpose of the course is to expand students' understanding of expression and to enhance the communication skills that are essential for teachers.

The course consisted of 15 classes held once a week. During the first half of the course, 7 lectures were given by a professional high school teacher, a laughter yoga instructor, a ceramic artist, and 4 performance artists, respectively. The lecturers told the students their own view on expressions by giving a performance and explaining about the motivation behind their works. During the second half of the course, the students formed groups of 10 to create original pieces of work using physical expressions. At the end of the course, all the students acted on stage.

2.2 Use of the LMS during the Course

The students were assigned homework with LMS (NEC Corporation's i-Collabo.LMS V4). They were asked to write a weekly essay reviewing what they had learned in class. The essays were written and submitted with the LMS. The themes were as follows:

- Something that you hope to learn from the course
- The most interesting topic of the class and your thoughts on the topic
- Something that you hope to learn from the group activity for planning a performance
- A plan of your group to perform on stage
- Feedback/comments on the group performances
- An evaluation of your own performance, of the group work done to create a piece of work, and of your self-understanding
- Your thoughts about what "expressions" are

2.3 Analytical Perspective

The student essays written with the LMS were analyzed according to the following aspects:

- Length (number of characters)
- The types of change that occurred in the students' thinking regarding expressive actions
- Lessons/activities that changed students' understanding of the concept of expressions

3 Results

3.1 Essay Length

Table 1 shows the length of the student essays, which were written after each class. The third set of essays was written by hand during class, in response to the lecturer's request. The midterm essays (7th) and final essays (16th) were essential tasks. The students were asked to write these two essays in approximately 1000 characters. Except for the handwritten and mandatory essays, the average length of the essays was 421 characters.

Table 1. Length of student essays

Week	Total character count of the essays submitted with LMS	Number of students who submitted an essay with LMS	Average number of characters per essay
1	30824	131	235.3
2	71759	151	475.2
3	-	-	-
4	63562	154	412.7
5	73723	161	457.9
6	62630	154	406.7
Midterm	179113	166	1079.0
8	50997	161	316.8
9	50781	159	319.4
10	51798	157	329.9
11	27729	96	288.8
12	91945	139	661.5
13	97653	160	610.3
14	76653	157	488.2
15	73867	157	470.5
Final	172936	164	1054.5

3.2 Types of Changes in Students' Thinking about Expressive Actions

Students' Understanding of Expressive Action at the Start of the Course. First, descriptions of expressive action were identified in the student essays written after the first class. They were divided into the following categories:

– Sending and receiving a message

  • Conveying ideas or feelings clearly
  • Understanding the right meanings of words, gestures, and facial expressions

– Teaching children

- Catching children's attention
- Motivating children to learn
- Giving understandable explanations
- Giving a proper response to a variety of children
- Encouraging children to express themselves

– Self-expression

- Expressing oneself in one's own way

Students' Understanding of Expressive Action at the End of the Course. Next, the students' descriptions of expressive action were identified in their final essays. Some of the new perspectives on expressive action fell into the following categories:

- Having an effect on others
- Identifying what I want to say
- Revealing one's personality and way of life
- Discovering an unknown self-disposition

The student essays from the start of the course had no mention of the audience. However, a number of students referred to the audience at the end of the course. ("*We need to care about the audience. Expressive actions are not meant to convey information in only one direction.*" "*A message can be understood by each audience member in a different way. The audience (receiver) is an integral part of the performance*"). Some students focused on expressive actions not just as a result but also as a process. ("*The process of creating the performance is an important part of expression. A performance is realized on the basis of the process of looking for a new way to express an idea and preparing for a good performance.*") Moreover, students' negative feelings about expressive actions turned into positive ones. ("*Expressing an idea is very enjoyable. I feel very happy when my message is accepted.*" "*Expressive actions are not extraordinary experiences. They are what we do every day.*")

3.3 Lessons/Activities That Changed Students' Understanding of the Concept of Expressions

Through the process of essay writing, the students associated their changes in thinking about expressive actions with their experiences in the class. Each student described the topic or activity that he or she had been most impressed with and that had influenced his or her understanding of expressive actions. Examples are as follows:

- An exercise to see how much the message was transferred
- A pantomime performance that expresses a feeling beyond words
- A performer's attitude of improvisation based on audience response

- An example of ceramic works that are given an entirely new meaning by a viewer
- An activity of creating a drama based on the theme, "my way of living"

4 Discussion

The analysis of student essays written with the LMS showed the following:

- Students wrote 400-character essays after each class. They were able to look back on their learning experiences and improve their understanding of expressive actions.
- Students' understanding of expressive action was expanded through the course. They found out that expressive actions consist of more than conveying information accurately.
- Through the process of essay writing, students related the changes in their thinking with regard to expressive action with their classroom experiences.

These effects may be attributed to both the activity of writing an essay after each class and use of the LMS. Compared with conventional handwritten reports in class, the LMS has two advantages for student learning. One is that students can write essays at their own pace. When students use the LMS outside class, they can take time to reflect on their experiences and to develop their thinking. Without the LMS, the students were forced to write an essay in just 10 minutes. The second advantage is that students' essays are accumulated automatically in the LMS, enabling students to review them at will and access their learning trajectories.

5 Conclusion

The study suggests the possibility of LMS as a tool for students' self-reflection. LMS is often used for providing learning contents. In addition, LMS may help students to reflect on their classroom experience and improve their understanding of the concept. By using LMS in combination with hands-on activities in class, educators would provide an enriched learning environment for students to learn.

References

1. National Institute of Multimedia Education: E-learning tou no ICT wo katsuyoushita kyouiku ni kansuru chousa houkokusho (2008)
2. Mogi, K., Ueda, N., Kariyado, T., Sato, Y., Miyata, Y. (eds.): Kyoudou to hyougen no workshop. Toshindo, Tokyo (2010)

The Impact of System Interactions on Motivation and Performance in a Game-Based Learning Environment

Erica L. Snow, G. Tanner Jackson, Laura K. Varner, and Danielle S. McNamara

Department of Psychology, Learning Sciences Institute, Arizona State University, Tempe, AZ, 85287, USA
{Erica.L.Snow,TannerJackson,Laura.Varner,Dsmcnama}@asu.edu

Abstract. The current study examined how students' frequency of interactions with game-based features impacted their system performance (i.e., total trophies won and achievement levels earned) and attitudes toward the game-based system, iSTART-ME. This study (n=40) was a part of a larger study (n=124) conducted with high school students. Results indicate that students' interactions with game-based features were positively related to both their system performance and their posttest attitudes toward the system. These findings provide further support showing that the integration of game-based features has positive effects on students within educational learning environments.

Keywords: Human-computer interactions, learning, motivation, educational technology, game-based features, adaptive environments.

1 Introduction

Learning scientists have begun to investigate how game-based features impact students' affect and performance within Intelligent Tutoring Systems (ITSs). When students interact with game-based features incorporated within an ITS, they report improved engagement and an increased likelihood of future system use [1-4]. Although previous work has shown a positive relation between the implementation of game-based features and student affect, it remains unclear whether students' system performance varies as a result of interactions with these features. The current study addresses this question by examining the relation between students' frequency of interactions with game-based features, their system performance, and their posttest self-reported attitudes toward the game-based system, iSTART-ME.

1.1 iSTART-ME

The Interactive Strategy Training for Active Reading and Thinking – Motivationally Enhanced (iSTART-ME) is an adaptive system that was designed to help students improve their reading comprehension ability by teaching strategies in a game-based virtual environment. iSTART–ME incorporates educational games and interactive features into an adaptive environment which allow students to practice reading comprehension strategies [5].

C. Stephanidis (Ed.): Posters, Part II, HCII 2013, CCIS 374, pp. 103–107, 2013.

Previous work has shown that the iSTART-ME system is effective at improving students' reading compression skills [6]. The addition of game-based features into the iSTART-ME system has been shown to increase students' engagement overtime [5]. The current study builds upon this previous work by examining students how the frequency of students' interactions with game-based features impacts system performance and posttest attitudes.

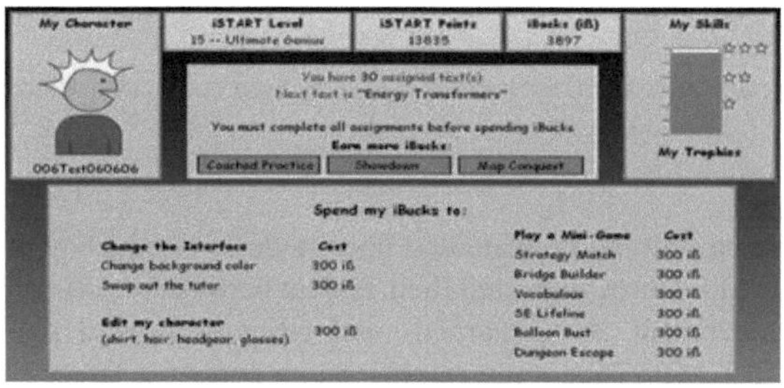

Fig. 1. Screen Shot of iSTART-ME Selection Menu

Inside of the iSTART-ME system, students choose to play games, check their progress in the system, or personalize interface elements (see Figure 1 for screenshot). Students earn points by playing practice games, which were designed to reinforce the iSTART-ME comprehension strategies. As students accumulate more points, they advance to higher achievement levels (maximum of 25), where they have more opportunities to interact with game-based features.

There are four categories of features inside of iSTART-ME: generative practice games, identification mini-games, personalizable features, and achievement screens. Generative practice games provide students the opportunity to write their own self-explanations, whereas the identification mini-games require students to recognize which strategies are used within example self-explanations. For both generative and identification games, students can win trophies based on their performance. Trophies are earned as students progress to varying performance thresholds inside of the generative and identification games. Personalizable features provide students a means to control and represent themselves within the environment. These features include a customizable avatar, a configurable background theme, and a variety of pedagogical agents. Students can also monitor their performance and progress through the system using achievement screens (e.g., points earned, achievement levels, and trophies won).

2 Method

High-school students (n=40) from a mid-south urban environment participated in an 11-session experiment consisting of a pretest, eight training sessions, a posttest, and a delayed retention test. This sample of students was part of a larger study (n=124) that compared three experimental conditions: iSTART-ME, iSTART-Regular, and a no-tutor control. The current study focused solely on those students who were randomly assigned to the iSTART-ME condition. These students had access to the full game-based system, including all personalizable features and games.

During the first session of the experiment, participants completed a pretest survey including measures of their attitudes, prior knowledge, and comprehension skills. Throughout the following 8 sessions, students freely interacted with the iSTART-ME system (at least 1 hour per session). At the tenth session, students completed a posttest, which contained measures similar to the posttest. Approximately 1 week later, students completed a delayed retention test that included measures of self-explanation ability and reading comprehension.

In the current study, students' attitudes toward the system were measured using posttest questions (see examples in Table 1). Additionally, system performance was represented through students' earned trophies and achievement levels. The total number of earned trophies reflected students' performance across both the generative and identification practice games. Similarly, students' achievement levels reflected the number of points received through interactions with all practice environments.

Table 1. Postest Measure of Student Attitudes

Dependent Measure	Response Statement	Response Scale*
Enjoyment	*"I had fun using the computer system."*	1 - 6
System Reuse	*"I would use this system again."*	1 - 6

*1 (Strongly Disagree) to 6 (Strongly Agree)

3 Results

The current study examined how students' interactions with game-based features impacted their system performance and posttest attitudes. A median split was con-ducted on students' total frequency of interactions to create two groups: high and low interactors. ANOVAs on the system performance variables revealed that high

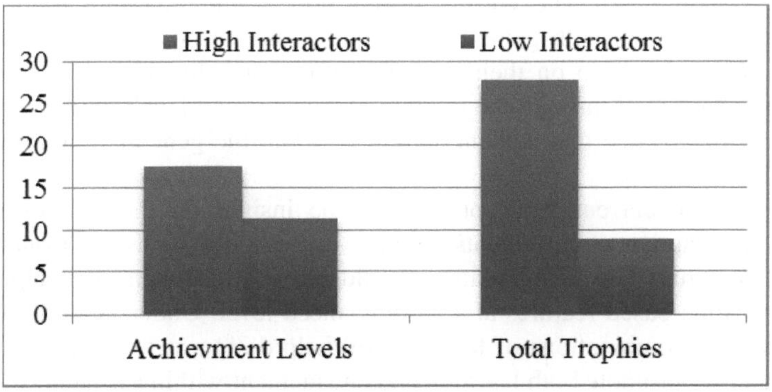

Fig. 2. System Performance Means for High and Low Interactors

interactors attained significantly higher achievement levels, $F(1,38) = 13.22$, $p < .001$, and earned significantly more trophies, $F(1,38) = 7.328$, $p < .001$, than the low interactors (see Figure 2 for means). These results indicate that students who interacted with the available features more frequently performed significantly better within the system than students who engaged in fewer interactions.

Similarly, ANOVAs on the posttest attitudes revealed that high interactors re-ported greater overall enjoyment, $F(1,38) = 5.59$, $p < .05$, and a higher likelihood to use the system again, $F(1,38) = 4.27$, $p < .05$, than the low interactors (see Figure 3 for means). These results suggest that when students engage with system features more frequently, they enjoy the system more and report a higher likelihood to return for future use.

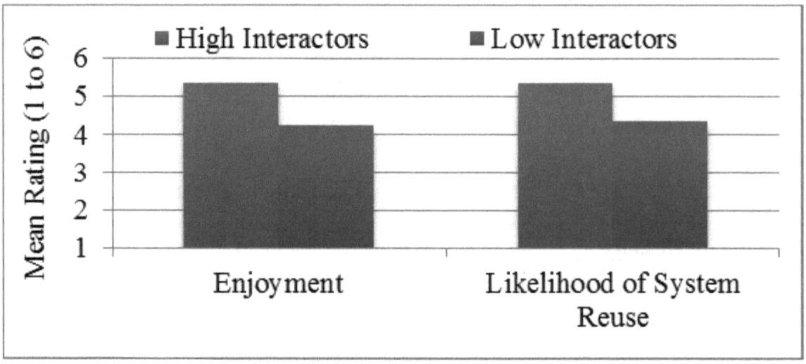

Fig. 3. Posttest Attitude Means for High and Low Interactors

4 Conclusions and Implications

The current work examined how students' total interactions with game-based features impacted their performance and attitudes toward the game-based tutoring system, iSTART-ME. Findings from this study are in line with previous work that has found increases in students' affect when game-based features are incorporated within a learning system [1-4]. The current results add to the literature by showing that students' interactions with game-based features have a positive impact not only on students' affect but also on their system performance. In this work, system performance was measured through the number of trophies and levels earned, which reflect the quality of practice that students produce within the generative and identification games.

Although the current work provides some insight on the role of game-based features in adaptive environments, future work should focus on isolating varying types of features. This manipulation would allow researchers to decipher the true impact of game-based features at a more nuanced level. Understanding the impact of individual and combinations of features will help designers to optimize systems that simultaneously promote both learning and engagement within a system.

Acknowledgements. This research was supported in part by the Institute for Educational Sciences (IES R305G020018-02; R305G040046, R305A080589) and National Science Foundation (NSF REC0241144; IIS-0735682). Any opinions, findings, and conclusions or recommendations expressed in this material are those of the authors and do not necessarily reflect the views of the IES or NSF.

References

1. Cordova, D., Lepper, M.: Intrinsic Motivation and the Process of Learning: Beneficial effects of Contextualization, Personalization, and Choice. Journal of Educational Psychology 88, 715–730 (1996)
2. Rowe, J.P., Shores, L.R., Mott, B.W., Lester, J.C.: Integrating Learning and Engagement in Narrative-Centered Learning Environments. In: Aleven, V., Kay, J., Mostow, J. (eds.) ITS 2010, Part II. LNCS, vol. 6095, pp. 166–177. Springer, Heidelberg (2010)
3. Malone, T., Lepper, M.: Making Learning Fun: A Taxonomy of Intrinsic Motivations for Learning. In: Snow, R., Fair, M. (eds.) Aptitude, Learning, and Instruction, Cognitive and Affective Process Analyses, vol. 3, pp. 223–253. Erlbaum, Hillsdale (1987)
4. Moreno, R., Mayer, R.E.: Role of Guidance, Reflection, and Interactivity in an Agent-Based Multimedia Game. Journal of Educational Psychology 97, 117–128 (2005)
5. Jackson, G., Boonthum, C., McNamara, D.: iSTART-ME: Situating Extended Learning within a Game-Based Environment. In: Lane, H.C., Ogan, A., Shute, V. (eds.) In Proceedings of the Workshop on Intelligent Educational Games at the 14th Annual Conference on Artificial Intelligence in Education, pp. 59–68. AIED, Brighton (2009)
6. Jackson, G.T., & McNamara, D. S.: Motivation and Performance in a Game-Based Intelligent Tutoring System. To appear in the Special Issue for Advanced Learning Technologies in the Journal of Educational Psychology (in press)

Pilot Study of an Educational Turn-Based Online Game for Formative Assessment in E-Learning Environment

Fu-Hsing Tsai

Teacher Education Center, National Chiayi University, Taiwan
fhtsai@mail.ncyu.edu.tw

Abstract. This study proposed an educational turn-based online game, called tic-tac-toe quiz (TRIS-Q), for formative assessment in a research-developed e-learning system targeting knowledge about energy education for elementary students. This game combines multi-player tic-tac-toe game and online test. To stimulate students' motivation toward the online self-assessment, this study proposed a new game rule in TRIS-Q. When players take their turn in game, they must respond to a random multiple-choice quiz which was constructed according to the e-learning contents. Also, the victory of game will be influenced by their response. According to the research findings, after using online learning and TRIS-Q, students' learning effectiveness was significantly enhanced. Most of students had positive attitude toward the game-based assessment.

Keywords: Turn-based online game, game-based assessment, formative assessment, e-learning.

1 Introduction

Assessments often can be divided into summative assessment and formative assessment. Summative assessment means the test after the finish of the whole learning activity. The purpose is to evaluate students' total learning effectiveness toward certain teaching material and their grades [1]. On the other hand, formative assessment means the evaluation in learning. Besides grading or evaluating learning effectiveness, it is mainly adopted to provide learning feedback, enhance learning performance and improve learning [2]. Thus, formative assessment is important for teachers and students. According to the outcomes of students' formative assessment, teachers can improve the instruction and conduct remedial instruction, while students can recognize learning flaws and have self-improvement.

In traditional classroom, paper-and-pencil tests were treated as the tool of formative assessment. However, with the maturity of network technology and prevalence of online learning environment, online formative assessment has been widely applied to e-learning courses. Online assessment is convenient test and learners can have the assessment without the limitation of time and space. Through online tests, it can provide learners with instant feedback [3]. Also, teachers can immediately understand students' learning progress and learning performance [4]. Thus, online assessment can

C. Stephanidis (Ed.): Posters, Part II, HCII 2013, CCIS 374, pp. 108–112, 2013.

help teachers properly manage and guide learners with inferior learning effectiveness, and enhance learners' interaction and feedback in self-directed learning to properly have self-management and self-improvement.

However, although online assessment is almost the essential functions in most e-learning courses, it cannot be ensured that every e-learner has the intention to actively conduct online formative assessment repeatedly. Hence, with current prevalence of game-based e-learning and in order to enhance learners' motivation to use online formative test, game-based formative assessment was proposed by some studies. For instance, Wang [5] applied a web-based quiz-game-like formative assessment in an e-learning environment. According to the Wang's research finding, the e-learning effectiveness with game-based formative assessment was better than the one with normal web-based test. Also, the game-based formative assessment enhanced online learners' intention to actively do self-assessment.

To date, the multi-player online games (MOGs) have become the dominant form of computer games. However, there are few research studies using online game for the formative assessment on e-Learning. Based on the above rationale, this study attempted to develop a turn-based online game, called tic-tac-toe quiz, for formative assessment in a research-developed e-learning system targeting knowledge about energy education for elementary students. It aimed to enhance effectiveness of e-learning and students' motivation to use online formative assessment.

2 The E-Learning System with Turn-Based Online Game for Formative Assessment

According to the curriculum guidelines in Taiwan, this study developed an e-learning system targeting knowledge of energy education suitable for elementary schools. When e-learners log in this e-learning system, they can start self-directed online learning activity through reading online learning contents related to energy knowledge. Noticeably, based on the learning contents, this study developed a turn-based online game, called tic-tac-toe quiz (TRIS-Q), in the system for learners to have online self-assessment at any time. The TRIS-Q combines online test and multi-player tic-tac-toe game. Students will see a game lobby shown as Figure 1 after logging in the game. Players can input texts here to interact with others, and join a tic-tac-toe game where is waiting for the second player, or create a new game and wait for the second player. As soon as two players join a game, the tic-tac-toe game starts shown as Figure 2. The game rule is similar to the traditional tic-tac-toe game, that is, the first person to place three tokens in a row, column, or diagonal is the winner. However, this game changes some rules of traditional tic-tac-toe. That is, when a player takes his turn, the game will randomly pop a multiple-choice quiz which was constructed according to the e-learning contents, shown as Figure 3. Since the victory always goes to the one who makes the first move in tic-tac-toe, in order to increase the difficulty and playfulness, the game rule is slightly modified. If the player responses the right answers, he can draw his token; otherwise he will draw his opponent's token. Thus, the new game rule could stimulate participants to seriously answer the questions in TRIS-Q. Also, this game provides every student's history of answering quizzes for the feedback of self-assessment. Students can obtain feedback and revise mistakes through checking the personal answering history. Moreover, this game also provides the high score list which presents the top ten player scores and names.

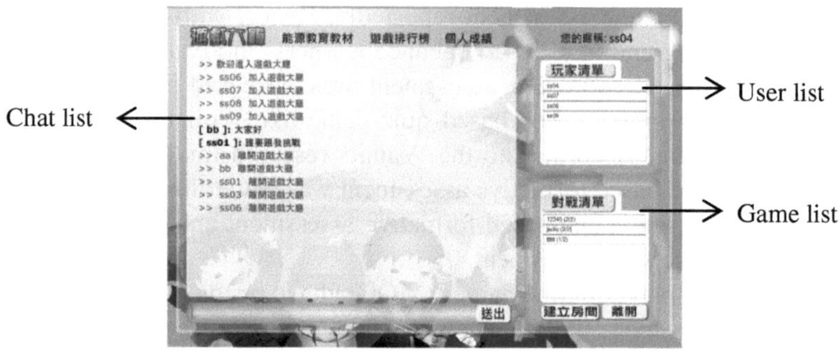

Fig. 1. The game lobby of game-based formative assessment

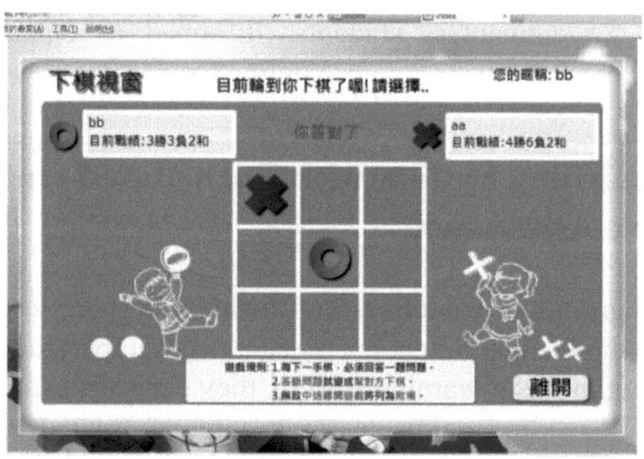

Fig. 2. Screen snapshot of playing online tic-tac-toe

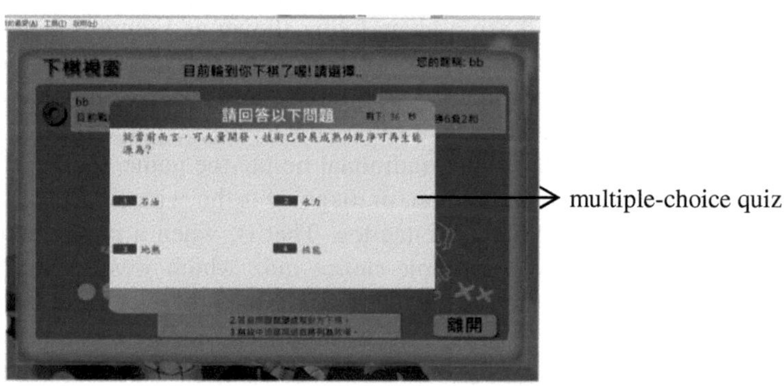

Fig. 3. Screen snapshot of answering quiz when playing game

3 Research Design and Finding

In order to find primary effectiveness of online game-based formative assessment, this study conducted quasi-experiment with pretest and posttest of single group and questionnaire survey to probe into elementary students' change of energy knowledge literacy and learning perception after using the online learning system. This study treated 23 Grade 5 students in one class of one elementary school at Chiayi County as subjects to conduct two-week online learning activity. Students were asked to use the e-learning course for two sessions (40 minutes each) evenly spread out over two weeks in computer classrooms. Moreover, within these two weeks, students also can proceed e-learning after school at any time. Before and after the experiment, the researcher conducted self-designed energy knowledge test (20 multiple choice questions. Difficulty and discrimination are 0.61 and 0.42 respectively) on the subjects. After the experiment, learning perception questionnaire (25 items of 5-point Likert-type scale, Cronbach α is 0.97 and there is one open-ended question) was conducted on subjects in order to find students' perceptions after using online game-based formative assessment.

According to the findings, this study found that before participating in this online learning, the subjects have average score of energy knowledge test as 45.43 and after the learning, their average score is 60.22. Based on t test of paired samples, scores of pretest and posttest reach statistically significant difference ($t=2.704$, $p=.010$). Thus, it means that the e-learning effectiveness of elementary students' could be enhanced through the online game-based formative assessment. Moreover, as to students' perception after using online game formative assessment, based on 5-point scale (strongly agree is 5 points, etc.), it demonstrates that averages of all questions are above 3.5. Thus, all students have positive attitude toward the tic-tac-toe quiz. Their positive comments are as follows: "the design of the game is good", "it was super cool", "it was fun", "I expected such game and I learned the principle and energy. I want to play it again", etc.

4 Conclusion and Future Work

This study proposed a game-based formative assessment in e-learning environment upon multi-user online game. The game is based on tic-tac-toe many young students are familiar with. In the game, e-learner must respond to one question related to the learning contents for students' game-based assessment. Thus, students can recognize their e-learning effectiveness in the game, enhance motivation to use online formative assessment and improve learning effectiveness. According to the findings, after using online learning and game-based assessment, students' learning effectiveness was enhanced. Most of students had positive attitude toward the game assessment. They suggested that it is easy and fun to operate the game and it increases their motivation to use online assessment. However, this study is a primary experiment and the findings should be validated by future experimental design with control group. Future studies can include single-player tic-tac-toe assessment game in online learning system. Thus, students can choose to play online or play with the computer, thereby satisfy students' preferences. The difference of learning effectiveness of different game assessment models can also be compared in the future.

Acknowledgements. The work was supported by the National Science Council of the Republic of China under Grants NSC 100-2511-S-415-015-, NSC 101-2511-S-415-018-.

References

1. Bloom, B.S., Hastings, J.T., Madaus, G.F.: Handbook on formative and summative evaluation of student learning. McGraw-Hill, New York (1971)
2. Sadler, D.: Royce: Formative assessment: Revisiting the territory. Assessment in Education 5(1), 77–84 (1998)
3. McKimm, J., Jollie, C., Cantillon, P.: ABC of learning and teaching: Web based learning. BMJ: British Medical Journal 326(7394), 870 (2003)
4. Liu, C., Wang, S., Zhang, C.: Comments on the Practice of Developmental Evaluation. Educational Research 20(3), 75–76 (1999)
5. Wang, T.H.: Web-based quiz-game-like formative assessment: Development and evaluation. Computers & Education 51(3), 1247–1263 (2008)

The Development of Interactive Book Apps to Teach Young Children Mathematical Concepts

Cathy Weng[1] and Apollo Weng[2]

[1] National Taiwan University of Science and Technology,
Graduate Institute of Digital Learning and Education,
43, Sec. 4, Keelung Rd., Taipei, 106, Taiwan
[2] China University of Technology, Digital Multimedia Design,
No. 56, Sec. 3, Xinglong Rd., Wunshan District, Taipei City 116, Taiwan
{cathyhaien,libanweng}@hotmail.com

Abstract. Many studies have shown positive effects of using storybooks to teach mathematics on young children's attitude toward mathematical learning as well as their abilities and skills to solve mathematical problems. As technology advances, interactive electronic storybooks are also playing as key tools to enhance students' learning. The purpose of current study is to explore how to combine the characteristics of storybooks and the interactive technology to develop a highly interactive e-storybook App on iPad to enhance preschoolers' learning in numeric concepts. It is believed that this study on interactive math storybook Apps will give numerous benefits toward many individuals such as children, parent and teacher, instructional designers.

Keywords: Interactive e-book, Mathematical storybooks, Book App design.

1 Introduction

Many children do not like Mathematics, find it to be a difficult subject to learn, and have poor performances in schools. Mathematics difficulties are especially pronounced in students from low-income families [1]. Researchers have found that children from low-income backgrounds enter school with much less mathematical knowledge and competence than their more affluent peers, and these early deficits tend to have long-term consequences. Early mathematical knowledge predicts students' math achievement test scores in elementary school, middle school, and even high school [2]. Some researchers even indicated the strong effect it has on a person's career advancement [3]. Moreover, according to Duncan et al. [2] the relationship between early and later mathematical knowledge is about twice as strong as that between early and later reading achievement. Thus, early Mathematical concepts and knowledge are so important in a person's life, and finding effective interventions to increase the impact and effectiveness of teaching and learning early mathematical knowledge presents an important challenge to researchers and teachers alike today.

In the past, cognitive scientists have argued that storytelling is the most natural way of delivering organized knowledge to human cognitive system, and when the

C. Stephanidis (Ed.): Posters, Part II, HCII 2013, CCIS 374, pp. 113–117, 2013.

information is presented within a story context, rather than in a decontextualized format, it usually can be learned and retained more effectively [4], and this effect is quite robust [5]. The use of storybooks to support children's learning, and the research that investigates this, generally focuses on learning related to language development, such as early literacy concepts [6]. However, in 1989, National Council of Teachers of Mathematics started to advocate the use of children's trade books (storybooks) as a way of introducing mathematical ideas [7], and linking mathematics instruction to children's literature has become increasingly popular since then. In fact, when linking up young children's love of fantasy to the learning of mathematics, teachers can make mathematics meaningful to them. Many empirical findings also suggested that it is useful to embed the mathematics in a story context, and to develop mathematical concepts through sequenced mathematics problems connected to the storyline and the pictures [4]. According to Schiro [8], with those stories and mathematical literatures, children can not only be provided with a context for making meaning of abstract mathematical concepts but also taught the importance of mathematics in their world and even changing their attitudes toward mathematic concepts. Thus, using stories to enhance students' Mathematical concepts is not something new, and it has been a widely accepted, sound strategy for the teachers.

As the technology becomes more and more advanced, storybooks can appeared as electronic books have interactive components that allow children to deviate from the story sequence by clicking on hyperlinks or hotspots that activate sound effects, oral reading, animations, games, music, or other interactive features. Electronic books can take many different forms from talking books to CD ROMs, or today as book apps. The word "app" is an abbreviation for "computer application," which is a computer program that is accessed through an icon on the tablet computer screens. Recently the term "app" has taken on a whole new meaning as Apple Computers have developed programs for their computers, iPads, iPods and iPhones that include everything from games, websites, television stations, and now books. Here, the book app is an interactive storybook used on mobile devices, and it is even more user friendly and allows more direct experience for the user through the touch of the screen with their fingers to control the device. In the past, learning software has been well recognized for its ability to increase a child's independence and sense of control over their learning, which increases motivation and self-esteem [9]. Nowadays, when the electronic storybooks are developed as book apps, they will give users even more possibilities, as they are more flexible and accessible.

Under this current study, the authors develop a book app that is "born digital" as compare to most of the electronic books are still digitalized form of the printed book. This means that more interactive multimedia features will be utilized. The book app wants to create mathematical connections to real world situation through an adventure story that teaches numerical concepts for preschoolers, and hope it will engage them and make them learn. In the following section, it would be focused on introducing how this book app was developed.

2 The Development of the Book App

The Model of the Instructional Design. The development of the book app was based on the backward design discussed by Wiggins and Mctighe [10]. It is a three-stage approach to planning, where at stage one, we carefully identify desired results. Various numerical concepts were identified for our target audience that is the pre-schoolers, following on the standards announced by the Ministry of Education in Taiwan. The second stage is determining acceptable evidence. At this point, we focused on how to measure student's successful learning of those concepts. Finally at the third stage, with clearly identified results and appropriate evidence of learning, it was then the time to fully think through the most appropriate instructional activities. Here will be the actual story content developed. In order to establish an interesting and comprehensible story to teach preschool numerical concepts, the story content developed are actually following Thorndyke's [11] story grammar (see Table 1) that is a framework of elements that helps to organize oral and written works of literature so that information may be stored and retrieved easily. These elements and their rules of combination comprise a framework or schema that describes the organization of most narrative texts. By including all the elements and grammar rules, the book app developed would be a more complete and motivating story.

Table 1. Grammar Rules for Simple Stories [11]

Rule #	Rule
1	Story -- Setting + Theme + Plot + Resolution
2	Setting -- Characters + Location + Time
3	Theme -- (Event)* + Goal
4	Plot -- Episode*
5	Episode -- Subgoal + Attempt* + Outcome
6	Attempt -- Event*/Episode
7	Outcome -- Event*/State
8	Resolution -- Event/State
9	Subgoal/Goal -- Desired State
10	Characters/Location/Time -- State

The symbol "+" specifies the combination of elements in sequential order. The parentheses around Event show that the element is optional and the asterisk (*) indicates that the elements may precede the statement of the goal.

The Developmental Platform of the Book App. The Book app was constructed on two multimedia book-app design platforms, Presentation and Mocol, by Chidopi Co., Ltd. in Taiwan. Presstation allows users to post stories, upload photos, videos, music, or website links to create interactive iPad ebook apps. It is a user-friendly tool and users do not need to have a programming background. On the other hand, MoCool is also an automatic app maker platform. It allows easily transfer of contents into App format. It allows digital contents to take full advantage of the finger-tap capabilities of the various mobile devices. The MoCool platform is using updated HTML5 as core technology presenting contents and effects efficiently and productively. The powerful effect engines and modules help content writer spread their creativity without knowing any technical codes. It can also support multimedia, rich interactions, and animations by uploading raw materials such as images, videos and texts [12].

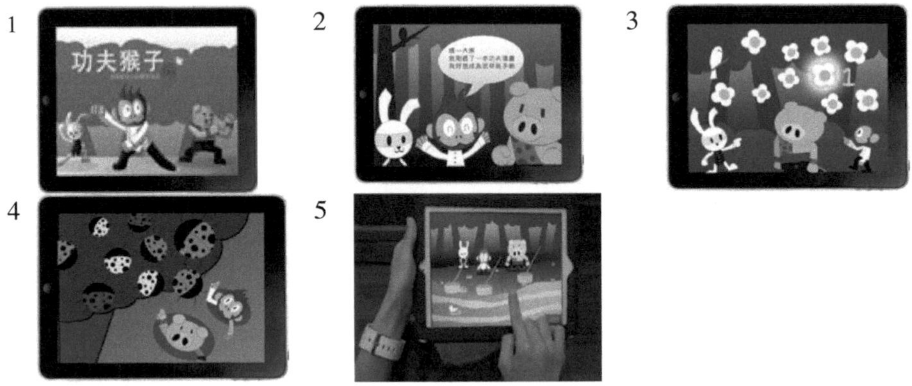

Fig. 1. The screen shots from the actual book app presenting numerical concepts

1. The title page of the book app, Kong Fu Monkey-The Development of numeric cognition.
2. Conversation will be shown with printed text as well as sounds in the dialogue boxes.
3. Blinking on the flowers leads the reader touching with their fingers, and it will count the flowers with the printed symbols.
4. Using objects appeared in kids' daily lives, it utilizes the familiarity to attract preschoolers' attention
5. Reader can use their fingers to swipe and flip to the next page

The Description of the Mathematic Content and the Story Covered in the Book App. What is innovative about the book app, "Kong Fu Monkey", is that the storytelling is in the form of an adventure story that starts with three friends who wanted to learn Chinese Kong Fu, so they follow a mysterious bird leading them to find the Turtle Master for the lessons. This format allows the numerical concepts to be taught in a systematic, hierarchical progression. The story is interwoven with the targeted numerical concepts (counting, number knowledge, number transformation, estimation, and number patterns) and extends over several lessons, so that they provide a medium for ongoing instruction and deepening mathematics understanding for the children. Through the animated pictures and hearing dialogues, the readers can comprehend the presentation and the analytic explanation of the involved basic concepts. In the story, the characters (the three friends) also encounter multiple obstacles, each building upon the previous, in terms of both story plot and math content. By teaching these skills in the carefully written story context including what is familiar, children would be able to make connections to the real world and daily experiences.

Each lesson is presented in the form of a new problem that the readers must follow the characters to solve in order for the story to progress. This draws the children into the action of the story, actively engaging them as critical participants as the drama unfolds. Therefore, they are more invested in solving the problems occur in each section and motivated to utilize their intellectual abilities in the acquisition of new knowledge and skills.

3 Conclusions

With carefully designed story and the interface of the book app, it is believed that the book app developed in the research will bring great benefits to the preschoolers' learning on numeric concepts. The present findings suggest a future direction for early childhood mathematics education. The use of a story context provides an important conduit for communicating mathematical ideas. However, in order to have empirical evidence on the effectiveness of this book app, further investigation is needed on some kind of experiment carried out with real preschoolers.

Acknowledgments. This work was supported by the National Science Council (NSC), Taiwan, R.O.C., under Contracts No. NSC101-2511-S-011-004.

References

1. National Assessment of Educational Progress. The nation's report card. Mathematics highlights 2003 (No. NCES2004-451). US Department of Education, Jessup (2004)
2. Duncan, G.J., Dowsett, C.J., Claessens, A., Magnuson, K., Huston, A.C., Klebanov, P.: School readiness and later achievement. Dev. Psy. 43, 1428–1446 (2007)
3. Jordan, N.C.: Early predictors of Mathematics achievement and Mathematics learning difficulties. Encyclopedia on Early Childhood Development (2010)
4. Schank, R.C., Abelson, R.P.: Knowledge and memory: The real story. In: Wyer, R.S. (ed.) Knowledge and Memory: The real story, pp. 1–85. Lawrence Erlbaum Associates, Hillsdale (1995)
5. Mishra, A.: Age and school related differences in recall of verbal items in a story context. Soc. Sci. Inter. 19, 12–18 (2003)
6. Anderson, A., Anderson, J., Shapiro, J.: Supporting multiple literacies: Parents' and children's mathematical talk within storybook reading. Math. Edu. Res. J. 16(3), 5–26 (2005)
7. National Council of Teachers of Mathematics: Curriculum and evaluation for school mathematics. National Council of Teachers of Mathematics, Reston (1989)
8. Schiro, M.: Oral storytelling and teaching mathematics: Pedagogical and multicultural perspectives. Sage Publication, Thousand Oaks (2004)
9. Moody, A.K.: Using Electronic Books in the Classroom to Enhance Emergent Literacy Skills in Young Children. J. of Lit. and Techf. 11(4), 23–52 (2010)
10. Wiggins, G., McTighe, J.: The Understanding by Design guide to creating high-quality units. ASCD, Alexandria (2011)
11. Thorndyke, P.W.: Cognitive structures in comprehension and memory of narrative discourse. Cognitive Psychology 9, 77–110 (1977)
12. Chidopi (April 10, (2013), `http://www.chidopi.com/site/services-2/mocool/?lang=en`, `http://www.chidopi.com/site/services-2/mocool/?lang=en` (retrieved)

Educational Character Recognition System Implementing an Interactive Visualization of Multi-dimensional Distribution

Takehiro Yamamoto, Nobuyuki Esaki, and Tetsuo Takeshita

Department of Information and Computer Engineering,
Toyota College of Technology, 2-1 Eiseicho, Toyota, Aichi 4718525, Japan
esaki@toyota-ct.ac.jp
http://www.ice.toyota-ct.ac.jp/experience/digit_recognition/

Abstract. In this paper, we propose visualizing multi-dimensional distribution used in pattern recognition system and construct a visualization system for multi-dimensional space which stimulates intuitive and visual understanding of pattern distribution for the purpose of education. We treat the method of visualizing the multi-dimensional vector data of each character on the handwritten digit recognition system. By applying principal component analysis, the original vectors are converted into principal components and three components. Ellipsoids of equal probability for each category are derived and visualized in the three-dimensional space shown in the visualization system. As a result, the boundary surfaces of each distribution of categories can be seen easily in the reduced three-dimensional space in spite of the fact that visualized vectors distributions do not represent all of vectors data. In conclusion, learners of pattern recognition can be stimulated their interest in and comprehension of multi-dimensional distribution through using this system.

Keywords: educational character recognition, principal component analysis, visualization of feature space.

1 Introduction

Pattern recognition systems including character or speech recognition systems are used in many places and occasions. They generally process multi-dimensional random vectors[1]. This makes it difficult for us to understand how the vectors are distributed in space because humans can imagine three-dimensional space at most. Furthermore, it is also difficult to compare mass and multi-dimensional vector data to recognize the objects. In this paper, we propose visualizing multi-dimensional distribution used in pattern recognition system and construct a visualization system for multi-dimensional space which stimulates intuitive and visual understanding of pattern distribution for the purpose of education.

In the previous paper, K. Yamamoto et al. proposed a visualization method for multi-dimensional data carrying out repetitive application of fuzzy clustering

C. Stephanidis (Ed.): Posters, Part II, HCII 2013, CCIS 374, pp. 118–122, 2013.

and fuzzy mlitiple discriminalt analysis[2]. And we, D. Mochizuki et al. created the character-recognition sysytem for education as shown in Fig. 1. The questionnaire result of a user shows the difficulty of visualization of feature quantity comparison on the weighted direction index histogram method[3]. N. Esaki et al. produced the visualization system using principal component analysis as an experiment based on the questionnaire result[4]. The system of this study further improves these prototypes.

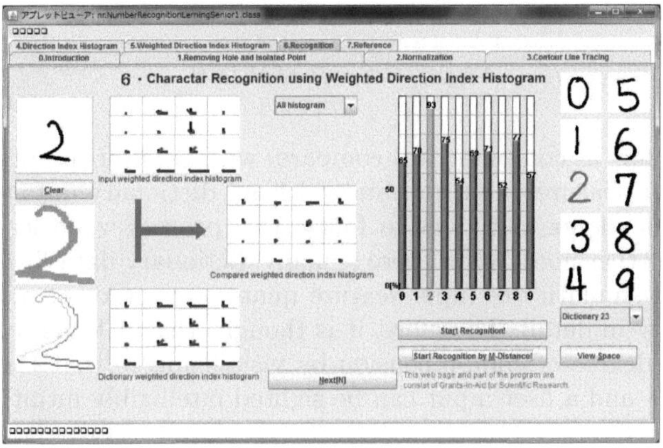

Fig. 1. Educational character recognition system showing a result of the weighted direction index histogram method. It is difficult to understand the process, although recognition is successful.

2 Methods

As a subject of study, we treat the method of visualizing the multi-dimensional vector data of each character on the handwritten digit recognition system. This system recognizes digits by using weighted direction index histogram (WDIH) that is a 64-dimensional random vector. WDIH vectors are processed dimensional reduction of random variables by using principal component analysis (PCA). In this section, we describe the feature space derived from WDIH method and give details of PCA to perform dimension compression of vector space easily.

2.1 Weighted Direction Index Histogram Method

In the educational character recognition system in Fig. 1, we can use the WDIH[5] as a useful recognition method. In process of recognition, the weighted direction index histogram is processed, where the 64-dimensional feature quantity can be obtained from a handwritten character. And the 64 dimensions consist of vertical four cell, width four cell, and four directions as shown in Fig. 2.

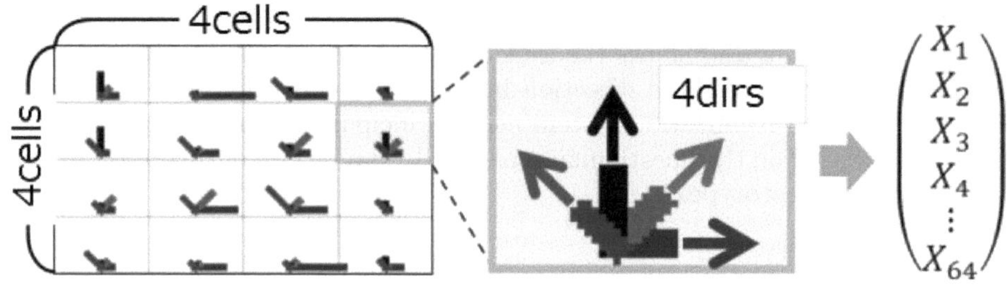

Fig. 2. Concept of WDIH

It is easy for a computer to compare with a user input each of the multi-dimension feature quantity obtained from dictionary data. On the other hand, it is difficult for a student to follow this process when learning pattern recognition. Furthermore, when there is many dictionary data, it is necessary to investigate the similarity of input feature quantity to a lot of multi-dimension feature quantity in detail. Therefore, it is thought that it leads to improvement in a student's degree of comprehension by visualizing so that the similarity of dictionary data and a user input can be sighted intelligibly intuitively.

2.2 Visualization for Multi-dimensional Data

Principal component analysis (PCA)[6] is originally a mathematical procedure that uses an orthogonal transformation to convert a set of observations of possibly correlated variables into a set of values of linearly uncorrelated variables, which are called principal components. To use PCA, we can collect multivariate distributed over many dimensional space to the eigenvalue of a large small number of dispersion. Therefore we reduce the dimension of feature space into three or less, where humans can imagine space.

Feature vectors are distributed over three-dimensional space. About the vector in the same category, distribution of a principal component score follows a normal distribution. Therefore we try to visualize the vector group in the same category with each equal probability ellipsoid.

3 Products

We implement interactive visualization as mentioned above. On our educational system, first, recognition processing is carried out to a user's input character by the WDIH method. Then in the feature space where recognition processing was performed, a feature vector is obtained from each dictionary data to a user's input character. Finally, each vector which carried out dimension compression is drawn to three dimensions by PCA.

On the system of the previous version[4], We have drawn the vector group in the scatter diagram simply, where data must be plotted according to the number of dictionaries as shown in the left part of Fig 3. On the other hand, in the system after improvement, in the right part of Fig 3, feature space is classified according to the equal probability ellipsoid, and it could be more familiar with a beginner.

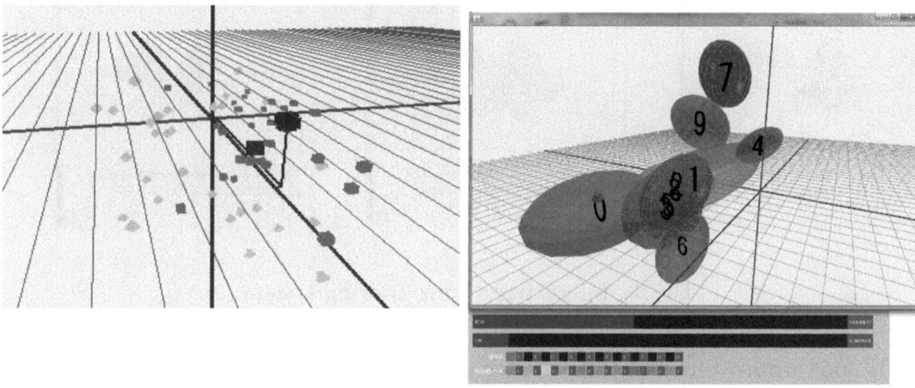

Fig. 3. The results of visualization for multi-dimensional data with the point diagram (left part) and with the probability ellipsoids (right part)

However, the size of the equal probability ellipsoids shown here is dependent on the Mahalanobis' generalised distance in fact. Figure 4 shows the equal probability ellipsoids which are not painted in the suitable size. At the present stage, this distance cannot be determined automatically but it has become the specification which a user defines free with a slide bar.

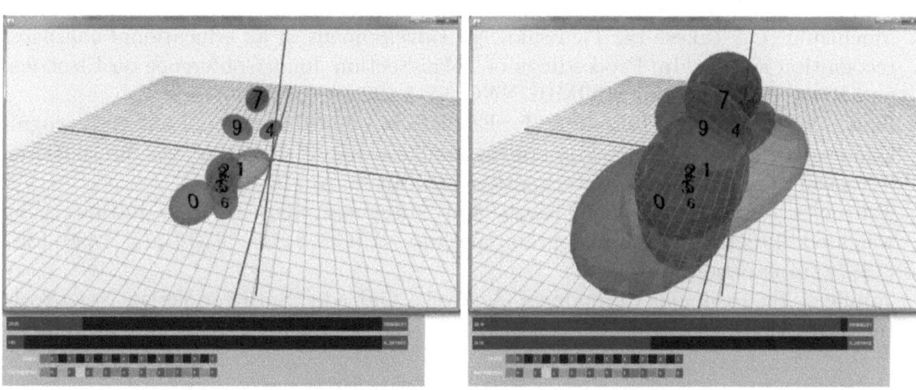

Fig. 4. The difference of the Mahalanobis' generalised distance to the same result

Furthermore, in order to give dialogism more, we improved the system to draw the vector corresponding to the letter which a user inputs on-line. Data is newly inputted interactively, while distribution of the feature space constituted with the data inputted once is drawn. Then the vector corresponding to the interactive inputting data is sequentially drawn in the visualized space.

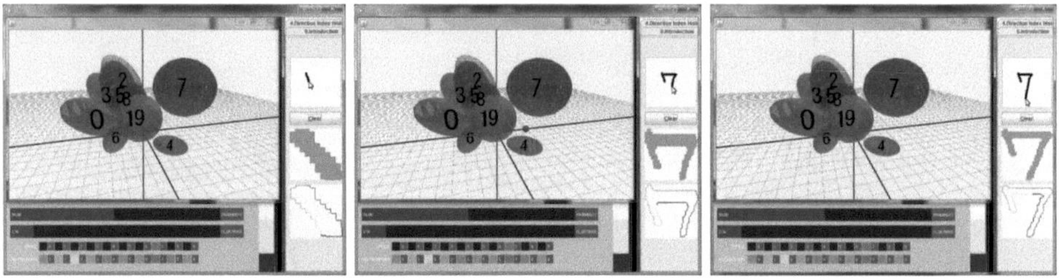

Fig. 5. Interactive vector drawing system

By this improvement, when a user does hand-drawn the same character as the recognized one, the feature vector approaches the classified feature domain until finishing drawing.

Evaluation experiments, such as a questionnaire, are future works.

References

1. Fukunaga, K.: Statistical pattern recognition, 2nd edn. Academic Press, Inc., San Diego (1990)
2. Yamamoto, K., Yoshikawa, T., Furuhashi, T.: A proposal of visualization method for multi-dimensional data using fuzzy clustering based on multiple discriminant analysis. IEICE Trans. J88-D-II(6), 975–984 (2005) (in Japanese)
3. Mochizuki, D., Takeshita, T., Esaki, N.: Development of an educational character recognition system. In: Proceedings of Tokai-Section Joint Conference on Electrical and Related Engineering, ROMBUNNO.N2-5 (2010) (in Japanese)
4. Esaki, N., Hisada, R., Takeshita, T.: Educational mutidimensional pattern recognition system using principal component analysis. In: Abstracts of 5th International Symposium on Advances in Technology Educaiton, p. 119 (2011)
5. Tsuruoka, M.: Handwritten Kanji and Hiragana character recognition using weighted direction index histogram method. IEICE Trans. J70-D(7), 1390–1397 (1987) (in Japanese)
6. Jolliffe, I.T.: Principal Component Analysis, 2nd edn. Springer-Verlag New York, Inc. (2002)

Part II
Health and Medicine

Persuasive Features in a Web-Based System for Weight-Loss Team Competition

Josipa Basic*, Borchuluun Yadamsuren, Dinara Saparova, and Yanfei Ma

School of Information Science and Learning Technologies,
University of Missouri, Columbia, MO
{jbyv7,ds754,ymyp6}@mail.missouri.edu,
YadamsurenB@missouri.edu

Abstract. Millions of Americans struggle to lose weight, and various online instruments have been developed to support them. Behavioral persuasion is an integral trait of online tools for weight loss. The goal of this study was to examine the effectiveness of persuasive features of the interaction design in a particular web-based system for weight-loss support using the Persuasive System Design (PSD) framework. In 2012, 1170 individuals competed in a web-based weight-loss challenge in a Midwestern city. Upon completion, 644 participants completed the survey to provide feedback about their experience in the competition. The survey data was analyzed to determine desired features of persuasive interaction design for weight-loss support in a web-based system. The findings of the study suggested that support in the primary task of losing weight, system feedback, and social interaction were the most preferred persuasive features that needed to be incorporated in online weight loss support systems.

Keywords: persuasive features, web-based system, team- based weigh loss competition.

1 Introduction

Obesity has attained epidemic proportions as a health problem in the United States. Millions of Americans struggle to lose weight, and various online instruments have been developed to assist with this challenge. These tools include various websites, online widgets, and smartphone applications making health information more accessible to everybody. According to Mobi Health News (2010), there are about 5820 medical, health, and fitness apps for smartphones with an estimated three million downloads. A number of persuasive strategies have been employed in the development of online health tools, including self-monitoring of daily physical exercise and caloric balance; social learning and teamwork to exercise and sharing health information with friends and families (Sundar, Bellur, and Jia, 2012).

* Corresponding author.

C. Stephanidis (Ed.): Posters, Part II, HCII 2013, CCIS 374, pp. 125–129, 2013.

2 Purpose of Study

The goal of this study was to examine the persuasive features of the interaction design in a particular web-based system for weight-loss promotion using the Persuasive System Design (PSD) framework (Oinas-Kokkonen & Harjumaa, 2009). This framework depicts the process of designing and evaluating persuasive systems and describes the type of content and software functionality to be included in the final product. The web-based system for weight loss promotion was used to support a 12-week team weight loss challenge started in May 2012 and ended in August 2012. The challenge took place in a Midwestern city and was offered to participants at no cost. Teams of four to six individuals competed to lose the highest percentage of weight-loss to obtain prizes. Players were required to use the system to create and regularly update their accounts.

3 Methodology

The participants of the competition were represented by individuals who were older than 18 years of age and pursued a weight loss goal. After four months of participating in the competition, all players were invited to take an online survey. The survey intended to provide information about participants' experiences with the competition and the effectiveness of the online weight loss support system. The survey was administered through Qualtircs, a web-based survey software. Survey data were analyzed both quantitatively and qualitatively: descriptive statistics of the quantitative data was generated through the Qualtrics; qualitative responses were coded manually for the occurrence of common themes.

4 Results and Discussion

Of the 644 participants who completed the survey, 86 percent were female and 71 percent were between 26 and 55 years old. Seventy three percent of the study participants have not achieved the weight loss goal set prior to the contest. The participants reported that their weight loss and overall experience interacting with the system would have been improved if the system provided more support in primary task of weight loss, system feedback, and social interaction. In addition to system credibility support, these categories are essential parts of the PSD framework.

4.1 Primary Task Support

The participants indicated a need for a system that would reduce their efforts with regard to performing the target behavior, i.e., weight loss. This could have been accomplished through offering a list of healthy and low-calorie foods and exercise plans on a regular basis throughout the contest. Relevant content, such as meal and exercise plans, news and notifications regarding their team activities should have been present in the prominent place on the website rather than in a random order.

Information provided by the system is more persuasive when it is tailored to its users' specific needs and interests (Oinas-Kokkonen & Harjumaa, 2009). To promote the weight loss, the system users expected it to provide exercise accommodation recommendations from experts to individuals with injuries, chronic pain or other health issues.

The participants expressed a need to be flexible in setting their own personal goals, including both desired weight loss and exercise level. They expected the system to provide features to allow tracking user performance or status in relation to predefined goals. This could have been accomplished by using graphical presentation of the user's weight loss progress and duration of the exercise over time. Survey respondents also wanted to have access to both personal and team performance metrics.

Providing simulations can persuade users to identify the link between cause and effect in regards to users' behavior (Oinas-Kokkonen & Harjumaa, 2009). For example, a system could have promoted weight loss by presenting its users with before-and-after pictures of people who have lost weight in the current or previous contests supported by the same system. The users also voiced an interest in features that could predict their weight loss based on certain calorie-intake or exercise plan.

4.2 Dialogue Support

According to the survey data, respondents expected the system to be more effective in providing weight loss support encouragement, like praise, rewards, reminders, and suggestions on a regular basis. Providing praise via words, images, symbols or sounds can make system users more open to persuasion (Oinas-Kokkonen & Harjumaa, 2009). Receiving automated messages as a reminder to perform a desired behavior and reach individual goals is likely to motivate system users to continue making healthy food choices and exercise during the contest.

Rewarding the target behavior by providing system users with virtual rewards could motivate them to continue carrying out a desired behavior (Oinas-Kokkonen & Harjumaa, 2009). For example, digital prizes could have been awarded to the individuals who accomplished the most significant weight-loss on a weekly or monthly basis. This way they would have been externally motivated throughout the contest.

Reminding system users of their target behavior during the contest could make them more likely to accomplish their predefined goals (Oinas-Kokkonen & Harjumaa, 2009). Notifications or emails containing their preset goals as well as exercise advice, healthy food suggestions, and healthy recipes could have been disseminated to the system users to keep them on track.

Finally, system could have provided users with suggestions regarding their target behaviors, which they could perform during the contest. These suggestions could have been disseminated to system users in the form of email notifications or text messages containing information promoting healthier eating habits and effective exercise plans.

4.3 Social Support

Social interactions among team members of the web-based weight loss contest could have been supported by incorporating content and features that facilitated social learning, comparison, normative influence, cooperation, competition, and recognition (Oinas-Kokkonen & Harjumaa, 2009). Observing other participants as they performed their target behaviors and outcomes of their behaviors could motivate an individual to perform that same behavior. Providing system users with a blog or a discussion board as a central space for sharing food consumption or fitness journal could have encouraged people to make healthy food choices and be more physical active. Enabling system users to compare their performance with the performance of others could have served as greater motivation on them to perform a target behavior. System users should have been able to share and compare their progress by using the system, including individual and team ranks in relation to other contest participants and teams.

The system could also have enabled contest participants to work towards the same goal by getting together to exercise. Creating this type of peer support has the potential to increase the likelihood that the person will adopt a target behavior, in this case lose weight. By providing means for collaboration, the system could have motivated its users to adopt a target behavior and consequently lose weight. Collaboration via web-based system could have been promoted by sharing motivational posts and pictures of individuals and teams as they were exercising, touching base regarding their progress, and planning face-to-face gatherings and team exercise.

The system should have provided means for competing with other teams and within teams to motivate contest participants in adopting a target behavior. To keep participants motivated throughout contest, weekly and monthly contests such as most percentage or pounds lost as well as nutritional and exercise trivia should have been organized.

Finally, the system should have provided public recognition for users who performed their target behavior and lost the most weight in a given time period. Names of individuals and teams who accomplished the most significant progress towards their weight loss goals could have been published on the web site. Email, text or system-based notification could have been sent when one of the team members weighted in and lost weight.

5 Conclusion

Participants expected more activities and features in the system to encourage weight loss, better system feedback to motivate them towards their weight loss goal, and improved support for social interaction with their own and other team members. These social interactions could have included challenges within teams and weight-loss comparisons between teams. Participants emphasized the value of recognition as a significant factor towards their weight loss goals. They wanted digital prizes and reminders from the web-based system for their weight-loss, such as exercises, healthy food suggestions, and recipes. Players emphasized the importance of features that supported community building, such as blogs or discussion boards to allow sharing their experiences, nutrition and exercise tips, exchange recipes and post motivational pictures of individuals and teams. Having these elements incorporated in the system would have helped online weight loss participants to be more successful in achieving their goal as well as overall improve their experience using the system and participating in web based weight loss contest.

References

1. Oinas-Kukonen, H., Harjumaa, M.: Persuasive Systems Design: Key Issues, Process Model, and System Features. Communications of the Association for Information Systems 24(28), 485–500 (2009)
2. Mobi Health News, The fastest growing and most successful health and medical apps (2010), http://mobihealthnews.com/the-fastest-growing-and-mostsuccessful-health-medical-apps/ (retrieved)
3. Mobi Health News, The world of health and medical apps (2010), http://mobihealthnews.com/research/the-world-of-health-and-medical-apps/ (retrieved)
4. Sundar, S.S., Bellur, S., Jia, H.: Motivational technologies: a theoretical framework for designing preventive health applications. In: Bang, M., Ragnemalm, E.L. (eds.) PERSUASIVE 2012. LNCS, vol. 7284, pp. 112–122. Springer, Heidelberg (2012)

Developing an Interactive Game System for Upper Limb Stroke Rehabilitation

Chun-Ching Chen

Graduate Institute of Interactive Media Design, National Taipei University of Technology
cceugene@ntut.edu.tw

Abstract. The number of cases of stroke has been increasing in Taiwan. Movement disorders such as hemiplegia occur commonly after stroke. Hemiplegic stroke patients are not able to control one side of their body, particularly upper limb. To help stroke patients recovery their lifestyles, rehabilitation plays an important role. This paper introduces the development of a digital system---a personalized interactive game, to help upper limb in hemiplegic stroke patients. Taking patients' needs and emotion into account, the system makes rehabilitation therapy more enjoyable. The results show that the system could help stroke patients alleviate mental fatigue and allow doctors to control and monitor the rehabilitation process of patients easily. Incorporating interactive game to stroke rehabilitation could be a feasible and acceptable way.

Keywords: Stroke rehabilitation, Upper limb hemiplegia, Human-computer interaction, Digital game, Interaction design.

1 Introduction

With the population aging, stroke becomes a major cause of disability in the elderly in Taiwan. The neurological symptoms of stroke differs from types of pathological lesion and severity of brain impairments, however, hemiplegia is the most typical symptom that can be found. Hemiplegia means the pathological region of brain causes one side of the extremity decay or disability on motor function. This will make the limb lack of strength and get out of control to lose functional ability of daily living. Among the stroke patients, upper limb hemiplegia is the most common – at a proportion of two-third (Gowland, deBruin, Basmajian, Plews, Burcea, 1992). Because brain impairment affects motoring skill, patients can only move their limbs in slow pace and unusually discontinuous way to execute goal-oriented tasks (Trombly, 1992). The patient always suffers weakness of muscle, abnormal tension of muscle, abnormal motor coordination, shoulder girdle and hip joint activity diminishing, and losing coordination of joints (Trombly & Radomski, 2002).

Different upper limb impairments might have various functional effects on movement control, particular for hands reaching, a basic movement for grasping objects, operating devices, even performing an action that requires some special skill and doing leisure activities. Therefore, this movement is frequently used to evaluate stroke

C. Stephanidis (Ed.): Posters, Part II, HCII 2013, CCIS 374, pp. 130–134, 2013.

patients' prognosis. In the daily life, many tasks require skillful operation and two hands working together. With normal central nervous system, individual muscle and joints can be well organized to lead to coordinate movement, and accomplish functional motion through normal motoring ability (Shumway-Cook & Woollacott, 2000). Hence it is crucial to effectively assess the patients and give treatment to recover stroke patients' upper limb function.

The rehabilitation for stroke patients aims to stimulate brain to recover the plasticity and reorganization. Therefore, the treatment will focus on motion training of paretic side extremity, e.g., the constraint-induced techniques proposed in past decade (Bonifer & Anderson, 2003, Taub, Uswatte, Morris, 2003). The constraint-induced technique is to restrain the activity of nonparetic side and constrain paretic side to make movement so as to activate the function of paretic extremity. This rehabilitation way has been frequently applied and studied; however, is more adaptive for cases with minor impairment, i.e., paretic side is still capable of basic motoring skill. For cases with severe impairment, scholars suggests bilateral movement training , which is to activate neural network by nonparetic side or produce interlimb coupling to stimulate the activity of paretic side (Mudie & Matyas, 2000, Cunningham, Stoykov, Walter, 2002).

Rehabilitation is a time consuming and boring process, either for patients or physical therapist. Stroke rehabilitation therapy mostly includes initial assessment of the doctor and therapist, planning of patients' activity and loadings, repetitive and continuous observation to record and adjust their tasks. Systematic, objective and reliable evaluation methods is critical for therapist to monitor and control patients' rehabilitation. For patients, it is important to ensure they are able to follow the therapy and continue the rehabilitation with patience so as to recover their ability to be back to normal daily life. Based on these requirements, digital technology may provide conventional rehabilitation new approach to enhancing the performance. Current state-of-the-art technology can provide more flexible, effective and efficient way for rehabilitation, through designer's efforts. Therefore, this study is to develop a tangible interactive game for upper limb hemiplegia patients' rehabilitation. The prototyping was finally evaluated by physical therapist and patients to identify its potential for future stroke rehabilitation.

2 Methods

Three critical steps to this study are: identifying system design requirements, prototyping and usability inspection and user's evaluation.

2.1 System Design Requirements

The system is divided into two parts, a digital game and an upper limb bilateral movement mechanism. The work to be done is to develop the content of the digital game and allow the patients to operate the mechanism to play the game, without using mouse and keyboard. The mechanism, developed by the Industrial Research Limited

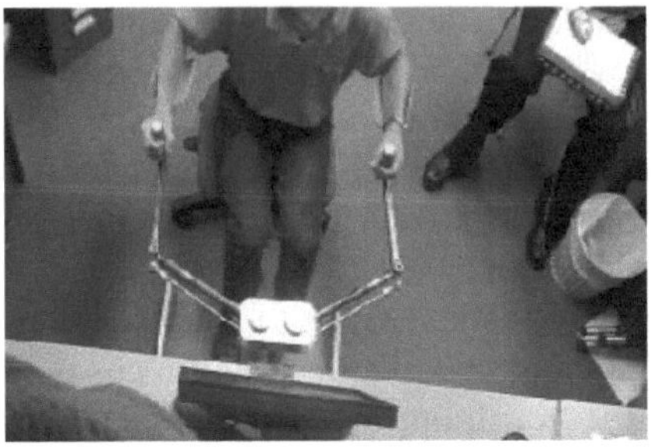

Fig. 1. Bilateral movement stroke rehabilitation mechanism

(IRL) of New Zealand, works bilaterally with two arm supports to provide severe upper limb stroke rehabilitation, i.e., through nonparetic side movement to bring paretic side (Fig. 1).

A series of interviews with technology experts and physical therapist were conducted to define the system design requirements. The main issues were addressed below.

- **Comfortable atmosphere to enhance patients' motivation**. The game should be warm, cozy, bright and natural, which makes them feel relaxed and comfortable. Light background music and encouraging voice are needed in the system to provide a positive environment for patients.
- **Designing difficulty levels based on rehabilitation progress**. Different stroke symptoms might respond differently to the game, so the level settings should be designed according to rehabilitation progress which allows the therapist to understand patients' ability simply from the level they can achieve.
- **Personal game training mode**. Besides normal game level setting, the game should provide training mode for patients to do training before they are able to start game level, in which the therapist should be able to define the training content.
- **Providing system feedback for both patients and therapists**. This includes two parts: for the patient, the system should provide how they interact with the system and remind them to correct their operation; for the therapist, the system should report all the pathologic data for them to monitor and evaluate patients' progress.
- **Allowing the potential of telemedicine development**. The system should provide online database to save and retrieve different users' profiles, including the therapist, patient and administrator. The therapist can remotely monitor patients' rehabilitation progress.

2.2 Prototyping and Usability Inspection

The system prototype was developed using Adobe ActionScript Version 3.0. When the patient operating the rehabilitation mechanism to interact with the game, the webcam grabs images and provides system feedback on the monitor (Fig. 2). The game prototyping was then evaluated by experts to improve its usability.

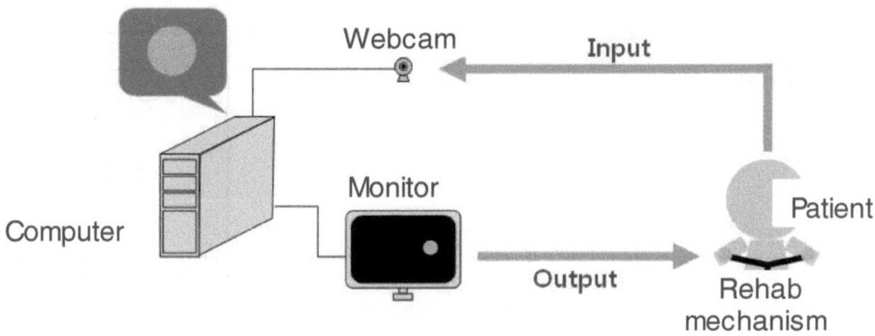

Fig. 2. Prototyping structure

2.3 Evaluation

The system prototype was evaluated by the patient and physical therapist to examine the feasibility and potential for future application. The system was set up in a room of the hospital in Taiwan (Fig. 3). Three stroke patients with upper limb hemiplegia, accompanying with their therapist, participated in the experiment and provided their feedback for the system. The process was also observed by the experimenter to observe and record all the interaction.

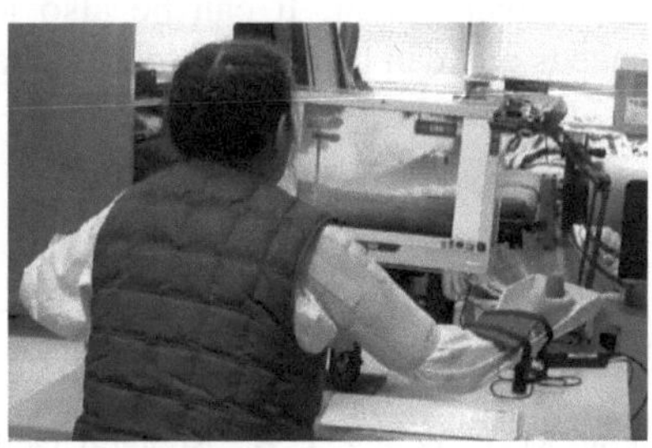

Fig. 3. The participants was interacting with the system

3 Results and Conclusion

The final game prototype used "animals and their home" as a story scenario, which is comprised of seven different levels, a "Trace Mode" for training, a "loadcell" to detect and remind patient's force, friendly user interface and the patient and therapist's database linked with remote server (Table 1).

The result of the experiment showed that all participants were interested in the system, mostly on playing the game. They indicated that the rehabilitation time elapsing faster than before. From the observation, it can be seen that participants keep good mood whether they can accomplish the task or not. All cases did not show their impatience or any rejection to all tasks.

Consequently, this study provides a potential for future stroke rehabilitation, particularly for upper limb hemiplegia. This study demonstrates the importance of incorporating different profession, e.g. design and medicine, in such a cross-field

Table 1. Game content

Image	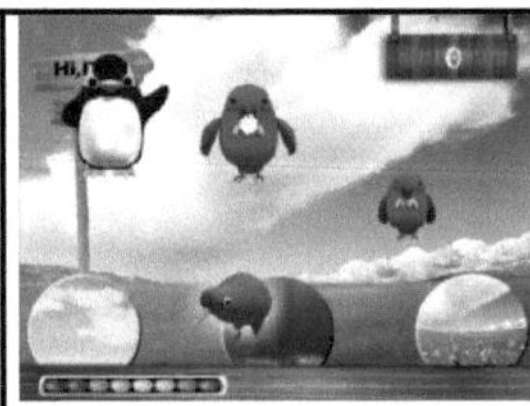	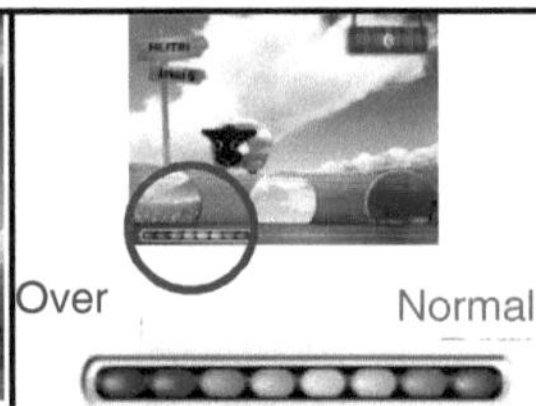	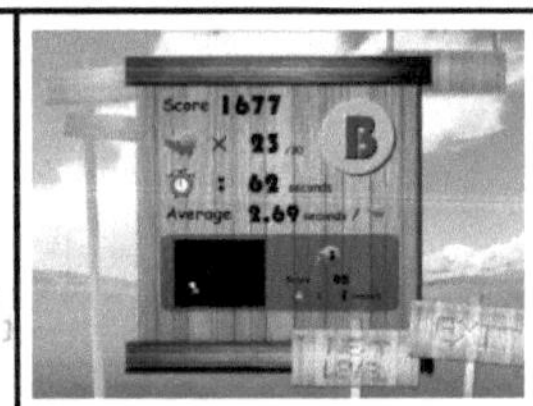
Function	A comfortable play atmosphere for stroke rehabilitation.	A "loadcell" indicator to detect and remind patient's force.	A user-friendly interface and information to provide patients' results.
Image	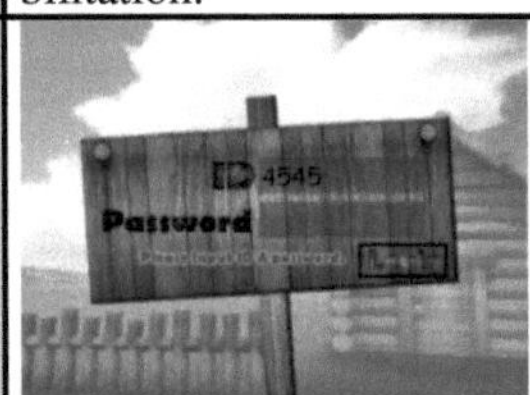	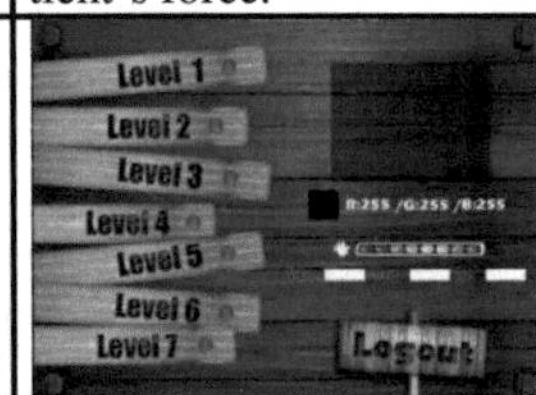	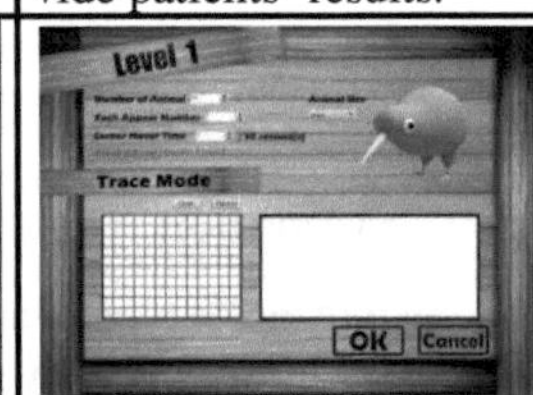
Function	The therapist can access to the game from personal computer or outside.	Seven different levels can show patient's progress.	"Trace Mode" for patient training, which can be set up by the therapist.

assisting technology system development. It can be also identified that interactive game provides emotional needs and can be applied to the rehabilitation.

References

1. Bonifer, N., Anderson, K.M.: Application of constraint-induced movement therapy for an individual with severe chronic upper-extremity hemiplegia. Physical Therapy 83(4), 384–398 (2003)
2. Cunningham, C.L., Stoykov, M.E., Walter, C.B.: Bilateral facilitation of motor control in chronic hemiplegia. Acta Psychologica 110(2-3), 321–337 (2002)
3. Gowland, C., de Bruin, H., Basmajian, J.V., Plews, N., Burcea, I.: Agonist and antagonist activity during voluntary upper-limb movement in patients with stroke. Physical Therapy 72(9), 624–633 (1992)
4. Mudie, M.H., Matyas, T.A.: Can simultaneous bilateral movement involve the undamaged hemisphere in reconstruction of neural networks damaged by stroke. Disability and Rehabilitation 22(1-2), 23–37 (2000)
5. Shumway-Cook, A., Brauer, S., Woollacott, M.: Predicting the probability for falls in community-dwelling older adults using the Timed Up & Go Test. Physical Therapy 80(9), 896–903 (2000)
6. Taub, E., Uswatte, G., Morris, D.M.: Improved motor recovery after stroke and massive cortical reorganization following Constraint-Induced Movement therapy. Physical Medicine and Rehabilitation Clinics of North America 14(suppl. 1), S77–S91 (2003)
7. Trombly, C.A.: Deficits of reaching in subjects with left hemiparesis: A pilot study. American Journal of Occupational Therapy 46, 887–897 (1992)
8. Trombly, A., Radomski, M.V.: Occupational therapy for physical dysfunction, 5th edn. Lippincott Williams & Wilkins, Philadelphia (2002)

A Sensor Glove System for Rehabilitation in Instrumental Activities of Daily Living

Aodhan L. Coffey and Tomas E. Ward

Department of Electronic Engineering, National University of Ireland Maynooth, Ireland
{aodhan.coffey,tomas.ward}@eeng.nuim.ie

Abstract. Paralysis with weakness on one side of the body is common after stroke, affecting over 50% of people and significantly impacting their quality of life. Research shows that high intensity, task-specific activities focused on the use of the affected limb are important for encouraging neuroplasticity. Unfortunately, due to the pressure on healthcare systems internationally, the length of stay at an inpatient rehabilitation facility is limited. Consequently, to maximise recovery it is critical that patients engage in their rehabilitation exercises both between sessions and long after the end of formal treatment. We describe here the design, development and test of an interactive sensor glove system capable of translating captured movements into hand gestures as a basis for augmentative control and rehabilitation function. The system described here is designed from an occupational therapy perspective where functional assessment and therapy requires an ecological validity and a context within activities of daily living.

Keywords: Stroke, Motor Rehabilitation, Occupational Therapy, Sensor glove, Augmentative control.

1 Introduction

Globally stroke is one of the leading causes of serious long term disability, with over four million stroke victims currently living in the United States [1]. Paralysis with weakness on one side of the body is common after stroke affecting over 50% of people. The increase in survival rates for stroke is testament to the advances in primary treatment made over the past decade. However, as a consequence the demand for outpatient services, especially rehabilitation is at an all-time high, putting tremendous pressure on healthcare systems. High intensity, task-specific exercises are known to be important for encouraging neuroplasticity [2-3]. Consequently, it is crucial that patients engage in continuous rehabilitation exercises long after the end of formal treatment. However, the debilitating physical deficit combined with the absence of trained supervision, often leads to a loss of motivation in patients resulting in poor therapeutic compliance which has a corresponding negative impact on recovery.

Many previous attempts have been made to address these problems. Virtual Reality (VR) and Augmented Reality (AR) are commonly used in an attempt to add an engaging context to rehabilitation training and to encourage and motivate patients to keep

C. Stephanidis (Ed.): Posters, Part II, HCII 2013, CCIS 374, pp. 135–139, 2013.

up their exercises. However, the reality is for each decade after age 55, the risk of stroke doubles[1]. Therefore, most stroke patients are 55 or older and have spent a considerable part of their lives without exposure to computers or video games. Furthermore, interviews show they have little or no interest in this form of therapy.

Our approach instead tries to engage the patient in activities identified as personally relevant (in this case to be able to control household appliances via a universal infrared remote control) while at the same time facilitating a suitable motor challenge and a measurement of movement ability.

2 Design Motivation

Studies of animal models of stroke-induced paralysis reveal that sessions of 400 - 600 repetitions are required for good recovery and that simple repetition of an exercise will have little benefit if it does not provoke motor learning [4]. Subsequently, our glove has been designed to encourage the user to perform gestures which are derived from therapist-specified motor exercises, the successful execution of which acts as control input to an environmental control system (ECS). Through interviews with careers and therapists it was determined that patients spend a considerable proportion of their day interacting with entertainment systems and that the interfaces to such devices can be very challenging to operate. Consequently we designed the ECS around an IR-based augmented controller for personal appliances (TV, DVD, radio etc.). Such a design places the rehabilitation process at the heart of relevant activities of daily living which are both personalized to the specific user and should elicit motivational engagement. A further design requirement is that the movement activity and operational context is recorded over time such that numbers of repetitions and performance scores can be reviewed by an occupational therapist at a later stage. A final feature is the inclusion of a dynamic task difficulty mechanism which increases or reduces the gesture challenge according to the user's performance. This feature is designed to provoke the necessary motor learning associated with effective therapy.

3 Hardware

3.1 Flex Sensor

The glove uses lightweight flex sensors to record the patient hand movement and gestures. A deflection-to-voltage conversion can be obtained using the flex sensor Rs in conjunction with a fixed resistor R_f. The output of this configuration is described by (1):

$$V_{out} = V_{in}\left(\frac{R_f}{R_s + R_f}\right) \quad (1)$$

In the shown configuration, the output voltage increases with increasing deflection. Although the flex sensors output is non-linear, a value for R_f can be chosen to maximize the desired deflection sensitivity range and subsequently the linearity of the corresponding results.

3.2 PIC Microcontroller

At the heart of our design is a microcontroller (PIC 16F688, Microchip Technology Inc, USA) which converts the analog sensor values into their digital equivalent. This device was chosen for its 8 analog to digital channels (10-bit resolution), five of which are needed, one for each finger. This device is also low profile (14 pins) and has High-Endurance Flash/EEPROM Cell allowing it to be reprogrammed up to 100,000 times, ideal for reprogramming new hand gestures.

We chose a lightweight flexible fabric for the glove which offers little resistance to movement to ensure no extra strain is put on the patient efforts by the device. A custom PCB was designed to house the microcontroller, voltage dividers, IR LED and power source. The flex sensors are connected to the PCB via flexible ribbon cables and are guided through loops at each segment of the finger. The flex sensor is only attached at the tip of the finger, allowing it to slide back and forward through these loops as the user flexes their fingers.

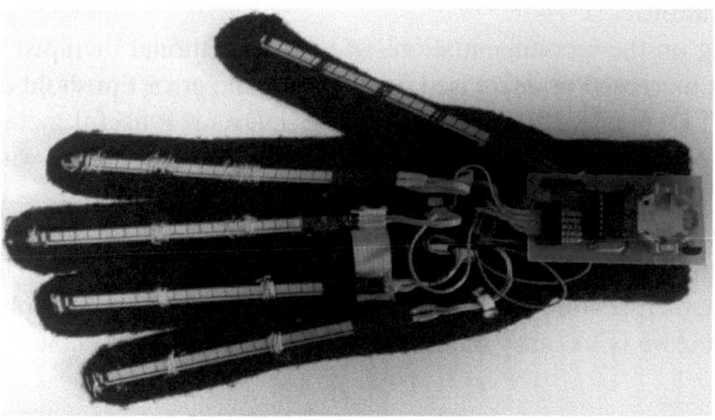

Fig. 1. The IR Glove

4 Software

4.1 Hand Gesture Recognition

By using a simple two stage calibration process we can determine an upper and lower threshold which will correspond to the hand being fully open (fingers extended) and closed (clenched fist) respectively.

The glove is easily programmed to allow an occupational therapist to define gestures suitable from the perspective of functional rehabilitation. A gesture is simply defined as a specific sequence of poses, $G=[P_S,P_M,P_E]$ taken from a predefined discrete set characterized by a pose vector $P=[p_1, \dots p_i, \dots p_N]$. In this case $N=5$ (one for each digit) and p_i is a dimensionless normalized scalar in the range [0,1] derived from the minimum and maximum deflections for each digit acquired during calibration. P_S, P_M and P_E corresponds to the beginning, middle and end poses of a gesture respectively.

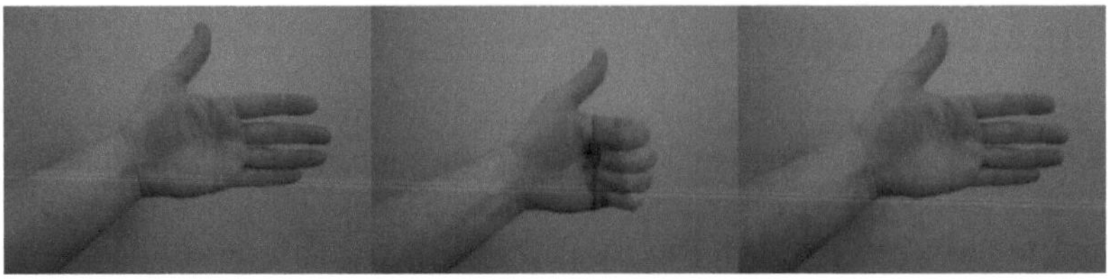

(a) (b) (c)

Fig. 2. Hand poses, (a) beginning pose, (b) intermediate pose, (c) end pose

A gesture is correctly identified when the glove detects each of the three poses that make up that gesture, in sequential order and within a defined time limit - *T*. Pose recognition is very simple and is based on the individual component differences d_i of the difference vector $D=P_T-P_U = [d_1,...d_{i,},...d_N]$. Where P_T is the target pose and P_U is the current pose. A pose is correctly identified if $\forall d_i \in D$: $d_i < e$ where *e* corresponds to a hard class boundary threshold which is interpreted as a task difficulty parameter in this application.

Depending on the recommendations of the occupational therapist, the difficulty of a task can be increased or decreased by changing the error threshold *e* or adjusting the time limit -*T*. Dynamic difficulty adjustment (DDA) is a useful method often used in gaming to optimize engagement through matching player's ability with an appropriate challenge [5]. We currently use a DDA approach which adjusts *e* or *T* based on a running average of the relevant performance measures (D_A or T_A) for the previous *M* gesture attempts. When D_A (or T_A) is greater than *e* (or T) we gradually increase *e* by an increment each gesture iteration until an appropriate balance is obtained and similarly if the gesture is too easy the difference measure is used to increase the difficulty level.

5 Evaluation and Discussion

The following data was downloaded from our glove after a preliminary test, in which the glove was worn by a healthy test subject and used to control a TV during a 10 minute session. The time limit chosen in which a gesture needed to be performed was 500 (ms) and an error threshold *e* was chosen to be 8%.

Table 1. - Results of preliminary test

Gesture (P_T)	**Attempts**	**Successful**	**Failed**	**Avg. Time (ms)**	**Avg. Difference (d_i)**	**Context**
1	15	14	1	443	5.3%	Channel Up
2	14	12	2	459	6.5%	Channel Down
3	6	6	0	462	6.1%	TV ON/OFF
4	20	19	1	426	5.5%	Volume Up
5	15	13	2	463	6.2%	Volume Down

From our preliminary results we can extract useful information such as how many times a gesture was attempted, and of these attempts how many were accurate and completed within the time limit. The IR glove is now under review for application in a clinical setting. Trials with stroke patients will help identify whether stroke patients benefit from an interactive form of therapy and if this concept will increase the amount of practise a patient engages in.

Acknowledgments. This work is supported by Science Foundation Ireland, grant number 09/RFP/ECE2376 and a John Hume Scholarship, National University of Ireland Maynooth.

References

1. American Heart Association: Heart Disease and Stroke Statistics - 2013 Update. American Heart Association, Dallas (2013)
2. Bowden, M.G., Woodbury, M.L., Duncan, P.W.: Promoting neuroplasticity and recovery after stroke: future directions for rehabilitation clinical trials. Curr Opin Neurol 26(1), 37–42 (2013)
3. Coffey, A.L., Ward, T.E., Middleton, R.H.: Game Theory: A Potential Tool for the Design and Analysis of Patient-Robot Interaction Strategies. International Journal of Ambient Computing and Intelligence (IJACI) 3(3), 43–51 (2011)
4. Kimberley, T.J., Samargia, S., Moore, L.G., Shakya, J.F., Lang, C.E.: Comparison of amounts and types of practice during rehabilitation for traumatic brain injury and stroke. J Rehabil Res. Dev. 47(9), 851–862 (2010)
5. Hunicke, R.: The case for dynamic difficulty adjustment in games. In: Proceedings of the 2005 ACM SIGCHI International Conference on Advances in Computer Entertainment-Technology (ACE 2005), pp. 429–433. ACM, New York (2005)

Apps for Rapid Epidemiological Analysis (AREA)

Joseph V. Cohn[1,*], Amos Freedy[9,**], Timur Chabuk[9], Gershon Weltman[9,**], David J. Combs[2,*], Antonio Anglero Jr.[3,***], Brian R. Johnson[4,*], David Rozovski[5,*], Stephen Eggan[6,*], Brennan Cox[5,*], Kirsten Carlson[7,*], and Elizabeth O'Neill[8]

[1] Office of Naval Research, Arlington, VA
[2] Naval Research Laboratory, Washington, DC
[3] Naval Safety Center, Norfolk, VA
[4] United States Air Force Academy, Colorado Springs, CO
[5] Naval Aerospace Medical Institute, Pensacola, FL
[6] Naval Medical Research Unit–Dayton, Dayton, OH
[7] Naval Air Warfare Center Aircraft Division, Patuxent River, MD
[8] Strategic Analysis, Inc., Arlington, VA
[9]Perceptonics Solutions, Inc, Sherman Oaks, CA
eoneill@sainc.com

Abstract. Communication is difficult in low income areas, given the lack of land based telecommunication and distances between population centers [1]. New methods to monitor/forecast epidemiological trends will enable our military to execute emerging operational requirements. Hand held devices, such as cell phones, smart phones and personal data assistants (PDAs) provide an effective source for collecting, analyzing and widely disseminating healthcare information, because of their widespread use in the very regions to which our military forces are, and will be, deployed. This effort develops handheld device applications that provide health surveillance, epidemiological analysis and forecasting capabilities.

Keywords: Mobile Device, Applications, Epidemiology, Data Collection, Forecasting, Military Health System, Medical Readiness, Humanitarian Aid, Disaster Relief.

1 Introduction

1.1 The Importance of AREA

The US Military is continuing to expand it efforts into non-kinetic operations to include emphasizing Stabilization, Security, Transition, and Reconstruction Operations (SSTRO) and Humanitarian Aid / Disaster Relief Operations. The

* Ph.D., Medical Service Corps, United States Navy.
** Ph.D.
*** Psy.D., Medical Service Corps, United States Navy.

C. Stephanidis (Ed.): Posters, Part II, HCII 2013, CCIS 374, pp. 140–143, 2013.

development and surveillance of the healthcare landscape forms a cornerstone of any strategy developed to support these actions (Figure 1). Hand held devices, such as cell phones, smart phones and personal data assistants (PDAs) provide an effective source for collecting, analyzing and widely disseminating healthcare information, because of their widespread use in the very regions to which our military forces are, and will be, deployed. For example, in Africa, over 75% of telecommunications are conducted using mobile devices [2]. Today's mobile devices have significantly expanded computational processing capability over earlier devices [3]. As well, the infrastructure for developing applications – "Apps"; a piece of software executable on a mobile device - is also rapidly maturing, with predictions of a threefold increase in the quantity of mobile apps by the end of 2012 [4]. Moreover, the types of information collectable by current mobile devices have expanded to include: high resolution pictures; video; text; geo location; and, in most cases, text-based annotations. The key to realizing this potential of mobile devices in supporting epidemiological efforts is to develop Apps that can fully exploit the various hardware and processing capabilities of today's mobile devices.

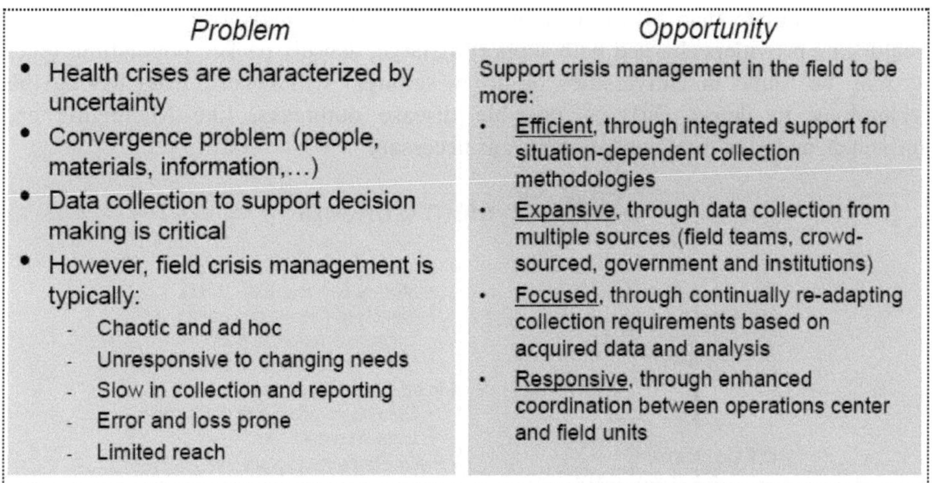

Fig. 1. Examples of current problems in epidemiological data collection/analyses and opportunities for improvement via AREA development. (Figure courtesy of Perceptronics Solutions, Inc.)

1.2 Primary Focus

This effort is focusing on developing apps that will enable: rapid data collection capabilities from multiple sources (e.g. web or text based files, manually input information and information collected using technologies inherent to hand held devices); artificial intelligence / machine learning approaches for data mining, analysis and forecasting; information visualization, to include geospatial localization for epidemiological pattern tracking; and real time capabilities for collaborative and interactive decision making. The output from these applications should enable users to better understand disease processes and progress; to map disease patterns; to better understand proximate and distal risk factors; and to develop effective courses of action. Ultimately, this technology will have broad application in commercial as well as military settings.

1.3 Field Use

The ability to develop assessments, forecasts and courses of action using real time epidemiological data collected across many different areas of operation will allow military decision makers to more effectively account for military medical readiness as part of their overall planning strategy. More locally, this technology should allow for faster and more accurate responses to potential disease outbreaks in the close-quarters common to military facilities, and ships. Commercially, this technology will provide similar levels of support, enabling health care providers, including Non-Governmental Organizations, charged with working in remote, impoverished and under-represented areas to better understand the moment-to-moment disease challenges they may encounter, and to plan effective treatments plans accordingly (Figure 2). As well, health care providers charged with supporting large, densely packed populations (such as may be found in Universities or urban settings) will benefit from having this technology to detect early-on possible disease outbreaks, like Meningitis and Influenza, and plan treatment strategies as necessary.

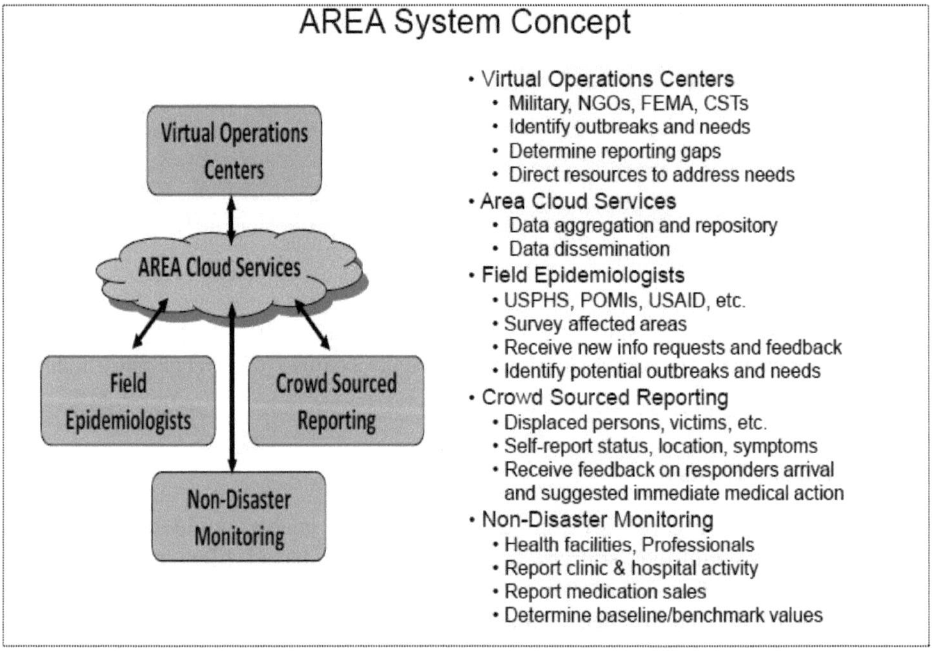

Fig. 2. Outline of AREA concept and capabilities (Figure courtesy of Perceptronics Solutions, Inc.)

Acknowledgements. Research and development of AREA by Perceptronics Solutions, Inc., has been supported by OSD through SBIR Phase I contract OSD11-H17 and funded by ONR BAA contract N00014-12-M-0108.

References

1. Tomlinson, M., Solomon, W., Singh, Y., Doherty, T., Chopra, M., Ijumba, P., Tsai, A.C., Jackson, D.: The use of mobile phones as a data collection tool: A report from a household survey in South Africa. BMC Medical Informatics 9, 51–58 (2009)
2. White, D.: Telecommunications: A dynamic revolution, `http://www.ft.com/cms/s/0/1868125e-6e5f-11db-b5c4-0000779e2340,dwp_uuid=1f2588a0-765d-11db-8284-0000779e2340.html?nclick_check=15`
3. Uti, N.V., Fox, R.: Testing the Computational Capabilities of Mobile Device Processors: Some Interesting Benchmark Results. In: 2010 IEEE/ACIS 9th International Conference on Computer and Information Science, pp. 477–481 (2010)
4. Horowitz, B.T.: Mobile health apps to triple by (2012), presenting challenges for mobile networks: Report, `http://www.eweek.com/c/a/Health-Care-IT/Mhealth-Apps-to-Triple-by-2012-Presenting-Challenges-for-Mobile-Networks-Report-869725/`
5. Anhøj, J., Møldrup, C.: Feasibility of collecting diary data from asthma patients through mobile phones and SMS (short message service): response rate analysis and focus group evaluation from a pilot study. J. Med. Internet Res. 6(4), e42 (2004)

Medical Modeling and Simulation Based Training Return on Investment Decision Model

Joseph V. Cohn[1,*], David J. Combs[2,*], Antonio Anglero Jr.[3,**], Brian R. Johnson[4,*], David Rozovski[5,*], Stephen Eggan[6,*], Brennan Cox[5,*], Kirsten Carlson[7,*], Meredith Carroll[8,***], and Elizabeth O'Neill[9]

[1] Office of Naval Research, Arlington, VA
[2] Naval Research Laboratory,Washington, DC
[3] Naval Safety Center, Norfolk, VA
[4] United States Air Force Academy, Colorado Springs, CO
[5] Naval Aerospace Medical Institute, Pensacola, FL
[6] Naval Medical Research Unit–Dayton, Dayton, OH
[7] Naval Air Warfare Center Aircraft Division, Patuxent River, MD
[8] Design Interactive, Inc., Oviedo, FL
[9] Strategic Analysis, Inc., Arlington, VA
eoneill@sainc.com

Abstract. This effort aims to develop a software-based decision tool for determining the actual return on investment of medical modeling and simulation based training technologies to provide acquisition decision makers with critical information for system design. This will ultimately improve the effectiveness and efficiency of current health services.

Keywords: Return on Investment, Modeling and Simulation, Training, Medical, Fidelity, Cost, Visualization Tools.

1 Modeling and Simulation Technologies

The military medical community faces a wide range of challenges to improve the effectiveness and efficiency of current health services and medical procedures' training from the medical corpsmen level to the emergency and trauma room nurses' and doctors' levels [1]. One approach that is gaining increasing popularity to ensure that all military medicine providers are able to stay current on medical knowledge – in light of rapidly evolving information, and the increasing pressure to move away from animal models- is the application of modeling and simulation technologies to medical training [1]. These tools can be expensive and, if mis-applied, can lead to ineffective or negative training. Ensuring that M&S based medical training systems are effectively developed requires a delicate balance between many variables, including

* Ph.D., Medical Service Corps, United States Navy.
** Psy.D., Medical Service Corps, United States Navy.
*** Ph.D.

C. Stephanidis (Ed.): Posters, Part II, HCII 2013, CCIS 374, pp. 144–147, 2013.

identifying current gaps, inefficiencies, redundancies and opportunities to improve upon training efficiency associated with training doctors, nurses, and corpsmen.

Numerous studies speak to the potential of M&S based technologies for enhancing training [2]. Nevertheless, there remains a lack of guidance on how to build systems that best support training specific skill sets, leading to an ever-increasing challenge for training designers to navigate the selection of technology components to provide the right balance between individual component fidelity, performance and cost. As might be expected, there are tradeoffs associated with finding the right balance between these three variables. As the fidelity of a system's components increases, so to do the costs as well as associated maintenance and support requirements, while the added performance improvements may be less than significant [3]. For this reason, it is critical that medical M&S training system implementers integrate system components at the level of fidelity that gives them the most value for the task that they are training.

2 Return on Investment Decision Support

To accomplish this, there is a need for a tool to guide designers on the fidelity level requirements and present trade-offs based on the task that is being trained, the desired level of performance improvement and anticipated return on investment in light of identified budget constraints (see Figure 1). This effort aims to develop a software-based return on investment decision support tool that: enables users to define critical variables for calculating return on investment; develops ontology linking these variables to each other, performance outcomes and return on investment; designs novel modeling and simulation-based tools to quantify the return on investment tradespace; and, interactively displays information, complex interactions or a visualization process that encourages designers to weigh the balance of improved performance versus the long-term cost consequences.

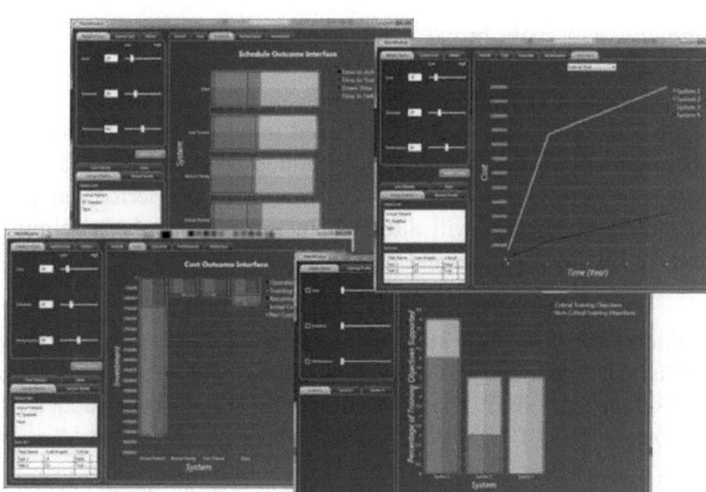

Fig. 1. ROTI Visualization Mode. Results are provided in multiple formats to facilitate tradeoff analyses and support effective decision making.

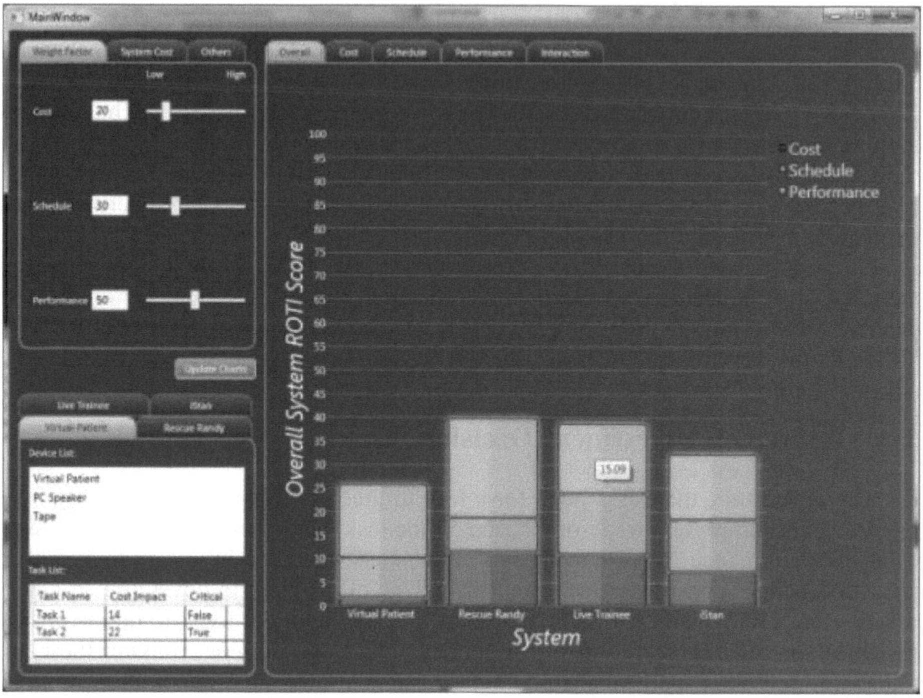

Fig. 2. ROTI Visualization Module, "Overall" display

3 Optimizing Training Cost, Time, and Performance

This technology will have broad application in commercial and military settings. Within the DoD, the ability to conduct return on investment analyses should generalize to other systems and platforms, including major acquisition programs of record. Commercially, modeling and simulation based training applications continue to form the cornerstone of a business's continuous training programs. Providing training managers with a tool for making informed decisions as to the performance-cost tradeoffs associated with a given tool will allow them to optimize their training dollars and maximize their employees' time and performance.

Acknowledgements. Research and development of Return on Investment Tool for Effective Medical Training (RITE-MT) by Design Interactive, Inc., has been supported by OSD through SBIR Phase I contract OSD11-H19 and funded by ONR BAA contract N00014-12-M-0105. We especially thank Dr. Meredith Carroll for her time and attention to this effort.

Distribution Statement A: Approved for Public Release, Distribution Unlimited. "The views, opinions, and/or findings contained in this article/presentation are those of the author/presenter and should not be interpreted as representing the official views or policies, either expressed or implied, of the Office of Naval Research or the Department of Defense.

References

1. Moses, G., Magee, J.H., Bauer, J.J., Leitch, R.: Military medical modeling and simulation in the 21st century. Stud. Health Technol. Inform. 81, 322–328 (2001)
2. Cohn, J.V., Stanney, K., Milham, L., Bell, M., Jones, D., Sullivan, J., Darken, R.: Training Effectiveness Evaluation: From Theory to Practice. In: Schmorrow, D., Cohn, J., Nicholson, D. (eds.) PSI Handbook of Virtual Environments for Training and Education: Developments for the Military and Beyond. Praeger Security International, Santa Barbara (2009)
3. Muller, P., Cohn, J.V., Nicholson, D.: Developing and evaluating advanced technologies for military simulation and training (CD-ROM). In: Proceedings of the 25th Annual Interservice/Industry Training, Simulation and Education Conference, Orlando, FL (2003)
4. Kaye, M.A., Sobota, M.S., Graham, D.R., Gotwald, A.L.: Cost As An Independent Variable: Principles and Implementation. Acquisition Review Quarterly (2000)

Dense Array, Low Field Magnetic Resonance Imaging Devices for Combat Casualty Care

Joseph V. Cohn[1,*], Masoud Radparvar[9,**], David J. Combs[2,*], Antonio Anglero Jr.[3,***], Brian R. Johnson[4,*], David Rozovski[5,*], Stephen Eggan[6,*], Brennan Cox[5,*], Kirsten Carlson[7,*], and Ms. Elizabeth O'Neill[8]

[1] Office of Naval Research, Arlington, VA
[2] Naval Research Laboratory,Washington, DC
[3] Naval Safety Center, Norfolk, VA
[4] United States Air Force Academy, Colorado Springs, CO
[5] Naval Aerospace Medical Institute, Pensacola, FL
[6] Naval Medical Research Unit–Dayton, Dayton, OH
[7] Naval Air Warfare Center Aircraft Division, Patuxent River, MD
[8] Strategic Analysis, Inc., Arlington, VA
[9] HYPRES, Inc., Elmsford, NY
eoneill@sainc.com

Abstract. Magnetic resonance imaging (MRI) is a non-invasive method capable of producing high spatial resolution images of body structures and identifying injuries. However, conventional MRI systems use large superconducting magnets ($\geq$ 1Tesla) that require high operating costs, long exam times, metal free environments, and are impractical to transport. Portable MRI systems using ultra-low magnetic fields in the micro- to milli-tesla range with superconducting quantum interference device (SQUID) technology have been developed, but these systems generate low signal-to-noise ratios (SNR), requiring very long averaging times to obtain modest spatial resolution. The initial phase of this project involved the development of a low field MRI system and resulted in the preliminary design of a transportable low-field (0.1 Tesla) MRI system, which has the advantages of ultra-low and high field MRI systems while avoiding their disadvantages. The current phase of the project is developing a small-scale portable low-field MRI system prototype of the full sized system. Development of this technology will have significant applications in both commercial and military settings.

Keywords: Magnetic resonance imaging (MRI), superconducting quantum interface devices (SQUIDs), ultra-low frequency (ULF), magnetic fields, signal-to-noise ratio (SNR), traumatic brain injury (TBI).

---

[*] Ph.D., Medical Service Corps, United States Navy.
[**] Ph.D.
[***] Psy.D., Medical Service Corps, United States Navy.

C. Stephanidis (Ed.): Posters, Part II, HCII 2013, CCIS 374, pp. 148–152, 2013.

1 Introduction

Magnetic Resonance Imaging (MRI) systems enable high resolution of the structure and function of the human body, providing a broadly effective means for diagnosing injuries. However, MRIs require high-powered large-scale magnets and electromagnetic pulse stimulation to produce these images, making them too large and too dangerous for use in metal-rich combat environments and preclude them from being used in synchrony with many other diagnostic technologies. Recent advancements in MRI technology have focused on reducing the magnetic field strengths needed to produce structural and functional images [1]. Using field strengths in the milli- and micro-tesla range, these ultra-low field (ULF) low-power consumption magnets have been coupled with superconducting quantum interference devices (SQUIDs) to produce MRI-like images [2-4]. Because these magnetic field strengths are so small, this technology is likely safe to use around metal [3,5] and should also be easily combined with other diagnostic tools like magnetoencephalograph (MEG), magnetocardiography (MCG) and even electroencephalography (EEG) to produce unparalleled functional imagery of the brain and body [2,3].

Currently, ULF MRI is limited to arrays of less than 10 SQUIDs, which cannot produce the high quality images or capture the large fields of view (FOV) typical of conventional MRIs. As well, image processing speed is increased at the expense of reduced signal to noise ratios (SNR) resulting in degraded image clarity. Finally, ULF MRI must average signals over multiple scans, which increases image processing time significantly over that needed for a single scan.

The objective of this effort is to develop and demonstrate a novel MRI system that combines low magnetic fields with dense-array SQUIDs to resolve issues involved with conventional MRI systems that require powerful magnets, making them costly to use and difficult to integrate with other imaging technologies, and undeployable to the battlefield (Figure 1).

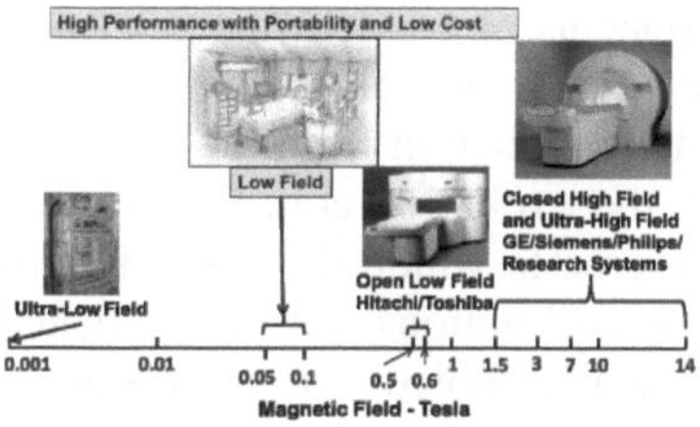

Fig. 1. Illustration of MRI systems ranging from ULF to high field. The proposed low field MRI combines the portability of ULF MRIs with the resolution of high field MRIs.

2 Technical Requirements

This effort focuses on developing and demonstrating a low field MRI system that incorporates a dense-array of highly sensitive sensors to produce conventional MRI-equivalent images from a single scan. The final system will demonstrate:

- A two-fold improvement in SNR over ULF MRI systems.
- An order of magnitude increase in sensor array density compared to ULF MRIs.
- The ability to build images from a single scanning trial.
- Significant reduction in size, weight, and power requirements compared to conventional MRIs.
- The capability to integrate other imaging technologies (MEG, MCG, and EEG) that are precluded from conventional MRIs.

3 Technical Approach

To achieve the required technical requirements, the objectives of the first phase of the research project were to establish 1) pick-up coil specification and design, 2) finalized and verified digital SQUID chip specification, design, and optimization and SQUID array configuration, 3) appropriate magnet size and type, 4) a suitable cooling system, and 5) available peripheral electronics including gradient and excitation coils and data acquisition and imaging software (Figure 2).

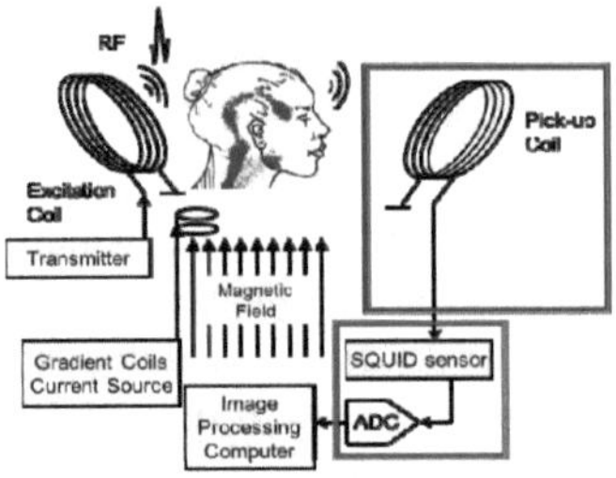

Fig. 2. Major components of an MRI system that were redesigned for the low field MRI. Components in the red and blue box require cryocooling.

One of the major components of an MRI that determines the quality of an image is the radio frequency (RF) receiver or pick-up coils. The pick-up coils detect the weak energy given off by magnetic induction from the precessing (spin) of hydrogen nuclei (MR signal) produced by the excitation coil. Pick-up coils also detect noise and are therefore limited by the degree to which the desired signal intensity exceeds the random noise. Several pick-up coil options were investigated and it was determined that cold copper coils (cryogenically cooled) with an optimum size of 3.5 cm in diameter would provide effective noise reduction and signal detection.

Analog SQUIDs have been shown to measure the very weak magnetic signals in ULF MRIs, which have poor SNR and spatial resolution. Resolution using analog SQUIDS could be improve by increasing the magnetic field strength or using large numbers of SQUID-based receivers (arrays >100); however, analog SQUIDs cannot operate in the presence of strong magnetic strengths and large arrays of analog SQUIDS greatly increase system complexity. Therefore, digital SQUID chips based on superconducting analog-to-digital converters (ADCs) that can operate at the desired low fields (0.05-0.1 T) and reduce system complexity were designed and the exact chip design parameters were finalized and verified. In addition a compact multi-SQUID design containing four digital SQUIDs per chip, multiplexed by a summing circuit was developed. These mulit-SQUID chips can be combined into a dense-array of 256 digital SQUIDs that will produce SNRs and image resolution typical of conventional 1.5T MRI systems (SNR=100) and combined with other imaging technologies (MEG, MCG, and EEG).

The magnetic field of MRI systems can be generated by superconducting magnets, electromagnets, or permanent magnets. Research into the magnet options eliminated superconducting magnets (used in conventional high field MRIs) and electromagnets (used in ULF MRIs) due to their large size, weight, and power requirements and because they require liquid cryogen (helium). It was determined that permanent Halbach magnets are the best choice for a low field transportable MRI because they are smaller, lighter, have been used in MRI systems, do not require liquid cryogen, and are available commercial-off-the-shelf (COTS) form several different vendors.

The required cooling of the superconducting chips as well as the pickup coils (Figure 1) will be achieved by using a commercially available cryocooler. The cryocooler is a closed-cycle refrigerator that uses helium gas as the refrigerant. Therefore, the proposed system does not require a liquid cryogen. The cryocooler system is self-contained in inside a standard wheel mounted instrumentation rack that can be easily transported and repositioned.

It was determined that for the final target low field MRI system, the gradient and excitation coils, as well as the data acquisition and imaging software do not need to be redesigned and can be procured COTS options from conventional MRI component vendors.

The initial phase resulted in the preliminary design of a transportable low-field (0.1 Tesla) MRI system that can be operated in the vicinity of metallic objects due to its low magnetic field (Figure 3). The system is compact, cost-effective, and projected to weigh less than 1,000 kg and require less than 2 kW power. The modular system consists of 1) a permanent magnet with gradient and excitation coils, 2) a helmet assembly with a dense array of cooled receiver coils, and 3) instrument control rack with cryocooler and dense-array of digital SQUID sensors. The system can be operated in the vicinity (within 3 ft) of magnetic metallic objects due to its low magnetic field, and is designed such that it can be used for magnetoencephalography (MEG), where the same digital

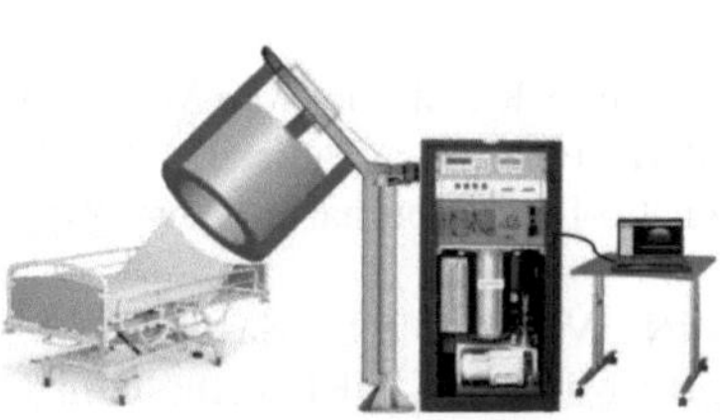

Fig. 3. Preliminary design of a compact, portable, low field (0.05-0.1 T) MRI system capable of image conventional MRI image resolution, but that can operate in the vicinity metallic objects

The technical objectives of the current phase of the project are build and demonstrate a small-scale portable high resolution MRI system at low field (0.05-0.1T) with all the features and specifications of the target system (except for the magnet and bore size). The imaging field of view will be 1cm x 1cm x 1cm, which will only require four channels of digital SQUIDs. This will require the acquisition of a commercial small magnet from Magritek, the development of a four SQUID digital chip, and the development of cryogenic packaging on a Sumitomo cooler.

The final phase of the project will focus on developing a 256 channel MRI system with a magnet bore diameter of 20 cm x 20 cm x 20 cm for human brain imaging.

4 Conclusion

This technology will have broad application in commercial as well as military settings. Low field MRIs will require less power, produce smaller and safer magnetic fields and have significantly reduced size and weight factors compared to conventional MRIs. As well, additional sensor technologies may be integrated. It will provide never-before achieved levels of injury resolution, significantly improving diagnostic accuracy and efficiency, optimizing the 'Golden Hour' during which critical lifesaving treatments are most effective. Commercially, this will enable greater levels of MRI access to a wider patient base not only in hospitals but in clinics and outpatient setting as well. First responders will be able to include this technology in their response kits to conduct on-site triage during mass-casualty events. Military applications include providing forward deployed surgical teams the ability to perform highly advanced diagnostic assessments before casualties are MEDEVACed to longer-term medical treatment facilities.

Acknowledgements. Research and development of Dense Array, Low Field Magnetic Resonance Imaging Devices for Combat Casualty Care by Hypres, Inc., has been supported by OSD through SBIR Phase I contract OSD11-H18 and funded by ONR BAA contract N00014-12-M-0103. We especially thank Dr. Masoud Radparvar for his time and commitment to this project.

References

1. McDermott, R., Kelso, N., Lee, S.K., Mößle, M., Mück, M., Myers, W., ten Haken, B., Seton, H.C., Trabesinger, A.H., Pines, A., Clarke, J.: SQUID-detected magnetic resonance imaging in microtesla magnetic fields. Journal of Low Temperature Physics 135, 793–821 (2004)
2. Zotev, V.S., Matlashov, A.N., Volegov, P.L., Savukov, I.M., Espy, M.A., Mosher, J.C., Gomez, J.J., Kraus Jr., R.H.: Microtelsa MRI of the human brain combined with MEG. Journal of Magnetic Resonance 194, 115–120 (2008)
3. Zotev, V.S., Volegov, P.L., Matlashov, A.N., Espy, M.A., Mosher, J.C., Kraus Jr., R.H.: Parallel MRI at microtelsa fields. Journal of Magnetic Resonance 192, 197–208 (2008)
4. Pruessmann, K.P.: Less is more. Nature 455, 43–44 (2008)
5. Mößle, M., Han, S.I., Myers, W.R., Lee, S.K., Kelso, N., Hatridge, M., Pines, A., Clarke, J.: SQUID-detected microtelsa MRI in the presence of metal. Journal of Magnetic Resonance 179, 146–151 (2006)

An App a Day Keeps the Doctor…Informed: User Evaluation of a Patient Mobile Health Application and Clinician Dashboard

Sarah Cook, Rita Sembajwe, Barbara Massoudi, and Amanda Recker

RTI International, Research Triangle Park, North Carolina, USA
{scook,rsembajwe,bmassoudi}@rti.org,
amanda.l.recker@gmail.com

Abstract. Data collection through mobile applications, or apps, is increasing due to the growing adoption of smartphones. The BreathEasy project used a smartphone application for collecting asthma patients' observations of daily living and a clinician dashboard to increase communication and understanding between patients and their clinicians. After a 6-month trial, these researchers collected evaluation data of these two systems from patients and clinicians through focus groups and the System Usability Scale. Here we present our findings on the user experiences of both patients and clinicians, as well as the perceived usability of the systems used. Their evaluations and recommendations will help improve future systems for these populations.

Keywords: Mobile Health Application, Dashboard, User Experience.

1 Introduction

Asthma is a common, chronic illness that affects over 23 million U.S. adults [1] who face daunting challenges in managing their disease conditions on a daily basis. In partnership with Virginia Commonwealth University (VCU), the authors developed and piloted a smartphone app, based on the latest clinical guidelines [2] for treatment and self-monitoring of individuals with asthma, to assist adults with asthma to better manage their care and disease condition.

BreathEasy, part of the Robert Wood Johnson Foundation's Project HealthDesign (www.projecthealthdesign.org), was developed through a user-centered design approach with iterative development and feedback cycles. Patients used an Android-based smartphone to record their observations of daily living (ODLs), including asthma and mental health symptoms, medication use, symptom triggers, physical activity, and activity limitations, among others. Clinicians (physician/nurse pairs) used a Web-based dashboard to review patient data and visualize trends and patterns in the ODL data on a regular basis in accordance with a disease management approach.

C. Stephanidis (Ed.): Posters, Part II, HCII 2013, CCIS 374, pp. 153–157, 2013.

2 Methods

Two focus groups consisting of 16 total patient participants were conducted in a conference room at a VCU medical facility to determine overall patient experiences using the BreathEasy app. All patient participants who completed the study (n = 29) were invited to attend, yielding a response rate of 55.1%. Of the 16 patient participants, 15 were female and 1 was male. A member of the research team who was not part of the patients' clinical team facilitated the focus group discussions. As an incentive for participation, patients were offered a $25 gift card and they were reimbursed for their transportation costs to attend. Because there were no contradicting responses between the two groups, findings for the focus groups are presented jointly, unless noted.

A clinician focus group was held with 10 clinician participants (5 nurses and 5 physicians), yielding a 50% response rate. A member of the research team facilitated this focus group as well. Clinicians offered feedback on the dashboard design and its impact on patient-physician relationships, care, and clinic workflow.

Patients and clinicians were asked to complete the System Usability Scale (SUS) at the end of their respective focus groups. The SUS is a 10-item questionnaire that evaluates perceptions of usability. Each question uses the same 5-item scale ranging from 1 (Strongly Disagree) to 5 (Strongly Agree). Scoring is completed by subtracting 1 from odd-numbered responses and subtracting the even-numbered responses from 5 [3].

3 Results

3.1 Patients

Patients unanimously agreed that the design of the smartphone app was simple, easy to use, and had a very small learning curve. A handful of participants commented on how they were not technically savvy but were able to use the app with no problem, even if they still did not know how to use the rest of the phone. One participant commented that it is easy enough that a child could do it, and participants unanimously agreed.

When asked about specific features that they liked about the app, patients cited the reminders for daily data entry. Some patients indicated that these reminders also made them remember to take their medications. A few patients said they found the reminders annoying but explained that they got annoyed because they had to go and put their data in, not because of the reminder itself; these patients still said that the reminder was very helpful. Participants also wanted a reminder added in if they had not put in the previous day's entry so that they would be reminded to go back in and enter the data.

When asked about things that they did not like or did not feel worked well, a few participants reported experiencing the following problems: The BreathEasy app would sometimes freeze and force close, which resulted in data not being saved. Another issue participants reported was that the app asked the same questions twice when they filled out their daily information. They said every day they would get some of the questions more than once. Some respondents thought it was a question about using their rescue inhaler they were seeing twice. Researchers believe these comments relate to the questions about using rescue medications and experiencing asthma symptoms, which both yielded a list of National Heart, Lung, and Blood Institute–specified asthma symptoms as answer options [2]. Because patients were seeing this list both times on days when they reported using rescue medications, they may have interpreted this as being asked the same question twice.

Overall, patients reported that the app was easy to use and had a small learning curve. Patients thought that the app was useful and shared many suggestions for items they would like to have added to it. They reported that they enjoyed tracking their ODLs because it made them more aware of everything they were doing as well as their surroundings and any asthma triggers they may have encountered. Patients also reported that knowing that their clinicians would be viewing their information made them more likely to adhere to clinical advice regarding medication use, physical activity, and other behaviors critical to self-management of asthma.

SUS Results

A total of 22 patients completed the SUS questionnaire. The mean score was 78.41 with a standard deviation of 14.13. According to Sauro, a mean score of 78.41 would be interpreted as a B+ if graded [3]. Question 8, stating "I found the system very cumbersome to use," had an average score of 2.82, where 1 (Strongly Disagree) was the desired score. This average score was furthest from the desired score of all 10 response averages.

3.2 Clinicians

BreathEasy included a clinician dashboard which allowed clinicians to view their patient's asthma-related ODLs—medication use, triggers, symptoms, physical activity, anxiety, mood, and smoking habits—through data submitted via the BreathEasy app utilizing a disease management approach.

Clinicians' feedback from the focus group indicated that the clinician dashboard was easy to use. They found that the design layout flowed well and was easy to understand at a glance. They especially appreciated the chart interface, which displayed ODL conditions and peak flow results.

Although the charting interface satisfied clinicians, the symbols used on the charts were not considered to be user-friendly. Clinicians felt the symbol color scheme (red and green) worked well, but the symbols themselves were small. Clinicians also felt that the red star representing an undesired health state and green star representing a desired health state could have been replaced by more universal symbols.

An automated alert system, initially presented as a need during the clinician dashboard requirements-gathering session but not integrated due to clinic security policies, was also mentioned as a desired key feature. Clinicians' feedback expressed the importance of an alert system via e-mail or messaging that would activate when significant changes in ODL conditions were detected. Their use of the system during the trial had required them to log in and check each patients' dashboard to identify any significant ODL changes.

In conclusion, there was highly positive clinician feedback related to BreathEasy's impact on clinic workflow, ability to offer access to clinically useful information, contributions to improved patient-physician relationships, and overall improvements to asthma care. The latter was attributed to increased patient empowerment and education, better medication management, and support for changes in clinical asthma diagnosis. A few challenges related to clinician liability and time reimbursement were discussed, but these were outside the scope of the user experience.

SUS Results

A total of 16 clinicians completed the SUS questionnaire. The mean score was 75.17 with a standard deviation of 9.66. A mean score of 75.17 would be interpreted as a B if given a traditional grade [3]. All 10 of the item response averages were closer to the desired score (1 for even items, 5 for odd items) than the undesired score. Question 6 had one of the scores closest to the desirable score with an average response of 1.40 (with a desired score of 1). Of the 16 clinicians, 10 reported strongly disagreeing with the statement "I thought there was too much inconsistency in this system."

4 Discussion

Overall results of focus groups and the SUS questionnaire among patients and clinicians using this asthma management mobile app and dashboard indicated satisfaction with the technology and its usability. Some specific issues encountered and reported during the patient sessions were related to the mobile smartphone usability itself as opposed to the app. These differences between the app and the smartphone were difficult to separate using the SUS questionnaire. However, given the acceptable score of the app, we are not concerned about difficulties with the smartphone affecting the results.

Through user evaluation of this app and dashboard combination, the researchers were able to better understand the users' experiences during the 6-month trial. Learning that the smartphone app was easy to use over a period of time will help us design future applications with a similar population. We also learned that more challenges lay on the clinician side of this initiative in the need to integrate an alert system when patient ODLs change significantly.

References

1. Strine, T., Mokdad, A., Balluz, L., Berry, J., Gonzalez, O.: Impact of depression and anxiety on quality of life, health behaviors, and asthma control among adults in the United States with asthma. Journal of Asthma 45(2), 123–133 (2006)
2. U.S. Department of Health and Human Services (2007) Expert Panel Report 3 (EPR3): Guidelines for the Diagnosis and Management of Asthma. National Heart, Lung, and Blood Institute (August. 2007), `http://www.nhlbi.nih.gov/guidelines/asthma/asthgdln.htm` (accessed April 5, 2013)
3. Sauro, J.: Measuring usability with the system usability scale (SUS). Quantitative Usability, Statistics & Six Sigma (2011), `http://www.measuringusability.com/sus.php` (accessed April 9, 2013)

Segmenting Instrumented Activities of Daily Living (IADL) Using Kinematic and Sensor Technology for the Assessment of Limb Apraxia

Charmayne M.L. Hughes[1], Manish Parekh[2], and Joachim Hermsdörfer[1]

[1] Institute of Movement Science, Department of Sport and Health Science, Technical University of Munich, 80992 Munich, Germany
[2] Electrical, Electronic and Computing Engineering, The University of Birmingham, Birmingham, B15 2TT, U.K.
{charmayne.hughes,joachim.hermsdoerfer}@tum.de, MXP534@bham.ac.uk

Abstract. In this paper we present a method of segmenting instrumented activities of daily living (IADL) using kinematic criterion coupled with sensor technology. To collect our training data we asked four neurologically healthy individuals to make a total of 60 cups of tea with a set order of ASs. We then evaluated our IADL segmentation technique in healthy individuals and patients with limb apraxia, and demonstrate that combining kinematic criterion with sensor data is provides an accurate means to segment IADL's into relevant ASs.

Keywords: action segmentation, apraxia, activities of daily living.

1 Introduction

After a stroke incident as many as 24% of patients suffer from persistent impairments of limb apraxia [1]; a cognitive-motor deficit characterized by impairment in the performance of skilled movement. Research has demonstrated that patients with apraxia have difficulty performing many activities of daily living (ADL), such as eating a meal or making a cup of tea or coffee [2-3], and have difficulty shaving or brushing teeth [4]. Despite these apparent difficulties, quantitative analysis of ADL performance is extremely rare and restricted to qualitative and/or temporal variables. There is, however, ample evidence that individuals with left brain damage (LBD) after stroke exhibit impaired movement kinematics during tool use [5-6].

Based on the kinematic analysis of tool use in patients with LBD, it is certainly a worthwhile venture to examine whether impaired movement kinematics are also observable during instrumented activities of daily living (IADL). We recently explored whether a complex IADL (i.e., preparing a cup of tea) could be segmented using kinematic criteria alone [7]. We found that action segment (AS) boundaries could be detected for neurologically healthy participants, but only if the task was performed in a prescribed order. However, it was not possible to detect AS boundaries when patients with apraxia performed the task, regardless of whether patients were

C. Stephanidis (Ed.): Posters, Part II, HCII 2013, CCIS 374, pp. 158–162, 2013.

free to choose the order of actions, or if action order was prescribed. Furthermore, the ability to detect AS boundaries was highly affected by the presence of irrelevant actions. In sum, it appears that segmenting IADLs using kinematic criteria alone is not an effective technique, as the kinematic profile of a movement differs depending on the order of action and irrelevant actions. In the present paper, we present an alternative technique which uses kinematic criterion coupled with sensor technology in order to segment an IADL (i.e., tea making) for later kinematic analysis.

2 Segmentation Technique

The tea making task was broken down to the following ASs: 1) Fill kettle, 2) add tea bag and sugar into mug, 3) Pour hot water from kettle into mug 4) pour milk into mug, and 5) stir mug contents. In order to detect these ASs sensors were integrated into the base and body of a kettle, a tea mug, and a milk jug. The instrumented objects hosted a 3-axis accelerometer and 3 force sensitive resistors (FSRs) which streamed data to a host computer via Bluetooth at 200Hz (with a 12bit analog to digital converter). The accelerometer monitored changes in the movement and orientation of the object, while FSRs monitored changes in weight of the object.

2.1 Sensor-Based Action Segmentation

The first step of segment parameterization was to determine the primary and secondary sensor characteristics for each AS, and then to infer the boundaries of each AS from the kinematic data. To this end, we collected training data from four neurologically healthy individuals, who were asked to make 60 cups of tea with milk and sugar.

From the collected data we were able to determine when sensor activity for each action segment begun and ended (Figure 1, top panel). The fillkettle AS was inferred from average of the kettle base FSRs, and the x and y axis kettle body accelerometers. Startfillkettle was determined by the first time point in the kettle base FSR series in which values exceeded +/-1 baseline values (~1700). Endstartkettle was defined by the first time point in which kettle base FSR values returned to baseline after fillkettlemaxima (≥3000), with a corresponding spike in both kettle body accelerometers (> +/-1 SD baseline value). The addteabagandsugar AS was inferred from the average mug FSR's. AS start and end was determined by calculating the first peak in the time series ≥ 1000 (addteabagandsugarmaxima), and then using a forward search from addteabagandsugarmaxima to the time point in which mug FSR values returned to median baseline values (500-600) within a period of 400ms, respectively.

The *addheatedwaterintomug* AS was inferred on the average of the kettle base FSR's, and the x and y axis kettle body accelerometers. *Startaddheatedwaterintomug* was determined by the first time point in which the kettle base FSR dropped and stayed below 200 for 700ms, and the x and y axis kettle body accelerometers increased to ≥ +/-2 SD of baseline values. *Endaddheatedwaterintomug* was determined as a return to baseline values (+/-1 SD) for all three sensors. The *pourmilk* action segment was inferred primarily from values obtained by the average milk FSR's by first locating *pourmilkminima*. A backwards search is then initiated along the time series to find the start of the *pourmilk* AS, defined when FSR values are < +/- 1 SD baseline (~ 800) for ≥ 100ms. *Endpourmilk* was determined using a forward search from *pourmilkminima* to the time point when FSR values were < +/- 1 SD baseline for > 100ms. The secondary characteristic of the *pourmilk* AS was based on average mug FSR values in which there was a >40-65N increase between *startpourmilk* and *end-pourmilk*. Lastly, the *stirmug* AS was inferred from the average of the 1mug FSR values. *Startstirmug* was defined as the first time point in which ≥ 3 peaks (with values ≥ 1000N) occurred within 100ms. *Endstirmug* was defined when mug FRS values returned to +/- 1 SD pre-peak baseline (940-960).

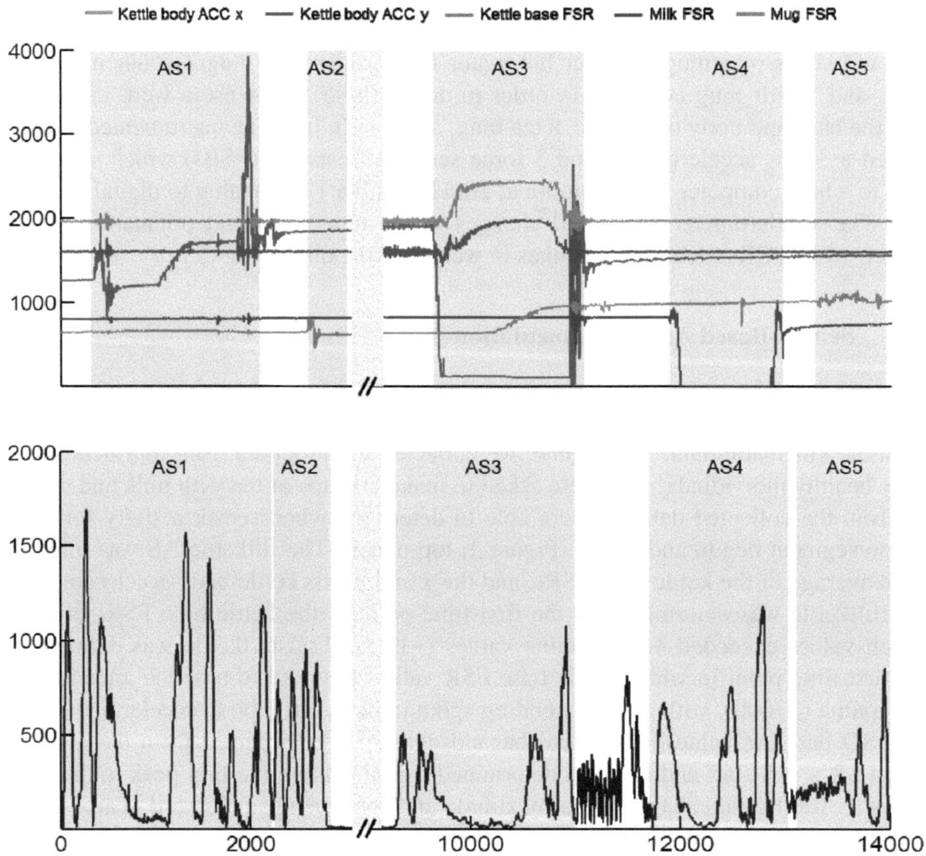

Fig. 1. Segmentation of a single tea making trial. The top panel depicts the data from the sensorized objects and the resultant classification of each action segment. The bottom panel depicts the kinematic data (resultant hand velocity) and the classification of the individual action segments. The shaded grey area depicts the time period in which the water was boiling and there were no hand or sensor actions.

2.2 Kinematic-Based Action Segmentation

Given our interest in the kinematics involved in each AS, the next step in the segmentation process was to link sensor activity and hand kinematics (captured from a five camera optical motion capture system [Qualisys AB, Gothenburg, Sweden] with 200 Hz temporal and 1 mm spatial resolution). Based on assumptions of motor control, we assumed that hand movements would precede sensor activity, and that hand movements would follow a straight path, with symmetric, bell-shaped, velocity profiles [8]. To this end, the kinematic onset of each AS was determined by taking the time point of AS onset from sensor data (e.g., *startpourmilk*) and performing a backwards search on the kinematic time series to the point that resultant hand velocity > 3% peak velocity. Kinematic offset for each AS was calculated using a forwards search from sensor AS offset to the time point in the kinematic time series in which resultant hand velocity dropped and stayed below 3% peak velocity. After segmentation, the following kinematic variables were calculated for each AS: movement time (ms), percentage total movement time (%), resultant peak velocity (mm/s), and time to peak resultant velocity (% AS).

3 Results

We evaluated our IADL segmentation technique in three healthy individuals and two patients with limb apraxia, who were asked to make 15 cups of tea with milk and sugar. Performance was analyzed by comparing sensor-based and kinematic-based action segmentation to video data captured during task performance (200 Hz), and determining the percentage of accurate AS onset and offset classifications.

Overall, we were able to successfully determine the pourmilk and addheatedwater ASs for all four individuals (>85% accuracy) using our combined sensor- and kinematic-based segmentation technique, as the FSR and accelerometers yielded the most consistent values across trials and participants. The performance of our technique to define the fillkettle AS was somewhat lower (60-85% accuracy across subjects), which was due to the presence of movement artifacts associated with the opening and closing of the kettle lid which occurred in earlier trials. The lack of consistent sensor data also influenced our ability to detect the addteabagandsugar AS. When the sensor and video data were compared it was observed that there was no noticable change in the mug FSR values when the subject added the teabag in some trials, which lead to a decrease in the ability to accurately detect addteabagandsugar AS offset. The ability to accurately classify the stirmug AS also differed across individuals (65-90% accuracy), which was primarily caused by individual differences in the force and length of stirring technique.

After segmentation, we evaluated the kinematic data to ascertain whether there were differences between healthy control and patients with limb apraxia. Overall, we found that the kinematics of the patient group exhibited greater inter-individual variability, specifically for the *addteabagandsugar* and the *stirmug* ASs. Furthermore, patients took longer to perform, and exhibited smaller peak velocities, for each AS, than healthy controls.

4 Conclusions

Our analysis indicates that kinematic analysis of IADLs is contingent upon effective segmentation techniques, which can be achieved through combined kinematic and sensor technology. After effective IADL segmentation, kinematic analysis revealed differences between the hand kinematics of healthy controls and patients with apraxia, specific to certain ASs. In future work this method will examine whether abnormalities differ depending on clinical variables (e.g., arm impairment, lesion volume, and lesion localization).

Acknowledgments. This study was supported by a grant from the European Commission (FP7-ICT-2011-288912).

References

1. Bickerton, W., Riddoch, M.J., Samson, D., Balani, A., Mistry, B., Humphreys, G.W.: Systematic assessment of apraxia and functional predictions from the Birmingham Cognitive Screen. J. Neurology, Neurosurg and Psychiatry 83, 513–521 (2012)
2. Foundas, A.L., Macauley, B.L., Raymer, A.M., Maher, L.M., Heilman, K.M., Rothi, L.: Ecological implications of limb apraxia: evidence from mealtime behavior. J. Int. Neuropsychol. Soc. 1, 62–66 (1995)
3. Ochipa, C., Rothi, L.J.G., Heilman, K.M.: Ideational apraxia: A deficit in tool selection and use. Ann. Neurol. 25, 190–193 (1989)
4. Hanna-Pladdy, B., Heilman, K.M., Foundas, A.L.: Ecological implications of ideomotor apraxia: evidence from physical activities of daily living. Neurology 60, 487–490 (2003)
5. Hermsdörfer, J., Hentze, S., Goldenberg, G.: Spatial and kinematic features of apraxic movement depend on the mode of execution. Neuropsychologia 44, 1642–1652 (2006)
6. Hermsdörfer, J., Li, Y., Randerath, J., Goldenberg, G., Johansson, L.: Tool use without a tool: kinematic characteristics of pantomiming as compared to actual use and the effect of brain damage. Exp. Brain. Res. 218, 201–214 (2012)
7. Hughes, C.M.L., Hermsdörfer, J.: Challenges and opportunities in measuring ADL performance in stroke patients with apraxia. Deutsche Vereinigung für Sportwissenschaft (dvs) Tagung der dvs-Sektion Sportmotorik (2013)
8. Morasso, P.: Spatial control of arm movements. Exp. Brain Res. 41, 223–227 (1981)

Supporting User's Continued Effort for Health by Estimating Mental Loads of Actions

Hitoshi Ikeda and Toshikazu Kato

Faculty of Science and Engineering, Chuo University 1-13-27 Kasuga,
Bunkyo-ku, Tokyo, 112-8551, Japan
kato@indsys.chuo-u.ac.jp, hitoshi1227@gmail.com

Abstract. Recently, lifestyle disease has become a social problem. It is difficult to improve exercise habits because people are hard to continue efforts for health. In previous studies for encouraging exercises, there are studies to improve user's motivation by visualizing exercise outcome. We should consider not only improvement of motivation but also lessening mental loads for exercises since improvement of exercise habits requires long-term continuation. This study estimates the low degree and gives suitable recommended information which prompts exercises. Therefore we propose health support which facilitates continuation of user's effort for exercise. We propose new approach method to prompt exercise. The experimental result indicated that a part of the approach method is effective. And we constructed KANSEI model, a correlation between degrees of each the feeling and the factors is revealed by data of each user than data of all users.

Keywords: Information Distribution, Estimate of Situation, Continual, Health Support System.

1 Introduction

Recently, lifestyle disease has become a social problem. It is difficult to improve exercise habits because people are hard to continue efforts for health.

In previous studies for encouraging exercises, there are studies to improve user's motivation by visualizing exercise outcome [1]. We should consider not only improvement of motivation but also lessening mental loads for exercises since improvement of exercise habits requires long-term continuation. This study estimates the low degree and gives suitable recommended information which prompts exercises. Therefore we propose health support which facilitates continuation of user's effort for exercise.

2 Approach

We describe an approach of this study. We assumed that users feel less the mental loads by incorporating exercise which relate to the actions in daily lives. We define

C. Stephanidis (Ed.): Posters, Part II, HCII 2013, CCIS 374, pp. 163–167, 2013.

feeling less mental loads of this action. As shown in Figure 1, we propose "Parallel Action", "Additional Action", and "Alternative Action" as a method which incorporates related exercise. There are the feelings for each action.

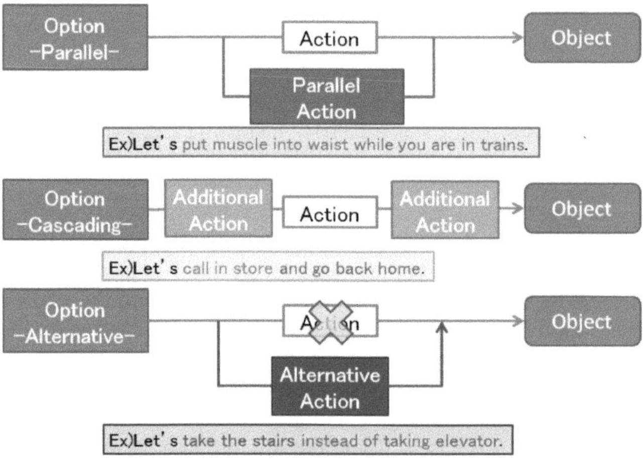

Fig. 1. Image of "Parallel Action", "Additional Action", and "Alternative Action"

A degree of defined feeling is different in user's state and situation of moment. As shown in Figure 2, we define factors giving the feeling to construct KANSEI model which measures the feeling [2].

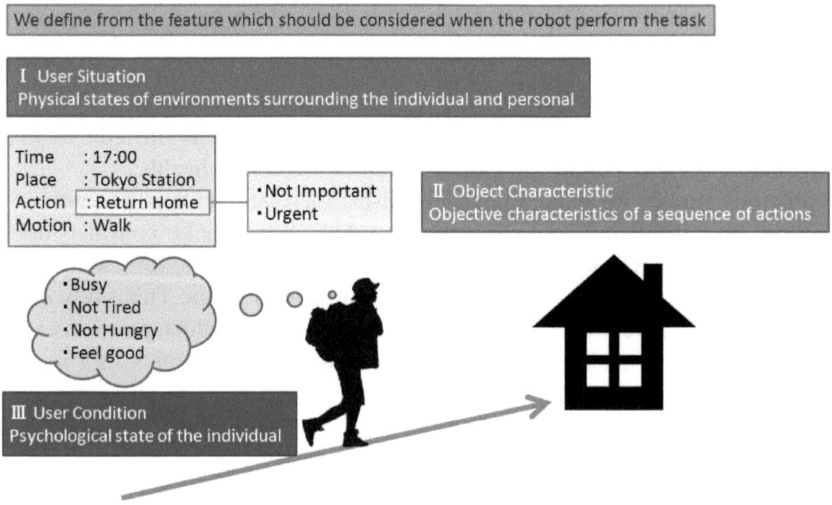

Fig. 2. Factors to construct KANSEI model

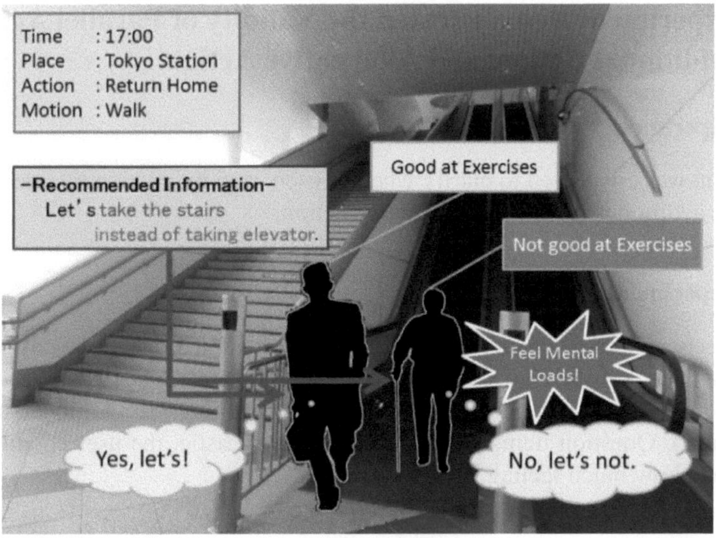

Fig. 3. A difference of feeling for recommended information by individual

Figure 3 shows one example about a difference of feeling for recommended information by individual. We develop the system which recommends related exercises (Parallel, Additional, and Alternative) as shown in Figure 4.

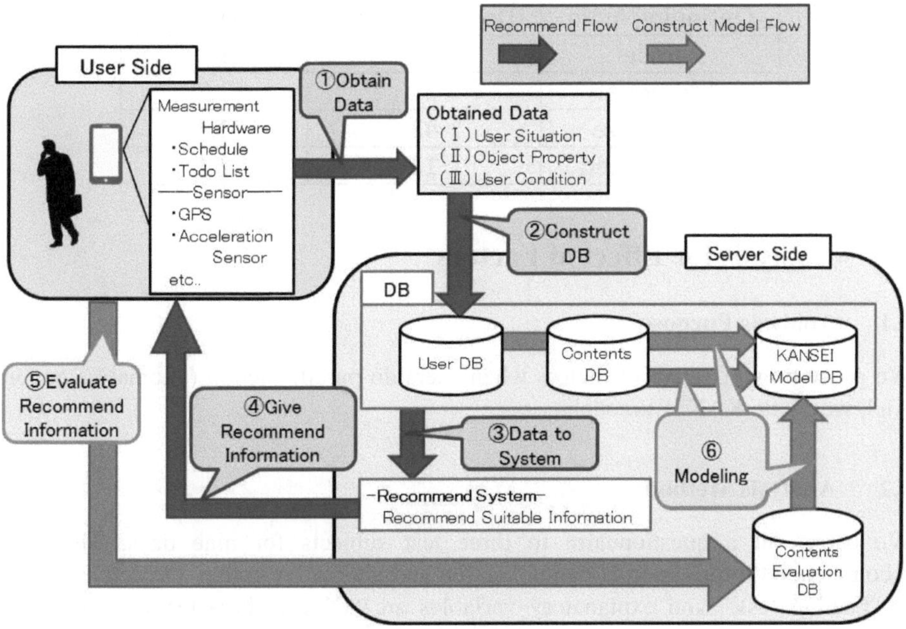

Fig. 4. Recommendation system summary

3 Experiment Demonstrated the Validity of Parallel Action, Additional Action, and Alternative Action

3.1 Experiment Purpose

Experiment was conducted to clarify whether users step into action by selecting parallel action, additional action, and alternative action.

3.2 Experiment Method

Test subjects are ten students in twenties. Each test subject has three day's questionnaire when test subjects go home. Test subjects make replies each recommended information. Recommended information is four types (parallel, additional, alternative, unconcerned). Question items are the object characteristic, the user condition, doing actually and how much feeling less (5 levels).

3.3 Experiment Result and Examination

Table 1 shows questionnaire result. As compared to Unconcerned, Do Actually of Parallel and Alternative is high. But Do Actually of Additional is 17%, and the rate is low. Recommended information of Additional needs to improve.

Table 1. Questionnaire result

Optioning Actin	Do Actually (%)	Feeling less
Parallel	51	3.8
Additional	17	2.7
Alternative	42	3.3
Unconcerned	13	2.1

4 Analysis for Effect of Factors

4.1 Analysis Purpose

We prove how effective of factors when users do parallel action (alternative action). And, we create KANSEI model.

4.2 Analysis Method

We carry out a questionnaire to three test subjects for nine days. This time, recommended information is parallel action and alternative action. Objective variable is "Feeling less", and explanatory variables are "Object characteristic" and "User condition".

4.3 Analysis Result and Examination

As a result of multiple linear regression analysis, table 2 shows multiple regression coefficient. For example, Feeling of test subject A affect objective variable materially. Therefore, effects on Feeling less vary widely among individuals.

Table 2. Individual model by multiple linear regression analysis

Parallel Action			Object Characteristic		User Condition			
		Constant	Importance	Urgency	Busy	Tired	Hunger	Feeling
A	Y=	-2.8		0.47	0.51	0.56		1.1
B	Y=	4.9	0.47	-0.39		-0.27	0.3	-0.13
C	Y=	5	-0.22	-0.11		-0.32	-0.12	0.49

5 Conclusions

Incorporating exercise which relate to actions in daily lives was found to encourage users to exercise. We create KANSEI model of the effect when users do parallel actions and alternative actions. In addition, we develop a system using the model and find out accuracy of the system.

References

1. Iio, J., Koyama, S., Hasegawa, Y.: Log-based Assessment for the Success and Failure of Dieting. IPSJ Journal 53(11), 2624–2634 (2012)
2. Tada, M., Kato, T.: Visual KANSEI Modeling Based on Focal Area Analysis and Hierarchical Classiflcation. The Transactions of the Institute of Electronics, Information and Communication Engineers D-II J87-D-II (10), 2004–2010 (1983)

A Support System for Healthy Eating Habits: Optimization of Recipe Retrieval

Yuma Inagawa[1], Junki Hakamta[1], and Masataka Tokumaru[2]

[1] Graduate School of Kansai University
3-3-35 Yamate-cho, Suita-shi, Osaka 564-8680, Japan
[2] Kansai University, 3-3-35 Yamate-cho, Suita-shi, Osaka 564-8680, Japan
{k470812,k531284,toku}@kansai-u.ac.jp

Abstract. In this paper, we propose a support system for healthy eating habits. Current methods of recipe retrieval generally rely on keywords or popularity. However, such approaches offer the same results to different users. In order to resolve this issue, we have developed a support system that incorporates nutritional management and preferential retrieval. In the preferential retrieval system, a recommender agent takes account of user tastes to extract and present menus. The user then, evaluates the menus recommended by various agents. Each recommender agents evolves on the basis of these menu appraisals. Over time, the preferences of the agents become similar to those of the users, resulting in menus that correspond to user tastes. This study thus utilizes an interactive immune algorithm (IIA) to optimize the preferential retrieval system. We tested the proposed system with a simulated user but genuine recipe data.

1 Introduction

It is difficult for cooks to device a new menus on a daily basis. Thus, cooks often consult Web sites when they need inspiration for their menus. However, contemporary recipe retrieval sites generally retrieve a recipe by using either a keyword or a popularity rank. Under these conditions, the taste preferences of a user are not considered, so the sites retrieve the same recipes for multiple users. Therefore, we propose a support system for healthy eating habits that considers the dietary needs and taste preferences of a user without prompting for keywords.

A preferential retrieval system was investigated in a previous study [1]. this conventional system learns user preferences through interactive genetic algorithm (IGA). However, when a user has a variety of preferences, the conventional system is hard put to learn the user's various preferences. In fact, the IGA of the conventional system converges to a single local solution. If the system continually makes recommendations that match one preference, the user may feel discontente. Thus, the system needs to recommend a variety of recipes that matches the breadth of a user's tastes.

In this paper, we propose a preferential retrieval system that employs an interactive immune algorithm (IIA). The proposed system can make recommendations

C. Stephanidis (Ed.): Posters, Part II, HCII 2013, CCIS 374, pp. 168–172, 2013.

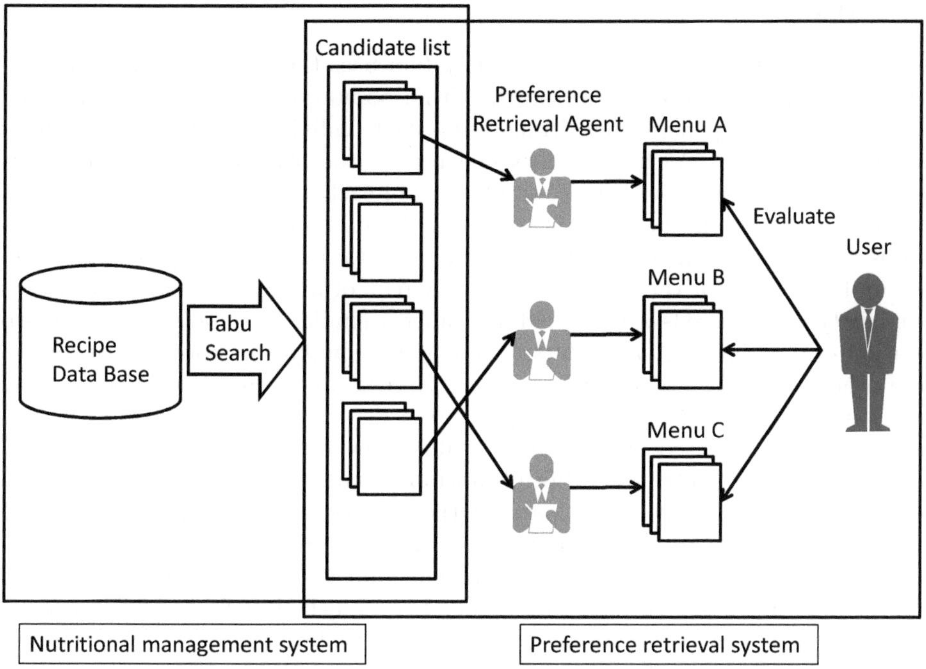

Fig. 1. Support system for healthy eating habits

to users in accordance with their preference. We focus on describing the preferential retrieval system and the simulations performed.

2 Support System for Healthy Eating Habits

2.1 System Framework

The support system for healthy eating habits is shown in Fig. 1. The support system consists of a nutritional management system and a preferential retrieval system. The nutritional management system was developed in a previous study [2]. Its database contains recipe data. The nutritional management system first uses the tabu search method to create nutritionally balanced menus that combine multiple recipes and then stores the generated menus in a candidate list. The preferential retrieval system recommends menus and learns user preferences. Its preferential retrieval agent uses the co-evaluation model and the only evaluation model proposed in a previous study [3]. Based on the stored information about user preferences, the agent searches the candidate list and selects a menu that the agent estimates will be approved by the user. The agent recommends the selected menu to the user. The user then evaluates the menus recommended menu by several agents. By repeating these operations, the agents can learn the various preferences of the user and recommend a greater diversity of appropriate menus to the user. In this manner, the agents evolve based on the evaluations by users.

2.2 IIA

In this study, the preferential retrieval system uses the IIA to learn the preferences of users [4]. The evolution starts with a population of randomly generated individuals. In a genetic algorithm (GA), each individual is represented by a so-called antibody. With every new generation, the fitness of each antibody is evaluated by the user, and the concentration of each antibody is calculated from the degrees of similarity between the pairs of antibodies. The degree of similarity is a measure of the extent to which the genetic information of one antibody is similar to that of the other antibody. A pair of antibodies with a degree of similarity that exceeds a threshold are called - similar antibodies. The concentration of a given antibody refers to how many similar antibodies exist among the other antibodies. The antibodies that exceed a concentration threshold are separated into memory cells and suppressor cells. Antibodies similar to the suppressor cells are erased. The expected value of each antibody is determined by its fitness and concentration. Multiple antibodies are stochastically selected from the current population on the basis of these expected values. In addition, the selected antibodies are modified by crossovers and mutations to form a new population, which is used in the next generation. The algorithm is terminated when the maximum number of generations has been reached. The well-known interactive evolutionary computation (IEC) generates solutions (antibodies) that are presented to the user. In other words, systems using IEC cannot learn preferences of users. Furthermore, systems using IEC require users to evaluate the evolving solutions repeatedly. Thus, increasing the burden that a user bears for evaluating will negatively affect the optimization performance. The preferential retrieval system can solve these issues using a preferential retrieval agent by the co-evaluation model and only evaluation model.

2.3 Preferential Retrieval Agent

The preferential retrieval agent implements a model to decode information about the user's preferences and retrieve a menu from a candidate list. That is, the agent can recommend menus for users according to their preferences. In this preferential retrieval system, the agent is optimized by including the IIA, which enable the agent to learn information about user preferences.

2.4 Co-evaluation Model

A preferential retrieval agent evolves by learning from a user's evaluation of a recipe that was presented to the user. However, an agent designed using the co-evaluation model also consider the evaluations of recipes presented by other agents. The agent evaluates all recipes that are presented to the user based on the information about the user's preferences. Conversely, the user evaluates all recipes that are presented by agents. The closer the evaluation by the user and the evaluation by the agent, the greater is the amount of consideration given by the agent. Using the co-evaluation model, the agent can obtain more information for its self optimization. Moreover, applying the co-evaluation model reduces the number of times that a users needs to evaluate data.

2.5 Only Evaluation Model

The optimization performance of the IIA can be improved by increasing the number of antibodies (agents). However, this increases the user's burden of evaluating recipes, because the number of recipes is the same as the number of agents. Therefore, this study uses an agent that employs the only evaluation model. Even though this agent is optimized using the co-evaluation model, it does not present menus to the user. Thus, by using the only evaluation model, the optimization performance of the IIA is enhanced without increasing the user's burden.

3 Simulations

3.1 Overview

In this section, we discuss the simulations that were performed to measure the optimization performance of the agent. The records of past evaluations by a user were exploited to improve the performance in the simulations. Thus, we replaced a real user with a simulated user. The simulated user was provided with some preferences to represent the variety of the real user's preferences. Hence, the simulated user evaluated the presented data using the same criteria as the real user. The most favorable evaluation was taken as the evaluation of the data presented. The number of generations of evaluation records was 20 when using the preferential retrieval system. We used 180 elements of the cooking ingredients as the recipe data. The output of each simulation was the error between the evaluations by the best preferential retrieval agent and the simulated user.

3.2 Results

The errors output by the simulation are shown in Table. 1, where GA denotes genetic algorithm, IA denotes the immune Algorithm, and NO denotes a nonoptimized agent. Table. 1 shows that the IA is preferable to the GA and the NO.

The simulation output related to learning a variety of user preferences is shown in Table. 2, which confirms that the GA can learn only a single user preference but the IA can learn a variety of user preferences.

3.3 Discussion

This study demonstrates how an agent in a preferential retrieval system can learn the preferences of a user. Such agents can thus recommend menus according to the preferences of users. In addition, this study demonstrates that the IIA can learn more of a user's preferences than the IGA. One limitation of this study is that all of the experiments were conducted with one simulated user instead of real users.

Table 1. Comparison of average errors of the IA, GA, and NO

Method - variety of poreferences	GA - 1	GA - 3	GA - 5	IA - 1	IA - 3	IA - 5	NO - 1	NO - 3	NO - 5
Average error	1.49	1.69	2.00	0.61	0.60	0.67	2.37	2.40	2.52

Table 2. Comparison of average learning

Method - variety of poreference	GA - 1	GA - 3	GA - 5	IA - 1	IA - 3	IA - 5
Average Learning variety of preferences	1	1	1	1	2.2	3.4

4 Conclusions

In this paper, we proposed a support system for healthy eating habits. We described not only the support system itself but also the simulations performed using this system. The preferential retrieval system learned the user's preferences using the preferential retrieval agent. Moreover, the preferential retrieval system exploited this information about the user's preferences to recommended menus that pleased the user. Through simulations, we confirmed the effectiveness of the optimization performance of the agent. In particular, we demonstrated that the IIA can learn more of a user's preferences than the IGA. As part of future work, we plan to test the effectiveness of this method further by applying it for real users instead of a lone simulated user in future.

Acknowledgments. This work was supported by Adaptable and Seamless Technology Transfer Program through target-driven R&D, JST.

References

1. Hakamata, J., Tokumi, Y., Tokumaru, M.: Development of a healthy eating habits support system that presents menus considering a user's taste and health: Optimization of Kansei retrieval system. In: 12th International Symposium on Advanced Intelligent Systems (ISIS 2011), pp. 479–482 (2011)
2. Tokumi, Y., Hakamata, J., Tokumaru, M.: Development of a nutritional management system for a healthy eating habits support system. Journal of Advanced Computational Intelligence and Intelligent Informatics 17(2), 324–334 (2013)
3. Tokumaru, M., Muranaka, N.: An Evolutionary Fuzzy Color Emotion Model for Coloring Support Systems. In: 2008 IEEE International Conference on Fuzzy Systems (FUZZ 2008), pp. 408–413 (2008)
4. Inagawa, Y., Hakamata, J., Tokumaru, M.: A framework of recommender system considering the variety of Kansei. In: Joint 6th International Conference on Soft Computing and Intelligent Systems and 13th International Symposium on Advanced Intelligent Systems (SCIS & ISIS 2012), pp. 197–202 (2012)

Wearable Health Monitoring System

Ali Mehmood Khan

TZi-Universität Bremen, Bremen, Germany
akhan@tzi.de

Abstract. One of the major scientific undertakings over the past few years has been exploring the interaction between humans and machines in mobile environments. In this work, we will examine how to utilize existing technology in order to build eHealth system for the heart patients. This system should be able to establish an interaction between patients and health physician so that patients don't need to visit clinic every time.

Keywords: Physical activities, emotion states, Physiological data, eHealth monitoring systems.

1 Introduction

Heart patients are supposed to visit their health physicians for a routine medical check-up on a regular basis. Sometimes, they come from long distance and sometimes they miss some events because of their medical appointment. Question is that why patients always need to follow this old tradition, cannot they just send all needed information to the health physician so that he could assess them? What kinds of information do health physicians need for assessing their patients' health conditions? In some cases, especially in heart diseases, physical activities and emotion states are also required along with the physiological information for the doctor in order to examine his patient's conditions when he is away from the doctor's clinic [1]. Researchers think that following information is needed for assessing heart conditions [1]

- Physical activities {sitting, standing, laying, walking, ascending/descending stairs, running, cycling, strength-training, swimming etc}
- Emotion states {sad, dislike, joy and stress}
- Physiological data {blood volume pulse, respiratory rate and ECG}

2 Related Work

A lot of research has been done for the recognition of physical activities using wearable sensor. Researchers have figured out several physical activities using wearable sensors like sitting [2,5,6,7,8,15], standing [2,5,6,7,8,15], laying [7,15], walking [2,3,4,5,6,7,8,15], climbing stairs [2,3,5,6,7,8,15], running [4,6,7,8,15], cycling [4,7,8,15], strength-training[7,16] and so on.

C. Stephanidis (Ed.): Posters, Part II, HCII 2013, CCIS 374, pp. 173–177, 2013.

Researchers already have identified some emotion states using sensors [9, 11]. In paper [9], a Bluetooth enabled skin conductance device was employed in gathering data in addition to the "blood volume pulse", "electromyogram" and "respiration". The researchers used the information obtained from the aforementioned techniques to mark the states neutral, anger, hate, grief, love, romantic, joy and reverence emotion states [10].

3 Hypothesis

The varying information (physical activities, emotion states) recognized by a wearable system along with the physiological data (blood volume pulse, respiration rate, body temperature and heart beat rate) pertaining to a patient can be transmitted to a physician, which he can then examine with the same efficiency as if the patient were physically present.

- ***First assumption***
  - The acceleration measured by a wearable device (3D accelerometer) indicates which activity the person is performing (lying, sitting, walking and running, ascending/ descending stairs, cycling, swimming and strength-training) with 100% accuracy.
- ***Second assumption***
  - The physiological data measured by wearable devices (EMG, blood volume, pulse, respiration and skin conductance sensor) indicate which emotion state the person is in (sad, dislike, joy and stress) with 100% accuracy.

4 Planned Research

In order to prove our hypothesis, we want to conduct a user study where we will hire heart patients and then following tasks will be performed as shown in Figure 1.

- Heart patients will do physical activities (Sitting, Standing, running, walking, ascending/descending stairs, cycling and strength-training) and meanwhile their physiological information will be recorded.
- We will change their emotions from Normal to sad, joy, dislike and Stress by showing IAPS images [12] and follow different experimental methodologies for changing their emotions [13, 14], we will use Lickert scale for measuring emotions. Meanwhile their physiological information will be also recorded.
- Patients' information (Anamnesis, physical activities, emotion states, physiological data) will be given to a physician and he will be asked to assess patients' health condition. (Indirect interaction)
- Same patients will be examined by a physician and he will assess their health conditions. (Direct interaction)
- Physician will be asked to give a feedback w.r.t direct and indirect interaction. (Evaluation)

- Later, we will do a comparison in order to know the difference between both datasets (direct interaction vs indirect interaction).

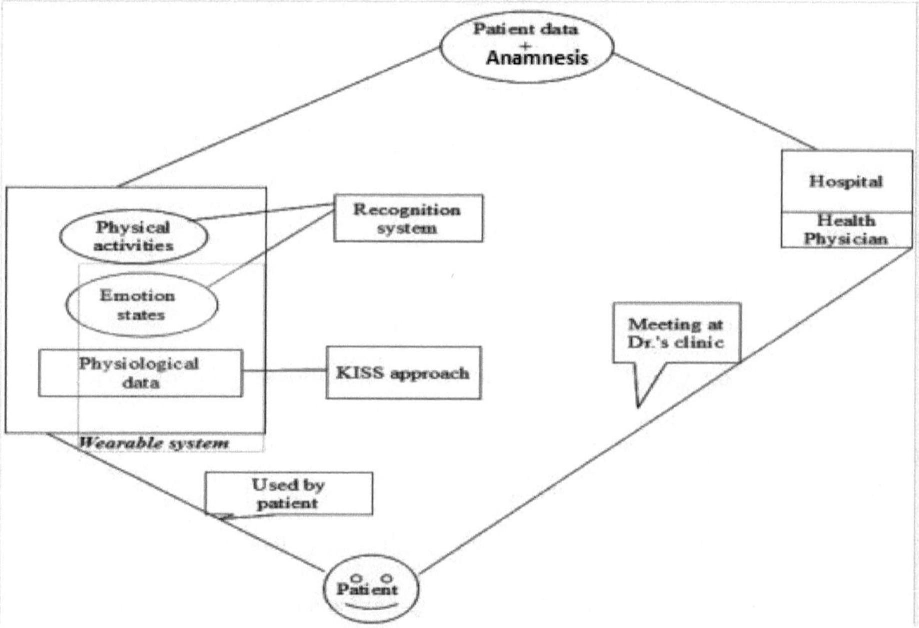

Fig. 1. Overall architecture

4.1 Test Case of our Plan

Name:			Anamnesis
Age:	Gender:	BMI:	

Physical activity	Time	Emotion states	Measurement (ECG, BVP, Body temperature, breath rate)
Sitting	09:00 – 09:02	Normal	~09:01– 09:02
Walking	09:05 – 09:07	Normal	~09:06 – 09:07
Lying	09:10 – 09:12	Normal	~09:11 – 09:12
Running	09:15 – 09:17	Normal	~09:16 – 09:17
Cycling	09:20 – 09:22	Normal	~09:21 – 09:22
Ascending stairs	09:25 – 09:27	Normal	~09:26 – 09:27

Descending stairs	09:30 – 09:32	Normal	~09:31 – 09:32
Standing	09:35 – 09:37	Normal	~09:36 – 09:37
Sitting	[Time]	to joy	[Time]
Sitting	[Time]	to sad	[Time]
Sitting	[Time]	to dislike	[Time]
Sitting	[Time]	to stress	[Time]

4.2 Physician's Room

Direct Interaction

Direct interaction between physician & patient

- Physician would assess patient's health conditions [Time]

Indirect Interaction

Results from test case with Anamnesis (without patient)

- Physician would assess patient's health conditions [Time]

Table 1. Feedback from Physician w.r.t direct and indirect interaction

Accepted (No difference)	**Accepted (Minor difference**	**Accepted to some extend**	**Acceptable (with some conditions)**	**Acceptable (for limited cases)**	**Rejected (No match)**

Comments from physician:

4.3 Target Group

- We want to target heart patients (with normal risk) from age 40 to 60 years.
- Would be great if we could get around 20 patients (negotiable).

References

1. Khan, A.M.: Personal state and emotion monitoring by wearable computing and machine learning. In: BCS-HCI 2012, Newcastle, UK (2011)
2. Lester, J., Choudhury, T., Borriello, G.: A practical approach to recognizing physical activities. In: Fishkin, K.P., Schiele, B., Nixon, P., Quigley, A. (eds.) PERVASIVE 2006. LNCS, vol. 3968, pp. 1–16. Springer, Heidelberg (2006)

3. Van Laerhoven, K., Aronsen, A.K.: Memorizing what you did last week: Towards detailed actigraphy with a wearable sensor. In: 27th International Conference on Distributed Computing Systems Workshops, ICDCSW 2007, pp. 47–47 (2007)
4. Choudhury, T., et al.: The mobile sensing platform: An embedded activity recognition system. IEEE Pervasive Computing, 32–41 (2008)
5. Kern, N., Schiele, B., Schmidt, A.: Multisensor activity context detection for wearable computing. LNCS, pp. 220–234 (2003)
6. Maurer, U., Rowe, A., Smailagic, A., Siewiorek, D.: Location and Activity Recognition Using eWatch: A Wearable Sensor Platform. In: Cai, Y., Abascal, J. (eds.) Ambient Intelligence in Everyday Life. LNCS (LNAI), vol. 3864, pp. 86–102. Springer, Heidelberg (2006)
7. Bao, L., Intille, S.S.: Activity recognition from user-annotated acceleration data. In: Ferscha, A., Mattern, F. (eds.) PERVASIVE 2004. LNCS, vol. 3001, pp. 1–17. Springer, Heidelberg (2004)
8. Khan, A.M.: Recognizing Physical Activities using Wii remote. International Journal of Information and Education Technology 3(1), 60–62 (2011) ISSN: 2010-3689
9. Strauss, M., Reynolds, C., Hughes, S., Park, K., Mcdarby, G., Picard, R.W.: The HandWave Bluetooth Skin Conductance Sensor
10. `http://affect.media.mit.edu/share-data.php` (January 17, 2010)
11. Kapoor, et al.: Automatic Prediction of Frustration. International Journal of Human Computer Studies 65(8), 724–736 (2007)
12. Lang, P.J., Bradley, M.M., Cuthbert, B.N.: International Affective Picture System (IAPS): Technical Manual and Affective Ratings. NIMH Center for the Study of Emotion and Attention (1997)
13. Vrana, S.R., Spence, E.L., Lang, P.J.: The Startle Probe Response: A New Measure of Emotion? Center for Research in Psychophysiology and Department of Clinical and Health Psychology. University of Florida
14. Bradley, M.M., Codispoti,M., Langa, P.J.: A multi-process account of startle modulation during affective perception. Center for the Study of Emotion and Attention, University of Florida, Gainesville, Florida, USA, Department of Psychology, University of Bologna, Bologna, Italy
15. Khan, A.M.: Recognizing Physical Activities Using Axivity device. eTELEMED, Nice, France (2013)
16. Khan, A.M., Kalkbrenner, G., Lawo, M.: Recognizing Physical Training Exercises Using the Axivity Device. ICT meets Medicine and Health, Bremen, Germany (2013)

Analysis on Drug Dosage Form Name Based on N-gram Technique and Network Analysis

Masaomi Kimura[1] and Fumito Tsuchiya[2]

[1] Shibaura Institute of Technology, 3-7-5 Toyosu, Koto City, Tokyo 135-8548, Japan
[2] International University of Health and Welfare, 2600-1 Kitakanemaru, Otawara City, Tochigi, 324-8501, Japan

Abstract. In this paper, we analyzed drug dosage form names. We created the network structure whose nodes are dosage form names. Its edges between dosage form names denote that they share some of sub-strings generated based on N-gram technique. We employed Simpson coefficient to define the weight of an edge. We proposed a new clustering method and applied it to the network. The results showed that "dosage forms" can be categorized based on not only physical form information but their application site,purpose,processing and so on.

Keywords: Medical safety, Dosage form, N-gram, Network analysis.

1 Introduction

Drugs have many kinds of forms, such as tablets, capsules, powder, intradermal injection and so on, which are categorized in "dosage forms". The information related to dosage forms is important to ensure the safety of medicinal usage, because the drugs with different dosage forms make their usage and effectiveness strength different, even if they have the same active ingredient.

Naively, we expect the word "dosage form" to indicate physical shapes of drugs. However, the names of dosage forms usually contain other information such as the routes of administration (*e.g.* oral powder) and properties (*e.g.* sustained-release tablets).

In Japan, there is a series of drug spec definition books called"Japanese Pharmacopoeia" [1]. It includes general rules for preparations, which define drug dosage forms. It is described that they are primarily categorized by the routes of administration / application sites of a body, and secondly categorized by physical forms, functions and properties. Though the categories are defined by medical experts but are not necessarily used as standard categories of dosage forms. In fact, there are no standard dosage form categories. This might originate in the variety of information contained in the names of dosage forms.

In this paper, we show the results of analyses applied to the names of dosage forms to identify the structures of the contained information. We employed the technique based on N-gram method and a novel network clustering technique.

We regarded the name of dosage forms as character strings and obtained a set of their sequential substrings. One reason why we used N-gram method is

C. Stephanidis (Ed.): Posters, Part II, HCII 2013, CCIS 374, pp. 178–182, 2013.

that the most of the length of each dosage form is short and, therefore, it can be regarded to carry much information per letter. Another reason is that the physical forms are usually expressed in short letter strings. Our strategy is to regard dosage form names as nodes in a network and the pairs of sharing the same sequential substrings as edges. We also introduced the weight of edges based on Simpsons coefficient.

The existing clustering methods have some difficulties. The traditional ones are maximization of modularity and spectral clustering. The difficulty of modularity maximization is known as resolution limit and the one of spectral clustering comes from the interpolation of discrete cluster label (integer) to real number. We propose the method that assigns the quantities to (nearly) diagonalize the adjacent matrix of a network. The nodes that have the same value of the quantities constitute a community of the network.

2 Target Data

We used 158 dosage form names listed in a code table used for Japanese drug approval, which is disclosed by Japanese authority, Ministry of Health, Labour and Welfare [2]. For simplicity, we omitted "日局" (official recipes for Japanese drugs), "その他の" (others) , and words in parentheses, which show additional information. We identified the same dosage form names after the omission, and separated plural drug names if they are bundled in one name. As a result, we obtained 119 target dosage form names.

3 Methods

We utilized N-gram method and extracted all substrings in each of dosage form names. Since a dosage form name consists of plural components which indicate physical forms, applied body parts and so on, we assumed that the more common substrings the dosage forms have, the more similar they are. Based on this policy, we propose the analysis method that connect a pair of dosage form names sharing the components with an edge and apply graph partitioning (community findings) to the resultant network [1].

Naive application of graph partitioning to the network does not reflect the commonality extent of components. Therefore, after connecting dosage form names with edges, we assigned weight to each edge. In order to measure the commonality, we used Simpson coefficient,

$$w_{ij} = \frac{|X_i \cap X_j|}{\min(|X_i|, |X_j|)}, \tag{1}$$

where X_i denotes the set of substrings generated by N-grams. We set $w_{ij} = 0$, if $\min(|X_i|, |X_j|) < \epsilon$ for some threshold ϵ.

[1] We should note that our target network is undirected and simple.

The standard methods of graph partitioning/community finding are Spectral clustering and Modularity maximization proposed by Newman et. al [3, 4]. The former needs to define the number of communities in advance and the latter has un-resolved problem, named as "resolution limit". We, therefore, propose another graph partitioning method. In order to get good partition, we arrange the well-connected nodes to belong to the same community. In terms of an adjacency matrix, its rows/columns corresponding to well-connected nodes should be neighbor, and this requires that non-zero elements of the adjacency matrix of the network get together to diagonal elements. In order to quantify this, we assigned the position x_i to Node i and defined covariance and variance of x_i as followings:

$$\sigma_{xx} = \sum_{i,j} \frac{A_{ij}}{2M}(x_i - \bar{x})(x_j - \bar{x}), \tag{2}$$

$$\sigma_x^2 = \sum_{i} \frac{k_i}{2M}(x_i - \bar{x})^2, \tag{3}$$

where A_{ij} is an adjacency matrix, k_i is the degree of Node i ($\sum_i k_i = 2M$), and $\bar{x} = \sum_i \frac{k_i}{2M} x_i$.

We assigned a series of $\{x_i\}$ to maximize the correlation coefficient,

$$r = \frac{\sigma_{xx}}{\sigma_x^2}. \tag{4}$$

As for the resultant series $\{x_i\}$, the value x_i for the well-connected nodes should be identical, since the position of non-zero elements of the adjacency matrix, (x_i, x_j), are almost along the line $y = x$, namely, $x_i \simeq x_j$. Therefore, after sorting the series $\{x_i\}$, we can find communities as "plateaus" of x_i values. We generalized this by utilizing weight matrix w_{ij} instead of adjacency matrix A_{ij}.

4 Results

Table 1 shows the resultant $\{x_i\}$. This shows that the similar dosage form names have similar values of x_i.

What is interesting is "絆創膏" (adhesive bandage) and "軟膏剤" (ointment) respectively belong to different clusters, though they share the Kanji character "膏" (plaster).

Contrary to this, "凍結乾燥注射剤" (freeze dry injection) and "粉末注射剤" (powder injection) belong to the same community but belong to the other community of liquid injections. It is interesting that the two dosage forms are in the same community, though they do not share the same substrings other than "注射剤"(injection). We note the fact that the word "性" (property) is contained in the dosage form names of liquid injections. This seems to divide liquid injection from other type of injections. This suggests that we can interpret the community which freeze dry injection belongs to as the community corresponding to the non-liquid injections.

Table. 1. The dosage form names and their x_i values. The values of x_i are normalized so that their maximum is 1 and minimum is 0. "Dosage Form (J)" in the header indicates original Japanese dosage form names, and "Dosage Form (E)" indicates corresponding English dosage form names.

Dosage Form (J)	Dosage Form (E)	x_i	Dosage Form (J)	Dosage Form (E)	x_i
気体	gas	1.00	腸溶性細粒	enteric-coated fines	0.08
液体	liquid	0.97	徐放性顆粒	extended-release granule	0.08
輸液	transfusion	0.93	腸溶性顆粒	enteric-coated granule	0.08
液絆	liquid plaster	0.87	注入剤	injectable filler	0.08
鉱物生薬	metal crude drug	0.83	浣腸剤	enema	0.08
薬品付絆創膏	medicated adhesive plaster	0.67	徐放カプセル	extended-release capsule	0.07
絆創膏	adhesive bandage	0.66	腸溶カプセル	enteric-coated capsule	0.07
ガーゼ付絆創膏	gauze plaster	0.64	コーティング細粒	coated fines	0.07
ハッカゴム膏	mint gum plaster	0.59	コーティング顆粒	coated granule	0.07
硬膏	emplastrum	0.57	徐放錠	extended-release tablet	0.07
軟膏剤	ointment	0.57	腸溶錠	enteric-coated tablet	0.07
軟稠エキス	soft extract	0.52	バッカル錠	buccal tablet	0.07
軟カプセル	soft capsule	0.52	内用細粒	internal fines	0.07
眼軟膏	eye ointment	0.46	コーティング錠	coated tablet	0.07
洗口うがい剤	mouth rinse collutorium	0.20	内用素顆粒	internal granule	0.07
洗浄・清拭剤	cleaner	0.20	かみ砕き錠	chewable tablet	0.07
洗眼剤	eye wash	0.20	重層錠	multi-layered tablet	0.07
尿道坐剤	urethral bougie	0.18	有核錠	pressure-coated tablet	0.07
膣坐剤	vaginal suppository	0.18	外用顆粒	external granule	0.06
肛門坐剤	rectal suppository	0.18	内用素錠	internal tablet	0.06
コロジオン剤	collodion preparation	0.18	内用発泡錠	internal effervescent tablet	0.06
グリセリン剤	glycerin preparation	0.18	顆粒	granule	0.06
乳剤性点眼剤	emulsion eye drop	0.17	外用発泡錠	external effervescent tablet	0.06
水性点眼剤	aqueous eye drop	0.17	外用錠	external tablet	0.06
非水性点眼剤	nonaqueous eye drop	0.17	内用	internal	0.06
懸濁性点眼剤	suspension eye drop	0.17	内用エアゾール	internal aerosol	0.06
懸濁剤	suspension agent	0.14	外用	external	0.06
芳香水剤	aromatic water	0.13	内用散剤	internal powder	0.06
皮膚用水剤	dermatological water	0.13	外用散剤	external powder	0.05
懸濁性注射剤	suspension injection	0.11	散剤	powder	0.05
非水性注射剤	nonaqueous injection	0.11	体外ガス剤	external gas	0.05
水性注射剤	aqueous injection	0.11	外用エアゾール剤	external aerosol	0.05
乳剤性注射剤	emulsion injection	0.10	組み合わせ剤	combination drugs	0.04
粉末注射剤	powder injection	0.09	噴霧・吸入剤	inhalation	0.03
凍結乾燥注射剤	freeze dry injection	0.09	ペンシル剤	pencil	0.03
粉末剤	powdered drugs	0.09	吸入ガス剤	inhalation gas	0.03
粉末状エアゾール	powdered aerosol	0.09	吸入型エアゾール剤	inhalation aerosol	0.02
乾燥エキス	dry extracts	0.09	綿吸着剤	cotton adsorbent	0.00
注射錠皮下埋没用	implantation injection tablet	0.09	紙吸着剤	paper adsorbent	0.00
注射錠	injection tablet	0.09	合成樹脂吸着剤	synthetic-resin adsorbent	0.00
徐放性細粒	extended-release fines	0.08	ガーゼ吸着剤	gauze adsorbent	0.00

We should also note another point. The community whose $x_i = 0.06$ contains several different physical dosage forms, such as tablets, capsules and fines. The dosage form names in the community commonly contain the substrings "外用" (outer) and "内用"(inner). This suggests that view points to categorize dosage forms are not necessarily limited to physical dosage forms but can be others, such as body parts which drugs are administered to.

These results suggest that Japanese dosage form names do not necessarily focus on drugs' physical forms. This is consistent with the categorization policy of Japanese Pharmacopoeia, primarily categorization by the routes of administration and secondly categorization by physical forms.

5 Conclusion

In this paper, we analyzed the dosage form name of Japanese drugs. We used the technique based on N-gram method and a novel network clustering technique.

We tend to associate the word "dosage form names" with physical form of drugs. However, our results suggest that dosage form names should be categorized by body parts which drugs are administered to or their properties prior to categorization by physical drug forms.

In future works, we will propose the coding system of dosage form names based on our results.

References

Ministry of Health, Labour and Welfare: Japanese Pharmacopoeia (2012), http://www.mhlw.go.jp/topics/bukyoku/iyaku/yakkyoku/

Ministry of Health, Labour and Welfare: FD Application Related to Approve of Drugs, Cosmetics and Medical Equipments (2012), http://web.fd-shinsei.go.jp/download/software/index.html

Newman, M.E.J.: Modularity and community structure in networks. Proc. Natl. Acad. Sci. 103, 8577–8582 (2006)

Newman, M.E.J.: Finding community structure in networks using the eigenvectors of matrices. Phys. Rev. E 74, 036104 (2006)

Integrating Potential Users Into the Development of a Medical Wrist Watch in Four Steps

Sylvia Kowalewski, Johanna Kluge, and Martina Ziefle

RWTH Aachen University, HCI-C, Theaterplatz 14,
52062 Aachen, Germany
{kowalewski,kluge,ziefle}@comm.rwth-aachen.de

Abstract. The focus of this study was on the integration of potential users into the development of a mobile medical device from the first idea up to a finished prototype. Apart from medical functions the special feature of this mobile small screen device is its completely icon based menu structure. In three consecutive studies the requirements concerning the design and usability of the wrist watch and its functionality were evaluated. A specific impact had the design of the, warning functions and the icon development that should be easily understood by affected users. In a fourth study, the developed prototype of the mobile small screen device was tested according to usability aspects and comprehensibility of the menu structure. Beyond chronically ill users, which were the target users, a group of healthy users served as control condition for evaluation purposes. Overall it could be shown that a completely icon-based menu structure on a small screen device is not only feasible, but also highly suitable if the design is following a completely user-centered development and evaluation procedure.

Keywords: Mobile devices, icon recognition, medical devices, hardware design, usability.

1 Introduction

Icon based menus have a lot of advantages compared to text based menus, especially in a medical context. Text-based menus are problematical for several reasons. The linguistic terms used to indicate an item's functions, such as their assignment to function classes (category headers) are oftentimes ambiguous and difficult to comprehend [1]. Furthermore, the representation of linguistic terms is space consuming thus wasting a resource of increasing scarcity and are, in addition, hard to read for vision-impaired persons [2]. Finally, text-based menu structures establish language barriers, a crucial disadvantage in times of increasing globalization.

In times of demographic change and the resulting increased demand for technical and medical assistance it is indispensable to integrate the needs of potential users in the design process of new (medical) devices. Moreover, everyday life is determined by globalization. It is thus important that persons with different linguistic and cultural backgrounds are able to understand the meaning of signs to gain access to a technical device [3]. Therefore, an icon-based menu-structure is favorable – provided the users

C. Stephanidis (Ed.): Posters, Part II, HCII 2013, CCIS 374, pp. 183–186, 2013.

are able to deal with it. For this reason it is most important to create a menu structure and a user-tailored icon design that are intuitively understandable. If this succeeds, a completely symbol-based navigation is space economical, intuitively understandable and independent of the linguistic background. To create such a menu, it is most important to have a good research base - especially for the healthcare context, in which medical necessity and critical time frames are crucial. The medical context is very sensitive. A healthcare device has to meet many more requirements compared to conventional ICT-devices. Medical assistance is often connoted with unpleasant attributes like vulnerability and illness. Devices equipped with medical monitoring functionality (e.g. monitoring cardio-vascular data anytime and anywhere) might cross personal intimacy boundaries, raising concerns about privacy, data security and maybe loss of control [4]. Also, users show a higher heterogeneity concerning their cognitive and physical abilities in this context [5]. This is another important point that has to be considered while creating a menu structure for a small screen device in the healthcare section. Considering the potential advantages of an icon-based menu over a text-based menu structure for small screen devices and the challenging requirements medical functionality implies in addition, it is indispensable to integrate users into the whole developing process of an icon based small screen device in order to understand needs, barriers, and usability requirements. Users are considered as experts for needs and concerns towards a (new) technology and novel device designs, because in the end, the success or failure of a product depends on the user's decision. Thus, our research focuses on the integration of the user into the developing process.

2 Method and Results

In this section the used methods and key results for each of the four steps are presented.

Step 1 – Understanding User Requirements Concerning a Medical Mobile Small Screen Device. The first step contained the development of a survey in order to get an understanding of the user's requirements on a mobile small screen device. A group of 64 people affected by diabetes or heart diseases (age 13-78 years) and a group of 30 healthy people (age 19-61 years) took part in this study. The aim of the survey was to evaluate disease specific user characteristics, special needs of ill users towards an "every day helper" and to answer the question which characteristics a "mobile small screen device" should have. Results revealed that diabetics have indeed other requirements than cardiac patients. Whereas reliability and safety aspects are most important for cardiac patients, diabetics emphasized design aspects of a mobile small screen device and the need for keeping control over their disease and not to relinquish it to a technical device. The stressed importance of design aspects in the diabetics group might be due to the younger age of diabetic participants (compared to the cardiac group).

Step 2 – Uncovering Users' Mental Representation of Navigation Items. In a second step, the sign production method was used to uncover mental representations of menu items [6]. A sample of 28 participants (age 17-55 years) was requested to draw suggestions for the graphical representation of 51 reference functions of a mobile small screen device half which contained disease specific functions. Based on the results, icons were developed and in a further study validated by asking users (N = 45, age 23 – 68 years) to label the symbols according to their function and to test whether the symbols are recognizable in different colors and sizes even on small displays. Based on these criteria a total of 42 icons were selected in the end.

Step 3 – Blink, Sound or Vibration? Thirdly, we conducted a computer based empirical testing to find out what an alarm design of a medical device should look and sound like (N = 36; age 21-72 years). In this step, different usage contexts were taken into account (at home, supermarket, work) and four different warning modalities (sound, color, luminance, movement) were evaluated. The main study objective was to find an appropriate way to warn the user in case of emergency and to remind the user of daily activities like medication. Results clearly revealed that user prefer context sensitive warning modalities that express the urgency of the warning through a specific color. In the working context all users emphasized the importance of a discrete signal with pulsating light and no sound signal with exception for urgent emergency cases in which a medium sound would be accepted. In contrast to that, a warning or reminder signal in a supermarket or at home should be in medium noise in any case. For simple reminders participants preferred green pulsating light and yellow for urgent warnings. Blink or flicker was never chosen as option for light movement whereas all participants valued a vibration as best modality in every context.

Step 4 – Ease of Use and Usability. The last step of the evaluation procedure was directed to the testing of the developed prototype of the mobile small screen device. The main focus was the comprehensibility of the menu structure and readability. The aim was to get a realistic idea of the ease of use and the usability of the icon-based menu structure. Within the usability test, we used thinking aloud as a method to understand participants' attitudes, feelings and cognitions when working on the wrist watch. The first half of the testing was free exploration and the second half required task solving. Additionally, participant observation by video was applied. A total of 20 people took part in this study (age 30-79 years). Participants got no instructions how to handle the device neither in the first part of the testing nor in the second in order to evaluate its self-explanatory character. In addition to the two practical trials participants were requested to fill in a questionnaire that contained several control aspects like technical experience especially with touch screen devices or whether one needs glasses. Altogether participants were able to handle nearly all functions of the device on their own. The sole exception were the two disease specific functions which half of the tested group did not understand until they got information from the experimenter on the disease specific purpose of these functions. Icons were, even for the oldest participant (79 years), readable and understandable. Generally no major age-related differences were uncovered and even experience with touch screens had no influence on the usability of the device. The most positive remarked characteristic of the device was its warning and reminder function as well as the touch screen.

3 Discussion

The outcome of our research showed that an icon-based menu navigation is easy to handle for users of all ages. All tested users appreciated the idea of a mobile small screen device for assistance and monitoring in case of diabetes or heart diseases and the finished prototype in the end was evaluated very positive regarding its functions. This fact might be the result of the detailed evaluation of user requirements from the early beginning of the design process. Through the extensive evaluation of the designed icons and their practicability on the base of the survey, a menu structure was designed which was easy to handle for the users. Nearly all icons showed little ambiguity when used in the context of the medical device. The participants were able to navigate through the menu successfully and showed a high comprehension of the structure and the meaning of the items although conditions in the usability test were really difficult due to the fact that participants got no instructions how to handle the device. Based on our findings it can be concluded that the integration of the user from the early beginning of a design process provides a guarantee for a device that meets the demands regarding usability and ease of use in all age groups. Also, the advantage of an icon-based menu over a text-based menu as mentioned in the beginning can be seen as being confirmed.

Acknowledgments. Authors thank participants for their willingness to share their expert view with us. Also, authors owe gratitude to Michael Diebold, Ines Lindner, Lena Taube and Philipp Brauner for research support.

References

1. Benbasat, I., Todd, P.: An experimental investigation of interface design alternatives: icon vs. text and direct manipulation vs. Menus. International Journal of Man-Machine Studies 38, 369–402 (1993)
2. Schröder, S., Ziefle, M.: Effects of icon concreteness and complexity on semantic transparency- Younger and older users. In: Miesenberger, K., Klaus, J., Zagler, W.L., Karshmer, A.I. (eds.) ICCHP 2008. LNCS, vol. 5105, pp. 90–97. Springer, Heidelberg (2008)
3. Pappachan, P., Ziefle, M.: Cultural Influences on the Comprehensibility of Icons in Mobile-Computer-Interaction. Behaviour and Information Technology 27(4), 331–337 (2008)
4. Wilkowska, W., Ziefle, M.: Perception of privacy and security for acceptance of E-health technologies: Exploratory analysis for diverse user groups. In: User-Centred-Design of Pervasive Health Applications (UCD-PH 2011), Held in Conjunction with the 5th ICST/IEEE Conference on Pervasive Computing Technologies for Healthcare 2011, pp. 593–600 (2011)
5. Gaul, S., Wilkowska, W., Ziefle, M.: Accounting for user diversity in the acceptance of medical assistive technologies. In: Full Paper at the 3rd International ICST Conference on Electronic Healthcare for the 21st Century (eHealth 2010) (2010)
6. Howell, W.C., Fuchs, A.H.: Population stereotypy in code design. Organisational Behavior in Human Performance 3, 310–339 (1968)

Factors Affecting Physician-Patient Communication in the Medical Exam Room

Jennifer Lyons[1], Ram Dixit[1], Colleen Emmenegger[1],
Linda L. Hill[2], Nadir Weibel[3], and James D. Hollan[1,3]

[1] Department of Cognitive Science
[2] Department of Family and Preventive Medicine
[3] Department of Computer Science and Engineering
University of California, San Diego, La Jolla, CA 92093, USA
{j2lyons,rdixit,cemmenegger,llhill,weibel,hollan}@ucsd.edu

Abstract. The recent push towards patient-centered health care has put a greater emphasis on patient health literacy. Health literacy is influenced by communication between physicians and patients. We conducted research at a local health clinic to examine communication between physicians, patients, and interpreters that were present to assist patients with limited English proficiency (LEP). We used the framework of Distributed Cognition to broaden our unit of analysis beyond individuals to include artifacts and the physical environment. We analyze three factors influencing communication: the availability of electronic medical records (EMR), the use of paper documents, and the presence of an interpreter. The physical space and artifacts are shown to impose constraints upon interaction and the flow of information throughout the exam room. We discuss implications for redesigning medical examination rooms and information technologies to create collaborative spaces that better support physician-patient communication, enhance patient understanding, and improve health literacy.

Keywords: Communication, health literacy, multimodal, Distributed Cognition.

1 Introduction

Health literacy is a key element of patient-centered health care that involves encouraging patients to take a more active role in understanding and managing their medical care [1]. An important contributor to health literacy is the communication that occurs between the physician and the patient [2].

In contrast to research in medical areas based on classical models of cognition, which focus primarily on the properties of single individuals, our research builds on the theory of Distributed Cognition [3,4]. Communication is seen as an emergent property of a system, which comprises not only of individuals, but artifacts, technology, and the sociocultural worlds in which activity is situated [5].

This exploratory pilot study investigates communication within the exam room of a local clinic serving LEP patients who often require interpreters. We explore the role

C. Stephanidis (Ed.): Posters, Part II, HCII 2013, CCIS 374, pp. 187–191, 2013.

of artifacts, interpreters, and the seating arrangement in communication. By highlighting ways in which communication is unsupported, our analysis can inform a redesign of the exam room to better support physician-patient communication and improve health literacy.

2 Methods

We collected data at a local community health center that provides comprehensive medical care for low income and multi-ethnic patient populations. The clinic provides interpreters in 8 languages to support physician-patient communication. EMRs have been used for all patient encounters since May 2010. The EMRs store patient medical history, and provide functions for note taking, preventative care, prescriptions, etc.

Two Microsoft Kinects were used to record multimodal data (body position, directional audio, video, depth-imaging) during medical exam sessions. We recorded visits with 12 consented adult patients (7 female, 5 male, half requiring an interpreter). Session lengths varied from approximately 5 to 13 minutes. The physician used a pause button to stop recording during physical exams.

To organize and analyze these data we employed the ChronoViz data analysis suite [6]. A group of 5 researchers analyzed the data from the 12 sessions, focusing on the general structure of each session and patterns of interaction. Two sessions (one English-fluent and one LEP) were selected for detailed analysis, which involved coding across the session for multiple modalities (head, body, hands, speech).

3 Analysis

The exam room system is a complex multiparty multimodal system. In our study, the physician sat in a rolling swivel chair side-by-side with patients seated on the edge of the exam table. When an interpreter was present, he/she sat across from the patient in a chair. The EMR rests on a mobile platform, positioned directly in front of the physician. In the following sections, we enumerate examples of emergent communication pathways, and ways in which the communication is supported or not.

3.1 Physician-Patient Interaction with EMR

The physician often references the EMR and moves it to be more accessible to the patient. In one instance, the physician asks the patient whether she remembered a recent blood test. The physician rotates the screen towards the patient and uses her index finger to highlight a test result on the screen. The patient puts on her glasses and leans closer to the screen (Fig. 1 a). This example shows the EMR serving as a material anchor where information is referenced by both the physician and patient.

Later in the session, we see the same patient making use of the EMR to highlight something on the screen for the physician. While the physician is speaking with the patient about the medications she is taking, the patient leans forward, reaches out with a piece of paper and points to the screen (Fig. 1 b). The patient says, "I just need two and you can take off this..." The use of deixis in her speech suggests that the meaning of her utterance is completed by the contents on the screen to which she gestures. Access to the EMR screen allows her to refer to the EMR, creating a common space for her and the physician to communicate.

While EMRs are primarily designed for use by physicians, it is clear from our observations that the EMR is being used as a tool to support physician-patient communication. The physician's interaction with the EMR is supported by her position in front of the EMR and the wheels on its platform. Patients' interactions with it are less supported, as patients were observed to lean in and put on glasses when reading and gesturing to the screen. The EMR is essentially effective as a communication tool, although ergonomic aspects of joint interaction with it are still poorly supported.

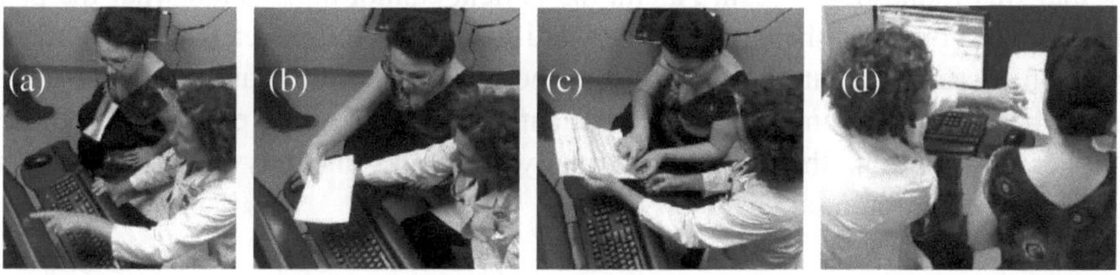

Fig. 1. Interaction with EMR: (*a*) physician, (*b*) patient, and paper: (*c*) patient, (*d*) physician

3.2 Physician-Patient Interaction with Paper

It is common for patients to bring in paper documents from visits to physicians outside the clinic. Of the twelve patients, five brought in such documents. It is important to note that the EMR does not contain all records of patient care received outside the clinic. Paper records are flexible and transportable, making it easy for the patient to carry a tangible history of a recent outside visit to supplement her verbal testimony.

In one instance, a patient brings a paper document with the results from a CT scan she had received outside of the clinic. She shows it to the physician and gives an explanation of what she understands about the scan, pointing at the paper as she speaks. The physician then takes the paper sheet, looks it over, and discusses the results with the patient (Fig. 1 c,d).

Paper is another resource that grounds the communication between the physician and patient. Both parties can refer to the content on the paper and apply their relevant knowledge: the patient applying an episodic report of history, and the physician applying her medical knowledge.

Paper also aids the physician in her medical decisions. The physician notes that the CT scan was insufficient for her to make a diagnosis, and orders an ultrasound for more information. Paper medical documents provide detailed records, are deciphered by the physician, clarified for the patient, and used in decision-making. The use of paper is well supported in this interaction, although there is still a wide range of limitations in incorporating paper information into EMR systems.

3.3 Interpreter Access to Artifacts (Paper + EMR)

Interpreter-mediated patient-physician communication dynamics were significantly different compared with patient-physician communication. Sitting across from the physician and patient, the interpreter has limited access to artifacts they interact with. This is an issue when access to these artifacts is important to understand their actions.

As we have shown, the EMR can be used as a communication tool allowing the doctor to reference or highlight relevant information to the patient. We see this again in a session with an LEP patient when the physician gestures to the EMR while explaining a breast imaging to the patient. The interpreter hears the physician's speech but cannot see the referenced image (Fig. 2 left). The patient is left listening to a foreign language and looking at a screen that may be difficult to understand.

Immediately after, the physician produces a pen and paper and draws an image of a cyst that was found in the scan. Again, the patient cannot understand what the physician is saying but nonetheless leans forward to look at the paper (Fig. 2 right). The physician gestures repeatedly, pointing to the picture she drew and mapping it to an area on her own body and then to the patient's body. When the physician is finished with her explanation, the interpreter finally translates the physician's speech and mimics her self-referential gestures.

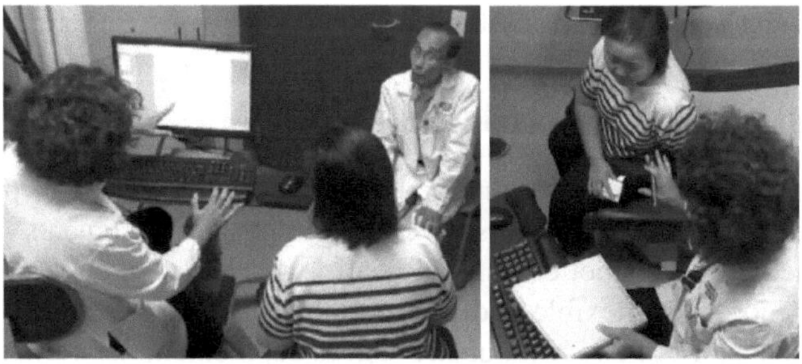

Fig. 2. (left) The physician points to the EMR. (*right*) The physician holds a drawing and gestures to the patient's body.

The interpreter cannot see the material anchors that provide context for the doctor's utterances. Thus, he cannot fully understand the physician's communication, which is tied to the artifacts she is interacting with. In effect the interpreter and the patient are only getting one of two mutually dependent parts (speech, artifacts) of the doctor's multimodal communicative actions.

The arrangement of the room influences the multimodal information available to each party. While the use of artifacts is somewhat well supported with English proficient patients, in interpreter-mediated interactions this kind of communication is poorly supported due to the constraints of the seating arrangement.

4 Discussion and Conclusion

Through our analysis, we discovered that the physical space and artifacts are factors that influence patient-physician communication. In this section, we discuss the implications for design that could improve unsupported pathways of communication.

The EMR's ability to display information augments patient-physician communication. The interface of the EMR however, designed for a user sitting directly in front of it, places ergonomic constraints on multi-party interaction with it. This is true for both patients (who must put on glasses and lean in), and interpreters sitting across the room with no access the EMR or other artifacts used in communication.

Paper is pervasive in physician-patient interaction. However, it is not searchable, and cannot mingle with digital information in the current system. Incorporating outside documents into EMRs is a time consuming and inconvenient process because it either needs to be entered by hand or scanned in at a later time.

These observations highlight the lack of support for collaborative multiparty interaction with artifacts in the exam room. To better support this kind of interaction we suggest redesigning the EMR as a collaborative communication tool. We envision a shared space in the exam room that allows all parties to have access to the EMR as well as paper documents. This system should also be able to integrate paper and digital documents in a way that supports clinical workflow. Having a common platform for the physician, patient, and interpreter to talk, gesture, or draw on would support multiparty multimodal communication. This would potentially reduce errors, enhance patient-physician communication, and ultimately increase health literacy. We feel that integrating our work on interactive paper [7] and interaction on and above the surface [8] will lead to novel and effective interfaces for interaction with EHRs.

References

1. Nielsen-Bohlman, L., Panze, A., Kindig, D.: Health Literacy: A Prescription to End Confusion. National Academies, Washington, D.C. (2004)
2. Williams, M., Davis, T., Parker, R., Weiss, B.: The Role of Health Literacy in Patient-physician Communication. Family Medicine 34(5), 383–389 (2002)
3. Hazlehurst, B., Gorman, P., McMullen, C.: Distributed cognition: an alternative model of cognition for medical informatics. International Journal of Medical Informatics (2008)
4. Hollan, J., Hutchins, E., Kirsh, D.: Distributed cognition: toward a new foundation for human-computer interaction research. ACM Transactions on Computer-Human Interaction 7(2), 174–196 (2000)
5. Hutchins, E.: Cognition in the Wild. MIT press (1995)
6. Fouse, A., Weibel, N., Hutchins, E., Hollan, J.D.: ChronoViz: a system for supporting navigation of time-coded data. In: Proc. CHI 2011 (May 2011)
7. Weibel, N.: A Publishing Infrastructure for Interactive Paper Documents: Supporting Interactions across the Paper-Digital Divide, Dissertation, ETH No. 18514, Zurich, Switzerland (2009)
8. Liu, Y., Weibel, N., Hollan, J.D.: Interactive Space: A Framework for Prototyping Multitouch Interaction on and Above the Desktop. In: Proc. CHI 2013 (2013) (in press)

Mobile Technologies and Its Advantages with Promoting Healthy Habits amongst Children

Monika Monk[1], D. Scott McCrickard[1], Adil Kadir[1], Brandon Dockery[1], and Kacie Allen[2]

[1] Department of Computer Science
[2] Department of Human Nutrition, Food, and Exercise, Virginia Tech, Blacksburg, VA 24061, USA
{mmonk90,mccricks,adilk,bsdocke,kacieal}@vt.edu

Abstract. This paper describes an app suite that consists of mobile games to encourage increased activity and healthier eating by children in fun and motivating ways. The apps include Scavenger Hunt, in which a user can take pictures of objects that match a specific color in a short amount of time; Fish Out of Water, that tracks the number of steps you take to "catch" the fish; Space Rayders, a mobile game similar to tag; and Health Attack, a memory game based off of the food pyramid. The paper describes how the apps help increase awareness of aspects important for living a healthier life for children, highlighting a plan for dissemination through youth clubs and mobile app stores.

Keywords: Mobile technology, interaction design, exergames.

1 Introduction

In today's society, there is an alarming number of people, especially children, who have life-threatening diseases and conditions. Several of these diseases and conditions, such as heart disease and obesity, can be "prevented or lessened with a healthy diet and exercise" [3]. In recent years, there have been several initiatives taken to help society live healthier lifestyles. One popular initiative is First Lady Michelle Obama's campaign to fight against childhood obesity [2,3]. The popularity of video games and mobile phones over the years opens a path to help address this epidemic.

Mobile technologies have become more integrated into today's society than ever before. From elders to young children, mobile technology has a range of users and is used for different purposes. One type of mobile technology that is becoming increasingly popular is called *exergaming*, defined as "video games that also provide exercise" [5]. Examples of popular mobile exergames that have had a positive impact on increasing activity amongst its users include the Wii Fit and the Kinect's Dance Central, both bringing positive attention to incorporating exercise into video games.

This paper describes our app suite, geared towards children, that includes different mobile games. The games increase the motivation to become more active by inspiring students to compete and cooperate at fun activities. The games have been deployed through the United States Boys and Girls Club with encouraging results [1].

C. Stephanidis (Ed.): Posters, Part II, HCII 2013, CCIS 374, pp. 192–196, 2013.

The ongoing effort described here shifts the game focus from a club environment with focused time periods, adult supervision, and a guaranteed multi-player environment to a broader use scenario in which anyone can download the games and will be motivated to use them.

2 Promoting Healthy Habits amongst Children

Each mobile game in the app suite was created from various different motivations, each geared towards healthy habits, including diet and exercise. Color Hunt, Space Rayders, and Fish Out of Water were mobile games for use by children from the local Boys and Girls Club [1]. The initial versions of these apps were used through the Boys and Girls Clubs of America in southwest Virginia. Over 30 young people played the games for 30 minutes a day, four days a week, for five weeks. Results from accelerometer data and student inquiry indicated that many of the games encourage a higher degree of physical activity, and many of the students enjoy the competitive, multimedia aspects of the games.

The versions of the games used by the Boys and Girls Club were targeted for specific session lengths, and they were intended to be used in supervised situations when an adult would configure the game to support multiple players. The games also collected data about game play, with permission from the children and their parents. Because of these complexities, each game was modified and updated so that they would be easy to use upon download in the android market. With several of these games, the initial versions involved very complex setup that wouldn't be suitable in a standalone app—most users who download apps from an app market want downloads that are simple and easy to use. The remainder of this section describes the apps, focusing on how they differ from the previous version.

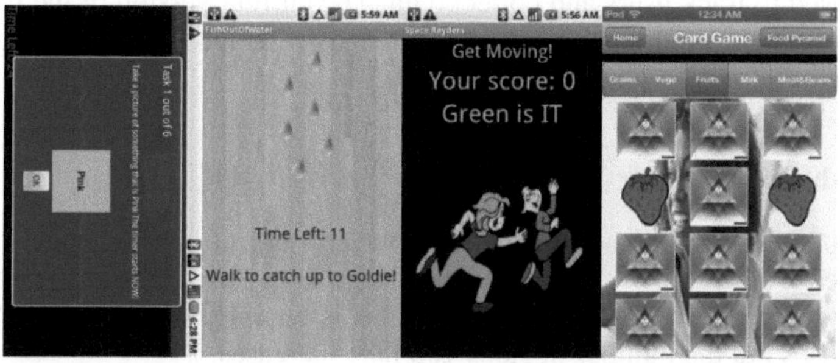

Fig. 1. Action shots of the games in our app suite (from left to right): Color Hunt, Fish Out of Water, Space Rayders and Health Attack

2.1 Color Hunt

Color Hunt (previously known as Scavenger Hunt [1]) is a game where the player's objective is to take a picture matching a target color that will be given in a random order. The user can choose between three different difficulty levels: easy, medium, or hard. As each level gets harder, the amount of time the user is given to find each color decreases. When the user matches each color correctly, they will be given points; if the user matches a color incorrectly, they will not receive any points. A screenshot of the game can be found in Figure 1.

The initial version of this game, known as Scavenger Hunt, involved the player taking pictures of different objects matching six preset colors. There was no time limit or scoring involved. When we were brainstorming ideas on how to make the game more interactive, we came up with several ideas. One idea involved adding a storyline to the game to make the player more engaged in the game; there would also be an incentive that the player would receive for completing each task correctly. Another idea involved having the picture of the item shown to the user in a pixelated picture to show the user how close he or she was to the target color. By showing the user just how close he or she was to the target color, they would be able to learn the different hex colors that a certain color can appear as. However, this idea was rejected because we felt as though this would confuse our target audience.

2.2 Space Rayders

Space Rayders is a "tag" game—a multiplayer game where each user is assigned a color. When the game begins, the person that is "it" is chosen, and they have to "catch" whoever is not "it". To catch another player, the "it" person comes closer to their target and the phones begin to light up and vibrate warning the target that they are about to be caught.

The current and initial versions of Space Rayders are very similar. The initial version, however, was too complex to distribute on the market: users would have a very difficult time trying to set up the game because they would have to follow a very complicated method so that each phone that was using the game would be connected that was used to track users and collect data. The current version of the game needs to only have the Bluetooth connected and minor user setup, with tracking and data collection removed.

2.3 Fish Out of Water

Fish Out of Water is a game in which the player's objective is to "catch" the fish that has escaped from its bowl. The player has to go a various number of steps in order to return the fish back to the bowl. As each task is completed, the time to "catch" each fish decreases but the number of steps you take increases.

Currently, this game has not been changed. Under consideration are changes to the background pictures to be more aesthetically pleasing to the user audience. This can be solved simply by uploading changes to the game through android market.

2.4 Health Attack

Health Attack is a memory game that incorporates different foods from each food group in the food pyramid. As each food is matched correctly to one another, an information pop-up will appear and give a fun fact about each food that is matched. This food is placed in a food pyramid diagram, which the user can find more information about the food. We are considering extending the platform set of Health Attack from iPhone to also include Android so that all the games in the app suite are more broadly available. This will allow us to view download data easier and provide updates when necessary.

Health Attack was not part of the game suite used in the Boys and Girls Club. It pre-dated the other games, and it was targeted towards the African-American community because of the increasing rate of obesity issues, particularly for this community [3]. When the design team developed Health Attack, they wanted to make the target audience children from ages 7-11 because of how influential children are around that age. The children would be able to play a video game but also learn about the different foods they were eating at the same time.

3 Dissemination and Analysis

To assess usage, the number of downloads and user feedback will be monitored and documented. A Facebook page -- www.facebook.com/ExergameAppSuite -- is used as the main advertisement source. This page is being publicized through email, Facebook messages, flyers given to elementary school teachers and various after school programs, and through word of mouth. Furthermore, the location of the App Suite in the Android Market will also be provided on all the advertisements. Based on the number of downloads, continual usage, and feedback, we can determine if our approach to using mobile games is effective or not. We will augment the games with "high score" pages to provide insight into the frequency and duration of play of users.

4 Conclusion and Future Work

With the rise in life-threatening diseases, such as obesity and heart disease, and the increased usage of mobile technology, different types of mobile exergames can be formed. Because more children are using the mobile devices, we have come up with a solution to help them become more active, learn about healthy lifestyles, and have fun all at the same time. In our app suite, there will be four games available to download. These games will be free and will be marketed through a Facebook page. The website can be found at www.facebook.com/ExergameAppSuite. For future work, we will expand the App Suite and monitor the Facebook page and App Suite to assess the needs and impacts of our work.

References

1. Allen, K.: Developing and testing smartphone game applications for physical activity promotion in adolescents. Ph.D. dissertation, Department of Human Nutrition, Foods, and Exercise. Virginia Tech. (2013)

2. Clark, D., Edmonds, C., Moore, A., Harlow, J., Allen, K., Winchester, W.W., Estabrooks, P.: Android application development to promote physical activity in adolescents. In: 2012 International Conference Collaboration on Technologies and Systems (CTS), pp. 566–568. IEEE (2012)
3. Hill, D., et al.: Mobile technologies for promoting health and wellness among African American youth. In: Stephanidis, C. (ed.) Universal Access in HCI, Part III, HCII 2011. LNCS, vol. 6767, pp. 36–45. Springer, Heidelberg (2011)
4. Payton, J., Powell, E., Nickel, A., Doran, K., Barnes, T.: GameChanger: a middleware for social exergames. In: Proceedings of the 1st International Workshop on Games and Software Engineering, pp. 36–39. ACM (2011)
5. Wylie, C.G., Coulton, P.: Mobile exergaming. In: Proceedings of the 2008 International Conference on Advances in Computer Entertainment Technology, pp. 338–341. ACM (2008)

Drug Name Similarity Index for Sound-Alikeness

Tomoyuki Nagata[1,*], Masaomi Kimura[2], Michiko Ohkura[2], and Fumito Tsuchiya[3]

[1] Graduate School, Shibaura Institute of Technology, Tokyo, Japan
ma12078@shibaura-it.ac.jp
[2] Shibaura Institute of Technology, Tokyo, Japan
{masaomi,ohkura}@sic.shibaura-it.ac.jp
[3] International University of Health and Welfare, Japan
iuhwfumito@gmail.com

Abstract. Drug name confusion is one of major medical errors. Some similar drug names can cause medical accidents. In order to solve this problem, the Ministry of Health, Labour and Welfare developed the drug name database system to prevent from authorizing drugs whose names are similar to existing drug names. Previous studies have been proposed the drug name similarity index based on look-alikeness. Despite of these efforts, the studies do not take account of drug name confusion caused by sound-alike. In this paper, we proposed the phonetic similarity index based on the features used in articulatory phonetics.

Keywords: Drug name confusion, Sound-alikeness, Name similarity index, Medical error, Human error.

1 Introduction

Though drugs are to promote people's health, they can be toxic if used improperly. People who use them are not perfect and can cause a medical error. One of the promising ways to prevent such an error is to device the systems which reduce human errors. Drug name confusion is one of major human errors related to safe use of drugs. Actually, some drug names are so similar that it makes medical experts confused unintentionally. For example, at some hospital in Japan, Succin, instead of Saxizon, was mistakenly administered to a patient and it unfortunately made him die. In order to prevent such accidents, the Ministry of Health, Labour and Welfare developed the system, Medicine Similar Name Search Engine, in order to prevent authorizing drugs whose names are similar to existing drug names. The system computes similarity of names based on character matching, such as edit distance and head and tail cosine similarity (htco). However, the system is inadequate to compute similarity more close to human sensitivity. Because the system computes similarity based on only matching character but without consideration the character shapes and the pronunciation. For example, ツルメリン and ソルノミン are also drug names in Japanese. The existing system computes the similarity of them low because the characters of them are almost different. However, because their shapes are very similar, people feel that

C. Stephanidis (Ed.): Posters, Part II, HCII 2013, CCIS 374, pp. 197–201, 2013.

these names are very similar in many cases. In order to solve this problem, Nabeta et al. proposed the drug name similarity index by improving the Letter-Sequence-Kernel (LSK)[1-2].

Despite of these efforts, the studies cannot perfectly prevent confusing drug names. This is because they only measure the look-alike similarity based on character matching. As Lambert et al. mentioned, drug name confusion can be caused by both sound-alike and look-alike similarity [3]. Doctors are often forced to do it in emergency, though they are prohibited from oral ordering. In such a situation, the drugs sound-alike with other drugs can cause mixing-up. We should also note that pronunciations can affect the name similarity, if we read them carefully. For this reason, in this study, we focus on drug name confusion caused by sound-alikeness and propose the phonetic similarity index of drug names.

2 Method

Before we define phonetic similarity index, we have to clarify the structure of speech sounds. Phonetics is the study of speech sounds and classifies speech sounds to three fields, articulatory phonetics, acoustic phonetics and auditory phonetics. Articulatory phonetics deal with how humans produce speech sounds on the basis of biological organ structures. Acoustic phonetics deal with how speech sounds is propagated in terms of frequency. Auditory phonetics deal with how humans hear speech sounds. Considering this, we might say that the similarity of speech sounds is consisted of the similarity of pronunciation, sound vibration, and perceptual process. In these fields, the considerable factor in first is similarity of pronunciation because if pronunciations of drug names are similar, these speech sounds are also similar in other fields. Thus, we just focus on articulatory phonetics and classify speech sounds based on their production process.

Articulatory phonetics defines speech sounds as a set of consonant and vowel. Consonant is a speech sound that is articulated with complete or partial closure of the vocal tract, and vowel is pronounced with an open vocal tract. These sounds are determined involved in the manner of articulation and the place of articulation. Manner of articulation describes how speech organs produce sounds, and place of articulation describes the points where block air stream. The International Phonetic Alphabet (IPA) defines speech sounds based on these features.

Especially, in Japanese, a character of Japanese phonetic alphabet consists of pair of consonant and vowel. Thus, we defined each similarity of consonant part and vowel part. When we defined the similarity of consonant part, we considered the similarity of each consonant because it is considered that a pair of characters which has similar consonant each other is more similar than the other pair. For example, Japanese character 'タ' (/ta/) is more similar to 'ダ' (/da/) than to 'マ' (/ma/). Since these characters have the same vowels, we can ignore the contribution of vowels to similarity in this case. This leads the fact that the consonant /t/ is more similar to /d/ than /m/. The difference comes from the features of pronunciations. For this reason, we defined the similarity of each consonant based on the IPA definition and classified them into some groups.

As for definition process of the similarity of consonant part, we defined the similarity of each consonant based on the features of consonant. We use this similarity to define phonetic version of Letter Sequence Kernel index.

In many languages, consonants are produced by discharging of the air from lungs. These are described by five factors: state of glottis, places of articulation, path of airflow, degree of occlusion, state of palatine velum. State of glottis is presence or absence of the vibration of vocal folds. The voiced sounds are the sounds which involve the vibration, and the voiceless sounds are the sounds which do not involve the vibration. Places of articulation are the places where block the airflow from lungs. We pronounce consonants by blocking the airflow by means of a combination of upper and lower speech organs such as bottom lip and upper lip, blade of tongue and teeth-ridge, and so on. For example, the consonant of 'パ' (/pa/x) in Japanese is pronounced by the combination of bottom lip and upper lip, whose sounds are called bilabial. If paths of airflow are not blocked, airflow runs through a center or edges of oral cavity to avoid tongue. Degree of occlusion can be expressed as a distance of two speech organs that block the airflow. Palatine velum is organ to regulate the airflow to nose. The sounds produced by the airflow flown to nose are called nasal sound. If the sounds are produced when palatine velum ups and blocks the airflow to nose, they are called plosive sound.

We defined the similarity index of consonants as the cosine value of the angle between the vectors representing whether the consonant has the corresponding feature.

By contrast, we defined the similarity of vowel part based on Letter-Sequence-Kernel.

3 Experiment

In order to estimate accuracy of the proposed similarity index, we conducted the experiment which compared it with the similarity of drug names based on human sensitivity. In this experiment, 20's university students answered the similarities of 20 pairs of drug names. For each pair of drug names, we played the subjects the sound of one of drug names, and after one-second pause, we played the sound of another. After subjects heard the sounds, they answered the similarity by means of Virtual Analogue Scale (VAS). VAS is a scale which measure subjective characteristics. The subject marks a point on the line between two end points, dissimilar and similar, to express the similarity that he felt. The response time was limited to 1.5 seconds for the reason to avoid the effects caused by memories. Figure 1 shows the correlation between the values of our similarity index and the averages of the subjects' answers.

The horizontal axis indicates the averages of the subjects' answers, and the vertical axis indicates our similarity index. This shows the tendency that the values of our index are higher than the similarities that the subjects felt.

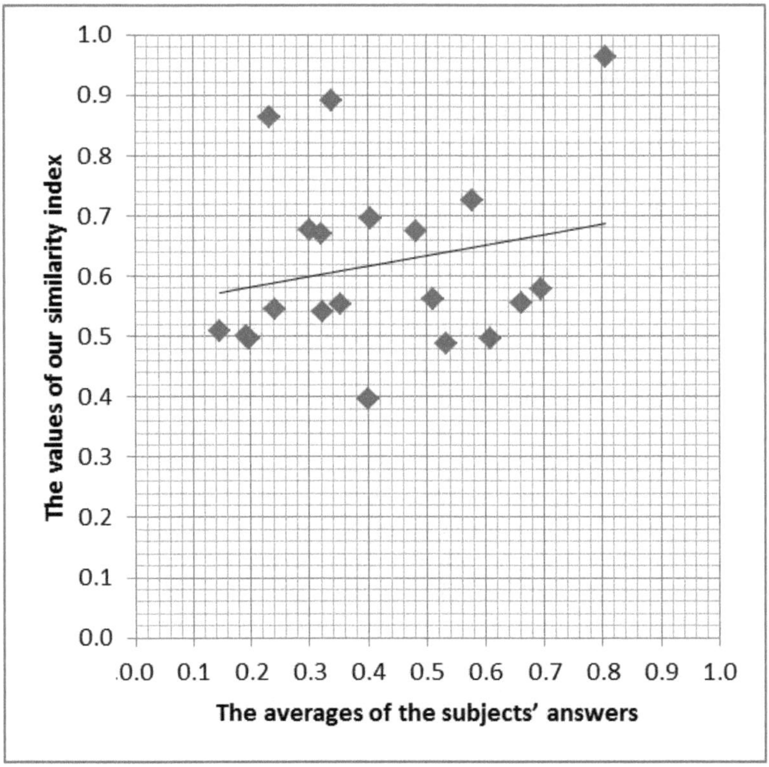

Fig. 1. The correlation between the valeus of our similarity index and the averages of the subject's answers

We investigated the cause of this problem and found that the contribution of consonant part generally gave high value to any pairs.

The consonant part of the proposed similarity is calculated based on the similarities between each pair of consonants included in the drug names. The cause can be our assumption that the phonetic features of consonants are equally taken in account to define the consonant similarity. We will investigate this in details in our future work.

In addition, the cause might originate in our definition of the similarity that was only based on consonant and vowel. The other factors which should be taken in consideration might be the coincidence of the characters at the head of drug names, the similarity of accent positions and so on.

4 Conclusion

In this paper, we proposed the similarity index of drug name based on sound-alikeness.

We used the property of Japanese letter sound, namely, each sound can be divided into consonant and vowel. We defined the drug name similarity index that consists of a consonant part and a vowel part. As for the consonant part, we employed the idea used in articulatory phonetics, classification of consonant based on the features of IPA. We used the similarity of consonants to define the consonant part of similarity. The similarity index of consonants was defined as the cosine value of the angle between the vectors corresponding to them. The elements of the vectors represent whether the consonant has the corresponding feature.

In order to evaluate the proposed similarity, we conducted the experiment where the subjects heard sounds of two drug names and answered the extent of their similarity. We investigated a correlation between the measured similarities in this experiment and the values of our similarity index. As a result, we found that the consonant part of our similarity index was higher than the subjects felt. Its cause can be our assumption that the phonetic features of consonants are equally taken in account to quantify the consonant similarity.

In the future, we need to improve the similarity by taking account of acoustic phonetics and auditory phonetics. Additionally, we will research the factor that affects a similarity of drug names, whose candidates are the positions of similar characters, prolonged sound, accents and so on.

References

1. Nabeta, K., et al.: The Similarity Index of Medicine Names Based on Character Shape Similarity. Transactions of Japan Society of Kansei Engineering 10(2), 287–294 (2010)
2. Nabeta, K., Hatano, A., Ishida, H., Kimura, M., Ohkura, M., Tsuchiya, F.: The Similarity Index of Character Shape of Medicine Names Based on Character Shape Similarity (II). In: Jacko, J.A. (ed.) Human-Computer Interaction, Part I, HCII 2011. LNCS, vol. 6761, pp. 628–636. Springer, Heidelberg (2011)
3. Lambert, B.L., Chang, K.Y., Lin, S.J.: Effect of Orthographic and Phonological Similarity on False Recognition of Drug Names. Social Science & Medicine 52, 1843–1857 (2001)
4. Tsuchiya, F., Kawamura, N.: Development of the System to Objectively Evaluate Similarities of Drug Names. In: Proceeding of APAMI – SJKMI and KOSMI Conference, pp. 348–351 (2003)

AR Dental Surgical Simulator Using Haptic Feedback

Katsuhiko Onishi[1], Kiminori Mizushino[2], Hiroki Ikemoto[1], and Hiroshi Noborio[1]

[1] Osaka Electro-Communication University
1130-70 Kiyotaki, Shijonawate, Osaka 575-0063, Japan
{onishi,t10007,nobori}@oecu.jp
[2] Embedded Wings Co. Ltd.
5-2-3 Ina, Minoh, Osaka 562-0015, Japan
k_mizushino@ewings.biz

Abstract. We describe about our dental surgical simulator which enable users to simulate dental surgical operation. Our simulator which enables the user to learn dental surgical methods through actual hand and body postures. The proposed system uses a display showing a virtual tooth model and real teeth and gums that are positioned close to the hands of the user, which allows the user to directly manipulate objects with haptic feedback. As a preliminary evaluation, in display system, we measured the deviation between real object image and virtual object image at user's view positions. And we confirmed the capability and the limitation of our system.

Keywords: Dental surgical simulator, augmented reality, direct manipulation.

1 Introduction

In dental surgery, most surgical training methods use plastic teeth or live patients. Although these methods are good for improving surgical skills, for example, the use of surgical tools and surgical procedures, task repetition is difficult because of the need for new plastic teeth or live patients for each task. Therefore, several types of dental surgical simulator have been proposed [1], [2], [3]. These simulators allow users to learn dental surgical methods using a unique interface. Most of dental surgical simulator use the haptic feedback interface for simulating dental surgical operation. However, most of these simulators use a typical computing display system, and so the user cannot experience the actual hand positions or body posture required during dental surgery.

In this paper, we describe about our preliminary work of a dental surgical training system for learning about real hand position and the body posture. To realize the practice of user's hand position and the body posture, our system set a display close to user's hand position and allows the user to operate surgical tasks directly. And it shows combined image with virtual teeth model as a surgical target and a real tooth model as other parts of the patient dental model. In order to adapt to any head position of the user, the system measured the head position of the user and the position of the real teeth model.

C. Stephanidis (Ed.): Posters, Part II, HCII 2013, CCIS 374, pp. 202–205, 2013.

2 Our Dental Surgical Simulator

In dental surgery, the surgical environment is usually such that a patient is lying in front of a dentist while the dentist operates. In such a situation, the positions of the dentist hands and the body posture of the dentist are different from those in traditional dental surgical simulation. For example, Figure 1 shows a typical hand position in dental surgical operation. It is needed strict movement to manipulate a dental tool for operating surgical tasks. The dentist put their hand on the patient teeth or gum as the fulcrum.

In order to realize manipulations with respect to user hand positions and body posture, the proposed system incorporates a half mirror placed horizontally between the head position and the position of the hands, as shown in Figure 2. The system then presents a combined image of the virtual teeth and the teeth model on the half mirror display. Furthermore, in order to adapt the head motion of the user for probing and confirming the surgical target, the system measures the head motion of the user and the teeth model. The virtual teeth are shown on an LCD display that can be adequately viewed by the user. The system uses a real teeth model around the surgical target teeth and the user is able to steady their hands against the model while performing surgical tasks, allowing the user to perform the surgical simulation tasks precisely.

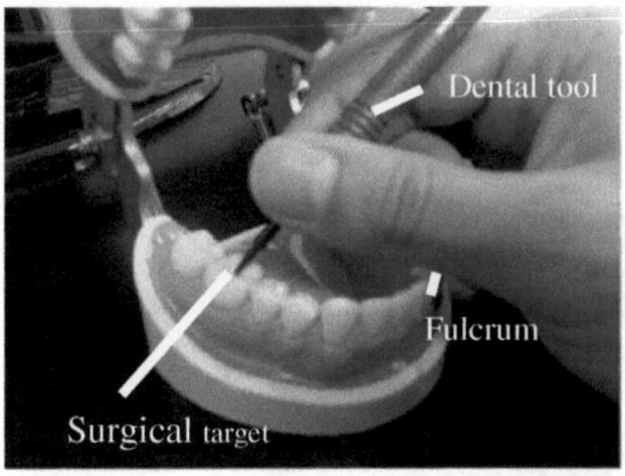

Fig. 2. An example of surgical hand position

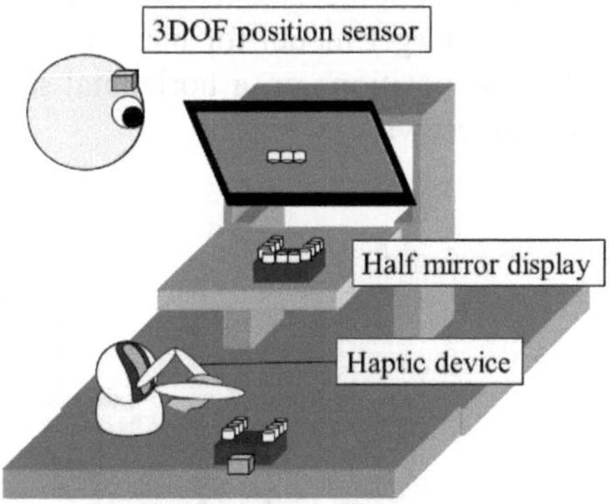

Fig. 1. Our dental surgical system

3 Prototype System

The prototype display is shown in Figure 3. The proposed system is implemented on a Windows PC, and the system measures the user's head position and real teeth and gum model position using 3DOF magnetic sensors. It shows the users a teeth model and virtual teeth reflected onto the display from the half mirror. Figures 4 shows virtual teeth model which our system uses. This model is created as a surface model by each parts and the system check the collision detection in real time between surgical

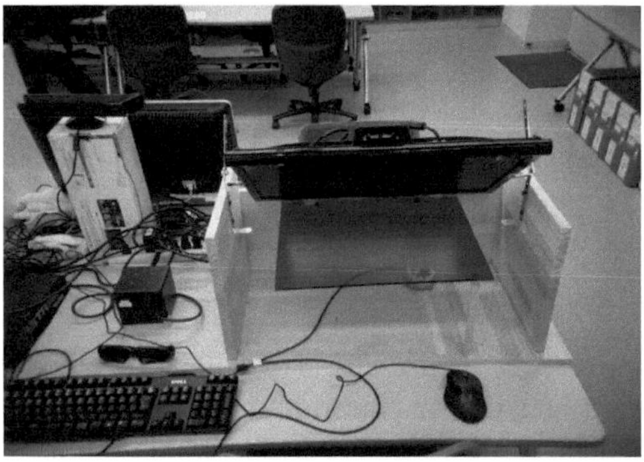

Fig. 3. Our prototype display

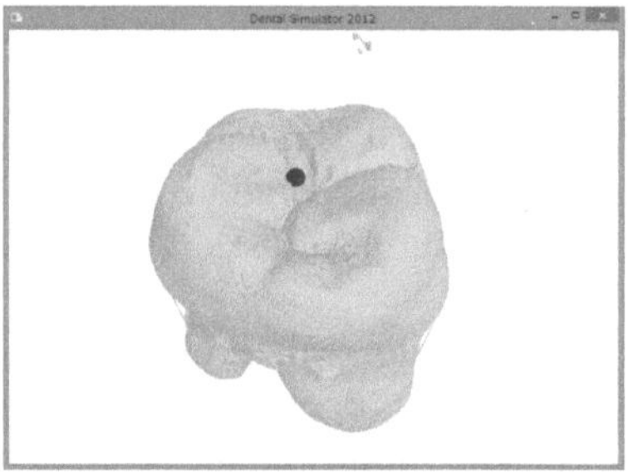

Fig. 4. Virtual teeth model

tools and the teeth model. And it is deformed the shape by user's surgical operation. Figures 5 is a usage image of our system. The system measures a viewing position of the user and shows the appropriate view based on that position. Then, the system allows the user to display the virtual and real teeth models simultaneously from any viewing position.

As a preliminary evaluation about the display system, we have measured the deviation between real objects and virtual objects in the user's view image. We use a cube model as the target model for measuring the deviation precisely. And it is measured from 8 view positions on a horizontal line. The deviation is about from 0.06cm to 1.00cm in these view positions.

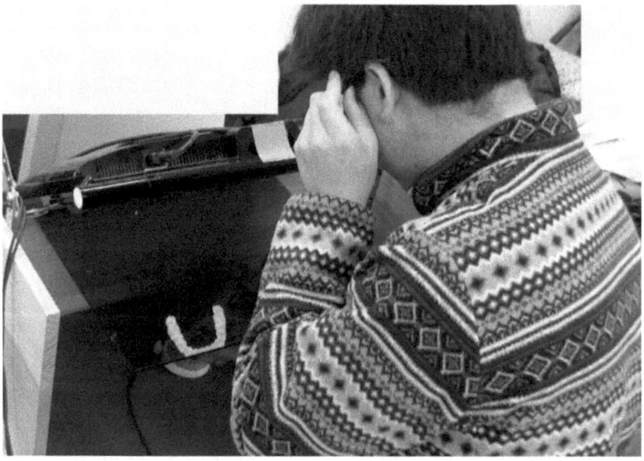

Fig. 5. An example of our display system

4 Conclusion

We proposed a dental surgical simulator system for a dental surgical simulator. The proposed system enables the user to view a combined image of virtual teeth and a teeth model. The user can see the combined image from any point of view by tracking his or her head position and the model position. We constructed a prototype system and confirmed the capability and the limitation of this system.

In future work, we will evaluate the haptic feedback module in this system. And we will improve the accuracy of the user's view image.

References

1. Rhienmora, P., Gajananan, K., Haddawy, P., Suebnukarn, S., Dailey, M., Supataratarn, E., Shrestha, P.: Haptic augmented reality dental trainer with automatic performance assessment. In: The 15th International Conference on Intelligent User Interfaces (IUI 2010), pp. 425–426 (2010)
2. Kim, L., Park An, S.: Efficient virtual teeth modeling for dental training system. International Journal of CAD/CAM 8(1), 41–44 (2008)
3. Yau, H., Tsou, L., Tsai, M.: Octree-based virtual dental training system with a haptic device. Computer-Aided Design & Applications 3, 415–424 (2006)

Combining a Tablet and an Electronic Stethoscope to Create a New Interaction Paradigm for Teaching Cardiac Auscultation

Daniel Pereira[1], Pedro Gomes[1], Élodie Mota[2], Emília Costa[2], Ricardo Cruz-Correia[3,4], and Miguel Coimbra[1]

[1] Instituto de Telecomunicações, Faculdade de Ciências da Universidade do Porto, Portugal
[2] Faculty of Fine Arts of the University of Porto, Portugal
[3] CINTESIS - Center for research in health technologies and information systems
[4] Faculty of Medicine of the University of Porto, Portugal
{danielpereira,rcorreia}@med.up.pt,
{ptmgomes,mcoimbra}@dcc.fc.up.pt,
{elodie.atom,emilia.d.costa}@gmail.com

Abstract. Learning cardiac auscultation is a fundamental but hard task for a medicine student, involving a combination of gesture mechanics and cardiac sounds interpretation. We aim to create a low cost simulator combining a tablet and an electronic stethoscope, thus defining a new interaction paradigm that al-lows a student to train auscultation when and where they want. In this paper we evaluate the usability of a first approach to this new paradigm using a high-fidelity prototype and its heuristic evaluation.

Keywords: Teaching, Heart Auscultation, User interface interaction, Electronic stethoscope.

1 Motivation

Cardiac auscultation is the difficult art of listening to heart sounds gathered via a stethoscope, which is routinely used for screening or diagnosis purposes. It requires not only interpretation skills (ex: murmur detection and characterization) but also mechanical ones (ex: where the stethoscope should be placed in the patient's chest). St Clair [1] and Mangione [2] have shown that the ability of medical students to recognize common cardiac murmurs is poor (approximately 20%) using traditional methods of learning. Barret [3] highlights the importance of repetition for effectively learning auscultation but all simulators that train both interpretation and mechanical skills are too expensive [4].

2 Aim

We aim to exploit the potential of the touch-based interaction offered by currently popular tablets to develop a cheap cardiac auscultation simulator for medical students,

C. Stephanidis (Ed.): Posters, Part II, HCII 2013, CCIS 374, pp. 206–209, 2013.

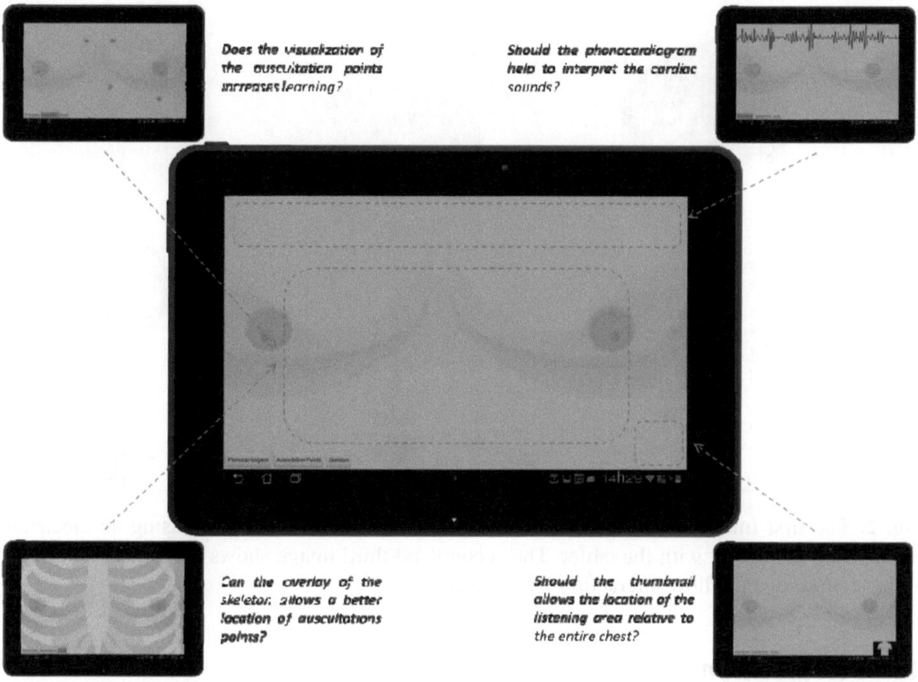

Fig. 1. Preview of the application showing the principal area of auscultation and some functionalities that we will explore

enabling them to train the mechanic and interpretation skills required by auscultation, combining it with a commercial off the shelf electronic stethoscope.

3 Prototype

Although developing a full medical student training system requires a multitude of disciplines (hardware, software engineering, pedagogy, etc.), in this paper we will focus on the interactive auscultation functionality. As such, we propose a vertical prototype for a 10 inches tablet that can be used for auscultation of the four principal cardiac focuses (aortic, pulmonic, tricuspid, mitral), combined with a wireless electronic stethoscope as its input/output interaction device.

In Figure 1, we propose a preview of the application and some functionalities that we will explore. The image A in Figure 2 shows the prototype who can allow an interaction using an electronic stethoscope and a high fidelity reproduction of cardiac sounds. The images B and C in Figure 2 show the adjustment made to the stethoscope to allow interaction with the tablet. This adaption was made using aluminum foil and making a slight cut in the plastic diaphragm to allow the passage of a contact point in aluminum in order to conducting electricity through the stethoscope chest piece.

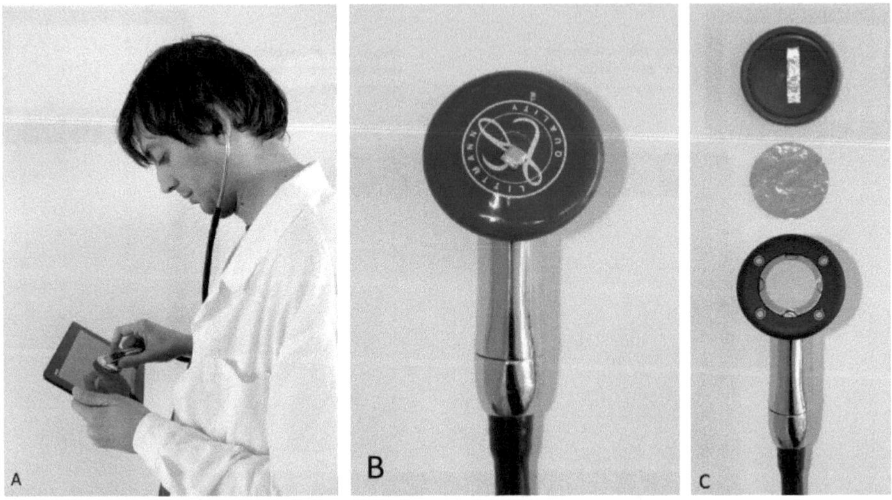

Fig. 2. The first image shows a medical student listening a cardiac sound using an electronic stethoscope to interact with the tablet. The second and third image shows the adjustment made to the stethoscope to allow interaction with the tablet.

4 Evaluation

We performed a heuristic evaluation following the principles proposed by Nielsen [5, 6]. We chose three senior students of the Faculty of Medicine of the University of Porto as evaluators because they represent the target audience of this project. The set of tasks performed by the evaluators is listed in Table 1. We developed a high-fidelity prototype intended to test the interaction paradigm between these two devices (tablet, stethoscope). The usability and pedagogical impact of a full interactive application intended to teach auscultation is not addressed in this paper.

Results highlighted four errors (Table 2). Three of them are related to the flexibility and efficiency of use and one to the visual clarity of the displayed information. All errors were easy to correct.

Table 1. Taks performed by the evaluators

Nº	Task
1	Enable the display of auscultation points
2	Enable visualization of the skeleton
3	Enable the visualization of phonocardiogram
4	Zooming in on the chest in order to view a large area plan
5	Zooming out of the chest to view the entire chest
6	After zooming in, slide by the image
7	Auscultate the chest with a stethoscope in order to hear a sound

Table 2. Detected problems with the heuristic evaluation

Nº	Heuristic	Severity	Description and Possible Solution
1	Flexibility and Efficiency of Use	3	The action to zoom in and zoom out is not obvious. It is suggested that it is possible to use the open pinch gesture. Another suggestion is to put a button to the zoom action.
2	Match Between System and the Real World	2	The swipe is too fast. Decrease the velocity.
3	Flexibility and Efficiency of Use	2	The timing of the double click is too long, which causes unexpected zoom out. Decrease the timing.
4	Match Between System and the Real World	1	The ribs of the skeleton are barely noticeable making it difficult to find the inter-costal spaces. Increase the skeleton contrast.

5 Discussion

The data collected with the heuristic evaluation allowed us to improve the high-fidelity prototype. However, we will continue working to improve the interaction between the user and the tablet using the stethoscope to provide a simulator that besides training the ear can also train the mechanics of auscultation.

Acknowledgement. This work was supported by FCT project PTDC/EIA-CCO/100844/2008.

References

1. St Clair, E.W., et al.: Assessing housestaff diagnostic skills using a cardiology patient simulator. Ann. Intern. Med. 117(9), 751–756 (1992)
2. Mangione, S., et al.: The teaching and practice of cardiac auscultation during internal medicine and cardiology training. A nationwide survey. Ann. Intern. Med. 119(1), 47–54 (1993)
3. Barrett, M.J., et al.: Mastering cardiac murmurs: the power of repetition. Chest 126(2), 470–475 (2004)
4. Karnath, B., Thornton, W., Frye, A.W.: Teaching and testing physical examination skills without the use of patients. Acad. Med. 77(7), 753 (2002)
5. Molich, R., Nielsen, J.: Improving a human-computer dialogue. Commun. ACM 33(3), 338–348 (1990)
6. Nielsen, J.: Heuristic evaluation. In: Nielsen, J., Mack, R.L. (eds.) Usability Inspection Methods, pp. 25–62. John Wiley & Sons, Inc., New York (1994)

Status and Problems of Computer-Aided Surgery in Japan

Kazuhiko Shinohara

School of Health Sciences, Tokyo University of Technology, Nishikamata, Ohta, Tokyo, 144-8535, Japan
kazushin@stf.teu.ac.jp

Abstract. Research and development (R&D) of computer-aided surgery (CAS) in Japan was started in the mid-1980s and has been progressing steadily through interdisciplinary collaboration. From the mid-1990s, many R&D projects on surgical manipulators and navigation systems for endoscopic surgery were started. In the early 2000s, a number of prototypes of master–slave tele-manipulation systems with navigational imaging were developed for robotic general surgery, cardiac surgery, orthopedic surgery, and neurosurgery. However, commercially successful cases such as "da Vinci™" are rare in Japan. Research into CAS developments revealed that limited R&D resources for human–computer interfaces, usability, regulatory affairs, and international marketing strategies might have been responsible for the commercial failure of Japanese CAS-related equipment. Taken together, further development of CAS requires interdisciplinary and international R&D cooperation.

Keywords: computer aided surgery, human-computer interface, R&D.

1 Introduction

Research and development (R&D) of computer-aided surgery (CAS) in Japan was started in the mid-1980s and has been progressing steadily through interdisciplinary collaboration. The main driving force for CAS was the rapid expansion of endoscopic surgery in the 1990s. However, commercially successful cases are rare in Japan. The status and problems of R&D of CAS were therefore investigated in this study.

2 Materials and Methods

Presentations and original articles on CAS presented in the Japan Society of Computer Aided Surgery (JSCAS) and the Japanese Society for Medical and Biological Engineering (JSMBE) journals from 1995 to 2012 were analyzed, and problems related to research and commercialization of medical devices of CAS were investigated.

C. Stephanidis (Ed.): Posters, Part II, HCII 2013, CCIS 374, pp. 210–214, 2013.

3 Results

Of 1503 presentations and original articles in the field of CAS presented at annual meetings and in the JSCAS and JSMBE journals, 550 (36.6%) involved surgical robotics, 784 (52.1%) involved imaging and navigation, 102 (6.7%) involved a human–machine interface, and 67 (4.5%) involved regulatory sciences. These results show a relative shortage of research on the human–machine interface and regulatory sciences. In Japan, many commercial imaging software applications and devices are available in the field of imaging and navigation systems. However, commercially successful cases are rare in Japan, and NaviotTM—a endoscope-manipulator for endoscopic surgery—is the only commercially successful case.

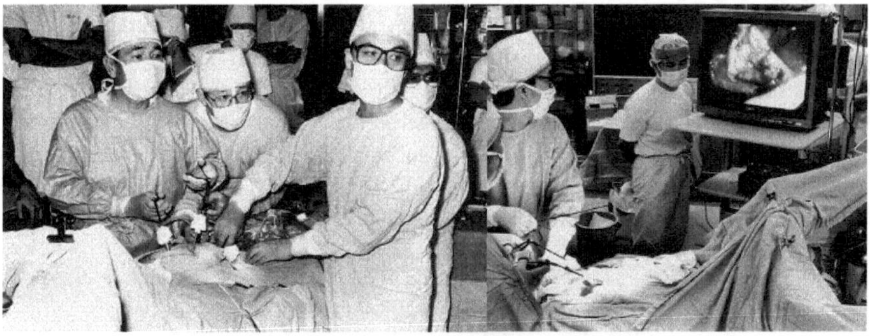

Fig. 1. A scene of endoscopic surgery in 1990

4 Discussion

CAS represents both a concept and associated methods and involves the use of computer technology for planning, navigation, and performing surgical operations. CAS developments run in parallel with the inauguration and development of endoscopic surgery. Endoscopic surgery is performed by small-diameter instruments under the image guidance of endoscopy. These instruments are inserted into the operation area with the endoscope via a few skin incisions of 5–10 mm diameter in the visceral wall.

Modern endoscopic surgery was started as endoscopic cholecystectomy by Mouret in France and by McKernan and Reddic in the United States in 1987. In Japan, the first endoscopic cholecystectomy was performed by Prof. Idezuki et al in 1990 and rapidly spread throughout the country. (Fig.1) In 1990, only 299 cases of cholecystectomy were operated by endoscopic surgery, comprising only 10% of all cholecystectomy operations. In 1995 more than 80% of cholecystectomy cases were operated by endoscopic procedures. Indications for endoscopic surgery, such as gastrointestinal surgery, cardiac and respiratory surgery, urology, and gynecological surgery, spread rapidly in Japan and in other developed countries. In 2011, 140 000 cases of endoscopic surgery were performed in Japan and included 25 000 cases of cholecystectomy. The main advantage of endoscopic surgery is minimization of skin incisions and pain; hence the term "minimally invasive surgery". However, surgeons must operate on internal organs via small-diameter access ports with limited tactile sensation and 2-dimensional imaging. In addition, the working space of endoscopic surgery is very small compared with conventional surgery, so the surgical skills and ergonomic stresses imposed on the surgeon have greatly increased. To overcome these technical difficulties of endoscopic surgery, many R&D trials were started in the 1990s to assist endoscopic operation by means of surgical robotics and imaging and navigation technology.

One of the original manipulators to work in the intra-abdominal cavity is AESOP™ (Computer Motion Co.), which manipulates the endoscope in the abdominal cavity by a voice-recognition interface. The da Vinci surgical system™ (Intuitive Surgical, Inc.) can be nominated as the most original device and succeeds surgical manipulators. The da Vinci™ is a master–slave manipulator for robotic surgery consisting of a surgeon–console with an ergonomic interface, a patient cart with multiple interactive robot arms, and a three-dimensional endoscope. The surgeon manipulates controllers on the surgeon–console by observing a three-dimensional image obtained via the endoscope. The da Vinci™ enables surgeons to perform complex procedures, like coronary bypass surgery and prostate surgery, through 1–2 cm incisions. As of the end of 2012, there were approximately 2500 da Vinci™ systems installed worldwide in hospitals. (Fig.2)

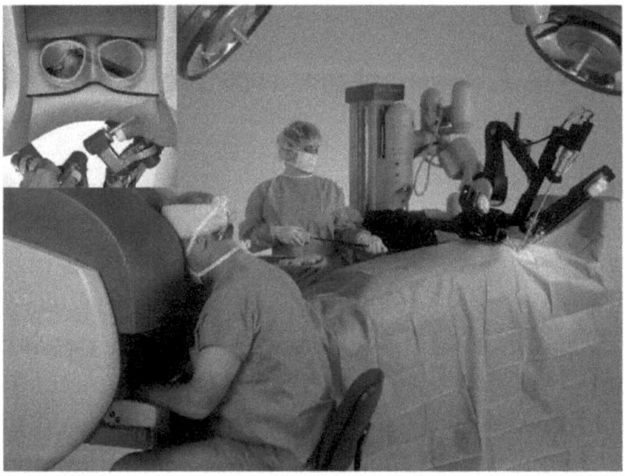

Fig. 2. da Vinci surgical system™ (first generation) from Surgical Intuitive Co

R&D of CAS in Japan was started in the mid-1980s. Initial developments included navigational aids for liver surgery which entailed three-dimensional reconstruction using computed tomography images. Then, many R&D projects on surgical manipulators and navigation systems for endoscopic surgery were started from the mid-1990s. In the early 2000s, many prototypes of new surgical robotic systems were developed and had advantages such as multi degree freedom, master–slave manipulation systems with navigational imaging and haptic sensation, and extensibility to telesurgery. In addition, a portable active-forceps with a deflectable and rotatable computer-controlled tip providing 6 degrees of handling freedom was completed. These surgical robots were developed for robotic general surgery, cardiac surgery, orthopedic surgery, and neurosurgery, and a manipulator for a rigid endoscope for laparoscopic surgery was developed and marketed as NaviotTM.(Fig.3)

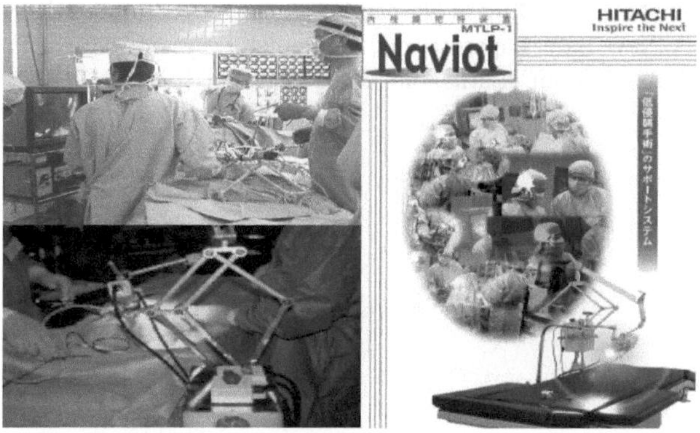

Fig. 3. NaviotTM, developed by University of Tokyo and HITACHI Co

From the perspective of commercialization and international export power, endoscopy and imaging technology are a strongpoint for Japan. However, commercially successful cases of surgical robotics such as da VinciTM are rare in Japan, with the exception of NaviotTM. Investigation of CAS developments revealed the following factors as responsible for the commercial failure of surgical robotics in Japan: limited R&D resources for human–computer interfaces, ergonomics and usability, regulatory affairs, and international marketing strategies of medical devices in the CAS field. Potential solutions to these problems include the establishment of interdisciplinary education and a research system for the CAS field (including medicine, engineering, ergonomics, regulatory sciences, and ethical issues), foundation of infrastructure elements (such as an animal experiment laboratory for venture companies), and training of coordinators and consultants on regulatory sciences, intellectual property, marketing, sales, and maintenance.

5 Conclusion

For smooth development and commercialization of surgical manipulators in the field of CAS, it is essential for R&D systems to adapt to social environments and global competition. Education on ergonomics and regulatory sciences is also necessary, in addition to computer information technology, as a component of medical and engineering education.

References

1. Shinohara, K.: Consideration of the human-computer interface in the operation room in the era of computer aided surgery. In: Stephanidis, C. (ed.) Posters, Part II, HCII 2011. CCIS, vol. 174, pp. 72–75. Springer, Heidelberg (2011)
2. Shinohara, K.: Implemantation problems of computerized physician order entry system in the operation room. In: Proceeding of Human Computer Interaction (CDR) (2009)
3. Kobayashi, E.: A New Safe Laparoscopic Manipulator System with a Five-Bar Linkage Mechanism and Optical Zoom. Journal of Computer Aided Surgery 4, 182–193 (1999)

Information for Supporting IBD Patients in Daily Life

Yusuke Takada, Yuki Kuri, and Naotake Hirasawa

Otaru University of Commerce, Hokkaido, Japan
{takada,kuri,hirasawa}@ouc-ux.org

Abstract. In this study the information necessary to support IBD patients in daily life was clarified and we developed the site to offer the information. The concept of the site was to offer three types of contents; the basic contents regarding IBD, the contents for the IBD patients and their family in order to live their stable daily life and the contents they referred habitually. Based on the concept we designed the information site and finished α version. The evaluation by the users in the system operation required some improvements of the contents, the trust of contents based on the support from medical institutions and the enhancement to communicate between the IBD stakeholders.

Keywords: IBD, Human-centred design, Web site.

1 Introduction

Inflammatory Bowel Disease (IBD) is a general term about chronic disease that causes inflammation of the digestive tract largely unexplained. It consists of two kinds of symptom; one is ulcerative colitis and another is Crohn's disease. It is a chronic sustained symptom and the cause of it has not yet become clear. In Japan IBD is acknowledged as intractable disease and the number of the patients is currently more than 170,000. When we think about the IBD patients, we can categorize them into two types based on the degree of severity; one is the patient who cannot live without the support of others and another is the patient who can manage his/her daily life like a healthy people corresponding to the symptoms. In Japan as for the former the support by the government is not always enough except for the support for working [1]. As the background of the situation, it is not revealed what kind of supports for daily life the patients need in order to keep their quality of life.

Therefore, in this study we aim at clarifying the information for supporting the patient in daily life and building an information site to offer it.

2 Site Concept

We began with envisioning the site concept before developing the site. To do it we carried out the following procedure.

First, we made a stakeholder map to identify the stakeholders involved in the site we planned to develop. Consequently we assumed the main users of the site were the patients and their family. Furthermore we categorized the patients by the degree of the

C. Stephanidis (Ed.): Posters, Part II, HCII 2013, CCIS 374, pp. 215–219, 2013.

symptoms and their activities in daily life. Secondly we analyzed 162 domestic sites related to IBD. We analyzed the site from the view of the site patterns [2]. As a result we could find there was no site that gathered and provided various kinds of information involved in IBD. Therefore we understood that the person who just had become the patient and his/her family was hard to look for basic information related to the disease.

Then our project asked the community of the IBD patient in Hokkaido to conduct the questionnaire survey and we had the effective response from 36 patients. After the survey we selected the six patients from the respondents of the questionnaire and carried out the interview in detail.

As a result of the investigation we could understand that most of the patients often felt anxieties related to their human relations, toilet support and their future life. In addition it was revealed that they tended to restrain communication with others because they are afraid of their sudden symptoms of the disease.

Consequently we set up three concepts related to the contents we planned to offer;

1. Basic contents regarding IBD,
2. Contents for the IBD patients and their family to live their stable daily life,
3. Contents the patients refer habitually.

3 Implementation

3.1 Site Design

In our project we carried out the site design based on human-centered approach [3].

We executed three design processes that consisted of concept building, low fidelity prototyping and high fidelity prototyping. In each process we followed the human-centered design processes, that is to say, understanding and specifying the context of use, specifying the user requirements in sufficient detail to drive the design, producing design solutions which meet these requirements and conducting user-centered evaluations of these design solutions and modify the design. The table shows the details of the processes.

Table 1. Development Processes based on the human-centered process

HCD processes	Design			Implementation		
	Concept Definition	LF Prototype	HF Prototype	α	β	Final
Context of use	CoU research	CoU research	-	-	-	-
User requirements	Service requirement definition	System and contents requirement definition	-	-	-	-
Solution	Service concept	Low Fidelity prototype	High Fidelity prototype	α system	β system	-
Evaluation	Concept evaluation	Prototype Evaluation	Prototype Evaluation	Operation test	Operation test	Audit
Outcome	Proposal of service	Basic service specification	Service specification	α system	β system	Final system

Through the design process we developed the contents like the following, corresponding to the site concepts as described above.

1. Basic contents regarding IBD

- Basic information of the diseases (including the summary, the causes, the symptoms, the cure and so on)
- Administrative support information for the patient
- Information related to the meal
- Information related to the exercise
- Book information involved in the disease
- Various links such as hospitals list for the special medical treatment, agencies for consulting service, communities for the patients, non-profit organizations for supporting the patients, personal sites of the patients, sites of the company related to IBD, research and educational institutions, and so on)

2. Contents for the IBD patients and their family to live their stable daily life

- Q&A
- Bulletin board system
- Experiences of the patient
- Restroom map
- NG food quick help chart

3. Contents the patients refer habitually

- Collections of recipe
- Q&A
- Bulletin board system
- Book review
- Life story introduction of the patient
- Off-line meeting information

3.2 Prototype Evaluation

We carried out the evaluation to the prototypes with usability inspection until high fidelity prototype design. After the evaluation we conducted the user test with the IBD patients during the high fidelity prototype. And then some contents were revised and alpha version was developed. Up to now we had conducted the operation test of alpha version to six informants with the diary method [4].

4 Evaluation

The results of the evaluation using the diary method showed 50% of informants judged the site available. On the other hands the others pointed out the problems to be sorted out such as the followings:

1. Basic contents regarding IBD

- Lack of information related to the latest social institutions and supports
- Lack of information related to about the working support
- Un-user-friendly descriptions about the disease

2. Contents for the IBD patients and their family to live their stable daily life

- Lack of information corresponding to the degree of the symptoms
- Lack of information related to the stoma and the medicines
- Lack of reference in order to recognize the degree of the symptoms for the patient
- Quite a few information of the other patients' daily life
- Lack of the trust of contents comparing the ones provided by doctors

3. Contents the patients refer habitually

- Lack of communication space between the users
- A few contents about the recipes
- Lack of new findings for the patients who have a long medical history
- A few spaces where the patients offer their information
- Lack of contents that make the patients excited and refreshed

4. Other

- Low usability related to navigation
- A few views from user
- Formal descriptions
- A lot of words
- A few photographs or illustrations

Consequently we could find quite a few information the patients needed in daily life such as a stoma, medicines, support systems, and so on. In addition we understood that many patients wanted to know the other's daily life. As a reason of it they could recognize themselves' situations by referring the other's life.

We recognized the requirement for increasing the trust with the support by medical institute. And then the need for setting up the space for communicating each other was revealed. Since the patients were forced to be restrained in their outside activities as described above, it seemed that they needed the additional and complementary communications as a reaction to the self-restraint in daily life. Furthermore the patients pointed out the problem of the usability of the site.

Thus we are planning to conduct the following improvements:

- The addition and improvement of contents,
- The collaboration with the medical institutions,
- The enforcement for offering the communication space,
- The improvement of the usability.

5 Conclusion

This study clarified the information necessary to support the IBD patients in daily life and we developed the information site to offer it.

The concept of the site was to offer the basic contents regarding IBD, the contents for the IBD patients and their family to live their stable daily life and the contents they referred habitually. Based on the concept we designed the information site and finished the evaluation to α version.

Considering the results of the evaluation by the users through the system operation, we are improving the contents and trying to find some medical institutions for supporting the reliability of the contents we offers. Furthermore we study the methods to enforce to communicate between IBD stakeholders such as patients, their family, medical staff, administration staffs, and so on.

References

1. IBD network and School of Public Health of Tokyo University, Research Report on the investigation for IBD patient's work situation. Hokkaido IBD Booklet 2, 29–32 (2006) (in Japanese)
2. Landay, D.K., Hong, J.A., van Duyne, J.I.: The Design of Sites: Patterns for Creating Winning Web Sites. Prentice Hall (2006)
3. ISO9241-210:2010, Ergonomics of human-system interaction - Part 210: Human-centered design for interactive systems (2010)
4. Usability Handbook, Kyoritsu Publishing (2007) (in Japanese)

The Use of Natural Interaction to Enrich the User Experience in Telemedicine Systems

Tatiana A. Tavares[1,2,3], Anna Medeiros[3], Rafael de Castro[3], and Eudisley dos Anjos[1,2]

[1] CI - Informatics Institute, Campus Castelo Branco, s/n, 58059-900 João Pessoa-PB, Brazil
[2] LAVID - Digital Video Applications Lab, Campus Castelo Branco, s/n, 58059-900 João Pessoa-PB, Brazil
[3] PPGI – Informatics Graduate Program, Campus Castelo Branco, s/n, 58059-900 João Pessoa-PB, Brazil
tatiana@lavid.ufpb.br, {linnamedeiros,rafaelhenriquec,guido}@gmail.com, eudisley@ci.ufpb.br

Abstract. Human communication always used gestures, movements and expressions as oral language support. Certain gestures are so commonly used around the world that are understood throughout different cultures and times, such as a wave or thumbs up. Natural Interaction is a way to apply this concept to user interfaces in computer systems. In this paper we discuss about the use of Natural Interaction features in a telemedicine system. More specifically, we demonstrate the use of natural interaction interfaces for control and manipulation of 3D objects inside Arthron tool. Arthron is a telemedicine tool used for surgery transmissions.

Keywords: Human Computer Interaction, Natural Interaction, Telemedicine.

1 Introduction

Making a brief retrospect we can identify the evolution of these devices through the command-based languages, through the graphical user interfaces (GUIs), and finally the direct manipulation with the advent of the use of the pointers (mouse). From the rise of touch screens, the use of cameras in the analysis of user actions and the creation of devices that allow us to use technology more easily. For example, the Kinect that enables us to think about the development of more sophisticated and natural user interfaces. The Natural Interaction (NI) studies ways that humans can interact through humans five senses, be that with gestures, voice commands, corporal expressions or human body parts detection and identification [1,2,3,4].

Natural User Interface or NUI is the used to refer to a user interface that applies concepts of natural interaction in its construction [5]. NUI is considered a new interaction paradigm, since the old and known WIMP (Window, Icon, Menu, Pointer) use concepts of interaction with devices themselves, i.e., there is the use of keyboard or mouse to access any part of the graphic interface, what is not considered as natural interaction, since using such hardware is not part of the naturalness of human being.

C. Stephanidis (Ed.): Posters, Part II, HCII 2013, CCIS 374, pp. 220–224, 2013.

Telemedicine or eHealth is one area that could benefit from this kind of technology. The widespread use of computer systems in healthcare is now a reality. Systems that can connect doctors, patients and students or make possible the evaluation of diagnostic tests from distance are good examples. Trends in telemedicine are systems that are capable of adding more advanced modes of interaction, such as three-dimensional interfaces and natural interaction.

2 Interaction in Telemedicine

It is clear from the literature [07] that the term telemedicine encompasses many different technologies, used in different ways. According to a review [07] that compares the provision of patients using face-to-face care with care using telecommunications technologies, sometimes telemedicine appliances make use of ongoing technologies or they are stimulated by enthusiasts more than clinical needs.

One example of technologies well-done applied in Telemedicine issues is the Virtual Reality. According with Gamberini (2001) the use of VE (Virtual Environment) lets users navigate and interact with a three-dimensional environment in real time. The use of VR features brought many real possibilities to Telemedicine systems, such as the remote manipulation of equipment, remote procedures training, interaction with anatomic models. This kind of feature is special useful for student training, surgery planning and also neuropsychological rehabilitation [08].

Telemedicine is a multidisciplinary field that can aid many aspects of health care, one of those is prevention. In this field, motivating factors and incentives are necessary to convince people to do sports, exercises, change nutrition type or composition and have a healthy lifestyle. This action can prevent diseases or obesity and cardio problems. To accomplish this task the serious games are an excellent opportunity, besides prevention they can also help with rehabilitation and therapy. Clinical feedback such as movement data can provide medical experts with useful information regarding patients' home training [09].

In order to use a more realistic game environment it is necessary to have some kind of equipment that provides for user a natural and transparent interaction. So that the experience is as natural as possible. In other words, we need to improve Natural Interaction (NI) features or using a Natural Interaction Interface (NUI). We have many options to develop this kind of features, different equipments and software. As a low cost alternative the Microsoft Kinect can be used as a full body input device. There are examples for telemedicine that uses NUI through Kinect, such as patient assistance and monitoring. In [10] is discussed a system that provides information about the exercises and gives feedback of the patient performance, also allowing the therapist to observe sessions remotely and recording them. Another example is discussed in [11], where the Kinect is used for improving stroke rehabilitation. This work shows different implementations using Kinect and evaluates them, showing the suitability of Kinect for being used in such application. González et al (2012) discusses the use of Kinect and Wii Balance Board as a low-cost alternative to estimate the center of mass of patients. This solution is closely related to human motion stability while walking and standing and it is very necessary in an increasingly older population. Otherwise, using Kinect and Wii, instead specific equipment, is a solution more accessible and portable. This solution can be also used for rehabilitation, motion stability assessment and balance training. Another telemedicine scenario that suits well with NUI through Kinect is the distance learning and training. For example, the use of NUI for better teaching-learning user interfaces. Medeiros et al (2012) presents a solution for enrich the user experience in a telemedicine system called Arthron as detailed in the next section.

3 IN Features in Arthron

The proposal of IN features for Arthron [18] was based in the need of a better user interface solution for 3D manipulation improved by our own experience in using Arthron for telemedicine activities. Besides, a "handless" user interface is very suitable for surgeries rooms and also telemedicine rooms.

The GTAVCS [19] developed Arthron tool which is a remote management tool for capturing and distributing multiple simultaneous streams of media to provide support for several video-collaboration scenarios, as broadcast surgeries in the context of telemedicine. The Arthron main feature is to offer the user a simple interface for handling different sources/streams of media simultaneously. Therefore the user can remotely add, remove, configure the presentation format and schedule the exhibition in time and space of media streams as shown in Figure 01-(a).

An innovation of Arthron is to provide the possibility to manipulate 3D objects, especially human anatomical structures, while viewing other streams, such as video. The addition of these 3D models is especially useful as a didactic resource focused to distance training and learning. Through this feature the physician-teacher can show students in an integrated manner to live video, models that demonstrate the normal organs function, tissues or structures of the human body. In Figure 01-(b) we present the integration of 3D models to Arthron tool.

(a)

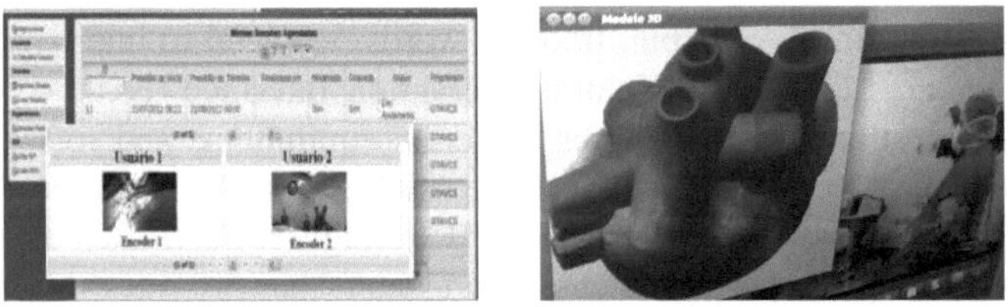

(b)

Fig. 1. Arthron User Interfaces. In (a) The interface for video manipulation and in (b) the 3D models used in a surgery transmission with Arthron.

In the 3D model manipulation section of this application was introduced the concept of natural interaction with the Kinect tool. This feature makes it easier the use and manipulation of the 3D models while viewing other flows managed by Arthron. After all in Telemedicine the using the hands and touch prevent simultaneous execution of medical procedures due to sterilization. In this sense the interaction without touching devices to manipulate 3D objects makes it possible that the physician can control and manipulate three-dimensional models during surgery.

As we mentioned before, the main goal of using IN features in Arthron was an alternative way to access the control functions used for 3D manipulation. So a gesture vocabulary was defined to identify the users modes of interaction. Figure 02 shows the main features which are used to interact with the application.

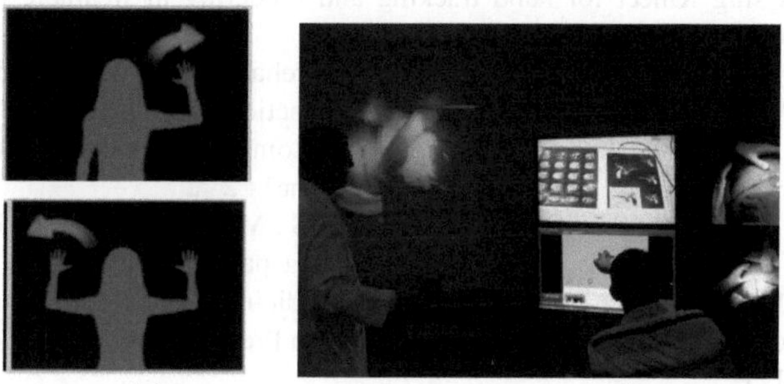

(a) (b)

Fig. 2. IN in Arthron. In (a) gestures vocabulary, where it shows how to start the both hands tracking, starting with the left hand. In (b) interaction with Kinect, the doctor is manipulating 3D models using Kinect. In this experience we are using a video wall with multiples video streams and the 3D models are loaded together.

For development IN features in Arthron we used the Microsoft Kinect to capture the depth image stream and the framework OpenNI to assist the depth stream processing. The Tracker component recognizes gestures and begins tracking the identified hand. The Renderer component then receives the hand tracking and decides how to manipulate the 3D object. To better understand the application you need to know that it was developed in a distributed manner. Components Screen, 3D Object and Gesture are used to interface with the user, access the 3D objects and interpret gestures, respectively.

4 Discussion

This work was developed focusing on the benefits that the use of Natural Interaction would provide for e-Heath or Telemedicine systems improvement. The Kinect was used to add movement detection to a preexistent tridimensional application, though OpenNI framework for Kinect. The primary results of user experiences figure that telemedicine systems as a large field of research and innovation for IN features.

So, IN is a "natural" user interface and it can improve, specially for complex systems, a easier way for interaction. On the current work stage it is possible to adapt the proposed solution for others scenarios of application, as training and remote manipulation.

Acknowledgments. We are grateful to the Lauro Wanderley Academical Hospital professionals for the partnership that made this work possible, specially Dr. Geraldo Almeida.

References

1. McCord, Charlotte. Gestures, Western Folklore 7, 290–292 (1948)
2. Frati, V.: Using Kinect for hand tracking and rendering in wearable haptics. In: World Haptics Conference (WHC) at IEEE (2011)
3. Researchers use Kinect gesture control in stroke rehab system. The Engineer (2012)
4. Hewett: Curricula for Human-Computer Interaction. The Association for Computing Machinery, Special Interest Group on Computer Human Interaction (2009), http://old.sigchi.org/cdg/cdg2.html#2_1
5. Vieira, E., Passos, M., Santos, B.A., Oliveira, S.S., Melo, E.A., Motta, G.H.M.B., Tavares, T.A., Filho, S., de Lemos, G.: Uma Ferramenta para Gerenciamento e Transmissão de Fluxos de Vídeo em Alta Definição para Telemedicina. Salão de Ferramentas do Simpósio Brasileiro de Redes de Computadores 2012, Ouro Preto. Anais do Salão de Ferramentas do SBRC (2012)
6. Rauterberg, G.W.M., Mauch, T., Stebler, R.: How to improve the quality of human performance with natural user interfaces as a case study for augmented reality. In: Smith, T.F., Waterman, M.S. (eds.) Identification of Common Molecular Subsequences (1996); J. Mol. Biol. 147, 195–197 (1981)
7. Currell, R., Urquhart, C., Wainwright, P., Lewis, R.: Telemedicine versus face to face patient care: effects on professional practice and health care outcomes. The Cochrane Collaboration (2010), http://www.thecochranelibrary.com/userfiles/ccoch/file/Telemedicine/CD002098.pdf (review)
8. Riva, G., Gamberini, L.: Virtual Reality in telemedicine. ch. 7. Communications Through Virtual Technology: Identity Community and Technology in the Internet Age (2001), http://www.neurovr.org/emerging/book1/1CHAPT_07.PDF
9. Wac, K., Hausheer, D., Fiedler, M., Bonato, P., et al.: Future Internet for eHealth. Report from Dagstuhl Seminar 12231 (2012), http://publik.tuwien.ac.at/files/PubDat_210335.pdf
10. Ni, B., Pei, Y., Winkler, S.: Kinect for Rehabilitation, http://vintage.winklerbros.net/Publications/iCREATe2012.pdf
11. LaBelle, K. Evaluation of Kinect Joint Tracking for Clinical and In-home Stroke Rehabilitation Tools. Notre Dame, Indiana. 2011. http://www1bpt.bridgeport.edu/jelee/courses/CS550_F12/Thesis/T3.Kinect%20Joint.pdf
12. González, A., Hayashibe, M., Fraisse, P.: Estimation of the Center of Mass with Kinect and Wii balance board. In: IROS12: International Conference on Intelligent Robots and Systems, Portugal (2012), http://hal-lirmm.ccsd.cnrs.fr/docs/00/73/46/29/PDF/IROS2012.pdf
13. Medeiros, A., Castro, R., Tavares, T.A.: Natural Interaction for 3D Manipulation in Telemedicine: A Study Case developed for Arthron Video Collaboration Tool. In: Workshop de Realidade Virtual e Aumentada, Paranavaí. Anais do WRVA 2012, vol. 1 (2012)

Healthcare System Focusing on Emotional Aspect Using Augmented Reality: Control Breathing Application in Relaxation Service

Somchanok Tivatansakul[1] and Michiko Ohkura[2]

[1] Graduate School of Engineering, Shibaura Institute of Technology, Japan
nb12505@shibaura-it.ac.jp
[2] College of Engineering, Shibaura Institute of Technology, Japan
ohkura@sic.shibaura-it.ac.jp

Abstract. We proposed a new healthcare system that focuses on emotional aspects to deal with negative emotional health in daily life. Our healthcare system integrates augmented reality to display virtual objects in real environments and Kinect, which allows users to freely interact with them. We also employ biological sensors to measure and detect user emotions, and provide three services based on their expected emotions: Relaxation Service, Amusement Service and Exciting Service. To implement a small prototype of this system, we have developed one application in relaxation service: Control Breathing Application. This application applied deep breathing techniques of stress management to supports users when they experience stress. This application displays a virtual music box to assist them perform deep breathing. Virtual objects and music can increase user relaxation and decrease their stress. The experiment is performed to measure the effectiveness of the application. From the result, our application can effectively decrease users stress when they experienced our application for short time.

Keywords: Emotion, Healthcare, Augmented Reality.

1 Introduction

In recent year, the design and implementation of ubiquitous system, intelligent space system and healthcare system are very popular. The basic idea of these systems is to automatically monitor the environment including human to provide assistance and services to them. Several systems are proposed to emphasize the support of the physical aspects at the expense of emotional aspects. However, emotional health is also important as much as physical health and negative emotional health can lead to such social and mental health problem as suicide problem.

We proposed a new healthcare system that focuses on emotional aspects using augmented reality to deal with negative emotional health in daily life. Our system provides services that allow users to interact with virtual objects in real environments to get different positive emotions and decrease their negative emotions. This system is

C. Stephanidis (Ed.): Posters, Part II, HCII 2013, CCIS 374, pp. 225–229, 2013.

designed to provide three services: Relaxation Service, Amusement Service and Exciting Service [1]. This paper focuses on Relaxation Service.

2 Relaxation Service Design

To implement a small prototype of this system, we have designed one application in relaxation service: Control Breathing Application.

2.1 The Design of Control Breathing Application

This application increases user relaxation with the deep breathing techniques of stress management [2]. The workflow of this application is shown in Fig. 1.

First, users can request this application in the relaxation service by web browser. Then they can start using this application by showing an AR marker to camera. The application detects the AR marker and displays a virtual music box, which slowly turns and plays music. The users inhale and exhale in harmony to the turning of the music box to control their breathing. While they are controlling their breathing, the ECG sensor on their chest records ECG signals to detect their respiration. If it isn't in harmony with the virtual music box, the application suggests that they breathe more shortly or deeply. The application continues to support users until they feel more relaxed. Our control breathing application is shown in Fig. 2.

3 Implementation of Control Breathing Application

Control breathing application synchronizes the results from augmented reality application which detect AR marker and display a virtual music box, and breathing detection which convert ECG signal to respiratory signal in order to detect inspiration and expiration. To implement control breathing application, we also need to implement augmented reality application and breathing detection as we describe below.

3.1 Augmented Reality Application

This application is implemented based on FLARManager [3] that build augmented reality applications for Flash more easily. The control breathing application will use this application to detects AR marker to render and display a virtual music box [4].

3.2 Breathing Detection

This breathing detection utilized ECG sensor to converts and analyzes ECG signal for detect respiration signal using ECG signal processing [5-6]. Our breathing detection derived the respiratory signal from estimation of the R-wave amplitude modulation [7]. This method performs low pass and notch filer to remove noise. QRS Detection is performed to detect QRS Interval. Then we remove baseline wander noise. After that,

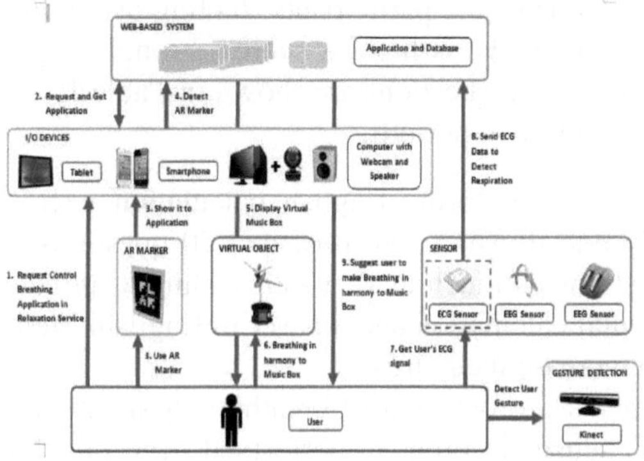

Fig. 1. The workflow of control breathing application

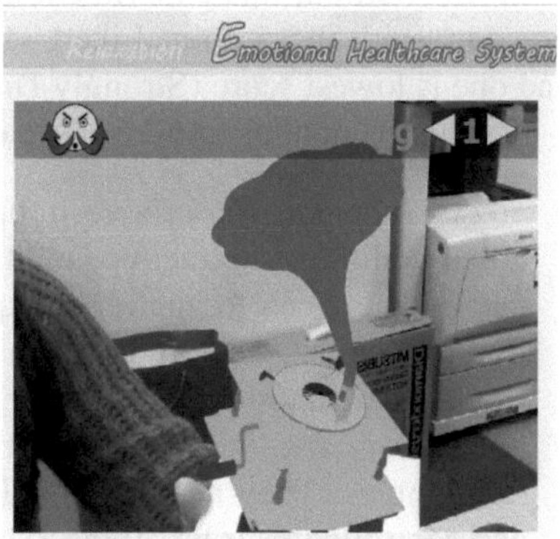

Fig. 2. Control breathing application

cleaned ECG signal is produced to detect peak amplitude and location of each RR-Interval in order to estimate respiratory signal. Then the interpolation is performed to smooth signal and down-sampled sampling rate in order to get respiratory signal. After that, we normalized the signal in order to easily detect inspiration and expiration signal and calculate time of inspiration and expiration. The control breathing application will use this application to detects users' respiratory signal and control their inhale and exhale in harmony with a virtual music box to increase their relaxation according to stress management technique.

4 Evaluation

We have performed the experiment with five young participants: four females and one male. This experiment is set to check this application that it can decrease stress effectively and to evaluate the participants' feeling when using this application [8].

4.1 Experiment

We have performed experiment to evaluate the effectiveness of the control breathing application by measuring stress of each participant using Cocoro Meter. This equipment measures the salivary amylase [KU/L] from saliva and classifies it into the stress

Table 1. Questions for evaluate user feeling

#	Questions
1	During using this application, you feel relax.
2	During using this application, you feel comfortable.
3	During using this application, you feel boring.
4	During using this application, you feel sleepy.
5	During using this application, you like it.

level. In addition, this experiment also evaluates the participants' feeling using questionnaire with the 5-point Likert scale where five is highest score (Strongly Agree) and one is lowest score (Strongly Disagree). The questions are shown in Table 1.

The experiment procedure is separated into two periods.

- *Stress Increase Period*: each participant performs English calculation exercise about addition, subtraction, multiply and division. We provided 70 questions; all participants need to answer the questions as much as they can within 20 minutes. The participants need to perform mental calculation and answer in English. Mental English calculation might be able to increase their stress.
- *Stress Decrease Period*: the participants use our control breathing application for ten minutes. They need to put ECG sensor in order to performed deep breathing and controlled their breathing. They listened to the classical music and watched the slow turning of virtual music box. The deep breathing techniques of stress management, the classical music and turning of 3D object might be able to decrease their stress.

The process to perform experiment is: firstly, the participants performed salivary amylase test to measure their current stress. Then the stress increase period is served to the participants for 20 minutes in order to increase their stress. After that, the participants performed salivary amylase test again. Then the stress decrease period is served to the participants for ten minutes in order to decrease their stress and increase their relaxation. Every five minutes past, the participant performed salivary amylase to check their stress. Finally, the participants answered the questionnaire to evaluate their feeling.

5 Result and Discussion

From the measured salivary amylase of all participants, if the measured data increases, it can indicate that the participants get more stress. If the measured data decrease, it can indicate that the participants get more relax. This experiment evaluate only the application can make user feel relax and decrease their stress. We calculate the percentage of users who got more stress after performing English calculation. We also calculate the percentage of users whose stress decreased while using our application for five and ten minutes. The percentage is shown in Table 2.

From the result in Table 2, after the participants used our application for five minutes, 80% of all participants feel more relax and their stress decreased. 40% of all

Table 2. Analysis Result of Effectiveness Aspect

	Stress Increase	Stress Decrease	Same Stress
After Stress Increase Period	60 %	20%	20%
After Stress Decrease Period 5 minutes	0 %	80 %	20%
After Stress Decrease Period 10 minutes	20%	40 %	40%

participants also feel more relax after using our application for ten minutes. However, some people didn't feel relax after using our application for five minutes but ten minutes pass, they feel more relax. Some people feel more relax after using application for five minute but they get more stress after using our application for ten minutes because they might feel tried when controlling their breathe for a long time.

From the analysis result of questionnaire, users agree that they feel relax, comfortable, boring and sleepy while using our application. However, they don't feel like or dislike when they use our application [8].

6 Conclusion

We proposed a new healthcare system that focused on emotional aspects for supporting adolescents and adults such as students and working people in daily life. The system can provide three services: relaxation, amusement and exciting service. This paper focuses on overall system design, the design, implementation and evaluation of control breathing application for relaxation service. From the experimental result, we can summarize that when users experience the application, they feel relax, comfortable and sleepy. However, they also feel boring. Moreover, we observed that our application can effectively decrease users stress when they experienced our application for short time. The improvement of relaxation service, the design and implementation of other services remains future works.

References

1. Tivatansakul, S., Ohkura, M.: Healthcare System Design Focusing on Emotional Aspects using Augmented Reality – Relaxed Service Design. In: IEEE Symposium Series on Computational Intelligence in Healthcare and e-Health (2013) (in press)
2. Antai-Otong, D.: Creative Stress-Management Techniques for Self-Renewal. Dermatology Nursing 13(1), 31–37 (2001)
3. FLARManager Augmented Reality in Flash, http://words.transmote.com/
4. Virtual Music Box: http://www.3dmodelfree.com/models/29549-0.htm
5. Vyas, M.P., Panse, M.S.: Various Methods to Detect Respiration Rate From ECG Using LabVIEW. In: International Conference on Biomedical Engineering and Assistive Technologies (2010)
6. Widjaja, D., Taelman, J., Vandeput, S., Braeken, M.A.K.A., Otte, R.A., Van den Bergh, B.R.H., Van Huffel, S.: ECG-Derived Respiration: Comparison and New Measures for Respiratory Variability. Computing in Cardiology, 149–152 (2010)
7. Arunachalam, S.P., Brown, L.F.: Real-Time Estimation of the ECG-Derived Respiration (EDR) Signal using a New Algorithm for Baseline Wander Noise Removal. In: Annual International Conference of the IEEE Engineering in Medicine and Biology Society, pp. 5681–5684 (2009)
8. Tivatansakul, S., Ohkura, M.: Healthcare System Design Focusing on Emotional Aspects using Augmented Reality - Re-Design of Control Breathing Application in Relaxation Service. In: 5th International Congress of International Association of Societies of Design Research (2013) (in submission)

mERlin: Development of an Emergency Department Tracking System

Jacob Towns[1] and John T. Finnell[1,2,3]

[1] School of Medicine, Indiana University, Indianapolis, IN, USA
[2] School of Informatics and Computing, Indiana University, Indianapolis, IN, USA
[3] Regenstrief Institute, Indianapolis, IN, USA
{jatowns,jfinnell}@iupui.edu

Abstract. In the United States, the Emergency Department (ED) represents a major portion of health care. The Institute of Medicine issued its report on Emergency Care entitled, "Hospital-based Emergency Care: At the Breaking Point" specifically calling for hospitals to adopt information systems to improve the safety and quality of emergency care. We describe the functional requirements, vendor development, and barriers encountered during creation of a system by an integrated, inter-professional team.

Keywords: Emergency Medicine, Electronic Health Records, Information Systems.

1 Introduction

In the United States, the Emergency Department (ED) represents a major portion of health care with 136.1 million unique patient encounters each year. One in every five encounters requires less than 15 minutes, and one in every eight results in an admission to the hospital. It is further expected that in the wake of recent healthcare reform, ED visits will continue to increase as access to healthcare grows. As a direct result of increased ED visits and decreased inpatient capacity, the Institute of Medicine issued its report on Emergency Care. The 2006 report entitled, "Hospital-based Emergency Care: At the Breaking Point" specifically calls for hospitals to adopt information systems to improve the safety and quality of emergency care. Additionally, EDs are mandated to submit the following "Core Measures" to the Centers for Medicare and Medicaid Services (CMS):

1. Median time from ED arrival to ED departure for admitted ED patients (Core Measure ED-1).
2. Admit decision time to ED departure time for admitted ED patients (Core Measure ED-2).
3. Median time from ED arrival to ED departure for discharged ED patients (Core Measure OP-18).

C. Stephanidis (Ed.): Posters, Part II, HCII 2013, CCIS 374, pp. 230–234, 2013.

4. Transition record with specified elements received by discharged patients (Major procedures and tests performed, principal diagnosis, patient instructions, plan for follow-up, new medications and/or changes to current medicines with quantity prescribed and instructions for each) (Core Measure OP-19).
5. Door to diagnostic evaluation by qualified medical personnel (Core Measure OP-20).
6. Median time to pain management for long bone fracture (Core Measure OP-21).
7. Left without being seen (Core Measure OP-22).

2 Hospital Setting

2.1 Physical Plant

Wishard Memorial Hospital is a level 1 trauma center with over 110,000 annual patient visits. The 80 beds are distributed across the following areas: 1) Shock/Resuscitation, 2) High Acuity, 3) Low Acuity-1, 4) Low Acuity-2, 5) Holding (for patients under arrest), 6) Annex (for psychiatric care), 7) Intake, 8) Rapid Sort, and 9) Back Assessment. Additionally there are several waiting areas distributed geographically.

2.2 Personnel

Wishard Memorial Hospital is a clinical training site for various providers at all stages of their careers. The Indiana University School of medicine requires all 4th year medical students to participate in an ED experience. Additionally, program requirements for Internal Medicine, among other programs, stipulate their residents have at least a one-month ED experience. Lastly, Indiana University is home to one of the largest three-year training programs in Emergency Medicine. Therefore, our setting differentiates us from non-academic institutions in that we have a constant influx of new providers of all fields on a yearly basis. As an example, in a single encounter within our ED, a patient may be assessed by a myriad of personnel including attending staff, residents, medical students, nurse practitioners, nurses, nursing assistants, techs, paramedics, consultants, admitting physicians/teams, interpreters, social workers, care managers, pharmacists, and physical therapists.

2.3 Patient Workflow

The vast majority (~70%) of patients enter the ED through the main entrance. They are greeted by a "Sort Nurse" who obtains the chief complaint (reason for visit), basic demographic data, and determines if the patient is either 1) "Sick" 2) "Not sick", or 3) "Critically ill," necessitating a Shock/Resuscitation room (Figure 1). If the patient is "Not sick," they are placed in an Intake room to be triaged and seen by a nurse and a clinician respectively. Once the patient has been assessed, they are moved from Intake to one of the other areas based upon clinician judgment.

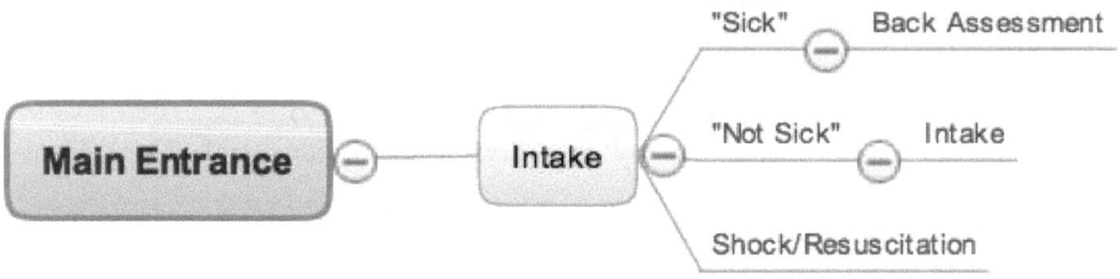

Fig. 1. ED Patient Flow from Main Entrance

The remaining 30% of patients arrive by ambulance or police. These patients as well as those sent from the Main Entrance/Sort Nurse as "Sick" are evaluated by the "Back Assessment Nurse". This nurse performs the same functions as the "Sort Nurse" in addition to an initial assessment. This allows the nurse to determine an appropriate care area within the ED for the needs of the patient.

3 Functional Requirements

We first began by analyzing our existing tracking system. We formed a workgroup to review the previous specifications and existing functionality, then reviewed commercial systems and had conversations with our peers to augment our specifications. This integrated, inter-professional team, physicians, nurses, registration, informaticians, and system administration, undertook the functional design of our system. The team met routinely over the course of months to create the tracking system.

After months of work, we finalized the design into the following content areas:

(a) An integrated system for all ED personnel- regardless of patient status (outpatient or admitted)
(b) Tracking
(c) System Reporting /Analytics
(d) Documentation
(e) Clinical Decision Support (CPOE/CDSS)
(f) Meaningful Use Criteria
(g) Interfaces / INPC
(h) Regulatory / Billing

Each of these content areas contains the required functional specifications. For example, under the Tracking category:

- Provide ability to assign same nurse to multiple patients in a single step.
- Provide ability to assign multiple physicians to a patient.
- Provide ability to assign multiple types of providers / levels to a patient.

- Support definition of "hall beds" in the system and ability to assign a patient to a hall bed. (e.g. multiple patients to a single location)
- Allow more than one user to access the same patient record at the same time (e.g. no record lock out).
- Automatically capture, time-stamp and track patient wait and activity times at each step of an ED visit to support analysis of throughput, workflow and potential bottlenecks.
- Capture time of triage.
- Capture time patient is in treatment room.
- Ability to hold a room for a patient prior to the patient's arrival (e.g. ambulance, helicopter, doctor's office).

After planning what functions and features were to be included, our committee worked closely with the software engineers on implementation.

4 System Build

We began with iterative mock-ups using existing data routinely collected by the nursing personnel and in situ "research" from the active use of the previous tracking system. These white board exercises allowed us to optimize content and placement of data within the system. We equipped our meeting room with several devices on the development side of the system to allow users opportunities to use and provide feedback to the steering group.

As the system started to mature we realized we would need a logical cutoff to roll out our first stable production version- 1.0. We reviewed the list of functional requirements and prioritized those that would be essential to the first release of the product.

Throughout the process, the entire ED was allowed to work with the system to learn how to use it. We had a technical "go-live" one week prior to our clinical "go-live," ensuring all the production systems would be functional. Additional testing was done by the super-user group during this one week period.

5 Lessons Learned

As with all system development, there were several "teaching" moments we would like to share. First, project management is critical. This sounds like a cliché, but it truly is critical. Second, we encountered significant delays in terms of user authentication. The hospital was undergoing a change in credentialing systems requiring all users to have an active directory account, and all access is required to be authenticated against this token. After assessing the personnel of all categories of users listed previously, there were over 500 users needing credentials to be added to the system and proximity cards issued. Lastly, there was a lack of personnel formally trained in designing the user experience. The clinical team signed off on what they believed was a rough version of the system that would undergo further polishing from the software engineers, but it was that rough version that was actually implemented. For example, the back button on the interface did not take one back a previous page. The user had to reload at times to return to previous screens. This created training issues as we tried to explain some of the design flaws. We eventually had faculty from the school of informatics and computing review the application and make several helpful suggestions to improve the user experience.

6 Summary

Emergency medicine requires unique technologic tools to provide outstanding clinical care. Systems developed for other environments may not naturally adapt to this clinical space. The way to design an optimal system is to have multiple users/roles input, seek outside advice from other systems/colleagues and create your own set of functional specifications. The functional specifications provide a framework for the system design and build. Additionally, we learned the value of requiring a resource for project management as well as having an expert in systems usability and design.

VR Tool for Interaction with the Abdomen Anatomy

Lizeth Vega-Medina, Gerardo Tibamoso, and Byron Perez-Gutierrez

Virtual Reality Center - Davinci Research Group
Nueva Granada Military University, Bogotá D.C, Colombia
{lizvega,gtibamosop,byron.perez}@ieee.org

Abstract. Due to ethical issues with the use of human and animal corpses in medical education, difficulty interacting with organs using sensory channels as sight and touch, and the possibility to have a tool compatible with low-cost equipment such as laptops and Novint Falcon haptic system, an interactive tool of the abdominal organs is being developed taking advantage of virtual reality tools that are increasingly available in the academic environment. The process of building this interactive system consists of the following steps: Source data are taken from images acquired by abdominal computed tomography (CT) or magnetic resonance imaging (MRI). Each selected abdominal organ (liver, kidney and spleen) is segmented by a semi-automatic process, from which a polygonal mesh is obtained to represent the 3D shape of the organ. Then the visual and mechanical properties of tissues, extracted from the recent literature, are associated to the polygonal representation with H3DAPI.

Keywords: H3DAPI, Haptic, Novint Falcon, Organ palpation, Simulation, Soft tissues.

1 Introduction

Every day is more complex to use human and animal corpses to learn anatomy. Ethical and legal aspects, besides the increase in the number of people that requires this kind of knowledge, has made that the use of appropriate academic methodologies for the teaching-learning process becomes more difficult. Thus, alternative methods are required to facilitate teaching and to approach the students to highly accurate, interactive computer models to have the same or similar results that are obtained with traditional methods.

Taking advantage of virtual reality tools that are increasingly available in the academic environment, an interactive tool of the abdominal organs is being developed. This library facilitates for medical students the learning process of anatomical structures, permitting to interact with the models in an affordable way, expanding the landscape that provides library resources and virtual applications currently available [1].

C. Stephanidis (Ed.): Posters, Part II, HCII 2013, CCIS 374, pp. 235–239, 2013.

2 Methodology

The process of building this interactive system consists of the following steps: Data acquisition of medical images, abdominal organs segmentation and 3D surface construction, and the integration to a visuo-haptic an interactive system.

2.1 Data Acquisition

Source data are taken from images acquired by abdominal computed tomography (CT) or magnetic resonance imaging (MRI).

2.2 Surface Delimitation

The liver, kidneys and spleen were segmented by a semi-automatic process, first the organ is selected as shown in Fig. 1(a), then, the organ is delimited in each image from the dataset shown in Fig. 1(b). Finally the segmentation organ is obtained as it can be seen in Fig1(c).

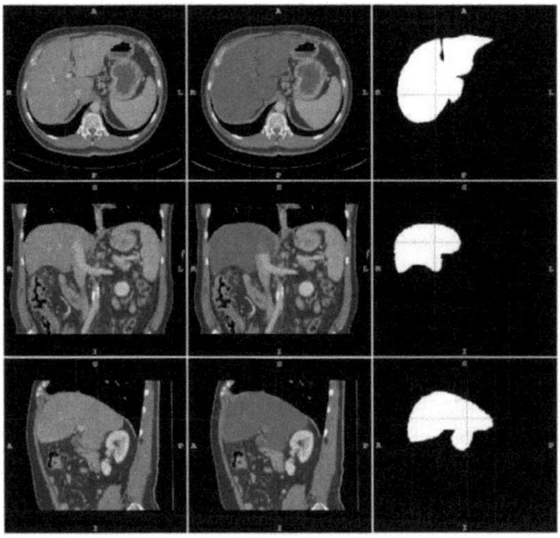

Fig. 1. Liver segmentation process using CT images

2.3 3D Surface Construction

After the segmentation is obtained, the next procedure is to construct a 3D closed surface using the algorithms based on Delaunay Triangulation [2]. This surface will behave as a solid because it does not have spaces or holes in it.

2.4 Haptic Interaction

After obtaining the 3D surface of the liver, spleen and right and left kidneys they are imported to H3DAPI[1] as shown in Fig. 2. There, the material properties of the surfaces as color, stiffness, damping, can be modified.

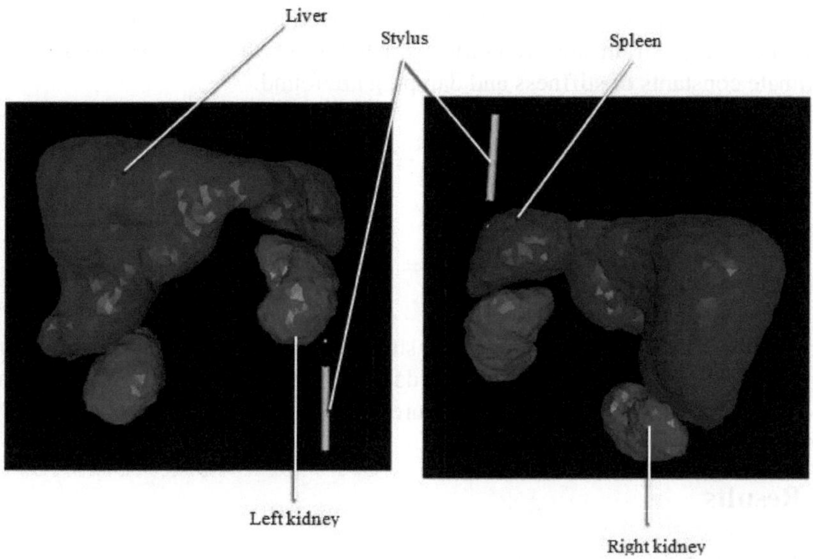

Fig. 2. Organs in H3DAPI

Then, the user is capable of feeling each one of the organs with the Novint Falcon Haptic Device. This permits the user to experience the shape, texture, stiffness, damping among others characteristics, in the simulated organ.

A basic spring-mass-damper model (Fig 3) were used to describe the behavior of a soft tissue and the interaction with the Novint Falcon. The model parameters were defined considering the experimental information of *in vivo* and *ex vivo* organs developed by Kerdok [3] and Rosen [4].

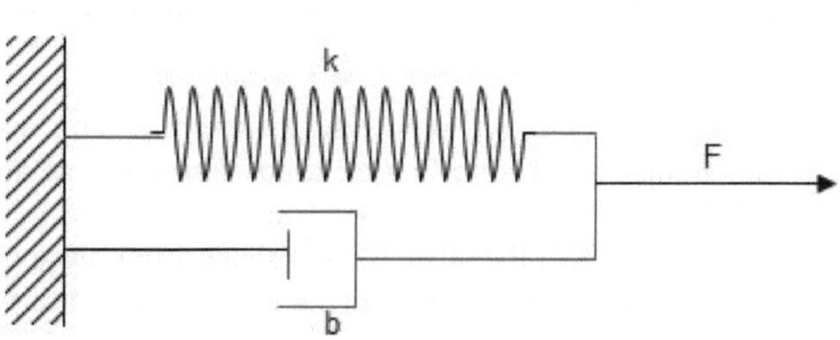

Fig. 3. Spring-mass-damper visco-elastic model

[1] `http://www.h3dapi.org/`

The model is represented by the equation (1)

$$F = F_s + F_d = kx + bv \tag{1}$$

Where F is the total force, F_s is the spring force, F_d is the damper force, k is the stiffness constant, x is the displacement, b is the damping constant and v is the velocity.

From (1) the parameters can be obtained to modify the material in H3DAPI, through the stress, strain and velocity extracted from the Kerdok and Rosen, the approximate constants of stiffness and damping are found.

$$\frac{F}{A} = \frac{F_s}{A} + \frac{F_d}{A} = Ee + \frac{bv}{A} \tag{2}$$

$$\sigma = \sigma_s + \sigma_d = Ee + \frac{bv}{A} \tag{3}$$

Where E is the Young's Modulus, e is the strain, σ_s and σ_d are the spring and damper stresses. The stiffness constant and the damping constant were found trough the stress-strain relations obtained from literature.

3 Results

An application was developed where the liver, spleen and kidneys were included using CT scans with resolution of 512x512x388 voxels and size of 0.58 x 0.58 x 1 mm. Each constructed mesh has different characteristics as shown in Table 1.

Table 1. Mesh description

Organ	Vertices	Polygons
Liver	2556	5108
Spleen	760	1516
Right kidney	596	1188
Left kidney	560	1114

It was necessary to make a scale to perceive the different textures according to the Novint Falcon characteristics, for this scale were used compact bone and oil parameters as the maximum value.

In this scenario the user can feel the stiffness and shape from these organs, besides seeing them and their spatial location between them, complementing this way the apprentice experience as shown in Fig.4.

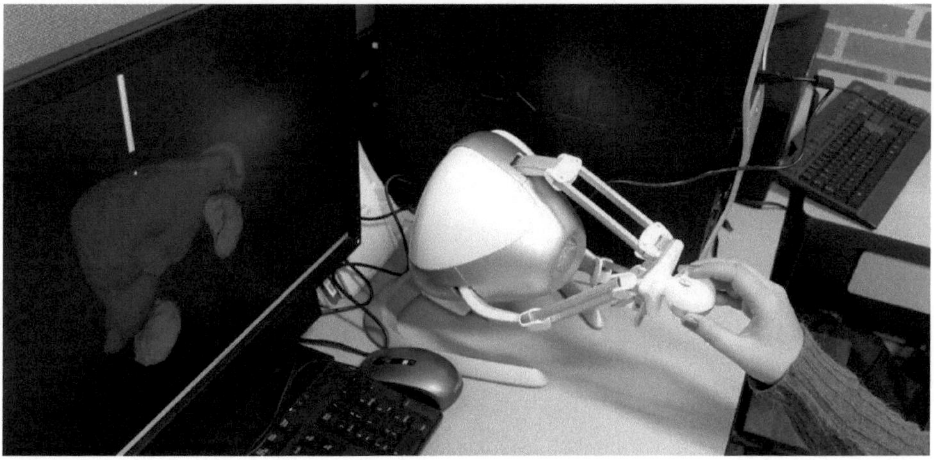

Fig. 4. Interaction system

4 Discussion

The Novint Falcon performance is suitable for shape, size and spatial location recognition by the user but is not a proper device for small displacements and forces because of its small dynamic range, which is why in some occasions the user cannot feel the proper feedback when touching the surface from any meshed organ. Also the Novint Falcon can be replaced by other haptic devices as the Sensable Phantom Omni[2] or Entact Robotics W5D[3] with more degrees of freedom and dynamic range that permits small displacements, force feedback and realism but increasing the cost of the overall system.

As a future work, another organs as stomach, small intestine, large intestine and bladder will be included in the same way to complete the abdomen anatomy.

References

1. Primal Pictures Anatomy TV, `http://www.primalpictures.com`
2. Tibamoso, G., Perez-Gutierrez, B., Uribe-Quevedo, A.: 3D Liver Volume Reconstructed for Palpation Training. Studies Health Technology and Informatics 184, 450–452 (2013)
3. Kerdok, A.: Characterizing the Nonlinear Mechanical Response of Liver to Surgical Manipulation. Harvard University (2006)
4. Rosen, J., Brown, J.D., De, S., Sinanan, M., Hannaford, B.: Biomechanical Properties of Abdominal Organs In Vivo and Postmortem Under Compression Loads. Journal of Biomechanical Engineering 130 (2008)

[2] `http://www.sensable.com/haptic-phantom-omni.htm`

[3] `http://www.entactrobotics.com/index.php/w5d-specifications`

Part III
Media, Art and Culture

Giving Form to the Voices of Lay-Citizens: Monumental-IT, an Intelligent, Robotic, Civic Monument

Tarek H. Mokhtar[1,*], Keith E. Green[2,3], and Ian D. Walker[3]

[1] Department of Architecture Engineering, College of Engineering, Al Faisal University, Riyadh, KSA
tmokhtar@alfaisal.edu, tmokhta@g.clemson.edu

[2] School of Architecture, College of Architecture, Arts, and Humanities, Clemson University, SC, USA
kegreen@clemson.edu

[3] Department of Electrical and Computer Engineering, College of Engineering and Science, Clemson University, SC, USA
iwalker@g.clemson.edu

Abstract. In an increasingly digital society, it seems only apt that lay citizens be afforded interactive systems in public spaces to give form to their thoughts and desires as a collective of individual voices. While civic monuments are largely static, petrified representations of the past, sponsored by institutions and political authorities, Monumental-IT is an open-source, physical-digital (robotic) environment reconfigurable in real-time by lay citizens. We elaborate a process for generating and evaluating design alternatives for Monumental-IT, a cyber-physical artifact. Results suggest that the four distinct configurations of the robotic, multi-sensorial Monumental-IT evoke four distinct emotions in users. As well, users interacting with the prototype evaluate the design as reflecting their sentiments concerning historical events. Finally, users evaluated Monumental-IT's design to be more apt for our increasingly digital society than conventional monument design. Monumental-IT serves as a guide for designing large-scale computational artifacts for the public domain.

Keywords: Robots for citizens, Design and Evaluation of Interactive and Responsive Environments, Human Robot Interaction, Architecture.

1 Introduction

Increasingly, computation is becoming embedded into the very fabric of our everyday, built environments at large-scale, impacting the ways in which we interact with each other and the things around us. Monumental-IT is an open, reconfigurable, and interactive monument designed to give form, color, sound and movement to users' feeling about a specified human event. We selected the history of slavery in historic Charleston, South Carolina [USA] in proximity to the old Slave Mart, where tourists and other individuals passing by the site could communicate their feelings [1]. Monumental-IT was designed through an iterative design process, (fig. 1). We elaborate the generation of alternative design concepts for Monumental-IT, the basis for their evaluation, and the critical process of selecting a final design.

C. Stephanidis (Ed.): Posters, Part II, HCII 2013, CCIS 374, pp. 243–247, 2013.

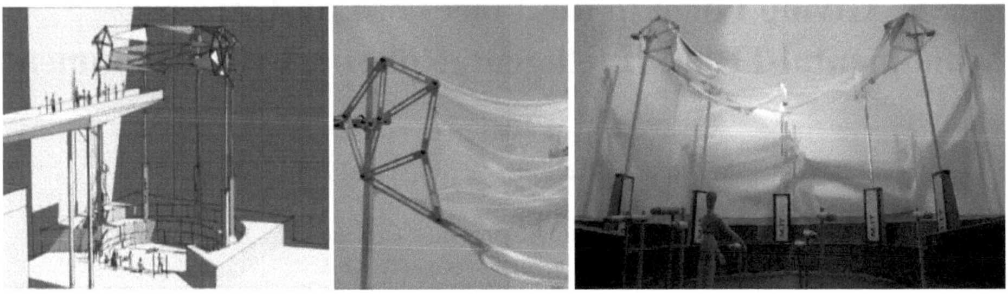

Fig. 1. Monumental-IT as a final conceptual design (left), and as a final to-scale prototype (middle and right)

2 Monumental-IT, Defined

This intelligent monument is comprised primarily of five tall masts terminated by actuated, hinged linkages; the movements of these scissor-like linkages reconfigure canopies of fabric tethered above the visitors (fig. 1, left). Microphones distributed across the physical site of the monument (fig. 1, right) invite users to annunciate what they feel in response to the history of slavery; this audio input then is "read" by the system for its emotive value, and translated by the system into a multi-modal, dynamic expression of sentiment, reflecting Fear, Anger, Sadness, or Happiness – our four characterizations of user sentiments concerning the history of slavery. As well, Monumental-IT affords remote users to access the Monumental-IT website and express their sentiments by way of responses (radio buttons) to a series of questions found there.

2.1 Conceptual Design Criteria

Inspired by the Italian artist Michelangelo's thesis of the "non-finito," in which parts of his statues were left incomplete for visitors to participate by their imagination in the making and completion of the statues, Monumental-IT is formally left "open" to user participation: internally, through a reconfigurable Wiki website that is open and available to all internet users to embody, in the monument, their thoughts, memories, and interpretation of the past; and externally, through a reconfigurable robotic body, that is open and available to people to retune it "collectively".

3 Process of Design: Six Stages

In developing a cyber-physical artifact of this scale and complexity, a human-centered "iterative design process" is critical. The iterative design process for Monumental-IT follows six steps: (1) *defining targeted users in the form of personas*; (2) *generating and describing numerous alternative design concepts*; (3) *subjecting the alternative designs to a conceptual screening process*; (4) *engaging in the concept resolution of fundamental components*; (5) *prototyping the selected design(s)*; and (6) *designing/establishing system behaviors*. By the sixth-stage in the process of design, a final, to-scale prototype has been identified as the concrete basis for realizing a full-scale, *in-situ* artifact.

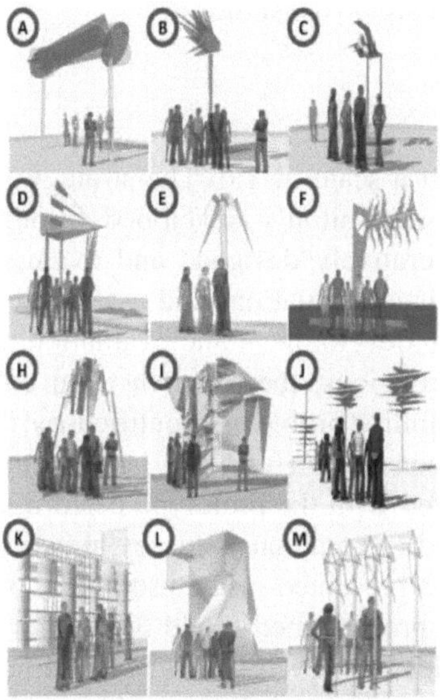

	Selection Criteria	A Rotating Tube	B Fan Leaves	C Waving Strips	D Solid & Void	E Flower Leaves	F Rotating Gears	G Muscle Body	H Spider Arms	I The Mesh	J Hydraulic Plates	K Strip Wall	L Skin Wall	M Skeleton & Skin
Design	Openness	-	-	0	-	0	0	0	+	+	+	0	0	+
	Configur-ability	-	+	+	-	+	0	0	+	0	-	0	0	0
	Structural Stability	+	-	-	+	-	+	0	-	+	+	+	+	+
	Aesthetics	-	0	0	0	-	0	0	0	0	-	0	0	0
	Techno. Viability	0	0	0	0	-	0	0	-	0	+	-	+	0
HCI	Legibility	-	-	+	+	0	0	0	+	-	0	+	0	+
	Impressio n-ability	+	+	0	0	+	+	0	+	-	-	+	+	+
Sum	Sum +'s	2	2	2	2	2	2	0	4	2	3	3	3	4
	Sum 0'S	1	2	4	3	2	5	7	2	3	1	3	5	3
	Sum -'s	4	3	1	2	3	0	0	2	2	3	1	0	0
	Net Score	-2	-1	+1	0	-1	+2	0	+2	0	0	+2	+3	+4
Rank	Rank (1=highest)	7	6	4	5	6	3	5	3	5	5	3	2	1
	Continue? No/Yes	N	N	N	N	N	N	N	N	N	N	N	Y	Y

Fig. 2. Twelve Alternative Design Concepts (Left), and Concept Screening Matrix (Right)

3.1 Concept Screening and Resolution

Our design chronology, in brief: we sketched more than 30 conceptual visions for Monumental-IT; from this field of 30 visions we cultivated twelve alternatives; we compared the twelve alternatives and selected the best two alternatives to physically prototype at 1:6 scale, after comparing the alternatives to the reference concept, two alternatives were selected for further development and prototyping, L: *Skin Wall* and M: *Skeleton and Skin,* (fig. 2), [3, 4]. Several aspects of the intelligent-monument concept required resolution, with three key aspects at the top of the list: (1.) the selection of hardware dedicated to actuating the robotic components, solved by using continuous rotation servomotors; (2.) the manner of mapping the audio inputs (human vocal effects) to human emotion, solved by employing Murray's vocal effects attributions to the four basic emotions [2]; and (3.) the manner of mapping human emotion to the colored lighting. As for the latter, with no evidence to inform this aspect of concept resolution, the design team reasoned to tentatively assign the "vibrant" color red to anger, the "cold" blue to fear, "multi-colors" red, yellow, green, and blue to represent happiness, and white to represent sadness. Some of these assignments were later changed to adhere to users' evaluations and feedback.

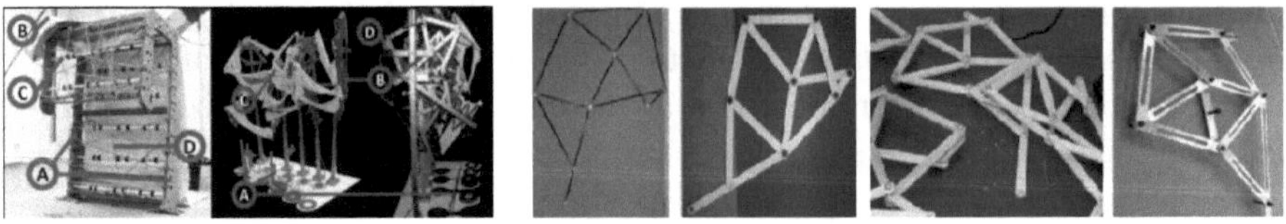

Fig. 3. Monumental-IT's Iterative Prototyping Process

3.2 Prototyping and Evaluations

The two selected alternatives were prototyped at a scale of 1:6. The strategy for the monument's movements, its "choreography," was initially developed through lab discussions. Both color and movement were iteratively designed and evaluated by user studies. Working from prototype "M", heuristic evaluations and usability evaluation techniques were employed for further design development and evaluation of Monumental-IT. From the completed heuristic evaluations, the research team collated, summarized and prepared a complete set of usability problems identified by the experts. Following the heuristic evaluations, sixteen users (from the larger university community – students and faculty) were presented with the prototype performing the four modes in succession. Users were then asked to complete a survey aimed at providing feedback about the monument's design as presented in the prototype, particularly with respect to verifying our mapping of programmed mode (color, form and movement) to emotion. We found that our modes, as initially designed, did not map well to the intended modes of "emotion" modes. These modes were later refined to better match users' preferences and feedback.

Table 1. Results on the effectivness of using Monumental-IT's assigned: colors (top-left), sounds (top-right), motion (bottom-left), and shadows (bottom-right) on the human-robotic interaction with it

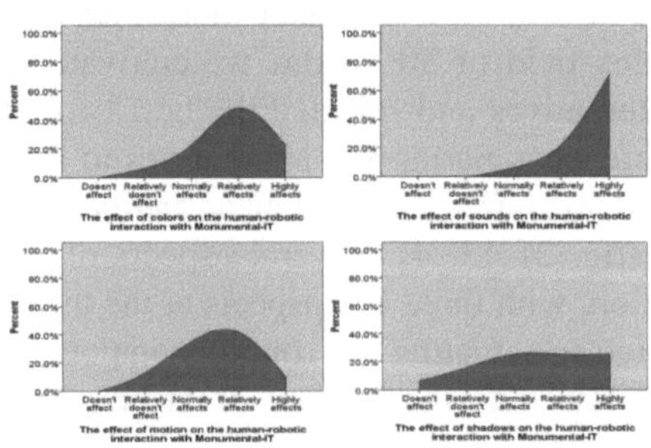

4 Final Prototype and Evaluation

The final 1:6 scaled prototype includes all physical and multi-sensorial features (color, material, texture, sound, and motion) following the lessons of the previous evaluations. In our final prototype, we used the same mixed UCD methods for evaluation:

heuristic evaluations, surveys in a lab setting, and quasi-experimental design (Separate-Sample Pretest-Posttest) to evaluate and validate the outcomes with lay-citizens. In the lab setting, we mitigated threats to internal, external and construct validity of the project. The results from these quasi-experimentation study show significant support for using colors (as M=3.87, SD=0.846, and Variance=0.716 on a scale from 1 (does not affect) to 5 (highly affects)); sounds (as M=4.65, SD=0.608, and Variance=0.37, on the same scale); and motions (as M=3.48, SD=0.851, and Variance= 0.725, on the same scale), as multi-sensorial features for Monumental-IT (table 1). Our results also suggest the effectiveness of Monumental-IT's reconfigurable multi-sensorial features (colors, sounds, motion) on the human-robot interaction were significant, with an overall improvement of 134.2%. "Motion" showed the highest effect on the human-robot interaction, with a treatment effect of 147.6%. Sounds likewise suggested a strong effect of sound on the human-robot interaction with Monumental-IT, with a treatment effect of 137.6%. The significance of the different color configurations was the lowest, with a treatment effect of 117.5%. Our results likewise suggest a significant effect for the use of multi-sensorial configurations on the human-emotion interaction with Monumental-IT. Finally, participants perceived Monumental-IT a monument for "all ages," as M=5.07 on a scale from 1 (for ages from 18-24) to 6 (for all ages), SD=1.72, and variance=2.958.

5 Conclusion

We presented the design and evaluation processes for a cyber-physical monument that is *literally* formed by public engagement. Monumental-IT represents one promising future for the HCI community with respect to: ubiquitous computing environments for public places; sentient, human-physical-digital interaction; and "robots for citizens." For any design activity, the earliest stages of generating and evaluating design alternatives, and ultimately selecting one or more for further refinement, is a complex undertaking. Finally, it should be evident that the realization of such an intelligent artifact, at full-scale and in-situ, is a costly and complex enterprise; as such, this ambition must begin, as does the monument-designer's work traditionally, with a to-scale prototype that adequately captures the complexity of the full-scale implementation.

References

1. Breazeal, C., Takanishi, A., Kobayashi, T.: Social Robots that Interact with People. In: Springer Handbook of Robotics. Springer, Berlin (2008)
2. Murray, I., Arnott, J.: Toward the Simulation of emotion in synthetic speech: A Review of the Literature on Human Vocal Emotion. Journal of Acoustic Society of America 2, 1097–1108 (1993)
3. Ulrich, K.T., Eppinger, S.D.: Product Design and Development. McGraw-Hill, New York (2000)
4. Stone, D., Jarrett, C., Woodroffe, M., Minocha, S.: User Interface Design and Evaluation. Morgan Kaufmann Series in Interactive Technologies. Morgan Kaufmann, San Francisco (2005)

To Decipher the Capital's Cultural Image Based on the New Generations' Perspectives on Action Figure Design

Kuo-Li Huang[1], Tsen-Yao Chang[2], and Ting-Chun Tung[1]

[1] Department of Visual Communication Design,
Southern Taiwan University of Science and Technology, Taiwan
{z3z,tungtc}@mail.stust.edu.tw
[2] Department of Creative Design,
National Yunlin University of Science and Technology, Taiwan
changty8908@gmail.com

Abstract. In this study, the population was based on the 585 works in a Nationwide Undergraduates Creative Action figure Competition which was themed "the capital image of Tainan", while the samples were based on the 43 elected works among them. A questionnaire on the capital's image was created, and then 300 copies of it were distributed to design departments in colleges and universities in eastern, southern, northern and central Taiwan. The capital's image in the undergraduates' eyes was deciphered by means of Kansei Engineering Theory, so that we could understand the historical changes in the capital's cultural elements as well as the correlation between action figure modeling and the capital's image in the new generation's eyes.

Keywords: capital image, action figure, Kansei Engineering, cultural design.

1 Introduction

Due to globalised markets, every country all develops its own unique cultural features, so as to pass on cultural features of local cultures through designs. "When Eastern National Palace Museum Meets Western Alessi", held jointly by National Palace Museum and foreign design "Alessi", was an event that integrates eastern cultures into action figure designs. Tainan City Government held local cultural activities that have cultural action figure, for combining local cultures with action figure designs. Such combination of cultures and action figure designs can attract young generations' attention. Through the works from Nationwide Undergraduates Creative Action Figure Competition, this study aimed to analyze new generations' action figure modeling design elements, the images and feeling expressed, and the correlations between action figure modeling designs and local images. Due to globalised markets, every country all develops its own unique cultural features, so as to pass on cultural features of local cultures through designs. "When Eastern National Palace Museum Meets Western Alessi", held jointly by National Palace Museum and foreign design "Alessi", was an event that integrates eastern cultures into action figure designs. Tainan City Government held local cultural activities that have cultural action figure,

C. Stephanidis (Ed.): Posters, Part II, HCII 2013, CCIS 374, pp. 248–252, 2013.

for combining local cultures with action figure designs. Such combination of cultures and action figure designs can attract young generations' attention. Through the works from Nationwide Undergraduates Creative Action Figure Competition, this study aimed to analyze new generations' action figure modeling design elements, the images and feeling expressed, and the correlations between action figure modeling designs and local images.

2 Research Methods

Through the practice of Kansei Engineering, the correlation between new generations' action figure modeling designs and the feeling for local image was analyzed in this study. Four stages were divided in this study: (1) Selection of the scope of experiment samples; (2) Abstraction of the elements of action figure modeling characteristics; (3) Undertaking of a questionnaire survey; (4) Analyses of survey results.

2.1 Selection of the Scope of Experiment Samples

In this study, the population was based on the works from the 2009 Nationwide Undergraduates Creative Action Figure Competition. The themes of this competition centered on the historical figures, cultures and local features about Tainan City, which conformed to the purpose of this study survey. This competition had 585 works in total. Among them, the 43 pieces of elected works, which were selected by the jury in the first stage and which expressed Tainan cultures, were the samples in this study for performing a kansei image survey.

2.2 Abstraction of Action Figure Modeling Elements

According to the studies made by Chen and Shen(2011), the categorization and definitions of traditional cultural action figure models were performed, while the table of cultural action figure modeling design elements was generalized primarily. Through Morphological Analysis, the samples were categorized according to their sample action figure models. They were divided based on 23 categories in 8 items: (1) Cultural Elements; (2) Accessories; (3) Model Lines; (4) Colors; (5) Postures; (6) Facial Features; (7) Facial Expressions; (8) Changes of Symbolic Patterns.

2.3 Questionnaire Survey on College Students of Design Departments

In this study, a questionnaire survey of the kansei image of "Tainan" was conducted for the samples. The 43 experiment samples were appraised based on 7-leveled Likert Scale. Attached with the pictures of these samples, a questionnaire survey of the action figure images was conducted for college students. According to the pictures of these action figure works, the subjects gave scores of 1~7, based on their feeling about each action figure sample. The subjects of this questionnaire were the college students of design departments respectively from northern, central, southern and eastern regions in Taiwan. Three hundred copies of this questionnaire survey were distributed, in which 268 copies were recovered. The statistic data of the survey results had been averaged, for performing Quantitative Theory Type 1 Analysis.

3 Results and Analyses

The analysis results of new generations' action figure modeling designs in terms of the kansei image of "Tainan" were listed as Table 1. The positive value of Categories Score (CS) represented positive image — feeling correlated with Tainan, while negative value represented the corresponsive negative image — feeling non-correlated with Tainan. In the item "Color Change", the category "7~8 colors" was 0.266, meaning that "7~8 colors" used in "Color Change" would be close to the image of "Tainan". Analyzed based on Item Partial Correlation (IPC), the results indicated that "Color Change" was 0.60 and "Facial Features" was 0.55, indicating higher IPC; their modeling would have greatest correlation and influence with Tainan image.

According to related studies made by Sugiyama & Inoue (1996), the correlation between Multiple Correlation Coefficient (R) and reliability was proposed. When Multiple R was 0.70~1.00, a very strong correlation was shown. When R was 0.84, it could be known that a very strong correlation was shown in the reliability of the predictive value. The survey results were sub-categorized into four different regions: northern, central, southern, and eastern regions in Taiwan. Such comparison results are listed in Table 2: In Northern Region, R was 0.77; in Central Region, R was 0.90; in Southern Region, R was 0.86; In Eastern Region, R was 0.82. As for the correlation analysis of the survey results of different regions, the students in Central Region would have higher correlation degree in terms of the feeling degree of modeling elements and Tainan image. The students in Northern Region and Eastern Region would have lower correlation degree in terms of the feeling degree of modeling elements and Tainan image. In this survey, because Tainan City in Southern Region was the main city of kansei image and it is nearer to Central and Southern Regions, we could infer that the students in Central and Southern Regions would have stronger correlative feeling in terms of the feeling and modeling elements about Tainan, compared with those students in Northern and Eastern Regions.

In terms of the CS in modeling elements, the categories of the highest scores and the lowest negative scores respectively corresponded to the image of "Tainan" in terms of kansei image. Listed as Table 3.The sequence arrangement of the optimized modeling elements of "Tainan" image was: "7~8 colors", "realistic", "simplification", "accessories-contained", "motion posture", "historic figures", "with obvious expression", and "geometrical— smooth".

The analysis results indicated: In terms of the manifestation ways used in new generations' Tainan cultural action figure designs, the color style of "5~8 colors" was the color effect that enables new generations to have greater feeling; in terms of the way to show facial features, they would have greater feeling about realistic practice; if local cultural elements were changed to be symbolic patterns in the applications of

Table 1. Quantitative Theory Type 1 Analysis

Item	Category	CS	IPC
Cultural Elements	(1) Historic figures	0.097	0.249
	(2) Historic spots and snack food	0.065	
	(3) Folk festivities	-0.104	
Accessories	(1) Accessories-contained	0.094	0.311
	(2) Non-accessories-contained	-0.175	
Model Lines	(1) Organic	-0.107	0.133
	(2) Geometrical– solid	-0.002	
	(3) Geometrical– smooth	0.056	
Color Change	(1) 3~4 colors	-0.482	0.601*
	(2) 5~6 colors	0.128	
	(3) 7~8 colors	0.266	
	(4) 9 colors and more	-0.099	
Posture Change	(1) Integration	-0.166	0.309
	(2) Motion posture	0.146	
	(3) Static front posture	0.065	
Facial Features	(1) Simplification - lines	-0.056	0.550*
	(1) Simplification - geometric ways	-0.202	
	(3) Realistic	0.783	
Facial Expressions	(1) With obvious expression	0.076	0.221
	(2) Without obvious expression	-0.087	
Changes of Symbolic Patterns	(1) Simplification	0.356	0.413*
	(2) Transformation	-0.044	
	(3) realistic	-0.279	
Constant Term		3.661	
Multiple Correlation Coefficient (R)		0.837	
Coefficient of Determination (R^2)		0.700	

Table 2. Comparisons of the Multiple Correlation Coefficients (R) in northern, central, southern, and eastern Taiwan regions

Item \ Region	Northern	Central	Southern	Eastern
R	0.77	0.90	0.86	0.82
R^2	0.60	0.80	0.73	0.68

modeling designs, the change practice of "simplification" would result in strongest feeling. The use of accessories for action figure models would enhance new generations' feeling about Tainan image. As for the motion changes of action figure extremities, obvious motions of extremities would enhance their feeling. In terms of their feeling about Tainan culture, they had stronger feeling and understanding about historic figures. If obvious expressions were applied in facial expressions, new generations would have better feeling about Tainan image. As for action figures' model lines, the manifestation of "geometrical– smooth" would result in enhanced feeling about Tainan image.

Table 3. Portfolios of the Optimized Modeling Element Designs

Sequence of the importance of modeling elements	Kansei image of "non-Tainan"	Kansei image of "Tainan"
1.Color Change	3~4 colors	7~8 colors
2. Facial Features	simplification - geometric ways	realistic
3. Changes of Symbolic Patterns	realistic	simplification
4. Accessories	non- accessories-contained	accessories-contained
5. Posture Change	integration	motion posture
6. Cultural Elements	folk festivities	historic figures
7. Facial Expressions	without obvious expression	with obvious expression
8. Model Lines	organic	geometrical— smooth

4 Conclusions

According to the analysis results, the portfolios of the optimized elements of new generations' Tainan cultural action figure designs were concluded. Future studies can be made to have further explorations of different groups and different local cultural features.

References

1. Sugiyama, K., Inoue, K.: The basic for Survey and Analysis by Excel: A Collection of Tools for Planning and Design. Kaibundo Publishing, Tokyo (1996)
2. Chen, C.-C., Shen, Z.-X.: The Study of Consumer Preference for Traditional Culture Creativity Design – A Case of Figure Designs. Journal of National Taiwan University of Arts (89) (2011)

A Museum Guide Application for Deployment on User-Owned Mobile Devices

George Kapnas[1], Asterios Leonidis[1], Maria Korozi[1], Stavroula Ntoa[1], George Margetis[1], and Constantine Stephanidis[1,2]

[1] Foundation for Research and Technology - Hellas (FORTH)
Institute of Computer Science,
N. Plastira 100, Vassilika Vouton, GR-700 13 Heraklion, Crete, Greece,
[2] University of Crete, Department of Computer Science
P.O. Box 2208, GR-714 09, Heraklion, Crete, Greece
{gkapnas,leonidis,korozi,stant,gmarget,cs}@ics.forth.gr

Abstract. This poster describes the design and development of a comprehensive Museum Tour Guide mobile application that can be installed on user-owned devices. The purpose of the application is to provide museum visitors with a device that can improve their experience through optimised planning of their visit and an always-available stream of information regarding the museum and its exhibits. The main goals, the design, as well as the implementation of the application are described and the main functions of the application are presented. Finally, conclusions are drawn and further development ideas are discussed.

Keywords: Mobile Device, Museum, Guide, Guided Tour.

1 Introduction

Although the use of mobile devices in museums was introduced over 60 years ago [1] and has been the norm -mostly in the form of audio guides- for decades, only recently has the advancement of technology allowed to have devices with full multimedia capabilities and adequate processing capacity and stamina resting at the palm of a hand. As a result of this advancement, combined with the widespread adoption of smartphones and tablets in the past few years, a large portion of the population nowadays always carries with them at least one smart mobile device with an impressive array of sensors and significant computing power. The work described here aims to take advantage of the near-ubiquity of such devices to create a rich mobile museum touring guide that can be installed on an average smartphone or tablet and escort the user during their visit to a museum, offering guidance and information whenever desired.

2 General Goals

The purpose of this application is to create a comprehensive, stand-alone mobile guide tool for the visitors of museums. The guide should offer services similar to

C. Stephanidis (Ed.): Posters, Part II, HCII 2013, CCIS 374, pp. 253–257, 2013.

those one would receive if they had a qualified guide constantly but unobtrusively escorting them around the museum during their visit. The major tasks the application should perform are:

- Area Information and Guidance: Offer location information for all exhibition areas, as well as any other places of interest; let visitors know with relative precision where they are located within the museum and enable them to easily find their way around it, whether they wish to visit a specific exhibition room or a utility area of the building.
- Thematic Information: Offer users detailed information with regard to the museum's permanent as well as any temporary exhibitions, its collections and its exhibits individually. Visitors should be able to use the mobile guide in order to access any information they may require, from simple descriptions to audio and video content.
- Tour Creation: The most prominent aspect of a tour guide is perhaps its ability to efficiently navigate and show the user around the museum according to their wishes. Options include tours focusing on specific collections or exhibits, choices based on how much time the visitor is willing to spend, but also extend to planning custom routes based on individual preferences and interests.

In addition to the application's key tasks, the following goals had to be achieved:

- Platform independence: As the application is intended to be installed on smart handheld devices owned by the users rather than provided by the museum itself, it was important that the application would be available for most major platforms and could perform well under different hardware specifications, from small mobile phones to large tablets.
- Accessibility: While this is a goal towards which all applications should strive, catering for users' potential disabilities has been part of the design process from the very beginning. Museums by their nature are institutions that should be fully accessible to everyone and a mobile museum tour guide can be an excellent tool towards improving overall accessibility. Currently, the implemented version offers a set of alternative colour themes that improve usability [2], while the future versions will integrate features such as UI resizing and scanning to facilitate mobility-impairments [3], TTS, etc.

3 Implementation

3.1 The National Archaeological Museum of Athens

The aim of the project is to create an application that can be integrated in almost any type of museum; this particular version has been tailored around the offerings of the National Archaeological Museum of Athens [4].

The museum building comprises three floors; all exhibition rooms are on the ground and first floors, whereas the basement only has some of the utility areas. There are several permanent collections, as well as a temporary collection available. For the optimal integration of the application with the museum's other online and interactive offerings, the museum's own segmentation and categorisation of exhibits and collections was followed; exhibition rooms were also grouped in accordance with the definitions of the museum map. Additional information regarding the exhibitions and exhibits has been collected from the Odysseus Portal, provided by the Hellenic Ministry of Education [5].

3.2 Features

The developed application can be deployed in three major mobile platforms (iOS, Android, Blackberry Tablet OS) and can escort users during their visit to a museum offering guidance and information. The implemented features of the current version can be found below:

Free Navigation. A fully interactive map that supports touch-enabled zooming and panning functions through pinching and dragging gestures is provided. Users have the option to select any particular Point of Interest (e.g., room, exhibit) on the map and gain access to more details concerning it. If they wish to ask for a route to a different location within the museum, they can simply state the starting and the ending point, and the application will calculate the most convenient path and display it on the map, including appropriate instructions where the floor level may need to change.

Guided Tours. The application's touring feature currently allows visitors to select from a set of predefined tours, from short to extensive, depending on how much time they wish to spend. A tour is passively location aware; by asking the user to confirm their location in a room, it paces itself and displays the correct information for every step. In more detail, when a user states their location, the map centers to the respective room and virtual pins that correspond to the exhibits that belong to the selected tour are displayed to facilitate their detection in the physical room.

If the user decides to deviate from the predefined route either physically or just on the device, the application will comply, supplying any requested content along the way; in addition, it offers the options to either return the user and pick up from the last visited point, or simply continue from the nearest not yet visited one that belongs to the tour.

Exhibit View. Offering information on the museum's exhibits is one of the most essential functions of a guide. Aside from the description of each artefact, the application also offers additional multimedia content for a richer experience semantically segmented to facilitate comprehension (e.g., material, date found, origin, periodisation, etc.)

QR Code Identification. In order to satisfy a set of identification requirements within the museum, the use of QR Codes [6] was adopted. Each accessible building area has been assigned its own code, as has each individual exhibit within the museum. Through the use of their device's built-in camera, a user can inform the application of their current location or identify an exhibit they may be interested in finding more about. Using the same method, the guided tour can be updated as to which steps have already been completed or whether the user has decided to stray from the tour's path.

Search and Save. A search function and the ability to select and save exhibits as favourites are also among the implemented features. The search function enables users to query the application for information in different ways and create their own custom tours; they can search for a specific artefact, a utility or exhibition room, and add it to their favourites from where they can later create a new tour tailored to their preferences.

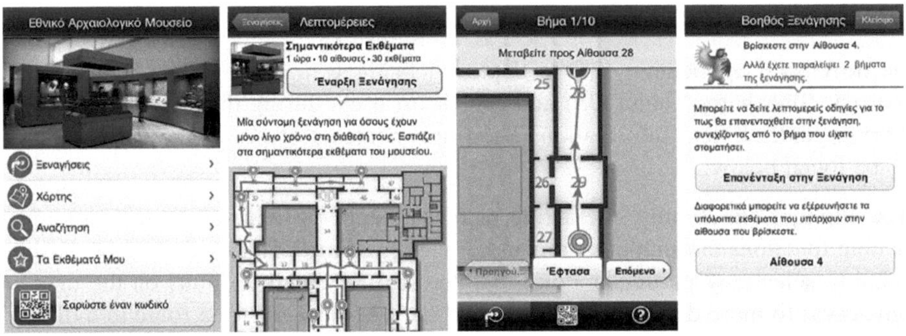

Fig. 1. Screenshots of different pages of the Museum Guide (from left to right): The main menu, a short tour of the main exhibits, confirmation of a completed step and the assistant indicating the omission of two steps in a in a preset tour

3.3 Implementation Issues

Regarding the application's internals, given that every archaeological site uses its own proprietary catalogue format, an extensible content categorization scheme was implemented to facilitate classification and discovery, where the application uses the appropriate query functions to discover relevant material.

In terms of storage needs, given that devices' capacity is limited and that free space is invaluable for smartphone owners, the application minimizes space requirements through caching. Whenever, a room is accessed, its exhibits and those of the surrounding rooms are dynamically loaded, while using an LRU policy [7] any past content is discarded. The selected approach apart from minimizing storage requirements also facilitates automatic content update without requiring from the users to update the application itself to get the latest content. However, to pre-empt network failures or unavailability, the guide also includes an "offline" mode where, if the user chooses to, content is permanently stored on the device which then periodically checks for updates.

Finally, to support content management and classification, an auxiliary editor was implemented to support developers in defining building maps and adding exhibits in the site's rooms.

4 Future Work

Although the application has already reached a satisfactory level of maturity, there are plans for the addition of more features. In particular, one of the current development priorities is the addition of background information collection from the application. In that way, data can be gathered relating to how each person uses the application and how they tend to interact with the museum's offerings and the museum itself. The collection of such data will enable a better understanding of users' needs and the corresponding improvement of the application. This could potentially be honed even further by categorising visitors according to information collected by the users in advance; age, nationality, professional background and other characteristics could be utilised to tailor a near-optimal tour for every individual.

5 Conclusions

This paper has introduced and described an application designed to act as a museum tour guide, which can be installed on a user's own mobile device. The current release of the application enables users to easily navigate themselves around the museum as well as follow predefined or custom tours. With always-available information and multimedia regarding all exhibits and other points of interest and the ability to tailor their experience to their needs, visitors are essentially accompanied by a comprehensive, intelligent guide that makes their museum experience not only richer, but also more efficient.

References

1. Tallon, L.: (May 19, 2009), http://musematic.net/2009/05/19/about-that-1952-sedelijk-museum-audio-guide-and-a-certain-willem-sandburg/
2. Doulgeraki, C., et al.: Methods and Tools for the Development of Unified Web-Based User Interfaces. In: Stephanidis, C. (ed.) The Universal Access Handbook. CRC PressI Llc (2009)
3. Ntoa, S., Savidis, A., Stephanidis, C.: Automatic Hierarchical Scanning for Windows Applications. In: Stephanidis, C. (ed.) The Universal Access Handbook. CRC PressI Llc (2009)
4. http://www.namuseum.gr/
5. http://odysseus.culture.gr/h/1/gh154.jsp?obj_id=3249
6. QR code. Wikipedia, The Free Encyclopedia (April 17, 2013), http://en.wikipedia.org/w/index.php?title=QR_code&oldid=550751789 (retrieved March 12-April 18, 2013)
7. Smith, A.J.: Cache memories. ACM Computing Surveys (CSUR) 14(3), 473–530 (1982)

Quantitative Analysis of Artists' Characteristic Styles through Biologically-Motivated Image Processing Techniques: Uncovering a Mentor to Johannes Vermeer

Minseo Kim and Jeounghoon Kim

Graduate School of Culture Technology, KAIST (Korea Advanced Institute of Science & Technology), 291 Daehak-ro, Yuseong-gu, Daejeon 305-701, Republic of Korea
{artmin,miru}@kaist.ac.kr

Abstract. This study was designed to improve the limitations of traditional analysis of artworks by quantitatively analyzing artworks through biologically-motivated image processing techniques that reflect visual information processing mechanisms of human vision. As the first step to achieve this goal, this study addressed one of the important questions in art history, uncovering a mentor for 'an artist who remains forever unknown' Johannes Vermeer, by adopting three interdisciplinary research methods of cognitive science, art history, and engineering. We performed orientation, radial frequency, and color analyses with the artworks for comparing the artistic styles of Vermeer and other artists who have been presumed to be his mentor. The results from three analyses have led us to the conclusion that a person who had the strongest influence on Vermeer is Gerard Ter Borch. This conclusion was strongly confirmed by verifying the research methods with an additional comparison of artistic styles between Rembrandt and Carel Fabritius, whose master-pupil relationship has already been revealed. This study is believed to provide a new perspective on uncovering previously unknown mentor of Vermeer, and the research methods adopted here can be applied to other related research issues in art history, such as authenticity debates on masterpieces, by quantitatively archiving artists' characteristic styles.

Keywords: Johannes Vermeer, Visual Information Processing, Orientation Analysis, Radial Frequency Analysis, Color Analysis.

1 Introduction

Artwork analysis requires a macroscopic framework and methodology, reflecting both art historical approach and scientific technique. Yet majority of artwork analysis relies heavily on either historical evidence or highly subjective appraisal, and many limitations have been addressed in appreciating artworks with conventional analytical methods. The scientific methods of investigation such as X-ray photography, infrared photography, pigment analysis, and radiocarbon dating have also limitations due to the possible danger of irreparable damage on the artwork. Artwork analysis, therefore, stands in great need of non-destructive analysis and objective methodology that can lend support to subjective appraisal, and moreover, collecting artist's distinct styles of

C. Stephanidis (Ed.): Posters, Part II, HCII 2013, CCIS 374, pp. 258–262, 2013.

painting and constructing a database are certainly needed for continuous application. We thus combined the traditional art appraisal with image processing techniques to standardize the artworks analysis. We defined the elements that most clearly manifest the artist's individuality and developed quantitative analysis of the elements and created a scientific reservoir of the individual artist's signature elements. As the first step to achieve this goal, we studied on uncovering Johannes Vermeer's mentor who remains largely unknown to art historians. Johannes Vermeer is well-known for highly realistic portraits and genre-paintings. However, his life and a question of who had the strongest influence on him still remains a mystery. Thus, this paper will focus on the study of the art historical background of Vermeer and other artists and provide a practical solution by introducing quantitative analysis of artists' painting styles through image processing techniques.

2 The Art-Historical Analysis of Johannes Vermeer

Johannes Jan Vermeer (1632-1675) is typical of the Delft School owing to his special techniques such as his expression of light, realistic interiors, and poetical descriptions of people. Presumably, he began his artistic training around 1645-47, later joining the Guild of Saint Luke as a master in 1653. The reason why this date is regarded as important is that Vermeer's early paintings are often embroiled in authenticity debates. Thus, it is important to identify who had the most influence on Vermeer because doing so helps to reveal Vermeer's stylistic development and distinguish replicas from original artworks. So far, five artists who are Abraham Bloemaert, Carel Fabritius, Gerard Ter Borch, Leonaert Bramer, and Rembrandt have been presumed to Vermeer's mentor through art historical records [2].

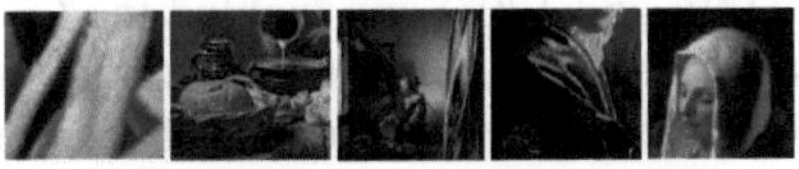

Fig. 1. Vermeer's artistic styles
(from left, sfumato, pointillès, depth, complementary colors, poetical face)

Vermeer's painting techniques are categorized according to the characteristics of human visual information processing. There are four components, which account for form (sfumato, pointillès), depth (various directions of lines), face, and color (complementary color) (Fig. 1). First, sfumato is a drawing style without lines or borders, in the manner of smoke or beyond the focus plane. Vermeer always regarded shadow is more important than lines for separating different objects. As a result, he mixed elaborative lines and blurry lines. Second, pointillès is a light expression technique in which points are formed on a polished or metallic surface. Vermeer specially used the pointillès technique on unreflecting surfaces, including bread, cloth, and baskets, showing clearly that he added new interpretations and appreciation to the usual pointillès method. Third, geometrical spaces made by various directions of lines – horizontal, parallel, and diagonal - give an illusion of space like a glimpsing through a keyhole. Fourth, complementary colors were used to emphasize the effects of light and to enhance the vividness of the quality of the materials. In particular, complementary pairings of yellow ocher and cobalt blue were the most representative characteristic of Vermeer. Fifth, Vermeer's faces in his artworks have been considered as poetical faces because they are involved in a type of mental activity. Vermeer tried to express important moral lessons or social critiques through his paintings. To do so, he always included a descriptive context.

3 The Quantitative Analyses of Artworks

For the quantitative analyses of Vermeer' artworks, an image dataset was built from the various websites. The main purpose of this was to minimize the source-dependency of the images and to verify that the images were analyzed and characterized based on the actual visual content rather than other artifacts which may be a feature of the image given its source [4]. As a result, the image dataset contains 535 images from six different painters, and each painting is normalized to 256 X 256 pixels without changing the aspect ratio. Also, most images were converted from color to grayscale except for those used in the color analysis.

3.1 Orientation Analysis

The orientation analysis was based on Vermeer's distinctive lines, including sfumato and pointillès styles and various directions of lines. This analysis compares and analyzes the styles of lines in the artworks of Vermeer and other artists who have been suggested as his mentors. To select artists' characteristic line styles quantitatively, line orientations were analyzed utilizing Gabor wavelets, which have been used to simulate configurations of the receptive fields of visual cells in human visual brain.

In this analysis, the Gabor wavelet applied four scales (2, 4, 8, and 16) and six orientations (0°, 30°, 60°, 90°, and 120°) and yielded the Gabor energy, which is defined as the sum of the squared values obtained by convolving Godd and Geven [3]. The Gabor energy refers to the average value which does not exceed the standard error (±2 SE) and is regarded as the representative value of each artist's style of lines. For a comparative analysis of the Gabor energy, a t-test was used to determine whether Vermeer's Gabor energy is similar to that of the other artists. The results showed that 'Gerard Ter Borch and Vermeer [t(29)=.537]' and 'Carel Fabritius and Rembrandt [t(22)=-.895]' are not statistically significant, unlike other relationships of artists. This result may therefore be considered as evidence that Gerard Ter Borch's artistic style is similar to that of Vermeer. Also, the result showing that Rembrandt and Carel Fabritius, who are known to have had a master-pupil relationship, have similar artistic styles verifies the reliability of these analyzing methods.

3.2 Radial Frequency Analysis

A radial frequency analysis exhibits and compares styles of faces in the artworks of Vermeer and other artists. To extract characteristic face styles of artists' works quantitatively, faces are analyzed by adopting radial frequency, which has been used in simulating configurations of the specialization of visual cells pertaining to curved shapes and actual faces. The use of radial frequency can create various closed circle figures by adding two or three circles or can abstract basic components by disassembling a closed circle figure. In this analysis, artist's faces are compared in terms of the distribution of the radial frequency components. As a result, 'Gerard Ter Borch and Vermeer [t(19)=-.948]', and 'Leonaert Bramer and Vermeer [t(19)=-.926] are not statistically significant, unlike other relationships of artists. This result may therefore be considered as evidence that Gerard Ter Borch and Leonaert Bramer have artistic styles similar to Vermeer's artistic style. Also, 'Carel Fabritius and Rembrandt [t(42)= .342]' and 'Leonaert Bramer and Rambrandt [t(49)= -1.628] ' additionally show similar artistic styles, these facts verify the reliability of these analyzing methods because they are known to have had a close relationship.

3.3 Color Analysis

A color analysis is valuable due to the fact that Vermeer used complementary colors to emphasize the effect of light in his paintings. Accordingly, this analysis exhibits and compares cobalt blue and yellow ocher in the artworks of Vermeer and of other artists. For the color analysis, RGB-coded images are transformed into the CIE L*a*b color space format because the CIE L*a*b corresponds very well to the perceptual differences of their appearances [1].

$$\Delta E = \sqrt{(p_1 - q_1)^2 + (p_2 - q_2)^2 + \cdots + (p_n - q_n)^2} = \sqrt{\sum_{i=1}^{n}(p_i - q_i)^2} \quad (1)$$

To discriminate the characteristic colors of artists' works quantitatively, colors were analyzed in terms of complementary color differences based on the Euclidean distance (ΔE)(1), which has been used when simulating configurations of opponent coding information processing in research on human color perception. Because the Euclidean distance is generally regarded as equal in terms of color within ΔE= 0.5-1.2, the analysis is judged by this criteria. The result of the analysis shows that 'Gerard Ter Borch and Vermeer' used perceptually equal colors in the 'Yellow ocher analysis [ΔE=0.8590]' and in the 'cobalt blue and yellow ocher analysis [ΔE=0.5276]'. Leonaert Bramer has also been presumed to be Vermeer's mentor by reason of the similarity of Cobalt blue, but this analysis shows that Vermeer's cobalt blue is most similar to that of Gerard Ter Borch, even if it does not show a perceptually equal color.

4 Results and Conclusion

This study offered important implications and gave direction to future research on Vermeer and the Delft School. First, the converging results of these three analyses (table 1) show that the most influential mentor of Vermeer is Gerard Ter Borch. In addition, the fact that Rembrandt and his pupil Carel Fabritius have a similar artistic style verifies the reliability of these analyzing methods. Actually, many studies shows that Vermeer was influenced by Gerard Ter Borch's genre scenes [5]. Second, the similarity of faces in radial frequency analysis between Leonaert Bramer and Rembrandt is full of suggestions in terms of their closeness. Finally, the difference between Leonaert Bramer's and Vermeer's cobalt blue will provide new implications for art history. Thus, this study provides a practical solution to the addressed issue in this paper by introducing quantitative analysis of artists' painting styles through image processing techniques.

Table 1. Results of analyses (✔: Similarities between the artistic styles of different artists)

	Orientation analysis	Radial Frequency analysis	Color analysis
	Bloemaert	Bloemaert	Bloemaert
	Bramer	**Bramer ✔**	Bramer
Vermeer	Fabritius	Fabritius	Fabritius
	Ter Borch ✔	**Ter Borch ✔**	**Ter Borch ✔**
	Rembrandt	Rembrandt	Rembrandt
	Bloemaert	Bloemaert	Bloemaert
	Bramer	**Bramer ✔**	Bramer
Rembrandt	**Fabritius ✔**	**Fabritius ✔**	Fabritius
	Ter Borch	Ter Borch	Ter Borch
	Vermeer	Vermeer	Vermeer

5 Implications

This study suggests a new vision for unsolved questions in art history as well as debates on the authenticity of masterpieces and offers a great potential to be applied for quantifying information on drawing styles into a database. An interdisciplinary approach of engineering, cognitive science, and art history adopted here by utilizing biologically-motivated image processing techniques is believed to contribute to a systematic analysis of artworks and would be very informative for future studies.

Acknowledgment. This research was supported by the Converging Research Center Program funded by the Ministry of Education, Science & Technology (2012K001342).

References

1. Berezhnoy, I.E., Postma, E.O., van den Herik, H.J.: Computer analysis of Van Gogh's complementary colors. Pattern Recognit. Lett. 28(6), 703–709 (2007)
2. Montias, J.M.: Vermeer and his Milieu-A Web of Social History. Princeton University Press, NJ (1989)
3. Johnson Jr., C.R., Hendriks, E., Berezhony, I., Brevdo, E., Hughes, S., Daubechies, I., Li, J., Postma, E., Wang, J.Z.: Image processing for artist identification: computerized analysis of Vincent van Gogh's painting brush strokes. IEEE Signal Process. Mag. 25, 37–48 (2008)
4. Shamir, L.: Computer Analysis Reveals Similarities between the Artistic Styles of Van Gogh and Pollock. Leonardo 45, 149–154 (2012)
5. Franits, W.E.: The Cambridge Companion to Vermeer. Cambridge University Press, Cambridge (2001)

New Service Design for Female-Twenties with Movie Enjoyment

Kazuhiro Kimura and Kazuhiko Yamazaki

Chiba Institute of Technology, Chiba, Japan
Kazuhiro19900804@gmail.com

Abstract. My study is inspired by human centered design (HCD) processing. My main target is aiming at twenties of Japanese female who don't like to go to movie theater often. In order to make them to be more positive to watch a movie, my design processes are starting from current investigation, user surveys, concept extractions, expanding ideas, mocking up, final products making and user evaluations. Therefore, I made an application (tablet) for this service design. What I concern about is, rather asking people to go to movie theater, I concentrate on information about actors/actresses. In additional from the results of user surveys, we can tell that people don't go to movie theater alone. In other words that we could use this key point, if we want to ask friends to go watch a movie, we can use the information that I created on my application and make good communication with my friends and share with them. Not only more young generation would like to go watch a movie eagerly, but also, help the movie industry get stronger.

Keywords: Human Centered Design, Service design.

1 Introduction

The film industry in Japan has deteriorated. One of the reasons is the problem that most of Japanese young people isn't interested in going to the theater to watch a movie doesn't solve.

The new way of enjoying a movie such as a 3D movie couldn't take root in their lifestyle and the trend quickly passed. If this situation continued, this kind of young people would increase and the film industry would follow a course of decline.

2 Purpose and Research Methods

2.1 Purpose

This research aims at Japanese women in their early 20's which there aren't many heavy users. Among them, we set the women who don't go to see a movie as a targeted user.

C. Stephanidis (Ed.): Posters, Part II, HCII 2013, CCIS 374, pp. 263–267, 2013.

Moreover the purpose of this study is proposing new service that makes these users raise the interest of films and enjoy films customarily.

2.2 Way of Research

We made prototypes in terms of user experience using Human Centered Design.

3 Design Process

3.1 Market Study

We widely investigated some services of enjoying a movie and decided point of focus in this research based on mapping the information of market study.

3.2 User Research

Interview and fieldwork was held for exploring user's value and problem.

3.3 Concept Making

To make what users desire1 clear, we made various user scenarios based on plenty of results from researches and created a concept figuring out how fascinate the scenarios have.

3.4 Create Idea

We ideated with many sketches based on several concepts. User interface was made by paper prototypes from a couple of these ideas and the direction of idea was decided focusing on function and scenario.

3.5 Draft Prototyping

Ideas were brushed up from improvements discovered by paper prototyping and new perspective. We created graphic with standard and showed it for real on a device such as a tablet to do prototype easily.

3.6 Prototyping

The problem was found out from draft prototype, function and graphic were improved more.

3.7 User Evaluation

The user evaluation was held for 5 people using a prototype and modified the design from this result.

3.8 Making a Final Product

The scenario and scene were improved from user evaluation's result. Moreover we created information architecture and user interface for new scenario as a final deliverable.

3.9 Improvement of a Product and Thesis Writing

I summarized these processes to write a thesis and created an application for tablets at the end.

4 Proposal

The proposal of this study is a tablet application "CASTY" that provides to enjoy a movie with cast centered.

We found a problem that Japanese women in 20's lost an opportunity to go to see a movie if they have an interesting film because the process of looking for a friend who wants to see the same one and inviting are quite bothering.

The biggest opportunity to see a movie is that their favorite actor appears on or not. It's more important than genre of films.

From this research, this application helps finding easily a friend who has the same favorite actor. We made a tablet which can show information such as photos of actor with a wide display as a targeted terminal.

4.1 Concept

This service has "enjoying a movie with cast" as a concept and 3 proposal values to users.

1. Value of finding information of favorite actor.
2. Value of sharing the favorite actor
3. Value of finding favorite actor and inviting you.

We made an image of red carpet of some gorgeous cinema exhibition as a concept of interface and aimed at making cast more attractive with simple and rich user interface.

4.2 Target User

College female students who don't often go to see a movie are a targeted user this time.

4.3 How to Use

It assumes that this service was used when user is on her own. First of all, user starts up the application to check her favorite actor and share it with her friends. After that, she will get information that a movie which the checked actor is in will be screened, and invites her friend who likes the same actor and you can make a plan in the same application.

4.4 Interface

This service has 4 respective interfaces.

1. News feed as a main page of this service shows updates what an actor your friend likes. (Fig.1) It gives an opportunity to get to know an actor you didn't know by displaying friend's update. Information of actors shows their names, pictures of them and what movie they are currently in.

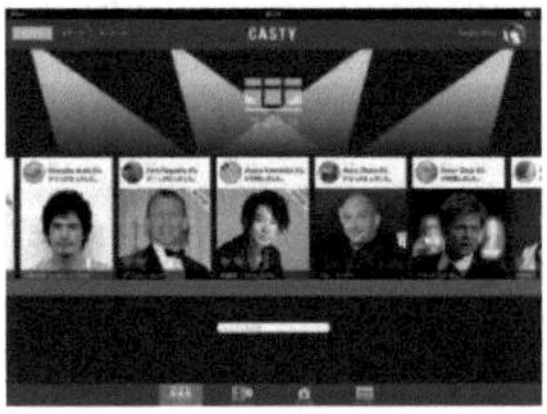

Fig. 1. News feed

2. If you had an curious actor on feed, it shows the actor's detail by tapping a picture of him. (Fig.2) You can LIKE the actor, share a picture of him with fans, and this application offers to show list of friends who LIKE the same actor.

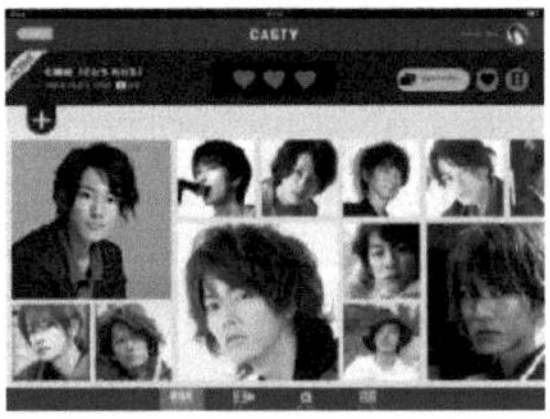

Fig. 2. Actor's detail

3. Movie detail on each actor's page shows cast and story. (Fig.3) Additionally as this content's feature, you can see the list showing whatactor your friends LIKEd and an amount of LIKE so that it describes how they have a motivation for watching a movie.

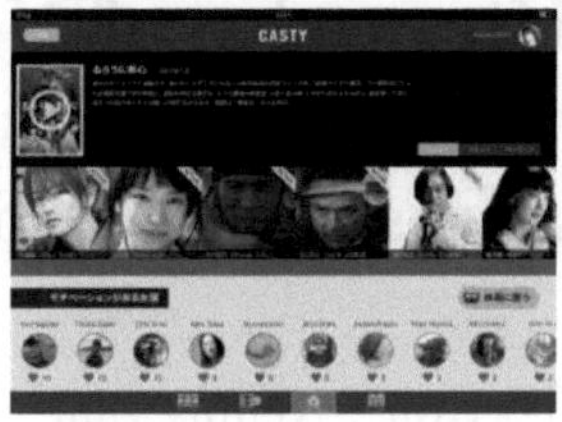

Fig. 3. Movie detail

4. If tapped a button of "Invite to the movies" on movie detail page, the invitation page comes out. (Fig.4)

This page offers 4 steps that is to choose a friend, a movie theater to go, the day and send a text to invite your friend.

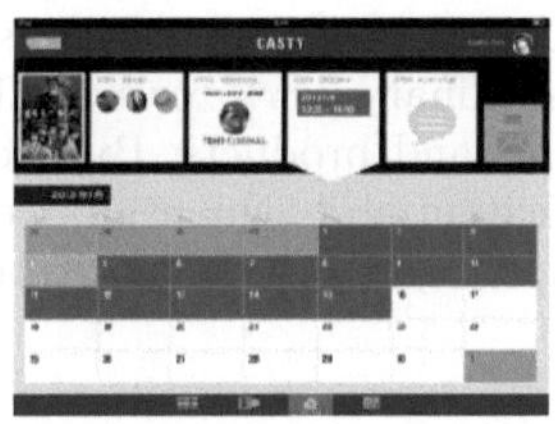

Fig. 4. Invitation page

5 Summary

Supporting to promote Japanese young women who basically don't see a movie to go to watch it through fun experience is important for moving into action by making feeling excitement. We were able to offer new movie style based on connections which those women place much value on. Improving repeatedly succeeded in showing attraction of films especially about GUI.

A Hierarchy of Needs for Developing Interactive Artworks, Systems and Products

Jeffrey Tzu Kwan Valino Koh[1], Kening Zhu[1], Roshan Lalintha Peiris[1], Mili John Tharakan[2], and Ryohei Nakatsu[1]

[1] Keio-NUS CUTE Center
NUS Graduate School for Integrative Sciences and Engineering
National University of Singapore
jtkvkoh@gmail.com
[2] Independent Researcher

Abstract. This manuscript attempts to address the need for discussion regarding the multidisciplinary work towards the development of interactive artworks, systems and products. By deconstructing the roles of technology, content creation and semantics, we attempt to understand the importance of each in regards to the motivation to develop interactive works.

1 Introduction

The main protagonist in Roald Dahl's Charlie and the Chocolate Factory [3], Charlie is faced with a difficult choice between choosing the very tangible benefit of feeding his family with the potential earnings through the sale of his newly discovered Golden Ticket to Arthur Slugworth, or to use his ticket to escape his hardships for a day to tour Willy Wonka's highly secretive and wondrous chocolate factory. After weighing the potential options, in Charlie's opinion there is nothing worth more to him then getting a chance to escape the banalities of his everyday life, if even for just a fleeting moment, and even when it means sacrificing a great source of sustenance for his entire family, and ultimately decides to experience a day with Willy Wonka in his factory.

The decision made by Charlie is a fitting metaphor to describe the binary choices we as a community of artists, technologists, researchers and practitioners face. Technology or content [20]? Invention or innovation [21]? Engineering or craft [22]? Aesthetics or functionality [5]? Tangibility or virtuality [17]? Analogness or digitalness [9]? Materiality or immateriality [6]? The question often appears in various forms within the many fields that ultimately make up the new media art, user experience, interaction design, and HCI communities. Is the development of more and more iterative technologies the ultimate means to benefit an audience? Or is the design of content more valuable?

At one point in the narrative of HCI as a developing field of expression, study and practice, the creation of newer, faster, smarter and better technologies seemed to be the means to unleash the human potential. The myth of

C. Stephanidis (Ed.): Posters, Part II, HCII 2013, CCIS 374, pp. 268–272, 2013.

technology as 'The Great Leveller' [13] was adopted by scholars, enterprise and policy makers alike. As such researchers and practitioners were interested in the development of novel interface technologies and their application. As soon as a methodological breakthrough was made, it was heralded as the future of interactivity. Tangible user interfaces [8], ubiquitous computing [23], affective computing [18], organic user interfaces [7], etc. have become almost biblical in terms of their reverence by the community, and directed most system, content and user experience development.

Yet even with these ground breaking epiphanies in the interactive research fields, we still use much of the same tools we used to work and play with as we did decades ago. We still type this manuscript on a keyboard using essentially the same metaphors as our precursors did years before [11]. Ishii and Ullmers seminal work on tangible user interfaces describes a world where digital data and analog life become one and the same. Yet at the time of this manuscript's authoring it has been about 15 years since their first work on Tangible Bits [19] was published, and it can be argued that tangible user interfaces are only just now becoming a viable way to interact with technology, though we are still far from the mainstream vision it set out to be.

Technologist soon realized that technology in of itself would not be the solution to all of lifes problems. Social scientists, designers and and other creative practices came into the forefront, and with it considerations of the audience, aesthetics and content became important [14].

Technological tools were now being described as platforms. Platforms such as YouTube allowed users to contribute immeasurable amounts of content [1]. Beyond the technology, the management of such content became a critical issue [12]. Along with the management of all this data, more importantly the deriving of semantic meaning from this content is quickly becoming a frontier of innovation. But what does this all mean to the interactivity researcher, creative practitioner and developer?

At the pinnacle of the motivational hierarchy of interactive systems development should be the user experience. More specifically we argue that the curation of technology and content, which enables users to derive meaning, is much more important to the user experience then both technology and content. Akin to Maslows Hierarchy of Needs [15] users of interactive systems also have a hierarchy of needs, namely technology at the base of the pyramid, followed by content, with meaning at its apex.

2 A Hierarchy for Interactive Systems Development

It can be assumed that a successful interactive product, artwork, design or installation requires a multitude of factors to make it succeed. At its absolute base, technology as a platform is needed to facilitate the possibilities of any work. Yet technology is empty unless it is filled with content. Content becomes the fuel to drive a meaningful technology. Without musical data, a compact disc is virtually useless. And even if content is present, this content is meaningless without the adequate semantics to make it at the very least comprehensible to the end user. If a non-Italian speaker attempts to read Dante's Divine Comedy [16] in the original language, the data that it contains would be meaningless. A parity between data and end user must be reached for it to be communicated.

2.1 At the Base of the Pyramid: Technology

From a technological viewpoint, material language plays an important role in the transmission and acquiring of meaning [10]. The semiotics of any piece of technology or material can offer a myriad of semantics. Take the example of silk. In many ways it has a widely different material language when compared to cotton. The material conjures all manner of context including that of ancient chinese royalty, down to the delicateness of the material when compared to cotton [2]. Likewise does porcelain possess a different semantic and contextual meaning when compared to clay, as does glass when compared to wood, and so forth. It is important for both the creative practitioner and technological developer to consider such contexts as it will ultimately affect the semantics of the final product they aim to develop.

When building new interactive works, we turn to the material language of the physical world, their meanings and contexts, and use them to leverage our interaction. Yet in fields such as HCI, we are still lacking a strong material language/semantics that will enable people to make meaning through the interaction with these interfaces [4]. We tend to see new interfaces as novel technology, instead of seeing it as materials to create meaning with. The next generation will see these interfaces as natural and normal, and will be able to see it beyond its wow factor to really use it in meaningful ways and to use these interface technologies as materials in their development of meaningful and useful products.

Every year we see more and more novel interfaces and interaction techniques unveiled. In some ways we need to allow all these new interaction techniques time to settle into the material landscape in order to allow it to propagate into everyday life so that people become familiar with it and over time, develop actual uses that will change and grow in relation to the meaning derived. Only through this use will we be able to actually have meaningful and semantic uses for these technologies.

2.2 In the Middle: Content

As was expressed in the preceding subsection, basic technology is needed to facilitate an interactive system, yet without content it is simply an empty shell. In order for meaningfulness to be derived, data or content is needed to be consumed, shared and interacted with by the end user. Content has primarily been within the domain of the designer.

If technology can be considered the material state of interactive systems, than content can be seen as a hybrid or transient state of both the material and immaterial [9]. Although not necessarily tangible when compared to technology, its material existence is there. Music produced from the playing of a compact disc embodies a state of sound, and travels in the material universe to the eardrum to be heard. The embodiment of this sound can be seen under a microscope on the surface of a compact disc, almost like bumps on a vinyl record.

Yet even though content is present, a semantic model is needed for it to be interpreted. Content without context and meaning is just as empty as a blank compact disc. This is realized and has given birth to fields of study such as big data or analytics research. Websites such as Twitter, YouTube and Facebook have a cornucopia of content, but the organization and interpretation of this data is just as important as the data itself.

2.3 At the Top of the Pyramid: Meaning

What both technology and content aim to ultimately support is the acquiring of meaning by the end user. The immaterial state of meaning is highly dependent on the end users interaction with a technology and understanding of its content [14]. In many ways an interactive artwork, product or system is not complete if there is no interactivity and semantic interpretation by the user. An interactive artwork, product or system is only halfway complete if an end user does not meet the combined effort of the technology and content in the middle. Because of this, communication of semantic meaning should be at the very forefront in directing the development of both technology and content. Without this complete cycle, the interactive product or system fails.

3 Conclusion

No interactive product, system or artwork is truly successful unless the above three requirements are fulfilled. Technology is needed at the very base to create a condition for any meaningful interaction with content by the end user to be successful. Content is needed for the end user to have data to interpret and interact with. Finally semantics and meaningful interaction by the end user completes an interaction cycle in order for the end user to be able to derive meaning, and should be the end result of the orchestration of the above described components.

Future explorations on this topic should include a deeper understand of each level of the pyramid. Discussion on the impact of materiality and immateriality of technology, content and meaning, and how it affects development of interactivity should also be explored. A thorough analysis of existing case study artworks, designs and technologies using the hierarchy would also reveal a better understanding of how the hierarchy could be applied.

References

1. Miller, E.: Community cleverness required. Nature 455, 1 (2008)
2. Baker, H.D.: Willmott, W.E. (ed.): Economic organization in chinese society. Studies in chinese society series, pp. xi, 461. Stanford University Press, OUP, London (1972); Journal of the Royal Asiatic Society (New Series) 106(1), 90–91 (1974)

3. Dahl, R.: Charlie and the Chocolate Factory. ePenguin (2010)
4. Dourish, P., Mazmanian, M.: Media as material: Information representations as material foundations for organizational practice. In: Proc. Int. Symp. on Process. Organization Studies (2011)
5. Dunne, A.: Hertzian tales. MIT Press, London (1999)
6. Fernaeus, Y., Sundström, P.: The material move how materials matter in interaction design research. In: Proceedings of the Designing Interactive Systems Conference, pp. 486–495. ACM (2012)
7. Holman, D., Vertegaal, R.: Organic user interfaces: designing computers in any way, shape, or form. Communications of the ACM 51(6), 48–55 (2008)
8. Ishii, H., Ullmer, B.: Tangible bits: towards seamless interfaces between people, bits and atoms. In: Proceedings of the SIGCHI Conference on Human Factors in Computing Systems, pp. 234–241. ACM (1997)
9. Koh, J.T.K.V., Peiris, R.L., Zhu, K., Polydorou, D., Nakatsu, R.: Uncovering analogness and digitalness in interactive media. In: Proceedings of the 30th ACM International Conference on Design of Communication, pp. 233–242. ACM (2012)
10. Krippendorff, K.: Product semantics: a triangulation and four design theories (1989)
11. Maes, P.: Why do we still use a keyboard and mouse to interact with digital information? Seminar (2011)
12. Manyika, J., Chui, M., Brown, B., Bughin, J., Dobbs, R., Roxburgh, C., Byers, A.H.: Big data: The next frontier for innovation, competition, and productivity, pp. 1–137. McKinsey Global Institute (2011)
13. Margolis, J.: Stuck in the shallow end: Education, race, and computing. MIT Press (2008)
14. Markussen, T.: Disciplining the body? reflections on the cross disciplinary import of embodied meaning into interaction design (2009)
15. Maslow, A.H.: Toward a psychology of being (1968)
16. Mazzotta, G., Alighieri, D.: Dante, Poet of the Desert: History and Allegory in the Divine Comedy. Princeton University Press (1979)
17. Milgram, P., Kishino, F.: A taxonomy of mixed reality visual displays. IEICE Transactions on Information and Systems 77(12), 1321–1329 (1994)
18. Picard, R.W.: Affective computing for hci. In: Proceedings of HCI International (the 8th International Conference on Human-Computer Interaction) on Human-Computer Interaction: Ergonomics and User Interfaces, vol. 1, pp. 829–833 (1999)
19. Redström, J.: Tangled interaction: On the expressiveness of tangible user interfaces. ACM Transactions on Computer-Human Interaction (TOCHI) 15(4), 16 (2008)
20. Setos, A.G.: The relationship between content and technology. In: Proceedings of the 4th ACM International Workshop on Contents Protection and Security, MCPS 2006, p. 1. ACM, New York (2006)
21. Staff, C.: Why invention and innovation diverge. Commun. ACM 52(8), 8–9 (2009)
22. Treadaway, C.P.: Hand e-craft: an investigation into hand use in digital creative practice. In: Proceedings of the Seventh ACM Conference on Creativity and Cognition, C&C 2009, pp. 185–194. ACM, New York (2009)
23. Weiser, M.: The computer for the 21st century. Scientific American 265(3), 94–104 (1991)

Digital Media Art Applying Physical Game Technology Using Gesture Recognition

Hae Young Lee, Han Moi Sim, and Won Hyung Lee

Department of advanced image Graduate School of Advanced Imaging Science, Multimedia and Film, Chung-Ang University #10112, HeukSeok - Dong, DongJak – Gu, Seoul 156-756, Korea
smallcrime.1@gmail.com, kmusic@naver.com, whlee@cau.ac.kr

Abstract. In this study, we propose Digital media art to experience a virtual reality applying physical game using gesture recognition technology and describe its application based on the concept. Gesture and gesture recognition refer to HCI (Human Computer Interaction) is an important concept. Therefore, we produce the Digital media art calls 'Thrill Seekers'. 'Thrill Seekers' is for simulating Experimental game interfaces which offers an amusement while experiment the virtual environment. The using device Kinect is a motion sensing input device. Existing Kinect game is already popular in physical interaction; action-based games, with its sensing technology. However, we use Kinect with open library program 'Processing' to create virtual game interface for people who enjoy thrills the most.

Keywords: Virtual interface, physical game, gesture recognition, Interaction.

1 Introduction

Gesture recognition is the most demand technology in HCI (Human Computer Interaction) application. There are many applications in game instead of using keyboard or mouse. The applications are becoming more physical and tangible. Kinect is the most affordable motion sensing device for physical game interface with wireless input by Microsoft for Xbox 360 video game console and Window PCs. It can detect user's information and motion with Kinect's built in RGB (Red, Green, and Blue) camera and depth sensor technology. The device can be separated from gaming console and the sensor data can be used as input for gesture recognition. To use this device as an application for physical game is able to raise game user's immersion although existing applications; keyboard and mouse, has a disadvantage to reduce the game user's immersion and physical method.

Therefore, in this study we use Kinect for the 'Thrill Seekers' as a new user interface for Digital media art. The theme of this project focused on thrill seeking behavior and extreme sports type people as a way of relaxation and relief from fatigue of routine everyday activities.

C. Stephanidis (Ed.): Posters, Part II, HCII 2013, CCIS 374, pp. 273–276, 2013.

Unlike many devices related to physical activity, our concept requires only subtle and constrained motion and the need to maintain balance while the user tilts the chest area forward and back or from side to side, which is monitored by the sensors.

2 Relate Works

2.1 Digital Media Art Implement Gesture Recognition Technology

Digital media art is a contemporary art due to the development of digital technology. Many artists implement the technology into their art works. The cutting edge technology and device is necessary for such an artist. For 'Thrill Seekers' we use Kinect as a cutting edge motion sensing device for the digital interactive media art. Gesture recognition can be seen as a way for computers to begin to understand human body language, this building a richer bridge between machines and humans than primitive text user interfaces or even GUIs (graphical user interfaces), which still limit the majority of input to keyboard and mouse.[1] We implemented gesture recognition system using Kinect, Processing code and Simple-OpenNI library.

3 Proposed Media Art

3.1 Concept

The first significant development in this work was the idea of moving human body which imposes specific physical requirements on their performance. This approach was based on the body movements and activities covered by our concept. We set out to find a suitable library example which could be extended and adapted to provide the desired user interface and visualization components. The used code is based on a Processing (www.processing.org) code by Ira and Danny Greenberg, providing the main visualization elements, which are combined with a number of functions incorporating the Kinect 3D control data. The mapping of the user's performance was developed in a bottom-up driven process, relying on practical experiments using the Kinect and observing the visualization.

3.2 The Process

3.2.1 The Interface

The physical interface that this project explores is based on movements of the upper torso aiming to stimulate user participation and ongoing interest by providing a visualization reflecting their performance. The Kinect enables the user to roam free from the computer, through a Bluetooth wireless connection and provides a very intuitive interface based on natural movements within a real world frame of reference. The main limitations in our project relate to the limited visual richness provided by the program.

[1] http://en.wikipedia.org/wiki/Gesture_recognition

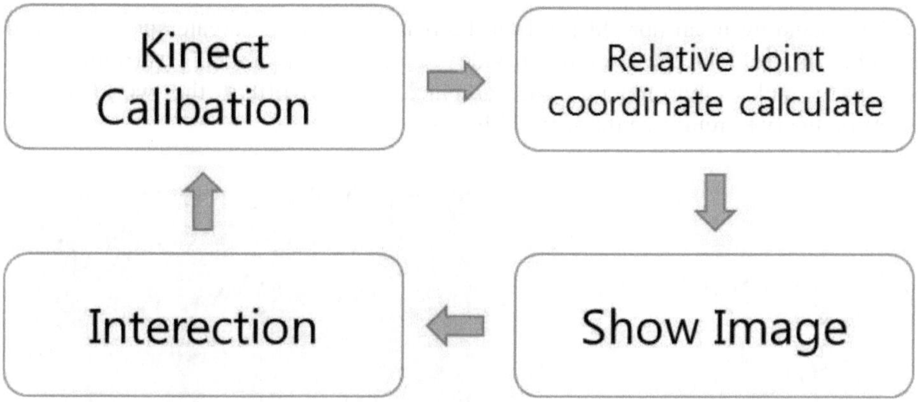

Fig. 1. The Process

3.2.2 How It Works

The user moves their body in front of the Kinect device. The visualization comprises a large number of cubes randomly distributed within a space resembling a wheel (rotating) with the viewer placed at the top and looking along the tangent of the circle. The table 1 is 15 joints defined by Simple-OpenNI. We can have the user's skeleton, location of the joint and Depth information through Simple-OpenNI. In this study, using torso information within these joints and read the axis's value in a real time.

Table 1. 15 Joints defined by Simple-OpenNI

Sensor	Joints	Sensor	Joints
0	Head	8	Right Hand
1	Neck	9	Left Hip
2	Torso	10	Right Hip
3	Left Shoulder	11	Left Foot
4	Right Shoulder	12	Right Foot
5	Left Elbow	13	Left Knee
6	Right Elbow	14	Right Knee
7	Left Hand		

When standing in an upright position the body movements create subtle shifts of the cubes in front of the user to provide an impression of being surrounded by the 'space junk' environment. The graphical visual offers the world moves correspondingly to reinforce the spatial illusion.

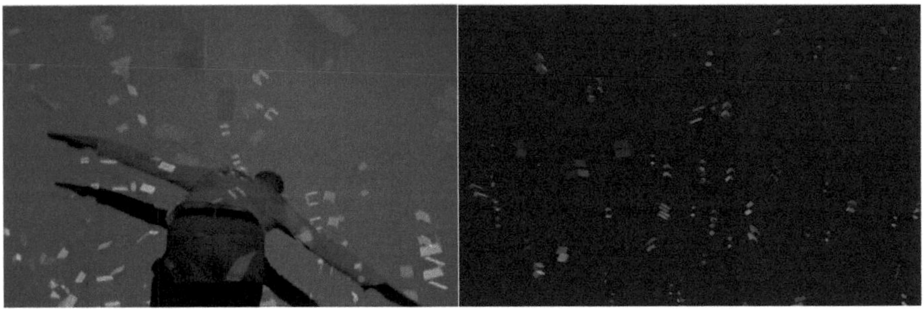

Fig. 2. Simulated Image

4 Conclusion

This study proposed the new way of interaction in digital media art adapting the method of game. In this study, we implement game elements using Kinect and its sensor. The change visual images by user's body movements through Kinect motion sensor offer relief feelings and relaxation to users. Not only use the hands but also use user's body for the most interesting digital media art also as a physical game. For the further study we should survey from more users and how they feel while they experience the 'Thrill Seekers' interface.

References

1. Cho, O.-H., Lee, W.-H.: Application of Reinforcement Learning System to Interactive Digital Art. Journal of Internet Technology 14(1), 99–106 (2013)
2. http://en.wikipedia.org/wiki/Kinect
3. http://medical-dictionary.thefreedictionary.com/Type+T+Personality

A Media Art Study Using Multi-Sensory Elements

Jaejoong Lee* and Jin Wan Park

117 Art Center, Chung-Ang University, 84 Heukseok-ro, Dongjak-gu, Seoul, South Korea
only104@navr.com, jinpark@cau.ac.kr

Abstract. This work will stimulate more than one sense. A lollipop is one of the world's most beloved snacks. Although it is common to normal people, a lollipop is not an affordable snack to poor children. This work expresses an imaginary lollipop by a user's drawing. The candy drawing is printed on a paper having a message on its backside. The message represents memories of childhood. The printer uses fragrance inks to print out an origami with a lollipop shape. The audience carries on art works which have a fragrance and lollipop shape. This is a fake lollipop, however it may represent a hope for everyone.

Keywords: Multi-Sensory, Aroma, Synesthesia, Processing.

1 Introduction

This paper is about "Scent of Lollipop," the art work chosen to be displayed in the SIGGRAPH Asia 2011 Art Gallery. The work was made with the theme of lollipop candy children favor. The printout of this work has the shape of lollipop candy, candy design familiar to us. The reason why I chose candy shape as the printout is that candy is sweets that can represent children. To some children who can procure it, candy is just common sweets. But, to others who cannot afford to buy it, it is the sweets of hope they want to have and eat. This work is designed to give spectators opportunities to make their unique candies, and through the process, create their individual identities, and, by letting them share the message of hope written on candy with other spectators, provide the opportunities to think of the real problems and future. And, by adding the element of fragrance, it tries to suggest a direction of artistic works which go beyond visual satisfaction and can stimulate multi-senses and induce synesthetic elements.

2 Study on Synesthetic Media Works

2.1 The Concept of Multi-senses and the Analysis of Works

Multi-senses is different from synesthesia which means two or more senses respond to a stimulus. It is senses responding to various stimuli.

* Corresponding author.

C. Stephanidis (Ed.): Posters, Part II, HCII 2013, CCIS 374, pp. 277–281, 2013.

In artwork and music piece, the communication between the artist and spectators is made through visual and auditory senses. Media art, however, by providing spectators with various sensory elements beyond the boundaries of visual and auditory senses, can make them have various experiences about the work.

Media art that communicates with the audience through multi-sensory experiences has existed continuously. Among numerous works, equipped with cutting-edge technology, and attracting eyesight of the audience, there have always been works which attract spectators' attention because of their analogue senses. "Water Lights" of Lee Jae-min which satisfies visual and tactile senses was a work displayed in SIGGRAPH 2006 Art Gallery. Sensor responding to water was installed on the panel on which over 300 LED light bulbs are densely attached. If a spectator dips his hand or brush in water and touches a LED light bulb with it, the light is on. Using such lights, a spectator can create various images. By touching the work, spectators communicate with the artwork.

"Hanahana" exhibited at the Ars Electronica 2007 is an interactive art which visualize aroma. The work was created by Kyoko Kunoh, Motoshi Chikamori, and Kakehi Yasuaki. If one sprinkles aroma on paper, and take the paper near the sensor of the work, the aroma sensor reads the value of aroma and visualize it by changing the size and color of the flower projected on screen. Hana of "Hanahana" means "nose" and "flower", and the work is a media art work which draws multi-sensory elements satisfying olfactory and visual senses.

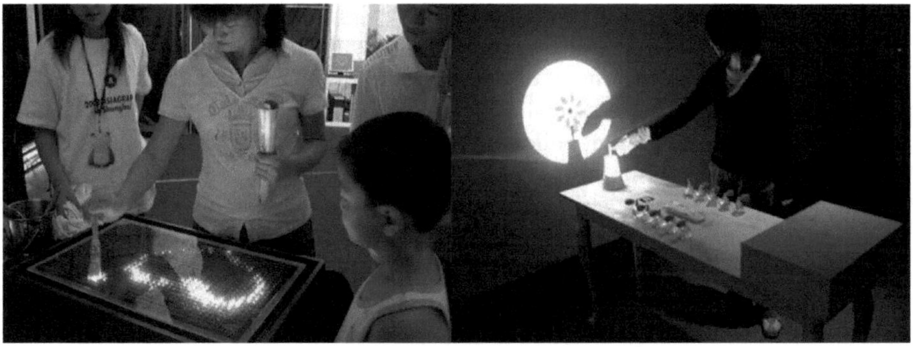

Fig. 1. Water Lights(left), Hanahana(right)

2.2 Embodiment of the Work

"Scent of Lollipop" is a work giving a message of hope. It changes the picture the spectator draws into a shape of lollipop candy. By letting spectators carry around lollipop candies, the message and meaning of "Scent of Lollipop" are communicated with others. And the aroma soaked in lollipop plays the role of catalyst maintaining the communication.

This work is what was embodied in Java-based processing language[1]. The Processing is the open source project of Ben Fry and Casey Reas that has been used by countless artists and designers across the world.

This work is a drawing system embodied by infrared tracking using Wii remote controller. The spectator can freely draw a picture in the designated space with infrared pen. Lines, planes, and colors of the drawn picture are mixed by rotation.

The mixed picture made out of the picture the spectator drew gets a shape of circle, which is printed out by printer.

If the circle-type printout is folded along dotted lines, it becomes like a virtual lollipop candy. On the back of candy, there are some sentences which can be shared with other people, along with a message of hope.

Interface

The input tool in this work is infrared pen. It is manufactured using TSAL6400 (IR Emitting Diode), and its operating voltage is 1.5v. By making basic calibration with infrared camera of Wii remote, and tracking infrared pen, the coordinates are changed into mouse coordinates. Pen interface allows the spectator to be able to use the pen as input tool, making the user feel more natural than the hardware like computer mouse. There is a circle at the center of the screen, and the user should draw the picture within the circle. The user can select colors from the color picker at the bottom.

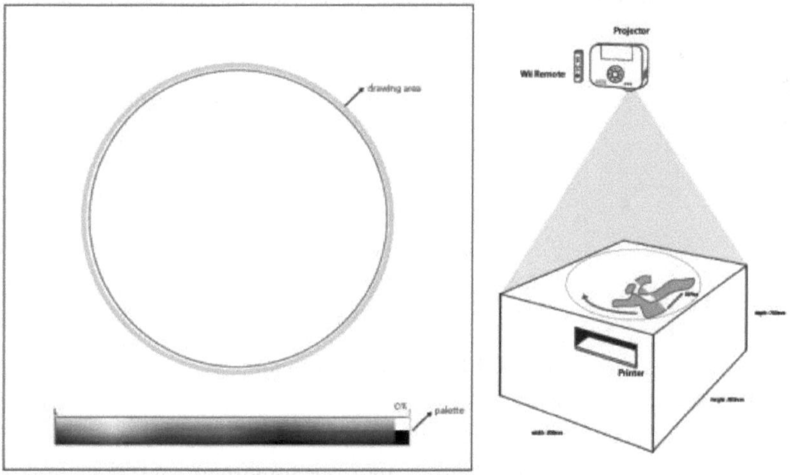

Fig. 2. "Scent of Lollipop" Interface

Rotation of Circle

Using the sine and cosine laws, the circle is made to become smaller and smaller, producing the spiral image. The spiral direction can be randomly chosen either

---

[1] `http://processing.org`

clockwise or counter-clockwise. And, to make the picture maintain a circular form, the radius of the circle becomes larger as it rotates, and when it finishes rotation, the radius becomes smaller, rather than it continues to be larger.

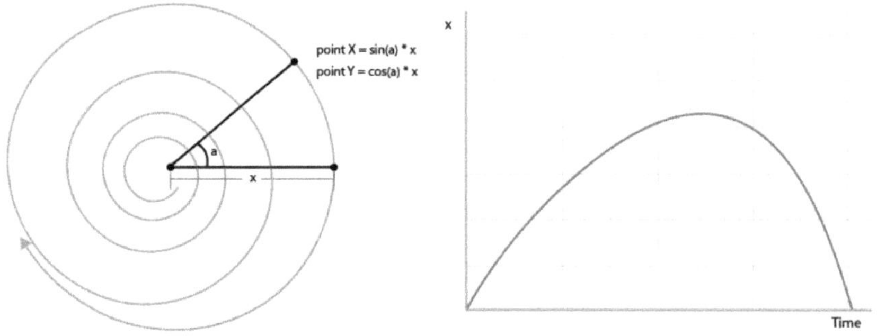

Fig. 3. The change of radius over time

Closed Curve Algorithm

To overcome the limits of the picture drawn only with lines, it is designed that, when the starting point and the ending point of the curve come close, the inside of the curve is filled. Through this process, one can get various results from simple interface.

If(dist(start_mouseX, start_mouseY, end_mouseX, end_mouseY) < 20)

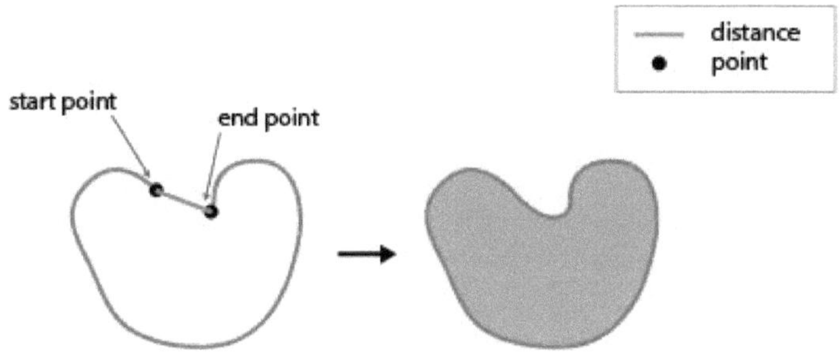

Fig. 4. Closed curve algorithm

Aroma

In this work, aroma, one of multi-senses, plays an important role. It is supposed to maintain the visually induced sense with olfactory sense. The printer used in the work is L200 of Epson which uses not cartridge exchange method, but large-volume ink injecting method. Using the characteristics of the printer in which the user can change ink freely, aroma of peach, apple, and lavender, etc. are added in 5 ink tanks. By such a process, it is possible to get printouts with various combination of the kinds of aroma depending on colors.

Image Printout

The result is printed on a square sheet of paper. To lead the spectator to make a lollipop form by folding the paper, the method of folding it is explained. The result is printed out by pushing the button connected to the Arduino board, or printout button marked on the screen.

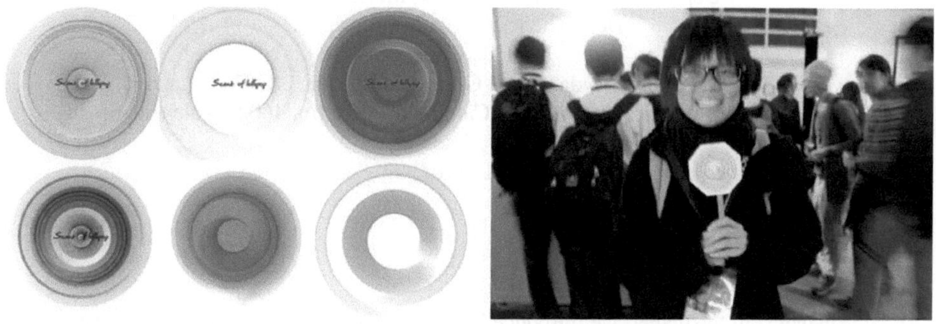

Fig. 5.

3 Conclusions

Unlike the cases of other SIGGRAPH exhibitions, at the SIGGRAPH Asia 2012 Art Gallery, Hong Kong, most of spectators were students. This artwork attracted more attention from female students who are more sensitive to colors than from male students, which seems natural. By adding elements which can stimulate multi-senses, this work intended to stimulate even emotion of spectators beyond the concepts of simple experience and game. Such aims were realized by the process which starts from tactile sense of pen and satisfies visual sense, and another process which stimulates multi-senses with olfactory aroma. And, the work was designed to make opportunities where people can communicate with each other through a medium called lollipop candy, and provide sustainable impression with the image which makes it possible to express one's identity with an uncopiable single result.

References

1. Reas, C., Fry, B.: A Programming Handbook for Visual Designers and Artists, 238. The MIT Press (2007)
2. Goodbye Privacy Ars Electronica 2007, pp.420–421. Hatje Cantz (2007)
3. Jung, H.J.: Desire Expression through the Drawings, Dong-Guk University pp.3–4 (2012)
4. `http://processing.org`
5. `http://johnnylee.net/projects/wii/`
6. `http://makeprocessing.com`

An Augmented Tourist Guide of a World Heritage City

Eulalia Rodríguez Fino[1], Jorge Martín-Gutiérrez[1], David C. Pérez López[4], M. Dolores Meneses Fernández[2], Vicente M. Zapata Hernández[3], and Felipe Monzón Penate[1]

[1] Dept. Expresión Gráfica en Arquitectura e Ingeniería,
[2] Dept. Ciencias de la Información,
[3] Dept. de Geografía
Universidad de La Laguna, Avda. Angel Guimerá Jorge s/n, 38202 La Laguna, Spain
[4] Universidad Politécnica de Valencia, Camino de Vera s/n, 46022 Valencia, Spain
{erfino,vzpata,fmonzon}@ull.es,
{jmargu,dmeneses}@ull.edu.es, dapelo@i3bh.es

Abstract. In this paper, we introduce the design and implementation of a tourist guide, using augmented reality technology, for visiting two of the most important routes in a World Heritage city. To produce this application, we used the augmented reality library, HumanAR, developed by our research group and created with the aim of integrating the applications we have developed. The application guides the user on a route across the town with a video of 3D animations of historic buildings along the way. The most symbolic buildings of the city are pictured and modelled on a walking tour across the historic site, designed to develop an interest in cultural tourism, keeping in mind the impact that this tourism may have on World Heritage cities.

Keywords: Augmented reality, world heritage, tourist guide.

1 Introduction

Augmented reality applications allow the introduction of additional information to our real view of the world, making it possible to superimpose virtual objects over real images captured by a camera. It's a technology that improves the experience of communication as well as that of human computer interaction. The AR environments have the following characteristics: they combine real and virtual environments; they are interactive in real-time; they are registered in four dimensions (three dimensional space and time), where virtual objects can be stationary or animated; there is interactivity between the object and the real world and abstract concepts can be made visible, in order to enhance the user's understanding.

These characteristics seem appropriate for producing a tourist route guide of the historic town of San Cristobal de La Laguna. In this paper, we justify the need for using such technological actions in the culture and tourism field and describe the completed application.

C. Stephanidis (Ed.): Posters, Part II, HCII 2013, CCIS 374, pp. 282–286, 2013.

2 Justification

There are many applications and benefits from using augmented and virtual reality technologies in activities related to historic heritage [1][2].

The augmented reality applications have several advantages over virtual reality environments including:

- The combination of real information and virtual elements, providing great realism over perceived information, avoiding the abstraction caused by virtual environments.
- The main added value of an augmented reality application is not based on the quality of their virtual models but on the viewing of dynamic information that is attractive and interactive in real time (images, videos, animations, 3D models, audio and text).
- The knowledge and tracking of the user's position eases the orientation and location of the places and elements of interest.
- The digital information is introduced in the real context, mixed with actual information captured by the senses and correctly referenced, respecting the user's position and point of view.

In the last few years, there has been rising interest in cultural tourism and its impact is huge on World Heritage cities [3] that are involved in creating tourist attractions. Through cultural activities and entertainment to promote the artistic and cultural heritage of the city, they seek to attract more tourists. This is the case in the city of San Cristobal de La Laguna (Tenerife, Spain), with its interesting past, historic buildings and street layout, making it a suitable town for trying to attract more tourists.

Tourist strategies show that a tourist who remembers his visit with enjoyment may return home and tell all his relatives and friends what a wonderful time he had. [4]. Bearing in mind that AR technology is growing, we may be able to create that enjoyment for the tourist, whilst viewing the places he will be visiting through AR. This may be the first approach to this technology for many of them and as we may already know, every time we experience it, we are often impressed.

On their arrival in the city, tourists will visit the tourist information office to gather information about the places they would like to visit. We have developed an AR application as an attraction for tourists, where they will be able to witness the city map becoming live on screen when it's using the computer's webcam, augmenting information already being viewed as 3D animations, with a musical background.

In this way, tourists may be able to know the path or route they may follow for getting to the buildings and other places shown in the guide. This could enable them to remember where there are places of interest to go on their visit.

3 Aim

It's necessary to keep in mind that tourism's purpose is to enhance new urban recovery processes [5]. In the case of the Canary Islands (Spain) and especially of San

Cristobal de La Laguna, tourism is one of the pillars of the economy and necessary for the future development of the town.

One of the key factors is the city's plain layout which has enabled the development of walking routes across it, improving the creation of commercial and private activities. This has brought about social and economic improvements for the city, including important developments on the political side.

The objective that made us create this tourist guide through augmented reality technology was the profile of tourists of this town. These include;

- Young visitors who travel as couples or with their families.
- Visitors of medium-high academic and cultural level.
- Visitors of medium-high economic possibilities
- Travel's motivation which is usually by recommendation
- Interests of visitors who know something about the city's culture, history and architecture.

The town was declared a UNESCO World Heritage city in 1999, which has led to some modernization, in keeping with the canary architecture and preserving its characteristic historical and cultural heritage. Alongside this, the rehabilitation, restoration and conservation of the town's most emblematic buildings, qualified by UNESCO as 'Cultural Interest sites', have led to considerable investment.

4 Work Description

As a starting point, a town map has been created where two routes have been drawn, one in red across the city centre and another in blue, around the town's outskirts.

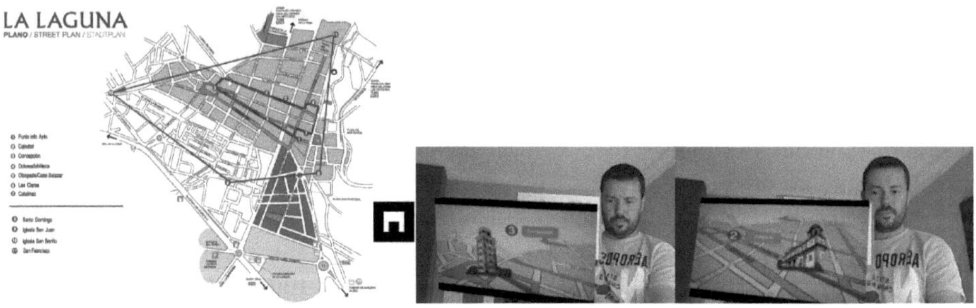

Fig. 1. Map of the historic La Laguna city with HumanAR markers. Implemented with Augmented Reality.

In the city there are several symbolic buildings, but over each proposed walking tour, the ones included in the Historic Building special protection plan have been underlined. Photographs of the buildings were taken and processed through image recognition software to obtain the correct perspectives.

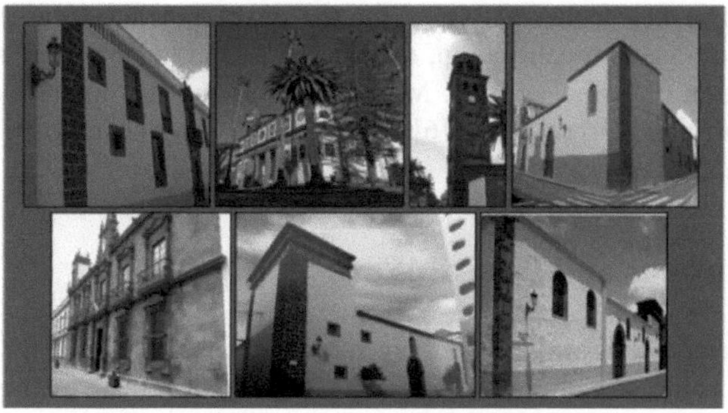

Fig. 2. Buildings of interest along the red route

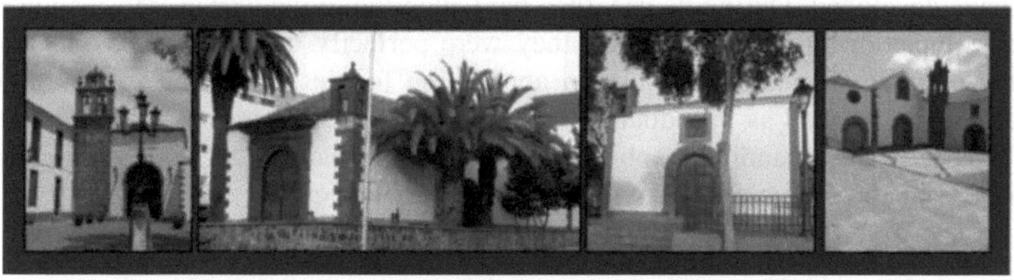

Fig. 3. Buildings of interest along the blue route

The red route walking tour proposes visiting seven points of interest whilst the blue route proposes visiting four. A Macromedia Flash animation was developed, where a virtual camera follows the path of the route until an interest point is reached, where a building's image rises perpendicularly over the plane, creating the sensation of fake 3D. A text tag shows the building's name and then the building fades while the line keeps its path, until the next point of interest, where the procedure repeats itself. When the seven points of interest on the red route are finished, the blue route starts. The multimedia element created has been an *.avi format video.

5 AR System: Software Library

Although there are several public libraries with AR capabilities, we have worked together with researchers of the Labhuman institute (www.labhuman.com) to create a software library called HumanAR, in order to assist the integration of Augmented Reality into our applications. HumanAR uses computer vision techniques to calculate the real camera viewpoint, relative to a real world marker, which calculates the integration of three-dimensional objects codified by the camera and captured by itself, in real time. When the marker enters the scene picked up by the camera, the fusion of the real world with the virtual object is shown on the screen. This requires the application to relate the two worlds (real and virtual) in a single system of co-ordinates. The key technical issues for the development of the AR library are; marker detection, camera calibration, calculation of marker position and orientation, and augmentation of virtual objects. More details about this library can be found by consulting Martin-Gutierrez et al. [6]. The graphics engine used to display three-dimensional models or video files was Game Studio A8.

6 Conclusions and Future Works

We regard augmented reality technology as a great potential tool for spreading and enhancing the value of Cultural Heritage, as it does not replace reality but improves its contents. It has established itself as a useful resource for the recovery and knowledge of heritage, because of its ability to add elements to an object's real view, offering different versions of it. Tourists have been impressed by the AR application we have developed. During its use, they paid attention to the virtual information and, after completion of the virtual tour, they were perfectly oriented for paying a visit to the city. We intend developing an application for describing the routes through smartphones, as well as introducing new functionalities over every point of interest, such as augmented audio, graphic and textual information, as well as interactive games, with all of them related to the town's history and culture.

Acknowledgement. The authors acknowledge the support received by Ayuntamiento de La Laguna, LabHuman, and Universidad de la Laguna.

References

1. Fritz, F., Susperregui, A., Linaza, M.T.: Enhancing Cultural Tourism experiences with Augmented Reality Technologies. In: Mudge, M., Ryan, N., Scopigno, R. (eds.) Proceeding of VAST 2005, Pisa, Italy, Eurographics Association Press (November 2005)
2. LifeClipper Project (2012), `http://www.lifeclipper.net/`
3. UNESCO. First Meeting of the Unesco/Unitwin Network. Report: Culture, Tourism and Development. Paris (March 2005)
4. Troitiño Vinuesa, M.A.: Estrategias sostenibles en los destinos patrimoniales: de la promoción a la gestión integrada e innovadora. Estudios Turísticos 172, 225–232 (2007)
5. Galdini, R.: Tourism and the City: Opportunity for Regeneration. Tourismos: an International Multidisciplinary Journal of Tourism 2(2), 95–111 (2007)
6. Martin-Gutierrez, J., Saorin, J.L., Contero, M., Alcañiz, M., Pérez-Lopez, D.C., Ortega, M.: Desing and Validation of an Augmented Book for Spatial Abilities Development in Engineering Students. Computer & Graphics 34, 77–91 (2010)

Interactive Art in the Age of Digital Reproduction

JeHo Oh and Chung-kon Shi

GSCT, KAIST, 291 Daehak-ro, Yuseong-gu, Daejeon 305-701, Republic of Korea
{anomewho,chungkon}@kaist.ac.kr

Abstract. The aim of this research is to study the features of interactive art in the age of digital reproduction. In the age of computer based digital technologies, interactive art will be changed by digital technologies. Interactive art consists of three factors: audience, installation, and content. Digital technologies have changed the installation of interactive art. In the age of digital reproduction, interactive art has the following seven special features: it is portable, it is private (not public), it represents realistic details, it has a kaleidoscopic orientation, it requires a network connection, it enables feedback/replies, and it can be archived.

Keywords: Interactive art, digital reproduction, interactive installation.

1 Introduction

The aim of this paper is to study the features of interactive art in the age of digital reproduction. In the age of mechanical reproduction, cameras and movies mediated by technology have transformed the artistic aura, according to Walter Benjamin [1]. Through technological development, art has become popular with the general public and artwork has become easy to reproduce. In the age of computer based digital technologies, where mechanical reproduction has been transcended, the concept of art has changed rapidly. In particular, interactive art is being changed through the use of nScreen, cloud computing, and smart devices.

This paper's research question investigates the ways in which digital reproduction has changed interactive art installation. For this study to be successful, this paper will analyze interactive installation. Since Marshall McLuhan first introduced the new media concept, which states that "the medium is the message," many researchers have been interested in media as an entity in and of itself. Interactive installation is media, and interactive art is included in digital media art. The primary question that needs to be answered is whether installation is media. From this point of view, digital media has changed, but the question remains: what is changing in interactive art through digital technologies? A complete picture of interactive art in the age of digital reproduction is needed. This research predicts impending changes to interactive art brought on by digital devices.

2 Literature Review

The issues surrounding previous forms of interactive art include audience participation, installation design, data programming, and a framework for the content mediated

C. Stephanidis (Ed.): Posters, Part II, HCII 2013, CCIS 374, pp. 287–291, 2013.

by new media. Research on interactive art has focused on the design approach of artwork and new installation devices [2][3]. Other research issues include the audience's experience and pleasure [4][5]. Previous research has categorized interactive art, but it has not studied the relationship between interactive art and digital reproduction. This research study, based on digital reproduction technologies, attempts to create a framework for new codes or designs for structures.

3 Study Aims

The aim of this research is to study the features of interactive art in the age of digital reproduction. As such, it aims to:

1) Categorize interactive art, subdivided by installation
2) Apply this new categorization to new media digital reproductions
3) Analyze the special features of new media interactive art
4) Predict the future of interactive art in the age of digital reproduction

4 Revised Categorization Method

The audience members experience the aesthetic content through the installation by their actions (the ways they interact with the art). The audience is the primary trigger of an interactive art installation. Consequently, communication between the audience and the art installation is an important issue. Through the development of computing science, the relationship between the audience and the installation is strengthened. Many research studies are defined by that relationship.

Fel's (2009) research forms the basis for this relationship. Fel defines the embodiment of interaction between the audience itself and the object. This communication is based on four factors: response, control, contemplation, and belonging. These categories help to formalize the relationship between the audience and the object.

Yun Zhang and Linda Candy's (2007) paper applies the information in this table to the focus of communication between humans and objects. As such, interactivities are classified according to type of communication and this coding scheme is used to analyze the view point of the relationship between participants and artifacts. In accordance with the degree of interactivity, the researcher proposes a variety of communication approaches and transforms the coding scheme: face-to-face communication, computer-assisted communication, proposal-assisted communication, drawing-assisted communication and interactive-artefact-assisted communication. The installation of interactive art has two basic requirements: a screen and an object. In this paper, these categories have been revised into an object, which consists of a screen, and an installation, from which the reference point becomes the relationship between the audience and the object.

5 Categorization: New Three Styles

Interactive art is defined as artwork that is created through audience participation using digital technology. Interactive artwork is composed of three factors: the audience, the installation, and the content. Research on interactive art considers these three factors simultaneously. The controversial issue is the role of installation. The audience does not communicate with the installation; instead, the audience communicates with the content by way of the installation. The installation is also the main trigger of interactive art. The installation is divided into categories. Consequently, that segmentalized installation plays a variety of roles based on the effectiveness of the content that is applied in the digital age. This paper examines three different categories based on installation: screen style, object style, and mixed style, and subdivides each.

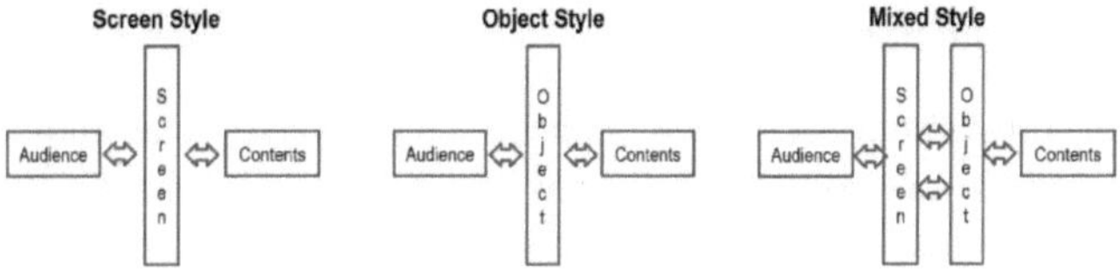

Fig. 1. New Three Styles

1) Screen Style
In screen style, the audience communicates with the content on the screen. The audience is represented on the screen by two figures: Image Type and Action Type. Image Type is when the audience is represented by the screen and watches its own image. Action Type is when the audience acts on the screen and performs actions.

2) Object Style
In object style, the audience communicates with the object of the artwork. The audience is represented in the artwork by two figures: Touch Type and Recognized Type (Sound/Smell/Taste/Perspective). Touch Type is when the audience engages with the artwork to touch an object. Recognized Type is when the audience does not engage with the artwork to touch an object, but rather recognizes the needs of the artwork.

3) Mixed Style
In mixed style, the audience communicates with the screen and the object at the same time. The audience engages in the art content mediated by the object and screen. The audience has an artistic experience by using the screen and applying that interaction to the object. The audience has an aesthetic moment by interacting with the screen through the object, and vice versa.

6 Application and Future

Current research on interactive art has not dealt with these three forms of installation, one-by-one. The installation of interactive art is a medium by which the audience relates to the content. However, installation is a form of live media in the digital age. We propose a new model for interactive art through digital reproduction. As such, interactive art will be changed by digital elements. Digital content is comprised of the following main elements: duplicability, random accessibility, manipulability, networkability, and multi-modality. We focuses on living installations using digital technologies. Currently, nScreen and cloud computing are two new forms of digital technology; As such, nScreen provides a variety of ways to interact with the screens on digital devices and cloud computing is delivered as a service over a network database, anywhere any time. In the age of digital reproduction, the object and the screen coexist with the installations. Users touch the screen display and perform various functions. The following are examples of interactive art in the age of digital reproduction:

1. Interactive art with nScreen

Using nScreen, interactive art screens can be very diverse. The audience can experience the interactive art contents by using the screen. The screen duplicates other screens and the audience's art experience becomes an unlimited reproduction.

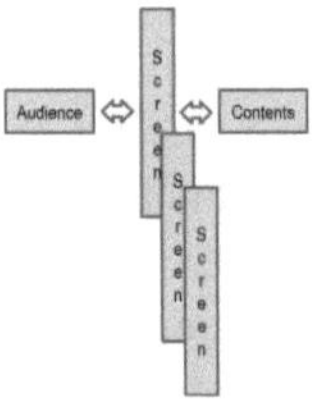

Fig. 2. Example of interactive art using nScreen

2. Interactive art with cloud computing

Using cloud computing, interactive art can be provided to an audience on a temporary basis beyond spatial boundaries. The audience experiences the artwork on the screen and creates aesthetic content. This art experience connects one device to other devices. Therefore, the audience enjoys its own artwork in clouding situations.

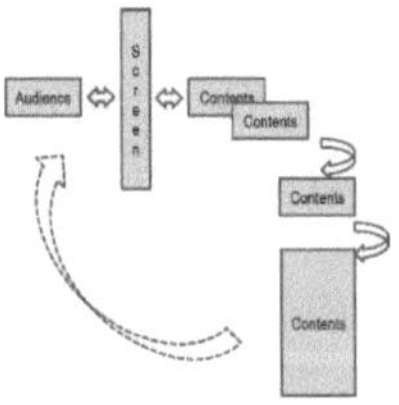

Fig. 3. Example of interactive art using cloud computing

Based on this research, interactive installation is changing through the use of digital technologies. This study applied digital features to categorize interactive art installation. Interactive art in the age of digital reproduction will have the following seven special features:

1. Portable art: new media interactive art will be portable and it can be taken anywhere.
2. Private art (not public): alternative interactive art will be private.
3. Representation of realistic details: interactive art with new media will be combined to produce exquisite detail and real-time artwork; it will be represented on an AR/VR/3D screen or on other digital devices.
4. Kaleidoscopic orientation: interactive art with new media will be kaleidoscopic.
5. Network connection: interactive art with new media will be available everywhere, without limitations of time and place.
6. Feedback/Reply: interactive art with new media will be simultaneously shared with the audience, and feedback and replies can be shared without the need for separate devices.
7. Archive: interactive art will be saved in archives and, thus, it will transcend previous limitations.

Based on these factors, interactive art in the age of digital reproduction will progress toward ubiquitous exhibition.

7 Conclusion

The installation of interactive art is being changed by digital technology reproduction, especially mobile devices. By categorizing the installations of interactive art, this research proposed a concept of new interactive art and offered predictions about changing the seven special features of interactive art by using digital devices. In the future, interactive art will be ubiquitously exhibited.

References

1. Benjamin, W.: The work of art in the age of its technological reproducibility, and other writings on media, CreateSpace Independent Publishing Platform (September 23, 2010)
2. Wong, C.-O., Jung, K., Yoon, J.: Interactive Art: The Art That Communicates. Leonardo 42(2), 180–181 (2009)
3. Haaslahti, H., Heikkila, S.: Space of two Categories. In: Interactive Installation with Shadow Projection, MM 2007. ACM (2007)
4. Costello, B., Muller, L., Amitani, S., Edmonds, E.: Understanding the Experience of Interactive Art: Iamascope in Beta_space. In: Proceedings of the Second Australasian Conference on Interactive Entertainment (2005)
5. Costllo, B.: A Pleasure Framework. Leonardo 40(4), 370–371 (2007)
6. Zhang, Y., Candy, L.: An In-depth Case Study of Art-Technology Collaboration. In: C&C 2007. ACM (2007)

Sequential Art in Real-Time 3D Applications

Jan Wojdziak, Dietrich Kammer, and Rainer Groh

Technische Universität Dresden, Department of Computer Science,
Institute of Software- and Multimedia Technology
{jan.wojdziak,dietrich.kammer}@tu-dresden.de

Abstract. A huge amount of data is produced continually in areas of application like entertainment, industry, and science. Contemporary technologies and three-dimensional computer graphics are qualified to process and to visualize this data. However, users are more and more faced with a flood of information, unable to efficiently process the information provided by three-dimensional computer graphics. Facing that problem, arrangement systems like typographic grids serve as an auxiliary layer to organize and arrange information units on a two-dimensional canvas. Due to the continually changing of interactive 3D scenes, there is no fixed order or priority of the visualized data in a projected image. Yet, in analogy to comic strips or comic books, frames that are organized in a grid can augment information visualizations. This contribution presents an approach to structure interactive 3D visualizations with the help of panels, whereby the user can recognize essential information in a given scene.

Keywords: HCI, real-time computer graphics, narrative structuring.

1 Introduction

The progress made in hardware technology allows today's computer systems to store and process very large amounts of data. Simultaneously, exploring and analyzing the vast quantity of data becomes increasingly difficult. For this purpose, information visualization and visual data mining help to deal with the flood of information. The advantage of visual data exploration is that the user is directly involved in the data mining process [5]. As a result, the availability of 3D visualization and interaction techniques is continuously growing. The widespread usage of interactive 3D graphics consequently results in a variety of systems. In standard 3D-applications, the user is enabled to change the parameters of a visualization by for instance adjusting the camera and can perform interactive operations in the presented views [1]. Due to this interactivity, the structure of the visualized content changes continuously and can hamper the visual data mining process [7]. A user-centered and task-dependent human-computer-interaction in interactive 3D-applications can be facilitated by providing an armature on which the content can be organized [3]. This can be reached by structuring the visualized information in an arrangement intended to convey information that is independent from the camera position and orientation.

Arrangement systems serve in comic strips and comic books as an auxiliary layer to organize and arrange information units on a two-dimensional canvas. Comparable

C. Stephanidis (Ed.): Posters, Part II, HCII 2013, CCIS 374, pp. 292–296, 2013.

arrangement systems are able to serve as a reference grid in space and thus structure three-dimensional content in visualizations. This contribution discusses the capability of two-dimensional panels as a reference grid in three-dimensional real-time applications. In analogy to comic strips or comic books, individual frames or multiple panels augment information visualizations by the implementation of concepts of sequential art in interface design of interactive real-time applications.

2 The Sequential Art – Comic

Our consideration is focused on providing interfaces that assist the user in perceiving spatial information as effectively and efficiently as possible [4]. We propose that design principles of comics are beneficial in enhancing interfaces as an efficient communication tool. Primarily, comics have a great capacity as a communication medium of images [2]. In spite of that, a precise definition of the medium in all its diversity is difficult. In [2] comics are described as sequential art. The crucial attribute of sequential art – the grid – is used to arrange pictures. The panel as the basic part of a comic is an individual frame and a single drawing within a grid. Each panel contains a picture that depicts a point in time within the story and is confined by using a grid as shown in Fig. 1. The whole story of a comic is narrated by the content and the sequence of pictures that constitutes a comic strip [8]. The grid delimits the images from each other and determines the order of the visual attention – the reading direction – of the observer. Therefore, it is important that obvious and intuitive arrangements of the panels guide the visual attention of the viewer subconsciously.

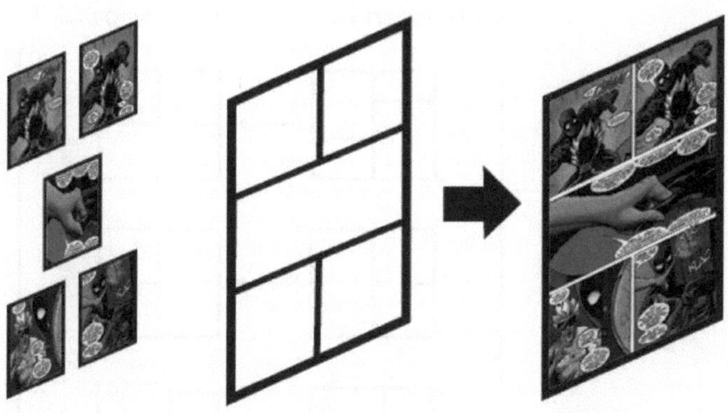

Fig. 1. Individual images, framed by panels are arranged by a grid and result in a comic strip (scenes from [6])

3 Structuring of Images

Comics enable an efficient perception of information with the aid of useful-structured content. Our aim is to adopt design principles of comics for computer generated images. By structuring the visualized objects of a virtual three-dimensional scene with the help of panels, a viewer can recognize essential information in a given context. Moreover, establishing a narrative structure by using panels allows guiding the attention of the observer. Prioritized objects of three-dimensional scenes are tagged appropriately to be detected faster. To this end, the properties of comics and its structure which lead to an intuitive understanding were analyzed. Especially the reading direction of panels in comics were considered. Yet, comics are read according to the reading direction in books, which cannot be directly applied to real-time computer generated images. The visual attention of users while observing pictures shift depending on characteristics shown in the image. Hence, the rules of sequential art are adopted and modified to visualize narrative structures of computer graphics images (Fig. 2):

- **Avoid Gaps**: Gaps in the horizontal adjustment have to be avoided. Straight lines navigate the attention intuitively and the natural reading direction is supported.
- **Intelligible Reading Direction**: A single panel can be subdivided vertically. Indeed, it is important to avoid ambiguous adjustments of panels to avoid ambiguity in the navigation. Subdivisions have to be carried out on the right side of the original panel only and should be maintained until the end of the line.
- **Depth by Overlap**: If the position of prioritized panels acts contrary to the reading direction, the grid is divided and a new level is generated. The grid receives a new dimension with the result of depth and therefore the metaphor of stacked comic pages. By a spatial arrangement of panels, the viewer reads the grid like pages of a book.

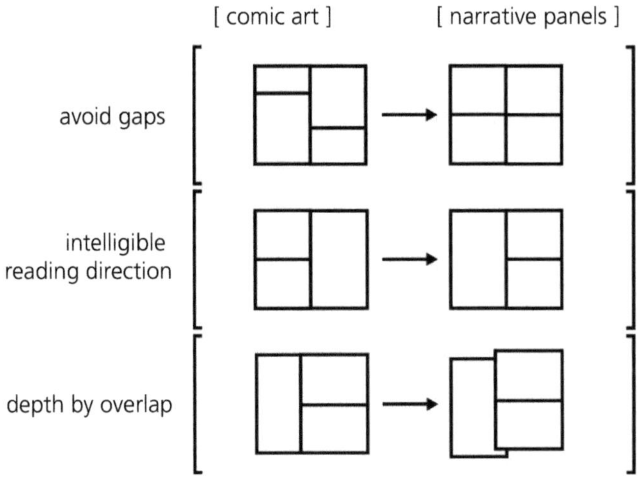

Fig. 2. Design principles to rasterize panels in (real-time) computer generated images

Henceforth, identified design principles of comics are transferred from comic books to narrative panels in computer graphics images. Building up on this design principles, arrangement systems can be generated to structure three-dimensional content in visualizations. The absence of a fixed 'reading direction' due to the interactive character of 3D-applications is counteracted by a priority-sustaining grid. The information value of the scene is clarified by panels and enhanced by defining a narrative structure of the projected scene. More precisely, the observer is supported in identifying relevant or prioritized information and its context, whereby the visual attention of the viewer in interactive computer generated images is guided.

4 Panels in Real-Time Applications

The implementation of the presented approach requires interactive computer systems. To this end, an application was implemented to realize the concept on the one hand and to verify the applicability of the interactive panels approach on the other hand [9]. Comparable with other 3D graphic applications, the interactive three-dimensional environment enable the user to navigate within virtual worlds and manipulate contained objects in real-time. The panels are created by framing the bounding box of the visualized three-dimensional objects or parts of the scene. Furthermore, the user assesses them by defining an order to serve as a reference grid in space. The panels are computed based on the rules of narrative panels as described in the last section. If the arrangement of the panels varies by changes in the virtual scene, the panels will be recalculated automatically. Therefore, a basic arrangement of the narrative panels as a reference grid is achieved. Fig. 3 shows the implementation of interactive panels in our real-time application. Crucial elements in this information visualization are accentuated with regard to the context, for example important elements of the molecule (Fig. 3).

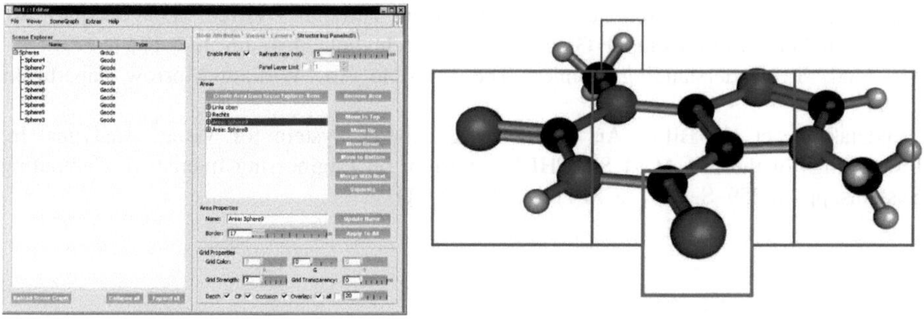

Fig. 3. The interface of the interactive 3D application visualizing a theobromine molecule structured by panels and an editor window for the panel management

5 Discussion and Future Work

This paper presents a novel approach to enhance visualizations of datasets. Panels act as a regulative approach to structure information in real-time applications. In spite of some elements of the scene being covered by frames, relevant information becomes accentuated. Additionally, a prioritization of the visualized objects is achieved, even though the objects are not centered in the image. Obviously, implementation of panels in real-time applications is an ongoing research topic.

With the foundation of narrative panels, different approaches for a more interactive use of panels can be developed. Multi-touch offers new styles of interaction and is therefore a technology with a great potential to enhance human computer interaction in combination with panels. For instance, the user groups objects in panels, presenting individual details of the framed part of the scene. Furthermore, panels as an interactive element are used to rearrange the scene context or to realize multi-views. Visualizations using panels with different perspectives on a dataset offer a better perception of details in context.

References

1. Dix, A., et al.: Human-Computer Interaction. Prentice-Hall (2003)
2. Eisner, W.: Comics & Sequential Art: Principles & Practice of the World's Most Popular Art Form. Poorhouse Press (2001)
3. Elam, K.: Grid Systems: Principles of Organizing Type. Princeton Architectural Press (2004)
4. Jokela, T., et al.: The standard of user-centered design and the standard definition of usability: analyzing ISO 13407 against ISO 9241-11. In: Proceedings of the Latin American Conference on Human-Computer Interaction, pp. S. 53–S. 60 (2003)
5. Keim, D., Andrienko, G., Fekete, J.-D., Görg, C., Kohlhammer, J., Melançon, G.: Visual Analytics: Definition, Process, and Challenges. In: Kerren, A., Stasko, J.T., Fekete, J.-D., North, C. (eds.) Information Visualization. LNCS, vol. 4950, pp. 154–175. Springer, Heidelberg (2008)
6. Kelly, J.: Deadpol, vol. 1(10). Marvel Comics (1997)
7. Mackinlay, J.D., et al.: Rapid Controlled Movement Through a Virtual 3D Workspace. In: Proc. 17th Annu. Conf. Comput. Graph. Interact. Tech., vol. 24(4), pp. 171–176 (1990)
8. McCloud, S.: Understanding Comics: The Invisible Art. William Morrow Paperbacks (1994)
9. Wojdziak, J., et al.: BiLL: An Interactive Computer System for Visual Analytics. In: Proceedings of the 3rd ACM SIGCHI Symposium on Engineering Interactive Computing Systems, pp. S. 259–S. 264. ACM Press, Pisa (2011)

Part IV
Transport

OnRoute: A Mobile Context-Aware Public Transportation Planning Application

Etienne Bertou and Suleman Shahid

Department of Communication and Information Science, Tilburg University, The Netherlands
e.m.bertou@tilburguniversity.edu,
s.shahid@uvt.nl

Abstract. In this paper we describe the design process of OnRoute, a mobile, context-aware travel application for managing navigation with public transport. The application uses an intelligent approach to using location data for easy step-by-step navigation in a more humane way. OnRoute incorporates all means of transportation, including walking, and consistently provides three views with increasing level of detail: a schedule overview, the current position in this step and the next possible action. Furthermore, individual preferences while travelling with public transportation are taken into account. The application learns from users' behavior and proposes better suggestions over time. User-evaluation of the final application design in a real-life setting showed users valued the user experience, design and unique features, and preferred OnRoute to existing smartphone travel applications.

Keywords: Public transportation, Route planning, User experience design.

1 Introduction

In the Netherlands an up-to-date collection of scheduling data for public transportation has become openly accessible via an open application interface of the travel information organization 9292 [1]. The data makes generating accurate and up-to-date schedules for travelling with multiple means of public transportation possible. When contextual information that becomes relevant during the navigation itself is not incorporated, a pre-defined route provides little benefit to the user. Our aim was to design a better solution for managing navigating with public transportation, focusing on 1) assisting users throughout all phases of travelling, 2) making navigation more user-friendly and 3) providing an overall better travel experience when using public transportation.

2 User Research

On different central train stations we interviewed twenty travellers that were waiting for their train to arrive. We discussed currently preferred information sources, problems experienced during navigation with public transportation and desired

C. Stephanidis (Ed.): Posters, Part II, HCII 2013, CCIS 374, pp. 299–303, 2013.

features of a possible solution for making travelling easier. In the Netherlands the railways and stations are all maintained by the Dutch Railways (NS). By interviewing NS-employees working at the station information was gathered on the frequency and nature of questions asked by travellers.

In our user research we identified two main users of public transportation planning applications: commuters and journeyers. Commuters use public transportation to travel along the same route frequently, whereas journeyers navigate along a relatively unfamiliar route to a possibly new destination. We learned commuters mostly value up-to-date information on delays and alternative route planning, while they deem locational information less important. As commuters are already familiar with their route, they prefer a clear overview of their schedule and an estimated time of arrival.

Journeyers, on the other hand, showed more interest in comprehensive route planning information. They would greatly benefit from step-by-step locational and contextual information to go with clear and more detailed instructions. During their trip, they continuously have to gather contextual information for correctly using their predetermined schedule. They are required to search for signs and information boards or ask personnel for information not provided by current route-planning applications. Walking from a train station to the appropriate bus stop or knowing exactly when to get off a bus or train, can be difficult on unfamiliar routes. This was found to result in a less comfortable travelling experience when having to follow a tight, predefined schedule. Users confirmed the importance of including all means of transportation in a travel application. This multi-modality is believed to lead to faster route finding and more comfortable journeys [2]. Accurate and up-to-date information on arrival- and departure times was also considered a primary requirement.

NS staff most frequently assisted travellers in finding the correct platform and confirming transit destinations. Travellers also ask about delays and route alternatives on a regular basis. The interviewed personnel considered answering these questions a major part of their work.

3 Conceptual Design and Prototyping

The primary user requirements for our travelling application were deduced from user research. Based on our analysis of the interviews, the process for managing navigation with public transportation could be separated into two major components: planning the initial route and assisting the user during travelling. For route planning many approaches have already been researched. Some schedule planners are able to incorporate much more contextual information [3], while other approaches advocate personalization [4]. For satisfying both commuter's and journeyer's requirements during navigation, we worked on a new solution. We created multiple scenarios and explored possibilities of different approaches to fulfilling user requirements. Examples are using smartphone camera's to overlay locational information or personalizing travel information on screens at train stations and bus stops.

After exploring multiple design alternatives, we decided on developing a smartphone touch-screen application using GPS – much like traditional navigation for cars – and a mobile data connection. The application would also feature maps of all Dutch train stations, which are already made available by the NS [5]. We designed an intelligent dashboard for a smartphone application that would use multiple views with an increasing level of information detail to assist both user groups during travelling.

The first dashboard-panel provided an overview of the schedule with the current step in the route being highlighted. It closely resembled the schedule overview of travel apps that are already available, with the exception that it would automatically adapt whenever the route scheduled would no longer be up-to-date or ideal. The second panel contained visual information on progress during the current step with estimated times of arrival and delays. Journeyers would be able to see exactly when and where they were expected to get off the train or buss, which would make travelling much more relaxed. The third and final panel showed specific locational information consisting of point-to-point navigation on how to get to the next point of relevance. Examples are how to get from one train platform to another inside a train station or where to walk after disembarking a bus.

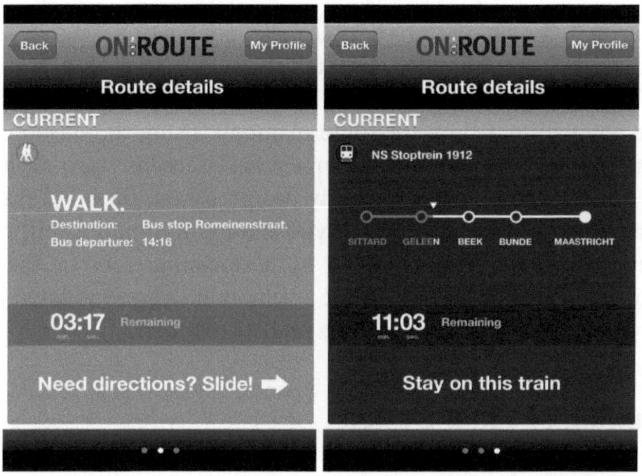

Fig. 1. OnRoute dashboard featuring progress and detailed travel information

OnRoute would personalize advice given during navigation to shift the focus from providing schedule information to creating a better travelling experience. Current route-planning apps rigidly provide the next point and time of departure in the set schedule. Waiting for the time of departure is a major part of travelling with public transportation and could be better spent. The application would provide suggestions based on user preferences and locational data. Instead of waiting at the nearest point of departure, users might prefer walking to the next bus stop in sunny weather and eventually board the same bus. Others might appreciate a cup of coffee or browsing a store. Users could add or remove means of transportation that were incorporated when suggesting routes. Also, they could set some initial customization regarding personal

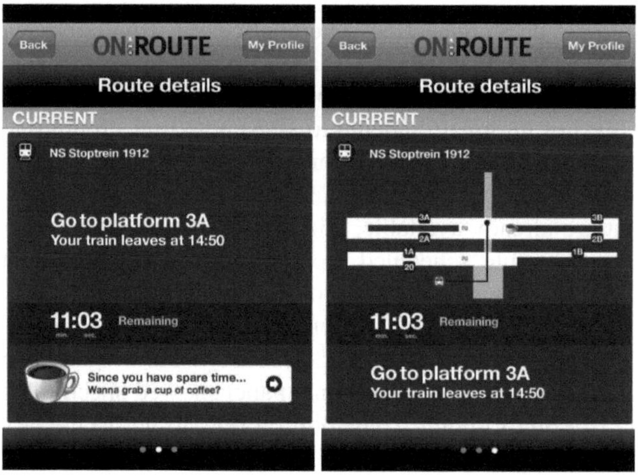

Fig. 2. OnRoute showing personalized suggestions and detailed information for navigation

preferences during navigation. Over time, the application would learn from the behaviour shown by the traveller and adjust suggestions for a pleasurable trip accordingly.

A complete navigational flow for route planning, using the dashboard and setting personalization was determined and all appropriate screens were sketched on paper. To allow task-based evaluation of the early design by the intended end-user, a paper prototype was created. After paper prototype testing, the high fidelity prototype was designed. Users evaluated the application by performing tasks on the actual device. By incorporating the mobile device in the evaluation, we revalidated design choices regarding layout and navigational flow in a realistic context.

4 Evaluation of Final Design

The final application was designed for iPhone. The fully working application was an extension of the high-fi prototype developed for specific stations and routes and it allowed user evaluation without designers' intervention. This way, we achieved realistic evaluation of the user experience in a real life setting. The application was evaluated by users at two train stations for planning their actual route. The results of early evaluation showed that users valued the overall user experience, minimalistic design and unique approach to assisting with navigating with public transportation. The consistency of separate levels of information on the dashboard panels, the clean interface layouts and the overall visual attractiveness were highly appreciated. All users preferred OnRoute for managing navigation with public transportation to other travel applications they had currently installed on their smartphones. The detailed qualitative and qualitative results of the final usability testing will be discussed in the extended article.

5 Conclusion and Future Work

In this paper we discussed the design process of OnRoute, a mobile, context-aware travel application for managing navigation with public transport. By incorporating the intended end-user early and often during the design process, we were able to design an innovative concept for managing navigation with public transportation.

Existing applications focus on route planning, whereas OnRoute also assists in managing navigation with all means of public transportation. It features are a dashboard with multiple levels of detail based on up-to-date locational information and personalizes travelling with public transportation with relevant suggestions. Users valued the comprehensive dashboard, maps of the train stations and natural way of making suggestions during navigation. Providing locational information in several levels of detail and personalizing the trip made navigating with public transportation easier and more pleasurable. Users preferred OnRoute to existing travel applications.

A limitation to our approach is the mobile data usage and use of GPS. Extended use of these features can be expensive and drain the smartphone battery. Alternative techniques for providing the required data are still being explored. Further improvements could be made by researching what specific personal preferences are desirable during navigating. Refining the suggestions provided by OnRoute requires further over-time analysis of actual use during travelling.

Acknowledgements. We would like to thank Eugene Houben, Jan Huntjens, Sylvie Bruys and Romy van Sambeek for working with us in designing the prototypes for OnRoute.

References

1. REISinformatiegroep B.V.: 9292 gelooft in open data, `http://9292opendata.org/` (retrieved)
2. Skoglund, T., Karlsson, M.: Appreciated – but with a fading grace of novelty! Traveller's assessment of, usage of and behavioural change given access to a co-modal travel planner. Social and Behavioral Sciences 48, 932–940 (2012)
3. Vaughn, K.M., Abdel-Aty, M.A., Kitamura, R.: A framework for developing a daily activity and multimodal travel planner. International Transactions in Operational Research 6, 107–121 (1999)
4. Letchner, J., Krumm, J., Horvitz, E.: Trip router with individualized preferences (TRIP): incorporating personalization into route planning. In: Proceedings of the 18th IAAI, vol. 2, pp. 1795–1800 (2006)
5. Nederlandse Spoorwegen: Informatie over station Sittard, `http://www.ns.nl/reizigers/reisinformatie/stationsvoorzieningen/stations/o-s/sittard` (retrieved)

Pilot's Interaction with a Glass Cockpit Navigation System

Ondřej Bruna, Tomáš Levora, and Pavel Pačes

Czech Technical University in Prague, Faculty of Electrical Engineering,
Department of Measurement, Technicka 2, 166 27 Prague 6, Czech Republic
{brunaond,tomas.levora,pavel.paces}@fel.cvut.cz

Abstract . Poster deals with interaction between pilots and navigation system of an ultra-light aircraft equipped with a glass cockpit. Glass cockpits are slowly replacing the gauges and dials used in small aircrafts and will play an important role in the future, because it is expected, it will replace them completely. Presented results are regarding the decision making, flight performance and pilot's justification of his choice. Data can be used to determine, if the pilots prefer to follow the navigator or independent flight, how they perform as pilots with and without navigation advisor. Based on this objective and subjective data conclusions are made. The outcome are suggestions for improvement of navigational instruments aboard and discussion focusing on how to help pilots in emergency situations stating both positive and negative opinions regarding use of glass cockpits.

Keywords: Emergency landing, navigation, ultra-light aircraft.

1 Introduction

Glass cockpit refers to a modern aircraft equipped with computers with LCD displays rather than with a usual dials and gauges [1]. Primary and secondary function displays provide pilot with all the information he needs to control the aircraft and to fly it along determined path. These systems are nowadays mounted in large aircraft such as Boeing 777 or Airbus 380. It also makes instrument flying easier. Computational power allows taking care of tasks which were not possible few years ago, for example an autopilot and flight management systems. It also makes it possible to incorporate special systems, which are not common. One of them is search for emergency landing site.

As electronics and microcomputers become cheaper and more powerful, glass cockpit is mounted to many light and to ultra-light aircrafts. This puts pilots of small aircraft in front of similar technologies as in large aircraft. Thanks to these technologies small aircraft have flight management systems of their own and also autopilot was incorporated [1]. There are also experiments with assistants which are supposed to help pilot to deal with unexpected or critical situations [2], [3] and displays are undergoing a long development with many different approaches [4],[5],[6],[7]. This will be also topic of this paper. Because pilots of ultra-light aircraft are not usually trained to fly under Instrument Meteorological Conditions, they do not train how to

C. Stephanidis (Ed.): Posters, Part II, HCII 2013, CCIS 374, pp. 304–307, 2013.

operate assistive systems. Emergency landing assistant, developed at Czech Technical University in Prague, helps to localize and lead pilot to safe landing place. This paper deals with pilots' reaction to emergency landing navigation assistant and states how pilots coped with the situation.

2 Methodology and Sample

20 pilots aged from 22 to 41 with average of 30 years were tested. Average number of flight hours was 200. Maximum amount of flight hours was 800 and least 50. Some subjects reported that they had previous experience with emergency landing. Most of the pilots had professional pilot license, but there were also some who had glider license as well. These pilots were extremely useful when stating the drawbacks of our emergency landing assistant. In the selected pilots who claimed to have previous experience with Garmin G-1000 or with other Integrated Flight Instrument Systems (IFIS). Some pilots reported that they use application in their tablets to serve the purpose of IFIS. Some applications are known to be able to emulate artificial horizon. Some pilots use tablets and smart phones in order to emulate IFIS.

The tests were performed on a 6 degree of freedom motion simulator. Before the test begun pilots had time to get familiar with the simulator and how it is controlled and how it behaves. The software used for simulation was FlightGear 2.4, which is considered as a suitable alternative among others [8]. To emulate IFIS our emergency landing assistant was used. During the flight it displayed the vital variables: indicated air speed, altitude, heading, pitch, roll, and horizon and in case of emergency it displayed flight director which led pilot to a safe landing site. The paradigms used were a "cross" and" tunnel". Pilot was supposed to keep the cross in the middle of the screen to stay on track. The cross moved on the screen in order to point out the direction of flight. Tunnel, on contrary, created a corridor of rectangles. The pilot always saw just 4 in advance and was supposed to fly through them. It lead pilot to a safe landing site as well.

The test had two phases. Firstly to see if there is a difference between the two approaches of guidance, the pilot was instructed to follow predetermined path as precisely as he could. He started with the plane already flying and the aircraft had still engine running. In this phase the only interest is to see, how pilot flies with a particular paradigm. Second phase was a task to fly certain trajectory from one point to another, and then return to the airfield and land. During this test the engine failed and the pilot was forced to perform emergency landing. But the pilot did not know in advance when this will happen. The pilot had available the emergency landing assistant. It was up to him if he/she decided to follow the suggested path or to perform landing on his own. The point is to evaluate how many pilots choose to follow. The ones who abandoned the guidance system are then questioned to get their explanation.

3 Results

The flight was evaluated using several metrics [9]. In first phase the focus was on error from predetermined flying path. Other important information was how many times the plane crossed the flight envelope and how many per cent of the flight was the plane out from the envelope. From the first phase was derived that pilots prefer the tunnel more than cross.

From 20 pilots only 13 were able to proceed to second phase. 7 had significant difficulties to follow the flight director. It has been concluded, that subjects were not able to cope with the simulator's behavior. Therefore they were not allowed to proceed to second phase.

Pilots selected navigation paradigm: 4 selected cross and 9 selected tunnel. From all performed emergency flights there were only 6 flights considered successful. All the pilots tried to follow the path from the beginning but only 6 pilots managed to maintain the trajectory. And even from this group all the pilots disobeyed the navigator in the final phase of flight – approach and landing.

When the flight was finished, the pilots were asked to compare whether they were more stressed with the navigation or without. The result is that seven pilots reported, that the navigation made them stressed and therefore they decided not to follow it. They also complained that it was not clear where the navigation led them and could not localize the landing place themselves. Some pilots decided to drop the navigation once the airfield was in reach and could see it. The did not follow the path for landing and stated, that it would be enough, if they just knew the direction, where the airport is, airport's heading, the distance and aircraft's potential altitude on the moment of arrival. They also noted that they would not trust the system, if it would not consider wind.

4 Conclusions

Authors realize that to provide more relevant results more subjects are needed. The expectation was that pilots will appreciate the navigation and in the subjective rating will mark flight with navigation as less stressful. Results seem to suggest that navigation under emergency circumstances can create a pressure on pilot resulting in even more stress. To gain pilots' trust the systems must prove itself in real emergency situations. Not considering a wind as an input is one of the major flaws for emergency landing. Wind can strongly affect the flight trajectory.

It seems that navigation systems will be much more likely used during a cruise than in case of emergency landing. Pilots suggest that system could point out the direction of closest possible landing site and should mark it on the screen, so the pilot could decide on the way of getting there himself, considering all circumstances that may occur.

Acknowledgements. This work was supported by the Grant Agency of the Czech Technical University in Prague, grant No. SGS12/193/OHK3/3T/13.

References

1. Technically Advanced Aircraft Safety Study, http://www.faa.gov/training_testing/training/fits/research/media/TAA%20Final%20Report.pdf
2. Shen, Y.-F., Rahman, Z.-U., Krusienski, D., Li, J.: A Vision-Based Automatic Safe Landing-Site Detection System. IEEE Transactions on Aerospace and Electronic Systems 49(1) (January 2013)
3. Frantis, P.: Emergency and precautionary landing assistant. In: 2011 IEEE/AIAA 30th Digital Avionics Systems Conference (DASC), Seattle (2011)
4. Sarter, N.B.: The Need for Multisensory Interfaces in Support of Effective Attention Allocation in Highly Dynamic Event-Driven Domains: The Case of Cockpit Automation. The International Journal of Aviation Psychology 10(3), 231–245 (2000)
5. Sarter, N.B., Woods, D.D.: Pilot Interaction With Cockpit Automation: Operational Experiences With the Flight Management System. The International Journal of Aviation Psychology 2(4), 303–321 (1992)
6. Sarter, N.B.: Pilot Interaction With Cockpit Automation II: An Experimental Study of Pilots' Model and Awareness of the Flight Management System. The International Journal of Aviation Psychology 4(1), 1–28 (1994)
7. Barrows, A.K., Enge, P., Parkinson, B.W., David Powell, J.: Flight Tests of a 3-D Perspective-View Glass-Cockpit Display for General Aviation Using GPS, ION GPS95, Palm Springs, California, USA (1995)
8. Yavracuk, I., Kubali, E., Tarimci, O.: A low cost flight simulator using virtual reality tools. IEEE Aerospace and Electronic Systems Magazine 26(4), 10–14 (2011)
9. Bruna, O., Holub, J., Paces, P., Levora, T.: Small Aircraft Emergency Landing Decision Support System – Pilots' performance Assessment. In: XX IMEKO World Congress, Busan, Republic of Korea (2012)

Road Accident Auto-dialer via Pressure Sensor

Kim Nee Goh, Yoke Yie Chen, and Davindren Arumugam

Computer and Information Sciences Department
Universiti Teknologi PETRONAS
Bandar Seri Iskandar, 31750, Tronoh, Perak, Malaysia
{gohkimnee,chenyokeyie}@petronas.com.my, ddmax90@gmail.com

Abstract. An accident sometimes goes unnoticed, for example, falling into a ravine. Thus no one is able to make emergency calls to the relevant authorities. Airbags in vehicles are designed to inflate when serious accidents occur. However, reliance an airbag alone may not be sufficient. This research explores developing a prototype using crash and pressure sensor as a parameter to trigger auto-dialer to call a pre-programmed list of numbers when an accident occurs. Global Positioning Satellite (GPS) and Global System for Mobile Communications (GSM) modules are integrated to track vehicle location and send information. A Short Message Service (SMS) will be sent containing the vehicle registration number and GPS location, to the authorities or even the insurance agent. This life-saving system which can be placed in the black box of a vehicle to report incidences and thus reduce the time needed to relay accident location information to the relevant authorities.

Keywords: Accident, airbag, pressure sensor, auto-dialer, GSM, GPS.

1 Introduction

In Malaysia, rate of road accidents, casualties and deaths have been increasing. Based on Malaysian Institute of Road Safety Research (MIROS) newspaper article released in 2009 [1], the number of crashes involving men drivers were 2.4 times more than women drivers. Men scored 1,351.74 crashes per 100,000 male populations, while women were 537.97 crashes per 100,000 female populations. Table 1 shows the number of accidents by year and gender, based on reports from Royal Malaysia Police Force, analysed by Malaysian Institute of Road Safety (MIROS) [1].

Table 1. Number of accidents by year and gender

	2006	2007	2008	2009
Male	145,502	161,763	190,788	244,336
Female	52,167	60,079	73,241	103,153

Some accidents need immediate medical attention. Delay in relaying information will delay medical attention probably cause deaths. Reducing the time taken from when the accident happened and for responders to be dispatched is crucial as it

C. Stephanidis (Ed.): Posters, Part II, HCII 2013, CCIS 374, pp. 308–312, 2013.

decreases mortality rate by 6% [2]. As stated by [3], each minute that an injured crash victim does not receive medical care, it widens the gap of their survival rate. Analysis showed that reducing accident response time by 1 minute, it correlates to 6% difference in the number of lives saved. Airbag technology does not efficiently curb fatalities. Also, drivers tend to panic and fail to handle the situation effectively.

We propose a system that is aimed to make them feel a degree safer when travelling. This research will develop a prototype that combines crash and pressure sensors with auto-dialer to allow the system to call a pre-programmed list of emergency numbers. GSM and GPS communication modules will send information and for track vehicle location. However, the scope of this paper is to develop a simulation system to simulate pressure sensor and trigger auto-dialer to call the authorities.

2 Related Work

This paper [4] researched on an in-car terminal, combining GPS, GSM and a control module to detect car incidences. CCTV is used to verify the incident when a report is obtained. In an accident, an alarm report is triggered and sent to the Transport Management Center (TMC) via GSM and GPRS. There are two ways incidences could be reported, manual and automatic incident detection. In manual incident detection, spectators, CCTV or the conscious driver can report the incident. The disadvantage is the accuracy of witnesses in relaying location information. This can be overcome using GPS module. In automatic detection method, when the driver is unconscious and no witnesses were around, the auto-alarm can be triggered by one of the in-car sensor, for example the airbag. However, it did not specify if any information was sent, but rather just an alert signal. It was also mentioned that GPS has the most accurate navigation system, but it does have problems in transmitting signal through large objects like buildings. Capacitive Sensing (CPS) Module was suggested as a solution as it is more widespread and has less blind zone. However, the positioning error is larger. Thus, they used these two technologies interchangeably. Our research will focus on using airbag as a main triggering mechanism to indicate that an accident has taken place and it is somewhat severe. In [5], the researchers researched on automotive airbag suppression based on occupant classification. It was mentioned by [3] that airbags will be triggered if acceleration is over 60G. Airbags can also cause fatal injuries if the occupant is a child smaller (in weight) than a normal size of a 6 year old. Using machine vision-based occupant classification system, with less than 5 seconds, it is able to identify whether the occupant is rear-facing infant seat, child, adult or an empty seat. Accuracy rate was approximately 95% which was extensively tested with 21,000 real-world images of occupants in vehicles.

White et. al. [2] introduced an approach to eliminate delay between accident occurrence and the first responder dispatch through in-vehicle automatic detection and notification system. Sensors are placed on smartphones to detect accidents and notify emergency personnel. G-forces acceleration experienced by the vehicle is recorded, which includes acoustic signatures from air-bag deployments or accident noises. By using a combination of data like sensor data such as accelerometer and acoustic information and intelligent sensor data filtering, the detection system could reduce false positive signals. It was reported that it is not able to detect minor accidents, as filters were used to reduce false positives. Valente et. al. [6] research on trucks transporting dangerous goods, such as radioactive chemicals, is monitored to ensure safety to the driver and other vehicles. Real-time monitoring of parameters inside the cargo bay (i.e. temperature, ionizing radiation level) using wireless sensors were used to detect and prevent dangerous situations. GPS is used to detect the location of the vehicle. These data are then sent via General Packet Radio Service (GPRS) to a main station, where it will monitor the mechanics of the trucks. General Motors Co., uses GM's OnStar [7] system to notify the relevant authorities about an accident that is triggered by in-vehicle sensors like airbag. Transmission of the accident information is through built-in cellular radios. If an accident occurred, OnStar will automatically place a voice call to the relevant authorities so that the authorities can inquire about the condition of the car occupants, provide guidance and predict whether an ambulance should be sent to the scene of accident.

Authors in [8, 9] defined situational awareness as a condition where a person is being informed of the environment in time and is able to predict the future outcomes within the environment. In fact, [10] claims that in times of mass emergency, people use Twitter to gather and disperse information. Context has to be placed for people to better understand their surroundings. Training machines are used to identify valid tweets and extract tweets that will contribute to situational awareness. This shows how important situational awareness is in times of an emergency. The novelty from our work is the use of auto-dialer after crash sensors are triggered. GPS module will capture the accident location and send an SMS containing car registration number and GPS coordinates.

3 Results and Discussion

Fig. 1 shows the process flow of the proposed prototype. When an accident happens, it will activate the auto-dialer. The auto-dialer will call a pre-programmed set of numbers through GSM network to inform of the accident via voicemail. An SMS will be sent, containing the car registration number and GPS location of car. Once a report is obtained, the phone operator receiver will have a system to display time/date record, car registration number and will show the location in a map for the operator to contact the nearest relevant authorities.

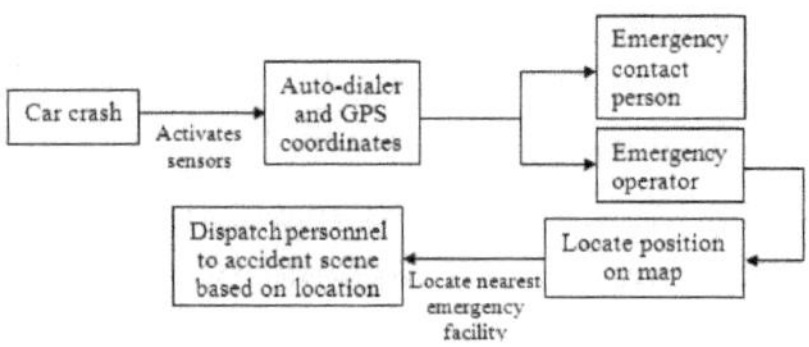

Fig. 1. Process flow

Our conceptual model has a little modification. An extra connection of pressure sensor will be fixed in addition to the crash sensor. The reason is to avoid any possible form of failure in the auto-dialer, which is directly affected by airbag function. This ensures only a defined amount of pressure is considered severe to demand for medical and emergency attention. This is to avoid activating the auto-dialer, for minor fender-bender incidences.

Fig. 2 below shows the conceptual design of our prototype. The pressure sensor will be set to a predefined threshold sensing level. Once the pressure sensed exceeds the threshold, it will trigger the auto-dialer. The auto-dialer is integrated with GSM and GPS modules. If that area has poor GSM network reception, the government allocated bandwidth for emergency calls can be utilized. Therefore, the emergency call number in the system can still go through but emergency contact person will not be reachable.

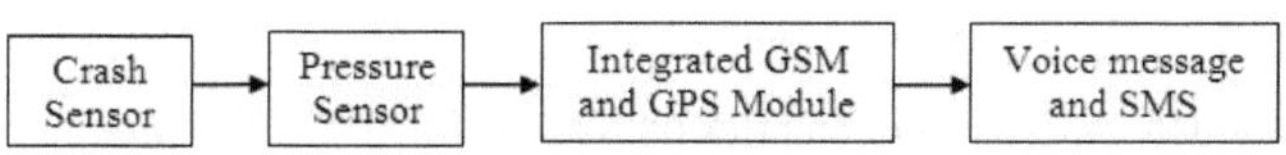

Fig. 2. Proposed design

For the proposed design, a computer application is developed to simulate such event (Fig. 3). The pressure level during idle is slightly above 5. The pressure threshold level is set to 6. Fig. 4 shows the event when pressure is above the threshold level of 6. Thus, the SMS is triggered to be sent to the two preprogrammed numbers. In our simulation, two numbers were pre-programmed. However, more numbers can be added depending on individual's need, whom some of them may include friends and insurance agents.

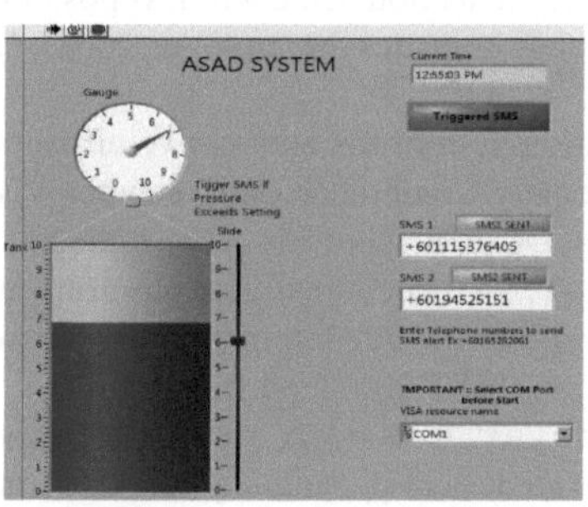

Fig. 3. Main system interface

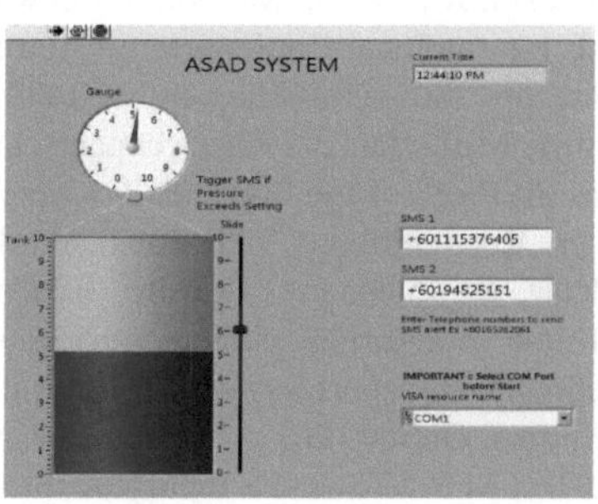

Fig. 4. Pressure level above treshold and Notification of SMS sent

In this simulation, we managed to get the SMS module to work properly. Our next steps would include developing a full scale prototype to be fitted in remote control cars for testing. The proposed system is aimed to provide quicker medical attention to the accident victim.

4 Conclusion

A conceptual model was proposed to include pressure sensor to trigger the auto-dialer when accident happens. A computer application was developed to simulate the proposed design. Only with predefined amount of impact will pressure sensors be triggered. SMS module has been developed and is fully operational. This invention would help to reduce the time taken for police or ambulance to receive information regarding accidents and improve the response time of relevant authorities. Our future works would include developing the complete prototype and placed it in remote control for real world test scenarios. Development of the full prototype will be discussed in future papers.

References

1. Mohd Sadullah, A.F.: Gender and risk on roads (March 20, 2011), http://www.miros.gov.my/web/guest/photo?p_p_id=101_INSTANCE_TmPd&p_p_lifecycle=0&p_p_state=normal&p_p_mode=view&p_p_col_id=rightbar&p_p_col_pos=1&p_p_col_count=4&_101_INSTANCE_TmPd_struts_action=%2Ftagged_content%2Fview_content&_101_INSTANCE_TmPd_redirect=%2Fweb%2Fguest%2Fphoto&_101_INSTANCE_TmPd_assetId=173379
2. White, J., Thompson, C., Turner, H., Dougherty, B., Schmidt, D.C.: WreckWatch: Automatic Traffic Accident Detection and Notification with Smartphones. Journal of Mobile Networks and Applications 16, 285–303 (2011)
3. Evanco, W.: The impact of rapid incident detection on freeway accident fatalities. Mitretek Systems, Inc. (2006), WN96W0000071
4. Li, C., Hu, R., Ye, H.: Method of freeway incident detection using wireless positioning. In: IEEE International Conference on Automation and Logistics 2008 (ICAL 2008), Qingdao, China, pp. 2801–2804 (September 2008)
5. Farmer, M.E., Jain, A.K.: Occupant classification system for automotive airbag suppression. In: Proc. of the 2003 IEEE Computer Society Conference on Computer Vision and Pattern Recognition (CVPR 2003), Washington, DC, USA, pp. 756–761 (June 2003)
6. Valente, F., Zacheo, G., Losito, P., Camarda, P.: A telecommunications framework for real-time monitoring of dangerous goods transport. In: 9th International Conference on Intelligent Transport Systems Telecommunication (ITST 2009), pp. 13–18 (2009)
7. Unknown, OnStar (2011), https://www.onstar.com/web/portal/home
8. Endsley, M.R.: Toward a theory of situation awareness in dynamic systems. Journal of the Human Factors and Ergonomics 37, 32–64 (1995)
9. Sarter, N.B., Woods, D.D.: Situation Awareness: A Critical but Ill-Defined Phenomenon. International Journal of Aviation Psychology 1, 45–57 (1991)
10. Vieweg, S.: Twitter communications in mass emergency: contributions to situational awareness. In: Proc. of the ACM 2012 Conf. on Computer Supported Cooperative Work Companion (CSCW 2012), pp. 227–230. ACM, New York (2012)

Developing Visualisation Techniques of Tasks in Air Traffic Control Work

Hajime Hirako[1], Toshiya Sasaki[1], Kazuhiko Yamazaki[1], Hisae Aoyama[2], Satoru Inoue[2], and Yutaka Fukuda[2]

[1] Chiba Institute of Technology, Chiba, Japan
{hrkhjm0508,toshiya.ssk1,designkaz}@gmail.com
[2] Electronic Navigation Research Institute (ENRI), Tokyo, Japan
{aoyama,inoue,fukuda}@enri.go.jp

Abstract. Air Traffic Controllers are expected to continue maintaining the safety of the air space and maintaining air traffic flow to run smoothly in complex systems in the future. In this research, we focused on task analysis of air traffic controllers in actual en-route ATC in an experimental activity based on a Human-Centred Design approach for designing the new concept user interfaces. We discuss the method of design to develop a system of human consciousness, especially for Air Traffic Controllers.

Keywords: User Interface Design, Human-Centred Design, Air Traffic Control, Experience map.

1 Background and Purpose

Air Traffic volume is predicted to be increasing in the future. Air Traffic Controllers will also have to handle more complex and heavier air traffic situations in the future. The tasks involved in ATC put heavy demands on the information processing capacities of air traffic controllers. To keep smooth and higher safe air traffic flow, future ATC systems need to be equipped with supporting functions or higher usability interfaces for assisting controllers work. In order to design a future system that can assure higher safety, enhance usability, and support human reliability, the idea of Human-Centred Design processes can help designers in understanding the features in the operations and intentions of the controller.

This research aims to propose a visualisation method to support the task analysis process for designing a new interface for the future ATC system. We believe that a visualisation process for analysis can contribute to the easy understanding of the essential meanings of subjects, when designers design a new interface concept which involves higher usability and efficiency for controllers in ATC work. Understanding user's behaviour is one of the important factors for considering interface design along with the Human-Centred Design (HCD) process.

C. Stephanidis (Ed.): Posters, Part II, HCII 2013, CCIS 374, pp. 313–317, 2013.

2 Approach and Design Process

Air Traffic controllers' work needs to get support from the systems in the future ATM concept such as a 4D-TBO. However, support tools should be user-friendly systems in order to maintain a good relationship between controllers and systems. HCD is one effective method to understand the users' requirements. In order to design a system that can assure safety, enhance usability, and support human reliability under the future concept systems, the idea of HCD processes can help an engineer or an designer in considering the features in the control system operations and the intentions of the controller. "Understanding and specification of a user's usage state" in the "Human-Centred Design process for interactive systems as defined in the Human-Centred Design process ISO9421-210 (Figure.1)". It can be said that this is a key item in the Human-Centred Design that works to visualise the usage state of the product and service being investigated to understand that the user's behaviour is basic for all of the processes of work afterwards. Regarding the observation survey technique, various forms can be taken depending on the purpose and the situation. Because it seeks to investigate how the user is using the product and service. The observation technique can be used to generally investigate a detailed understanding of the usage state and potential needs. However, it requires a lot of time and the workload is huge. In this paper, firstly, we propose an observation survey technique that can obtain survey results of high effectiveness, with a process of Human-Centred Design that can be executed simply compared with conventional techniques.

3 Method of Analysis

Setting of Analysis. To analyze how air traffic controllers work, we built an experiment system for collecting data through simulator experiments (Figure 2). The radar controller and coordination controller, who take charge of en-route ATC, frequently monitor the display of the radar control interface and the data of flight strips, and carry out controlling tasks while exchanging information. For instance, when the radar controller projects the existence of a related aircraft from the radar monitor, a series of instructions from the radar controller are directed to the pilot through communication with the aircraft to avoid conflict. The controllers then input the contents of these instructions into the RDP (Radar Data Processing) system, and input data to the flight strip.

Preliminary Case Study of Task Visualisation. As a preliminary analysis, we tested 5 types of analysis techniques to develop a task visualisation method for analysing Air Traffic Controllers' work as shown in Table 1. The first one in the column is the mapping which focuses on eligible important situations. In this technique, an analyst makes the list of screen shots which were first selected as critical or important situations. And then, they add analytical annotations in each eligible situation on the map by using memo pads. This map can assist in the understanding of the flow of

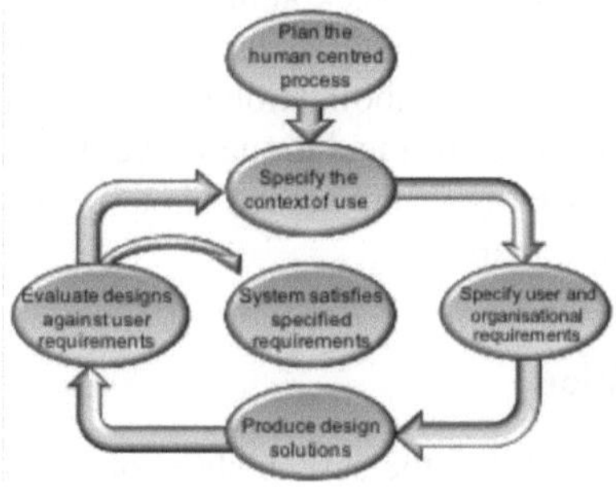

Fig. 1. The Human-Centred Design process ISO9421-210

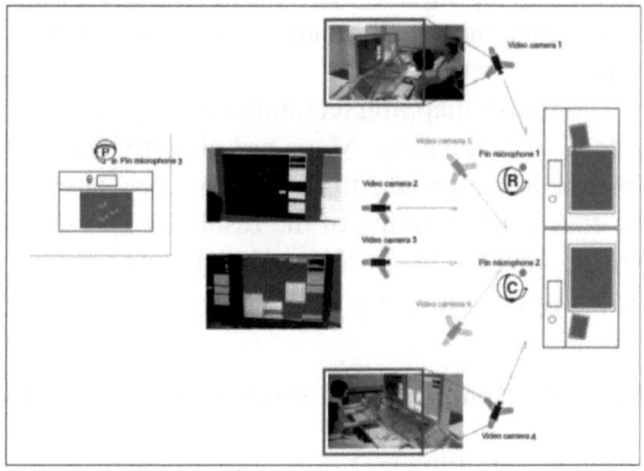

Fig. 2. Setting up a Simulator Experiment

Table 1. Five types of test visualisation methods

	Advantages	Disadvantages
The first mapping technique 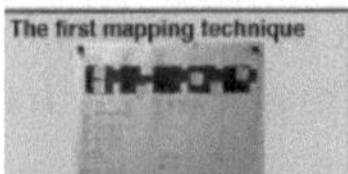	This map can assist in the understanding of the flow of critical situations in the scenario.	To line-up maps along with timeline is difficult because the temporal intervals of capturing screenshots are different.
The second mapping technique 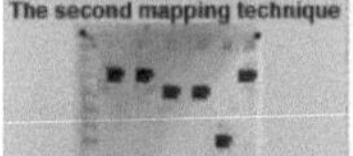	This map can describe in detail each task.	To make this type of map takes long time.
The third mapping technique 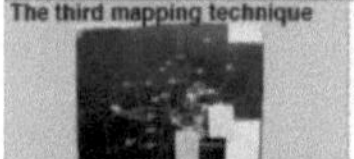	Trajectories of the cursor can help understand idea the controller' s actions.	To detect the timings when the controller use pull-down menu contents is difficult.
The fourth mapping technique 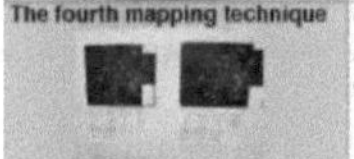	This map can assist in the understanding of each aircraft movements along with timeline.	Task symbolisation is not effective support in understanding of the results of task analysis.
The fifth mapping technique 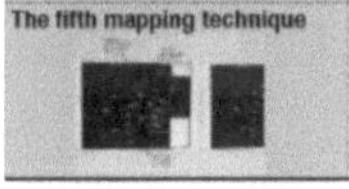	This map can assist in the understanding of each aircraft movements along with timeline.	The visibility of annotation sentence written by black letters has problems because some of them appear on the black background of the rader screen.

critical situations in the scenario. However, it is difficult to line-up maps along with timeline. Because the temporal length of the screen shot is different in each situation.

The second mapping technique plots the screen shot based on each task onto the timeline. An analyst adds some annotations on these screen shots from an analytical perspective. This mapping can describe in detail each task. On the other hand, it takes longer time to make this type of map. The third mapping technique focuses on the cursor trajectory and pull-down menu contents. In this technique, the screen shot has trajectories of aircraft and the cursor movement by the controller on the radar screen for every one minute in the observation scenario. Each screen shot is lined up on the timeline on the map. Trajectories of the cursor can help understand idea the controller's actions.

The fourth mapping technique uses symbols of task process to explain the situation instead of annotating. Maps are also divided into every 1 minute screen shot on the timeline as well as the third mapping. We attempt that task symbolisation can assist in the easy understanding of the results of task analysis. The fifth technique is the direct writing annotation. In this technique, an analyst annotates to the screen shots of the radar display which are lined up every 1 minute on the map.

3.1 Preliminary Case Study of Task Visualisation

From the preliminary 5 types of case studies, we found that the screen shots of maps should be displayed for each 1 minute. However, the black background of the radar display shows hard-to-read annotation sentences which in black letters on the map. Therefore, we developed our task visualisation method in which screen shots of radar display are divided into each 1 minute on the timeline of the map (Figure 3). It helps understand the task-flow of the controllers' work. And annotation spaces are also appropriate for writing sufficient information to understand situations. The contents of aircraft are shown by using a memo pad. And an analyst can write annotations such as interview and trajectory of the cursor position on the map which has a white background.

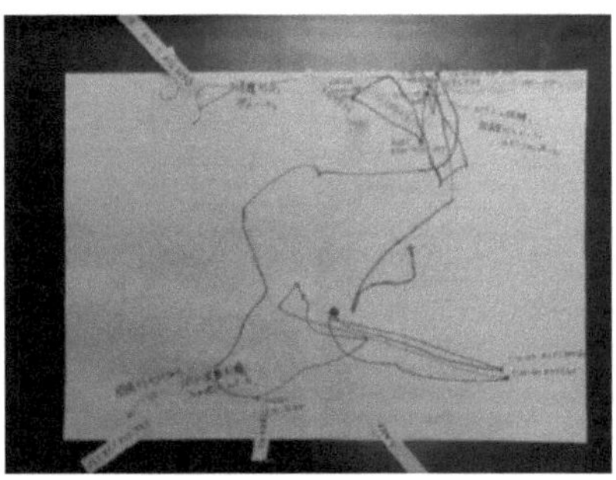

Fig. 3. Prototype of Task Visualisation technique

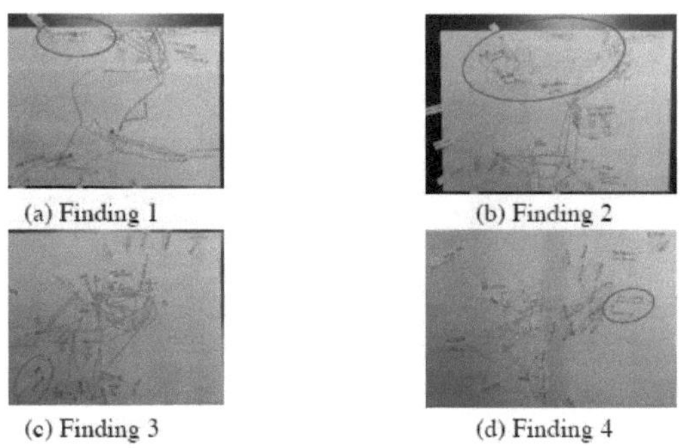

(a) Finding 1 (b) Finding 2

(c) Finding 3 (d) Finding 4

Fig. 4. Simulator observation

4 Case Study of Observation and Analysis

Simulator Observation. As a case study, we observed the working process of a radar controller. We carried out observations during 30 minutes in a time period of main traffic that imposed a certain level of workload on the ATCs. We observed that there are some specific features in the work of the ATCs; in particular, the basis of that work is prediction and instruction, to secure and maintain a safe traffic situation.

Analysis. From the analysis based on our method so far, we acquired the following findings.

1. The Air Traffic Controller starts to think of a strategy of arrival approach order regarding the target aircraft before entering to his/ her handling area. (Figure 4a)
2. The Air Traffic Controller is also aware of aircraft existing in the area to where the controller doesn't move the cursor of the mouse. (Figure 4b)
3. The Air Traffic Controller considers the relative aircraft for crossing as a group. (Figure 4c)
4. The Air Traffic Controller reassigns the route to the aircraft which is getting vectoring instructions after maintaining separation. (Figure 4d)

5 Proposing a Prototype Design of the Radar Screen

From the analysis, we proposed a prototype concept design of the user interface which focuses the spotlight on aircraft related with crossing in the future on a route. Under the conventional systems, Air Traffic Controllers need to search for crossing routes for the relative aircraft by themselves. Therefore, we expect this system will be able to assist in reducing the searching task to find crossing routes for relative aircraft by using our new concept.

References

1. ISO 9241-210:2010. Ergonomics of human system interaction - Part 210: Human-centred design for interactive systems (formerly known as 13407), International Organization for Standardization (ISO), Switzerland (2010)
2. Air Traffic Services Department Civil Aviation Bureau Ministry of Land, Air Traffic Services System in Japan (2006)
3. Handbook of fiscal 2010 Electronic Navigation Research Institute (2010)

Seamless Mobility: Individual Mobility Profiles for a Better Usability of Shared Vehicles

Moritz Küemmerling[1] and Christian Heilmann[2]

[1] German Research Center for Artificial Intelligence (DFKI)
Trippstadter Str. 122, 67663 Kaiserslautern, Germany
Moritz.Kuemmerling@dfki.de
[2] University of Kaiserslautern
Institute of Production Automation (PAK)
Gottlieb-Daimler-Str. 42, 67663 Kaiserslautern, Germany
cheilman@rhrk.uni-kl.de

Abstract. The shared use of vehicles, upon which many popular new mobility concepts like Car Sharing rely, pushes traditional interaction concepts to a limit. The amount of driver assistant and comfort features in modern vehicles is of high value for the driving experience. However, most of these features require substantial manual adjustments of settings according to the individual preferences of the driver. In temporarily used vehicles the feature adjustment will most likely become an annoying, time consuming recurring process that increases the risk of driver distraction. Hence, it is time to rethink the design of efficient human-vehicle-interfaces. Standardized, platform independent mobility profiles, accessible via the driver's personal mobile device, could be used to automatically adjust the vehicle features thus increasing the safety, comfort and usability of shared vehicles.

Keywords: Mobility, Profiles, User Modeling, Personalization, Human-Machine-Interaction, Intermodality.

1 Introduction and Motivation

"Kuruma banare", a Japanese expression often translated with "demotorization" [1], captures a lifestyle choice of especially younger generations who feel owning a car in congested and expansive urban areas such as Tokyo is more trouble than it is worth, and choose other mobility solutions instead [2]. New mobility concepts like Car Sharing are gaining popularity and represent a fast growing market. Such concepts offer individual mobility as a service without the costs and responsibilities of ownership [3]. Meanwhile, modern vehicles provide the driver with numerous driver assistant, personalization, infotainment and connectivity features. Although these features are of high value for the driving experience, they require substantial manual adjustments of settings.

From a usability point of view, scenarios, in which a car providing numerous adjustable features is shared by many people with different likings and preferences, present a

C. Stephanidis (Ed.): Posters, Part II, HCII 2013, CCIS 374, pp. 318–322, 2013.

new type of usability challenge for the design of efficient human-vehicle-interaction. Hence, we developed a new concept to ease the human-machine-interaction in case of shared vehicles. The concept is based on the platform independent modeling of user preferences to allow the automatic adjustment of vehicle settings thus saving time and avoiding driver distraction. A driver can use his mobile device with NFC technology to establish a connection between the vehicle and a cloud server where his personal mobility profile is stored. To proof the feasibility of the concept und to evaluate the approach, we designed a use case and are currently about to implement it on a hardware-platform composed of real car parts.

The paper is structured as follows: First we summarize some of the major findings of a user survey among frequent drivers. In section 3, we then give an overview and a brief description of the concept of profile-based human-vehicle-interaction. The paper ends with a short summary and a conclusion in section 4.

2 User Survey among Frequent Drivers

We conducted a survey among frequent drivers first to analyze the needs of people who are used to frequently switch vehicles and second to gather their opinions on our concept of individual mobility profiles.

In total we questioned 54 people (44 men and 10 women, 39 years average age) on three days during an automotive supplier business to business fair in Wolfsburg, Germany in October 2012. The average amount of vehicle-kilometers per year in our test group was 29.500 kilometers, which his more than twice the average amount of vehicle-kilometers per driver in Germany (13.000 kilometers per year [4]). Every interview partner owned at least one personal vehicle and frequently used rental cars and/or company cars for business purposes.

Among the top findings, the survey revealed the following:

- Every interview partner was familiar with the concept of car sharing, but only 10.4 % stated that they have already used car sharing in the past.
- 61.1 % of the test persons were willing to give car sharing a try in future.
- 51 interview partners answered that they would welcome and use a solution to faster adjust the features of shared vehicles.
- 11 interview partners additionally commented that such a solution would be of value not only for rental cars or car sharing services but also for families and companies where one or more vehicles are shared by several drivers.
- Three persons rejected the concept of mobility profiles and stated privacy matters like the possible misuse of personal data in the mobility profiles as their reasons for rejection.
- Over 50 % of the questioned frequent drivers identified personal information such as previous navigation destinations and personal setting of connectivity features to be a potential risk when such data is left behind by the driver in a temporarily used vehicle.

- 79.6 % of the interview partners were of the opinion that although infotainment systems in modern cars provide a good usability, their handling differs too much from brand to brand.
- The entry of the navigation destination and corresponding route options were considered to be the settings taking the longest time to adjust.
- When questions about the vehicle parts for which an automatic user-adaptive solution would be the most desirable, 72.2 % named seat and mirror adjustments.

3 Concept of Individual Mobility Profiles

Existing solutions for automatic feature adjustment in vehicles, such as programmable car keys or brand specific web platforms for the online configuration of a car, are not suited for new mobility concepts like Car Sharing. Whenever the physical platform is of less interest for the travelling person than the mobility service it actually provides, any limitation to a certain platform or brand would reduce the flexibility of the travelling person.

With regard to that different context of use, we developed an architecture allowing the platform-independent modeling of preferred vehicle settings as an individual mobility profile. The profile is stored and maintained in a cloud-storage. An online profile editor that can be accessed by any computer, smartphone or tablet, is used to create and edit the profile. The underlying dynamic user model distinguishes between general long term user-preferences and settings that are only of temporary use, like preselected navigation destinations for an upcoming journey. General preferences are, for example, favorite radio stations, audio and climate settings. Since there are some settings that cannot be modeled in a car-independent manner, like seat and mirror adjustments, the user model is extended by a database containing a growing list of platform-specific settings for every vehicle that the user has ever used. Each time the user drives a car for the first time, all settings that were manually adjusted by him (e.g., side mirrors) are updated in his user model together with a reference to the respective car model. The next time the user drives a car of the same model, the corresponding platform-specific settings apply automatically.

Furthermore, the user model contains a digital logbook that is updated when leaving the vehicle with information that would normally remain in the vehicle's storage, like the total and average fuel consumption, the kilometers driven, the driving time or the average and maximum speed. An automated digital logbook is useful in various ways. It eases for example the recording of private and professional use of company cars, which was mentioned by several interview partners in our user survey.

To proof the feasibility of our concept and to evaluate the profile-based human-vehicle-interaction, we set up a hardware-platform composed of real car parts (e.g., dashboard, infotainment system and electrically adjustable comfort seats). Additionally, we equipped the platform with a NFC-Smartcard and a Wi-Fi-Module. We then developed a native application for NFC-ready mobile devices with Android as operating system. Starting the app the user is asked to identify himself by entering his username and his password[1]. By simply tapping the mobile device to the NFC-Smartcard of the vehicle prototype, a Wi-Fi-Connection between the mobile device and the vehicle prototype is established. The application on the mobile device then retrieves the vehicle model reference that is sent in combination with the user-ID to the profile server where the mobility profile is generated as an XML-file out of the corresponding user model. The profile server sends the mobility profile file back to the mobile device from where it is transmitted to the vehicle prototype. A special application that extends the vehicle's architecture processes the received mobility profile and transforms the information into hardware-specific control commands. Invalid data of the mobility profile or settings corresponding to non-existing features are simply ignored. The normal functionality of our vehicle prototype is not affected by the additional application. The use of a mobility profile is not mandatory and each feature can still be adjusted manually.

Whishes the driver to leave the car, he must log out of the application on his mobile device and decide if he wants the application to update his mobility profile and log book and/or if the application should restore the factory settings for the car, thus erasing all personal data from the car memory.

4 Summary and Conclusion

In this paper we presented the concept for a new way of human-vehicle-interaction that is designed to meet the requirements arising from new mobility concepts like Car Sharing. Core element of the concept is the platform independent modeling of a driver's preferred set of vehicle settings. Being transmitted to a specific vehicle, the profile enables the automatic adjustment of settings in the vehicle, thus saving time and avoiding driver distraction. The overarching goal is to achieve more flexibility in the use and transfer between mobility platforms since flexibility is the key factor in successful intermodal passenger transport. The more intermodal mobility establishes in our society, the more it underlines the importance of a concept that eases and fastens the interaction with shared vehicles.

However, the benefits and consequently the success of the concept depend on a wide-scale adoption of the mobility profile protocol among multiple stakeholders (vehicle OEMs, authorities and service providers). A promising approach could be the collaboration with aspiring mobility platforms such as Daimler's project moovel[2] or MyCityWay[3] to which the presented concept could be a valuable complement. These platforms are specialized on gathering all sorts of traffic information and providing various ways of getting from A to B by selecting always the best and most efficient connection and transport (e.g., trains, shared cars, busses).

---

1 The username and password need to be entered only on the first time when the application is configured. Afterwards, the app can be unlocked by entering a shorter pin code.

2 `http://www.moovel.com`

3 `http://www.mycityway.com`

Acknowledgments. The research presented in this paper was supported by the Center for Commercial Vehicle Technology at the University of Kaiserslautern.

References

1. Winterhoff, M., Kahner, C., Ulrich, C., Sayler, P., Wenzel, E.: Future of Mobility 2020: The Automotive Industry in Upheaval? Arthur D. Little (2009), http://www.adlittle.com/downloads/tx_adlreports/ADL_Future_of_Mobility_2020.pdf
2. Kalmbach, R., Bernhart, W., Grosse Kleimann, P., Hoffmann, M.: Automotive landscape 2025: Opportunities and challenges ahead. Roland Berger Strategy Consultants (2011), http://www.rolandberger.com/media/pdf/Roland_Berger_Automotive_Landscape_2025_20110228.pdf
3. Shaheen, S., Sperling, D., Wagner, C.: Carsharing in Europe and North America: Past, Present, and Future. Transportation Quarterly 52(3), 35–52 (1998)
4. Radke, S.: Verkehr in Zahlen 2011/2012. Deutsches Institut für Wirtschaftsforschung. DVV Media Group, Hamburg (2012)

Influence of Repeated Experience on Unsignalized Intersection Crossing Behavior of Drivers without Right-of-Way

Toru Kumagai and Akihiko Takahashi

National Institute of Advanced Industrial Science and Technology (AIST), Tsukuba, Japan
{kumagai.toru,a.takahashi}@aist.go.jp

Abstract. The change of *start position*, where drivers step on the gas pedal just before entering unsignalized intersection within a residential area, through repeated experience was examined. The relationship with Driving Style Questionnaire (DSQ) was discussed. The results showed that subjects who decrease the distance from the edge of a cross lane to start position through experience had tendency to step on the gas pedal only just before entering intersections. The opposition was also true. These subjects had high scores in the following scales of DSQ: Methodical driving, and Preparatory maneuvers at traffic signals. The change of start position through experience also correlated with start position. For instance, start positions of these subjects were relatively small, and they were negative for some intersections.

Keywords: Driving behavior, habituation, adaptation, unsignalized intersection, Driving Style Questionnaire (DSQ).

1 Introduction

Intersection related crashes account for more than 50 percent of the total traffic accidents in Japan [1], and the most common causes are human error. Understanding the nature of driving behavior at intersections is essential for developing and implementing prevention measures.

In this study, the influence of repeated experience on crossing behavior of drivers without right-of-way at unsignalized intersections was examined. Concretely speaking, the change of *start position*, where drivers step on the gas pedal just before entering intersections, was examined, and the relationship with Driving Style Questionnaire (DSQ) [2] was discussed.

Repeated experience often leads to habituation, and driving behavior is not exception [3]. For instance, many drivers get driving faster a narrow street with experience [4]. Meanwhile there is a real possibility that drivers acquire proficiency through experience. The aim of this work is to describe the change of driving behavior through repeated experience and contribute to traffic safety.

C. Stephanidis (Ed.): Posters, Part II, HCII 2013, CCIS 374, pp. 323–326, 2013.

2 Methods

2.1 Data Preparation

A vehicle equipped with sensing devices [5] was used to measure driving behavior. Sensing devices included those for driver's operational behavior, such as steering wheel operation, and those for the vehicle condition, such as vehicle speed. This study used vehicle speed and pedal strokes of the acceleration and brake pedals. Pedal sensors attached to the pedals detected the pedal strokes. The speed signal was obtained from the front wheel speed sensor.

After outlining the experiment and obtaining the subjects' consent, crossing behavior of subjects without right-of-way was recorded at unsignalized intersections in a residential area of Tsukuba, Japan (Table 1). Eight subjects drove the vehicle on each intersections sixth a day six straight weekdays. All subjects were asked fill out the Driving Style Questionnaire (DSQ) after the experiment.

The data that were not influenced by other traffic were used in the following analysis. The ethics committee of National Institute of Advanced Industrial Science and Technology (AIST) approved this experiment.

Table 1. Properties of intersections. All intersections are cross roads. Fair visibility means that drivers have some visibility by the setback of the building on the left or right corner.

Intersection	Visibility Left	Visibility Right	Road width [m] Own	Road width [m] Cross	Distance from the nearest edge of the cross lane to stop line [m]
I1	Bad	Fair	5.	6.4	3.8
I2	Fair	Bad	5.	6.4	2.7
I3	Bad	Bad	5.	6.4	3.0
I4	Bad	Bad	5.	6.4	4.6
I5	Fair	Bad	5.	6.4	4.7
I6	Fair	Fair	6.4	6.4	10.8

2.2 Analysis

Intersection crossing behavior consists of *deceleration*, *safety confirmation*, and *acceleration* [6]. Drivers sometimes do not enter the intersection by the first acceleration, but deceleration again for safety confirmation after the first acceleration. In this study, *start positions*, where drivers step on the gas pedal just before entering intersections, were examined. Start position was defined as the distance from the nearest edge of the cross lane.

In addition to that, *pedal operation pattern*s were examined. Four patterns were defined here: PS, PL, PD and PR. PS means that drivers release brake-pedal, move their foot on the gas pedal, and step on the gas pedal only once before entering intersections in the most case. PD means that drivers step on brake-pedal once at least after moving their foot on the gas pedal. PL means that drivers change their pattern from PD to PS through experience. PR means that drivers change arbitrary their pattern between PS and PD.

3 Results

Table two shows averaged start position of the last three trials for each intersection. Inside of parentheses are correlation coefficients of each start positions and number of experience through experiment. Only coefficients greater than 0.6 are shown. A positive value means that start position was increasingly distanced from a cross lane through experience. The opposite is also true.

Table three shows pedal operation patterns for each intersection.

Table four shows categorization results of repeated intersection crossing behavior with start position and pedal operation pattern.

Table 2. Averaged start positions [m] (the distance from the nearest edge of the cross lane) of the last three trials. Inside of parentheses are correlation coefficients through experiment of each start positions and number of experience.

Subject	Intersection					
	I1	I2	I3	I4	I5	I6
S1	n/a	1.3(0.9)	2.7 (0.8)	2.3	2.7	3.8
S2	0.8	0.0	1.6	0.9	0.4	2.8
S3	-0.2	0.0	1.0	0.3	-0.6	1.1
S4	0.1	-1.0(-0.8)	0.7	-0.7(-0.7)	-0.6	2.8
S5	2.1	1.0	3.0(0.7)	1.3	1.7(0.8)	4.5
S6	2.1(0.6)	0.7(-0.6)	3.0	0.9	1.0(-0.7)	2.8
S7	0.8(-0.6)	1.0	1.0	0.9	1.0	4.8
S8	1.5	2.0	2	0.9	1.0	1.8

Table 3. Pedal operation pattern through experience

Subject	Intersection					
	I1	I2	I3	I4	I5	I6
S1	n/a	PL	PS	PL	PS	PL
S2	PR	PR	PR	PR	PR	PR
S3	PS	PS	PS	PS	PS	PS
S4	PS	PS	PS	PS	PS	PS
S5	PR	PR	PR	PR	PR	PD
S6	PS	PS	PS	PS	PS	PL
S7	PS	PL	PL	PL	PL	PL
S8	PS	PS	PS	PS	PS	PS

Table 4. Categorization of crossing behavior with start position and pedal operation pattern

Distance from the cross lane to start position	Pedal operation pattern PD or PR	PL	PS
Increase with Experience (IE)	S5	S1	
Not change	S2	S7	S3 S8
Decrease with Experience (DE)			S4 S6

4 Discussions

Subjects were categorized into three groups according to the change of start position through experience: Increase with Experience (IE), Not Change (NC), and Decrease with Experience (DE). Subjects were also categorized into three groups according to pedal operation pattern: PS, PL, and the rest (PR or PD).

The above two categorization had correlation (Table 4). All subjects in IE did not appear in PS, and all subjects in DE belonged in PS. Those two groups would be based on some style of driving behavior.

Score of DSQ scales given by each subjects were examined between IE and DE using linear regression. The result showed that drivers belonged in DE gave high score in the following scales: Methodical driving, Moodiness in driving, and Preparatory maneuvers at traffic signals.

The change of start position through experience also correlated with start position in reason. For instance, start positions of S4, who belonged in DE, was relatively small, and they were negative for some intersections.

The intersection I6 gave relatively greater start position for all subjects because the own road width was wide, and the distance from the cross lane to the stop line was relatively longer [7].

References

1. Analysis of Human Factors in Crossing Collisions. ITARDA Information No. 56. Institute for Traffic Accident Research and Data Analysis (ITARDA), Tokyo (2005)
2. Ishibashi, M., Okuwa, M., Doi, S., Akamatsu, M.: Indices for characterizing driving style and their relevance to car following behavior. In: Proceedings of SICE Annual Conference 2007, pp. 1132–1137 (2007)
3. Summala, H.: Accident risk and driver behavior. Safety Science 22, 103–117 (1996)
4. Kumagai, T., Takahashi, A.: How does repetitive experience influence driving behavior around on-street parking? In: Mobile Symposium 2013, pp. 89–92. Society of Mobile Interactions, Kobe (2013)
5. Akamatsu, M.: Measuring Driving Behavior, Detecting Unusual Behavior for Driving Assistance. In: SICE Annual Conference 2002 (2002)
6. Kumagai, T., Akamatsu, M.: Prediction of human driving behavior using dynamic Bayesian networks. IEICE Trans. Inf. & Syst. E89D-2, 857–860 (2006)
7. Takahashi, A., et al.: Naturalistic Driving Analysis of Crossing Non-signalized Intersections without Right-of way. In: The JSAE Annual Congress (2013) (in Japanese)

Diagnostic System Simulator of Honker Vehicle

Pawel Mikolajczak, Arkadiusz Rychlik, Piotr Szczyglak,
and Jaroslaw Szuszkiewicz

University of Warmia and Mazury in Olsztyn, Faculty of Technical Sciences, Poland
{pawel.mikolajczak,rychter,szczypio,jerry}@uwm.edu.pl

Abstract. The paper is dedicated to the issues concerning the on-board diagnostic system of the Honker military vehicle and simulator of the system. Purpose, architecture and used diagnostic monitors have been presented. One stressed that it is important that an operator should acquire the knowledge prior to working upon the real technical object. In the final part of the paper the diagnostic system simulator was described. It lets train drivers in the stress – free conditions which is a tool to gain experience characteristic for typical and exceptional operation situations.

Keywords: Simulator, diagnostic system, vehicle.

1 Introduction

Described in the paper the on-board diagnostic system and its simulator are dedicated to the military version of the Honker SUV [3]. It might serve as an ambulance, mean of transportation for up to 10 passengers, transport of technical equipment depending on a model or accessories. Despite variety of applications of these cars they have a common feature in the military conditions – information on the technical state at whatever time should be so precise to enable quick and adequate evaluation of the status of the vehicle. It has many a time important influence on the safety of soldiers serving in given conditions.

Owing to the diagnostic analyses identification of the research object was done taking under consideration five levels of decomposition. The detailed description of the decomposed structure of the researched object was included in the work [4]. Level five is a set of the basic elements; on this level identification of damages of certain parts or units, which will not undergo further decomposition, like an alternator, battery, clutch, transmission, etc., is carried out. A set of the basic elements was created under the rule that diagnosing of all the elements of the vehicle is possible but groundless. Two - state classification was applied in the developed diagnostic system (operating state, non-operating state).

The works [1] and [2] presents the methodologies of building the diagnostic parameters vectors, description of information models and their characteristic features for the subject under research.

C. Stephanidis (Ed.): Posters, Part II, HCII 2013, CCIS 374, pp. 327–331, 2013.

2 Diagnostic Monitors

In the presented system there might be distinguished 10 independent diagnostic monitors. Each of the monitors handles only one system influencing the functional and object state of the vehicle. When starting up the system the self-diagnostics is carried out – tests of measuring and executing elements are carried out.

The vehicle systems are considered to be damaged if describing them feature or set of features exceeds allowed value. Functionally, it means limitation or prevention of execution of a task. The monitors of the on-board diagnostic systems were divided into noncontinuous (conditional) and continuous (unconditional) – table 1.

Table 1. List of monitors used in on-board diagnostic system of Honker vehicle

Number	Distinguishing feature of diagnostic monitor	Kind/Description - use
1	System temperature monitor	continuous – temperature identification, identification of its limit and permissible values
2	Operating fluid level monitor	continuous – identification of volume levels of consumables
3	Monitor of engine cooling	noncontinuous – identification of thermal state of engine
4	Monitor of battery and wiring state	noncontinuous – identification of battery technical state and charging parameters
5	Monitor of fuel consumption and fuel level	continuous – identification of fuel consumption and vehicle range
6	Monitor of engine power	noncontinuous – identification of momentary and computational engine power
7	Monitor of drive system	noncontinuous – identification of wear (clearance) of drive system (clutch, transmission, reduction gear, driveshaft, main transmission)
8	Monitor of skid	continuous – identification of relative skid
9	Monitor of tire pressure	noncontinuous – identification of pressure drop in pneumatic tires
10	Monitor of transmission ratio	continuous – optimization of ratio in drivetrain system

3 Architecture of Diagnostic System

The RS-485 transmission system of linear construction based on half-duplex mode was used to build the communication and data transmission system. In the fig. 1 there was presented the functional structure of the developed diagnostic system along with the topology of diagnostic data transmission.

The structure of the developed modules was based on Atmega 2560 8-bit processors. The particular modules (transmitting and receiving devices) realize data exchange on the basis of the measurements results by the internal communication protocol. Graphical interpretation of the data protocol for module number 1 was presented in the fig. 2. The detailed description of the system structure can be found in the work [5].

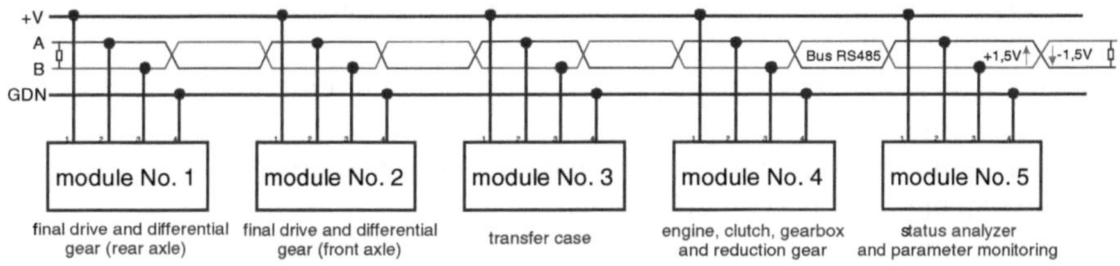

Fig. 1. Functional structure of diagnostic system and data transmission system: +V – 12 V power supply, GDN – ground, A,B – RS485 bus signal line [5]

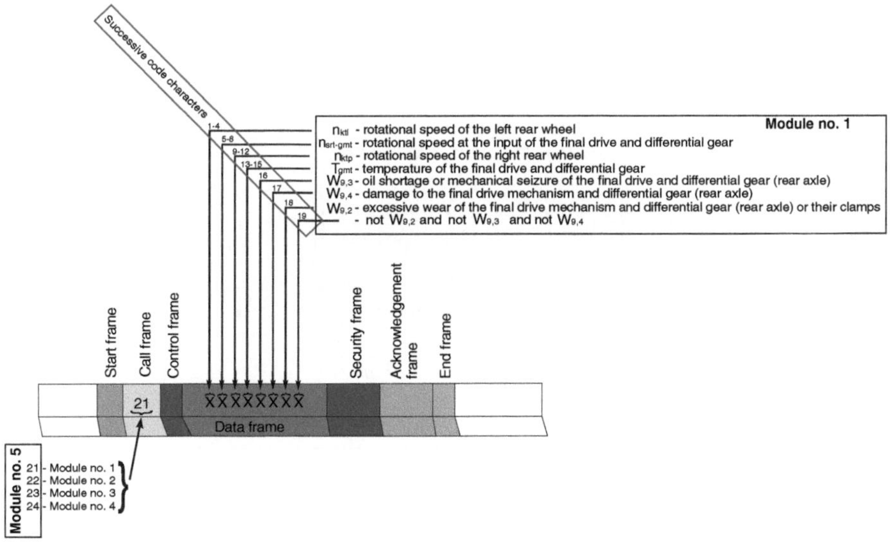

Fig. 2. Fundamental structure of data protocol generated by number 1 module [5]

4 Simulator

The purpose of building the simulator was to train drivers of a honker vehicle within operating the real on-board diagnostic system, to interpret messages showing changes of the vehicle state and to take decisions. It is worth admitting that the main reason of making mistakes is human behavior in situations unknown, when one has to perform complex thought processes, e.g. to diagnose an arising problem on the basis of available circumstances, carry out the comparative analyses, develop a procedure of actions suitable for a situation, perform these actions, evaluate their effects, etc. The more complex problem, the more time is needed for an operator to react and the bigger probability of making a mistake.

The simulation program includes the following modules:

- main page (starting),
- main control panel,
- engine – gears – reduction gear,
- sensors – signals,
- temperatures,
- states,
- configuration.

The main control panel (fig. 3) is an imitation of the real diagnostic panel. An operator can sequentially observe ten screens:

- GPS indications,
- Rear axle,
- Front axle,
- Transfer case,
- Transmission,
- Driveshafts,
- Monitored parameters 1,
- Monitored parameters 2,
- Event log.

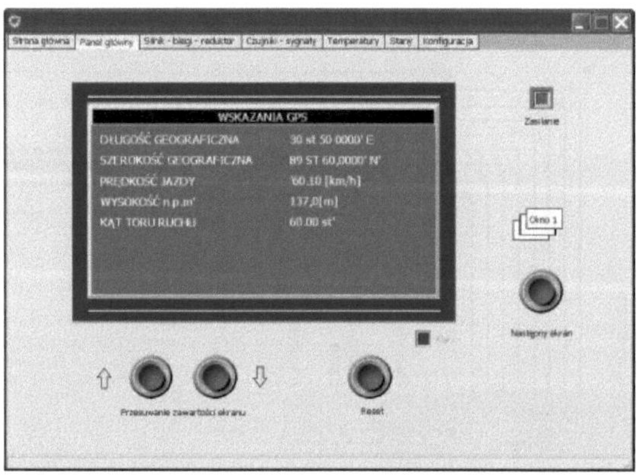

Fig. 3. Main control panel of diagnostic system

The engine – gears – reduction gear module is assigned to choose a ratio of the transmission and reduction gear. Additionally, a being trained operator can watch values of the rotational speed of the controlled shafts. In the "Sensors – signals" tap a trainee can choose binary values for the following signals: contacts of the vibration sensors in the main transmission, differential mechanism (front and rear axle), transfer case, transmission and reducing transmission, consumables levels and pressure in the oil system. The "Temperature" module is provided for simulation of temperature values of the cylinder block, engine and transmission oils, coolant, etc. If the limit values are exceeded then automatically window number 9 in the main panel will turn on informing on non-operational state. In the "States" module it is possible to choose non-operational states with division to vehicle systems included in the diagnostic model. The last module is "Configuration", which enables observation and change of start-up values.

5 Conclusions

- Within the confines of the research the prototype of the on-board diagnostic system was developed, which was installed on the Honker vehicle.
- The system was based on transmitting and receiving modules hooked up in the communication network in compliance with the RS-485 standard.
- The system is fully independent on the internal circuits of the vehicle and as a result of system defect or lack of its activation this does not influence the tasks realized by the vehicles.
- The performed verification investigations confirmed usefulness and functionality of the developed system both in utilitarian aspect and durability one.
- The diagnostic system simulator of a Honker vehicle enables carrying on trainings for drivers of that vehicle in stress-free conditions and it is a tool to gain experience in very often operation situations as well as in very exceptional ones.
- The simulator accurately reflects actions of the real system with few exceptions, which are supposed to improve the training process (e.g. occurring suggestions).

References

1. Kościelny, J.M.: Diagnostyka zautomatyzowanych procesów przemysłowych. Akademicka Oficyna Wydawnicza EXIT, Warszawa (2001)
2. Młokosiewicz, J.R.: Metoda wielopoziomowego badania stanu obiektów technicznych i synteza systemu diagnostycznego. Nr 1734/87, Wojskowa Akademia Techniczna, Warszawa (1987)
3. Niziński, S., et al.: Systemy diagnostyczne wojskowych pojazdów mechanicznych. ITE Radom (2011)
4. Niziński, S., Rychlik, A.: Hierarchiczny model diagnostyczny wojskowego pojazdu mechanicznego. Biuletyn WAT LX(1), 196–209 (2011)
5. Rychlik, A., Szczyglak, P.: Method of diagnosing the power transmission system in a Tarpan Honker military vehicle. Journal of Polish CIMAC 7(2), 175–182 (2012)
6. Michalski, R., Wierzbicki, S.: An analysis of degradation of vehicles in operation. Eksploatacja i Niezawodnosc – Maintenance and Reliability 1(37), 30–32 (2008)
7. Jasiulewicz-Kaczmarek, M., Drożyner, P.: Maintenance Management Initiatives towards Achieving Sustainable Development. In: Golinska, P., et al. (eds.) Information Technologies in Environmental Engineering. Environmental Science and Engineering, pp. 707–721. Springer, Heidelberg (2011)

Developing a User Interface Design of ATM Systems

Toshiya Sasaki[1,*], Hajime Hirako[1], Kazuhiko Yamazaki[1],
Hisae Aoyama[2], Satoru Inoue[2], and Yutaka Fukuda[2]

[1] Chiba Institute of Technology(CIT), Chiba, Japan
{toshiya.ssk1,hrkhjm0508,designkaz}@gmail.com
[2] Electronic Navigation Research Institute (ENRI), Tokyo, Japan
{aoyama,inoue,fukuda}@enri.go.jp

Abstract. Air Traffic Controllers are expected to continue maintaining the safety of the air space and maintaining air traffic flow to run smoothly in complex systems in the future. We discuss the method of design to develop a system of human consciousness, especially for Air Traffic Controllers. In this research, we proposed a prototype of the user interface which focuses the spotlight on aircraft related with crossing in the future on a route and Air Traffic Controllers specify when receive the information of the aircraft. Under the conventional systems, Air Traffic Controllers need to search for crossing routes for the relative aircraft by themselves. Therefore, we expect this system will be able to assist in reducing the searching task to find crossing routes for relative aircraft by using our new concept.

Keywords: Air Traffic Control, User Interface Design.

1 Introduction

Air Traffic volume is predicted to be increasing in the future. Air Traffic Controllers will also have to handle more complex and heavier air traffic situations in the future. The tasks involved in ATC put heavy demands on the information processing capacities of air traffic controllers. To keep smooth and higher safe air traffic flow, future ATC systems need to be equipped with supporting functions or higher usability interfaces for assisting controllers work. In order to design a future system that can assure higher safety, enhance usability, and support human reliability, the idea of Human-Centred Design processes can help designers in understanding the features in the operations and intentions of the controller.

The purpose of this study is to propose efficient and easy-to-use for air traffic controller, the new interface for the future ATC system. By analyzing the problems of the current ATC system.

* Please note that the LNCS Editorial assumes that all authors have used the western naming convention, with given names preceding surnames. This determines the structure of the names in the running heads and the author index.

C. Stephanidis (Ed.): Posters, Part II, HCII 2013, CCIS 374, pp. 332–336, 2013.

2 Visualization of Tasks

2.1 Observation

To analyze how air traffic controllers work, we built an experiment system for collecting data through simulator experiments (Figure 1).

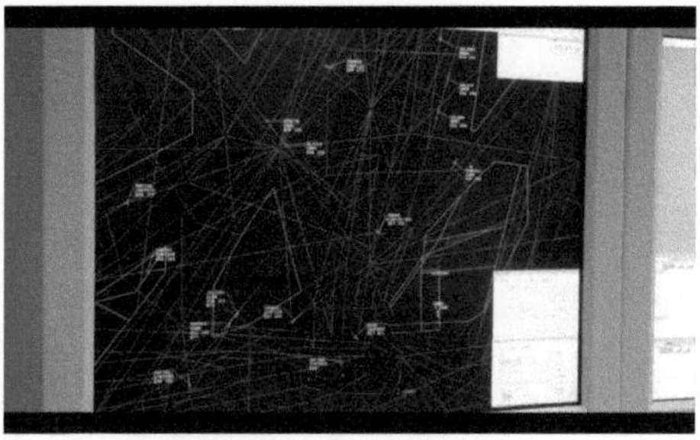

Fig. 1. Simulator of ATC system

2.2 The Method of Visualization Tasks

We developed our task visualisation method in which screen shots of radar display are divided into each 1 minute on the timeline of the map (Figure 2). It helps understand the task-flow of the controllers' work. And annotation spaces are also appropriate for writing sufficient information to understand situations. The contents of aircraft are shown by using a memo pad. And an analyst can write annotations such as interview and trajectory of the cursor position on the map which has a white background.

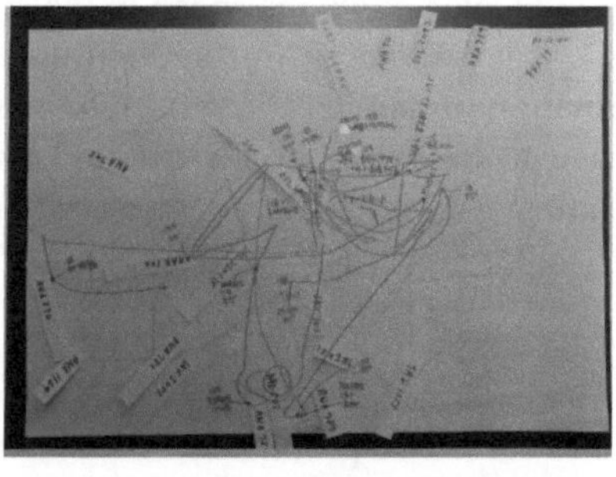

Fig. 2. The map of visualization tasks

3 Analysis of the Problems

3.1 Extracting Problems

About 30 problems were raised from a map to visualize tasks. The problem is summarized in items of time, scene, problem, cause of a problem and screen (Table 1).

Table 1. Problems raised from a map to visualize tasks

時間	シーン	気づき		原因	画面
		問題	違い		
03:00;00	AFR278,DLH710,UAL888の3機の到着順位を予測 管制が始まって間もなく、入ってきた航空機（AFR248、DLH710、UAL888）に対して到着順位を予測していた。	操作画面と到着予測を分けて整理しなくてはならない。 画面操作している間、航空機の情報を入力している間、別の航空機の到着順位を予測するためそれぞれ整理しなくてはならない。		別の航空機を操作していても、その後に新しい航空機が入域してくる。入域してきた航空機について把握しておく事によって先の業務の効率化につながる。そのため、操作した機体と考えている機体を別々で考えなくてはならないと考える。	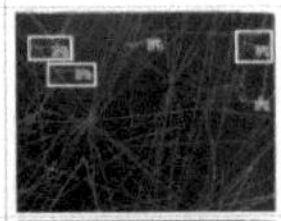
03:00;40	MAP機能「3」を使って日本列島を表示 DCP1のパネルに入ったマップ機能で日本列島について確認をしていた。	マップ表示は最初に確認してあとはほぼ使わない。 前半だけで、マップの表示をよく使い、後半はほぼ使っていない。		マップ機能は最初の確認の為にある機能ではないかと考える。後半は、指示が多くなってきたため余計な表示は見せないようにしている。	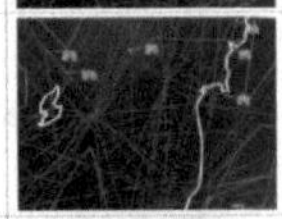
03:01;00	新しく入域してきた航空機に指示は行わないが意識をしていた。 新しく入ってきたDLH275など入ってきたがセクター内に入ってきた事により管制官は意識をするが指示はまだ行わない。	操作画面と到着予測を分けて整理しなくてはならない。 画面操作している間、航空機の情報を入力している間、別の航空機の到着順位を予測するためそれぞれ整理しなくてはならない。		別の航空機を操作していても、その後に新しい航空機が入域してくる。入域してきた航空機について把握しておく事によって先の業務の効率化につながる。そのため、操作した機体と考えている機体を別々で考えなくてはならないと考える。	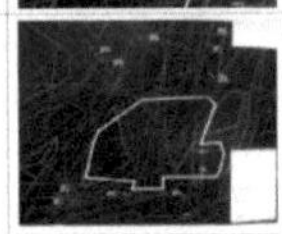

3.2 Consider of the Problem to Solve

In order to examine the priority of the problem to solve, the problems were divided. Result of categorize, the problems to be solved were down to two.

The first problem is that "the number of instructions is increased by inducing the aircraft." The reason for first problem is affecting the other aircraft to guide the aircraft and increasing instructions to return the aircraft to the original route when the separation can not be secured even down the speed of the aircraft.

The second problem is that "While air traffic controllers instruct the aircraft, they have to obtain the information of another aircraft." The reason for second problem is air traffic controllers have to be aware of the timing of instructions to the aircraft while they adjust the heading and altitude of another aircraft.

4 Ideation

In ideation, each of idea to solve two problems was developed (Figure 3). Ideas were developed in the direction of "reducing the number of instructions" and "easy to guide the aircraft" to solve the first problem that "the number of instructions is increased by inducing the aircraft."

And Ideas that air traffic controllers obtain the timing of Hand off, instructions of heading to induce the aircraft and instructions of altitude were developed to solve the second problem that "While air traffic controllers instruct the aircraft, they have to obtain the information of another aircraft."

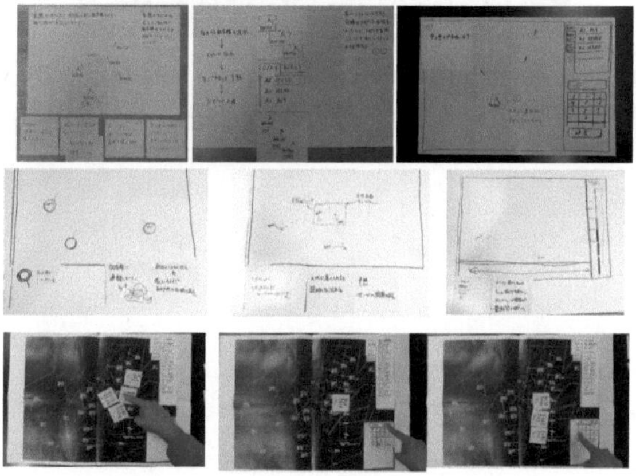

Fig. 3. Ideation and paper prototyping

5 Proposing the User Interface Design

From paper prototyping, we proposed the user interface which focuses the spotlight on aircraft related with crossing in the future on a route to solve the first problem "the number of instructions is increased by inducing the aircraft (Figure 4)." We expect this user interface will be able to assist in reducing the searching task to find crossing routes for relative aircraft.

And we proposed the user interface which air traffic controllers are able to specify when to receive the information they want to know about the aircraft in advance to solve the second problem "While air traffic controllers instruct the aircraft, they have to obtain the information of another aircraft (Figure 5)." We expect this user interface will be able to reduce the burden of air traffic controllers.

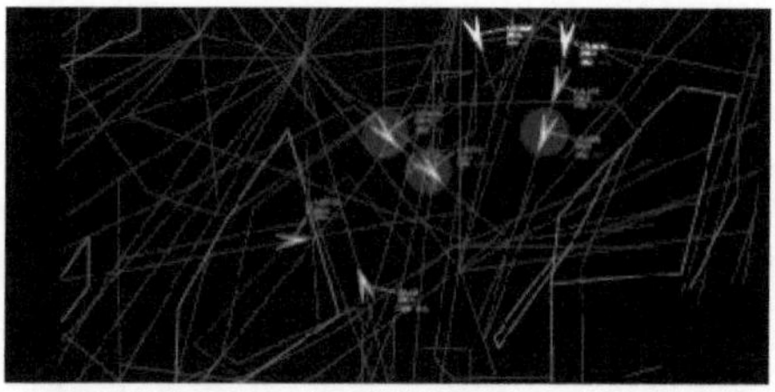

Fig. 4. The user interface which focuses the spotlight on aircraft related with crossing in the future on a route

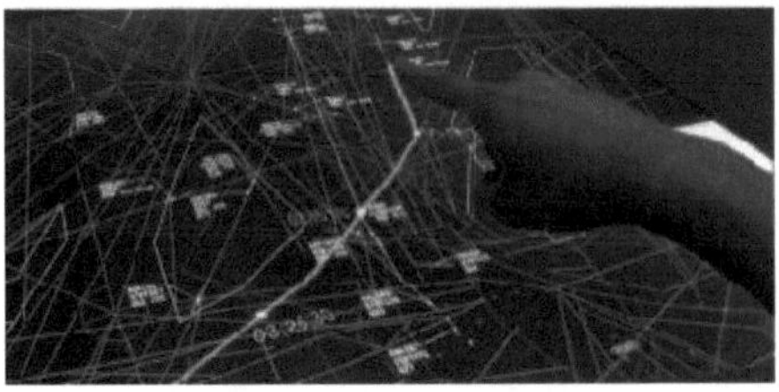

Fig. 5. The user interface which air traffic controllers are able to specify when to receive the information they want to know about the aircraft in advance

Discomfort in Automated Driving – The Disco-Scale

Felix Wilhelm Siebert, Michael Oehl, Rainer Höger, and Hans-Rüdiger Pfister

Leuphana University of Lüneburg, Institute of Experimental Industrial Psychology, Wilschenbrucher Weg 84a, 21335 Lüneburg, Germany
`{felix.siebert,oehl,hoeger,pfister}@uni.leuphana.de`

Abstract. Due to the increasing amount of automation in vehicles the role of the driver changes from having an active part in the driving of the vehicle to a reactive monitoring task. Since there is currently no method to measure subjective comfort or discomfort we developed a 14-item scale to measure the discomfort of a driver. Research suggests that it is easier for users to sense the lack of comfort and because of this we used experienced discomfort as an indicator for the absence of comfort. The questionnaire was applied in an experimental driving simulator study and proved to have a high internal consistency (r = .91). Results suggest that this questionnaire is a useful tool for assessing discomfort in automated HMI. This first version is focused on, but not limited to, automation and advanced driver assistance systems in vehicles.

Keywords: Automated Driving, Human-Machine Interaction, Discomfort, Questionnaire.

1 Why Measure Discomfort

Due to the increasing amount of computerization and automation in vehicles, driving is no longer a completely self-paced task. In highly automated vehicles, the driver's role in the human-machine interaction (HMI) changes from actively choosing the vehicle's speed and direction to a reactive monitoring task. Research in the field of vehicle automation and fully automated driving primarily focuses on the effects of the change of task on driving safety. Often, human factors issues, for example complacency [1] or situation awareness [2] and their relation to the monitoring quality are investigated. While the ability of a driver to monitor the automation is legitimately the first concern of research, it is also important to evaluate the comfort of the driver for three reasons:

The comfort of the driver determines the acceptance of the automation, and therefore how frequently it is used. Comfort should be high to achieve acceptance and usage of the automation and thus higher passenger safety [3].

Drivers in non-automated vehicles try to stay in a comfort zone [4] through the regulation of several crucial variables. In automated driving, drivers can only influence these variables by completely taking over control of the vehicle. It is therefore important to define and evaluate automation specific variables dependent on experienced comfort of the driver for different driving situations. This could prevent the

C. Stephanidis (Ed.): Posters, Part II, HCII 2013, CCIS 374, pp. 337–341, 2013.

driver from taking over control only for minor adjustments that are not critical to the safety of the vehicle.

The comfort of the driver during the automated drive is important to car-manufacturers for economic reasons. Customers are more likely to buy a car they feel comfortable in.

2 How to Measure Discomfort?

While these arguments indicate the importance of assessing the comfort of the driver during an automated drive, research is missing a specific tool to measure comfort in human-machine interaction, and especially in the car environment. Why is that? Comfort is defined [5] as "[...] a general mood, or emotion which is pleasant but not especially aroused, tense, or activated." Due to the weak nature of the mood or emotion comfort, it might be hard to observe subjectively. Hence, Seidl [5] proposes to measure discomfort - the deviation from the normal un-aroused state that is defined as comfort. But what leads to the deviation of the normal comfort state? In the context of driving, Summala [4] defines four variables that need to be above a certain threshold for the driver to feel comfortable in non-automated driving. The variables are vehicle-road-system, rule following, good progress of the trip, and safety margins. The variable vehicle-road-system is influenced by the road and vehicle condition. Thus, it is not changed by driving highly automated, since an autonomous car drives on the same streets as a non-automated car. The variable rule following shows no variance in automated driving because the automated vehicle is programmed to always follows the traffic rules. Similarly, the good progress of the trip does not rely on driving automated or non-automated, but on traffic conditions. The progress of the trip is therefore not influenced when driving automated. The main variable for Summala, and also for this research is the safety margins. They are defined as the time and space margins around the vehicle, i.e., the distance to other vehicles and objects on and around the road and the amount of time the driver has to react to these objects. These margins are an individual variable that can differ individually for different drivers [4]. In an automated drive these margins are fixed for every driver regardless of a driver's subjective safety margin.

Consequently, the goal of the present research was on the one hand to translate and empirically evaluate Summala's Safety Margin Model for automated driving, and on the other hand to develop a questionnaire that measures the discomfort in drivers of automated vehicles based on the safety margins of the automated vehicle. This could give researchers and manufacturers a tool to assess individual safety margins that an automated vehicle has to keep for the driver to feel comfortable. While up to know researchers use single items to assess comfort [6], the goal of this study was to focus the assessment of comfort on the comfort of the driver towards the safety margins kept by the autonomous car. Since developers are not only interested in situational comfort arising from the safety margins, items measuring the comfort of using the automated system in general are also integrated into the questionnaire.

3 Development and Experimental Validation

The items of the questionnaire were derived from Summala's theory of safety margins. Questions targeting the car's performance in the situation (situational component) and the general automation performance (system component) were also integrated. Questions were answered on a five-point Likert-scale with the poles strongly disagree vs. strongly agree. An example for an item measuring situational safety margins is "With more clearance distance my journey would be more comfortable". An example for an item measuring the system component is "I feel endangered by the system".

To evaluate the discomfort-questionnaire, we conducted a laboratory experiment. N = 32 participants (21 female) with a mean age of M = 22.97 years (SD = 2.90) were asked to drive a route in a state-of-the-art driving simulator running Stisim Drive (Version 2.08.06) by System Technology Inc. that simulated an extensively automated car.

Participants were told that the car automatically steered, regulated the speed, and kept enough distance to road obstacles. The task of the participants was to monitor the automated drive and to intervene if they felt that the automation was not safely steering or keeping the distance to obstacles. In a first training scenario, participants were asked to intervene on purpose by breaking to test if they were able to control the simulation, e.g., reach the pedals. In the second training, participants were told not to intervene so that they could get used to the automated drive. Thereafter, participants drove through six different driving situations. The situations were approximately three minutes long and the order was randomized for all participants. In all situations, the automated vehicle approached another vehicle that was driving ahead. The driving situations represent three types of roads: a country road, a country road with a construction site narrowing the driving lane, and a highway exit. The distance kept by the automation was varied twofold, either half of the speed in meters (uncritical condition), for example 50 meters (slightly over 160 feet) distance when driving 100 km/h (slightly over 60 mph), or a quarter or less of the speed in meters (critical condition). The uncritical condition corresponded to the legal regulation for German passenger cars with regards to distance between vehicles. The critical condition undercuts this regulation by about 50%.

Directly after each situation our 14-item questionnaire to assess discomfort was completed by participants. We were therefore able to derive the discomfort level during the automated drive in relation to the situation and the general discomfort for high and low distance over all situations combined.

4 Key Findings

The results show a difference in subjective discomfort measured by our questionnaire for different distances kept by the automation between vehicles on the road. This effect can be observed over all three different situations (Fig. 1).

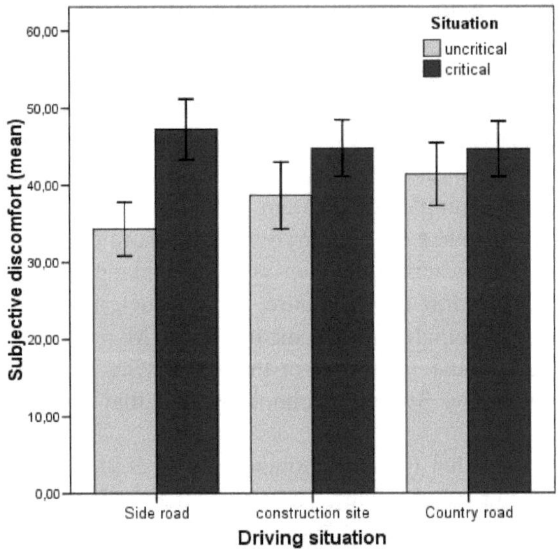

Fig. 1. Mean sum score of the subjective discomfort for all situations and conditions

Subjective discomfort is higher in situations in which the automated car maintains a small distance. This finding for automated driving is consistent with Summala's theory of safety margins [4] for non-automated driving. Independent of the distance kept by the automation, the different driving situations have a further influence on the discomfort, as can be seen in Fig. 1. The observed effect does not translate to a statistically significant difference between the situations and the subjective perceived discomfort. No main effect was found for the type of situation ($F_{(2,186)} = 0.70$; $p = .50$).

Independent of the situation, the distance kept by the automation in general seems to influence the subjective discomfort measured by the Disco-Scale. A main effect in condition "uncritical vs. critical" was found to be significant ($F_{(1,186)} = 23.23$; $p < .01$).

5 Future Work

Although the Disco-Scale already yielded a high internal consistency it is still a work in progress and is continuously improved. The questionnaire is going to build the basis of extensive studies on HMI in automated vehicles. An increase in the number of participants through further experiments is needed to validate the questionnaire, and items that may yield a lower corrected item-total-correlation will be exchanged.

Once the final set of questionnaire items has been determined and the questionnaire has been proven to have good psychometric properties, different variables of automated driving will be evaluated to determine their impact on subjective discomfort felt by the passenger. Relying on Summala's [4] theory of safety margins, further variables will include curve radii selected by the automation, side clearance, time to collision, time headway, as well as different road conditions that could influence the comfort/discomfort of the passenger during automated driving. The discomfort questionnaire could help to determine how automation parameters in the HMI must be adjusted for different conditions and situations. This would lead to the driver trusting the automation and feeling comfortable using it, and thus keeping the driver from taking over the control of the car. The questionnaire might also help researchers as well as practitioners to test non-invasive physiological measurements, for their validity to detect discomfort. This could allow for the real time adjustment of driving parameters of the automation according to the comfort state of the driver.

References

1. Russell, J., Barrett, L.: Core Affect, prototypical emotional episodes, and other things called emotion: Dissecting the elephant. Journal of Personality and Social Psychology 76(5), 805–819 (1999)
2. Ma, R., Kaber, D.B.: Situation awareness and workload in driving while using adaptive cruise control and a cell phone. Int. J. of Industrial Ergonomics 35(10), 939–953 (2005)
3. Parasuraman, R., Riley, V.: Humans and Automation: Use, Misuse, Disuse, Abuse. Human Factors The Journal of the Human Factors and Ergonomics Society 39(2), 230–253 (1997)
4. Summala, H.: Towards Understanding Motivational and Emotional Factors in Driver Behavior: Comfort through Satisficing. In: Cacciabue, P. (ed.) Modelling Driver Behaviour in Automotive Environments: Critical Issues in Driver Interactions with Intelligent Transport Systems, pp. 189–207 (2007)
5. Seidl, A.: Gestaltung von Ergonomietools zur prospektiven Komfortanalyse. In: Bubb, H. (ed.) Ergonomie und Verkehrssicherheit: GfA-Konferenzbeiträge der Herbstkonferenz 2000, 12-13 Oktober 2000 an der Technischen Universität München (Ergonomics and Traffic Safety), pp. 179–202 (2000)
6. Lewis-Evans, B., De Waard, D., Brookhuis, K.A.: That's close enough—A threshold effect of time headway on the experience of risk, task difficulty, effort, and comfort. Accident Analysis & Prevention 42(6), 1926–1933 (2010)

Sequence of Visual Behavior during Parking

Akihiko Takahashi

Natl. Inst. Advanced Industrial Science and Technology, Japan
a-takahashi@aist.go.jp

Abstract. The change of a driver's viewing direction during parking was investigated by studying the driver's focus points in each parking phase. Skilled drivers tend to observe the parking place to prepare the next motion even when the vehicle is not approaching the place; unskilled drivers look a long time in the vehicle's direction of travel to avoid contacting obstacles. This result suggests that helping a driver recognize the location of a parking place and a future position of the vehicle in the preparatory phase can be an effective parking assistance system.

Keywords: Parking, Visual Attention, Parking Support System.

1 Introduction

Parking and starting a car are among the most worrisome tasks for drivers. When parking a car, we must be careful not to collide with parked cars, passing vehicles, or obstacles around the car. The potential contact points or collisions change with time, making parking more difficult. Drivers should thus pay continuous attention to the moving locations in limited periods.

Considering such high mental loads, parking support devices are desired. Although low-velocity parking tasks do not cause serious accidents, various devices that support parking, such as rear-view monitors and proximity-warning systems, are actually being marketed. Automatic parking systems have also recently been marketed. It is not apparent, however, that such parking assistance devices provide real safety or assurance to drivers. To realize such assurance for drivers, the parking support devices should be well coordinated with the driver's natural attentive activity, including locations and moments where attention is focused. Knowledge of these locations and moments enables providing effective information to drivers to assist with parking and relieve the driver's anxiety.

It is difficult to directly grasp the sequence of a driver's changing focus points, but glancing directions and time length can be used as indexes. Glance activity itself is essentially random and sometimes lacks attention, so estimating a driver's focus of attention through glancing activity is difficult. To overcome this difficulty, glance directions from a number of parking trials were accumulated in order to cancel the randomness of eye motions in this study.

The following three parking/starting patterns are the most difficult tasks: backing into a parking space, backing out of a parking space, and parallel parking. This study

C. Stephanidis (Ed.): Posters, Part II, HCII 2013, CCIS 374, pp. 342–346, 2013.

concentrated on backing into a parking space, which is more common than parking nose-first in Japan.

2 Experimental

Figure 1 depicts the parking space used in the experiment trails (symbols in the figure will be explained later). Obstacles were formed with urethane-foam blocks and pylons with heights exceeding 1.0 meter so the driver could see them whenever the vehicle drew near. Those easily visible obstacles facilitated determining the driver's focus of attention. The parking space was narrow enough that drivers always had to reposition the vehicle into the final parking position.

Twenty participants, aged 21 to 74 (mean 42.5), tried the parking tasks. They drove cars routinely and they were not professional drivers such as taxi drivers or truck drivers. The drivers tried the task twice; the last trials were analyzed.

A sedan passenger car with a steering wheel on the right side was used in the trials. Vehicle velocity was measured using an acceleration sensor, and glancing activity was recorded using eye-mark recorder nac EMR-8.

Figure 1 presents details of the parking sequence. Backing into a parking space includes four different phases separated by vehicle direction (forward and backward); the phases are also shown in Fig. 1. Phases of the backward approach and retrying forward motion can be repeated in one trial because of the task difficulty. The transition between backward approach and position adjustment is defined as the moment when a rear bumper passes through the entry point of the parking space in the last backward approach. Labels of objects (explained later) are also shown in the figure.

The experiment trials were managed by an experimenter in the rear seat, and trials could be stopped whenever the participant wanted. The purpose and details of the experiment were explained to the participants by oral explanation and documentation, and informed consent was obtained. The experiment procedure, including a method of agreement of participants, was approved by the AIST ergonomic experiment committee before the experiment.

3 Method of Analysis

In this study, glance time length was measured in order to estimate focal points of attention. The eye-marks recorded were labeled with object labels (Fig. 1). A sequence of glances can be described as a transition of ratios of glancing time at objects in each phase, and again at each moment of a phase. The latter sequence of ratios indicates a continuous transition of attention in a phase and is expected to reveal subphases within a phase. The time length of the same phase differs from trial to trial, so time spans were normalized to 1.0 (100%). Glancing time lengths and locations of trials were accumulated in 2% time bins, and thus ratios of glancing locations of bins were obtained.

4 Results

4.1 Forward Approach Phase

The obtained transition of glancing ratio is presented in Fig. 2(a). When beginning the approach, drivers stared intently at entrance points (a) and (b). After that, drivers watched the road edge in front of the vehicle (f). Finally, drivers refocused on entrance points (a) and (b). This sequence suggests that drivers recognize the target parking location and plan a future vehicle track by first glancing at the entrance points. The driver should avoid contacting the front edge of the road, and, at the same time, should position the vehicle in a planned location to make the next backward approach easier. In the last step, the driver understands well the location of the front obstacle and refocuses attention on the entrance location to prepare the next backward move.

4.2 Backward Approach Phase

In the backward approach (Fig. 2(b)), the driver still stares at entrance points (a) and (b), and glances to the opposite side from the driver increase later, suggesting that avoiding contact with the vehicle opposite the driver imposes a greater visual workload. In this phase, several retries of one trial are accumulated.

4.3 Retrying Forward Motion

When retrying forward motion (Fig. 2(c)), the driver looks forward (f) first and then refocuses on entrance points (a) and (b), similar to the early approach phase. Several retries are accumulated in this phase.

4.4 Final Position Adjustment Phase

In the last backward approach and position adjustment phase (Fig. 2(d)), the driver looks in several directions in a short time. This phase can be divided into two subphases. The driver pays more attention to entrance points (a) and (b) in the earlier subphase and focuses on objects behind the vehicle in the later subphase. These visual activities are for avoiding a collision and position adjustment.

5 Discussion

Drivers can have several strategies for determining and confirm the location of the parking space and the future track of his/her vehicle for preparation. It is plausible that such differences of strategy affect parking efficiency. The difference between a strategy that results in quick and smooth parking and a strategy that causes several retries can suggest a good design principle for parking-assistance technology, since such a support device enables the driver to control the vehicle as a skilled driver.

In the following analysis, a skilled driver's trial is defined as a trial in which there was just one retry in backing a vehicle into a parking place. Since one participant provides only one trial, this definition contains both the driver's natural skill and an occasional strategy taken in a trial.

Figure 3 presents visual attention ratios of two groups, skilled drivers and unskilled drivers (more than two retries). The phases shown are the approach phase (with three subphases) and the beginning of the backward approach phase. In the earlier approach, attention of skilled drivers seems to confirm the entrance point (b) while unskilled drivers spend less time looking at the entrance points. In addition, in the final subphase of approaching, skilled drivers look at the entrance area, while unskilled drivers watch the front of the vehicle. This suggests that unskilled drivers were too cautious of contacting front obstacles and failed to confirm the target location, which is necessary to plan a future track.

For designing parking support systems, the result suggests that it is important to give information for early confirmation of a future parking position and a track to it.

6 Conclusion

This study investigated the transition of driver's visual attention when backing into a parking space. In each phase, a driver focuses attention on collision avoidance, preparatory target position recognition, and adjusting his/her vehicle positions, and the ratios of these visual activities varied with time. Preparatory visual attention was also found to play an important role for smooth parking. In order to assist parking by offering information at appropriate times, we should also clarify triggers or conditions for attention changes. Another problem is whether offering such information at appropriate times really provides assurance to drivers, and this should be clarified in human-machine interaction studies.

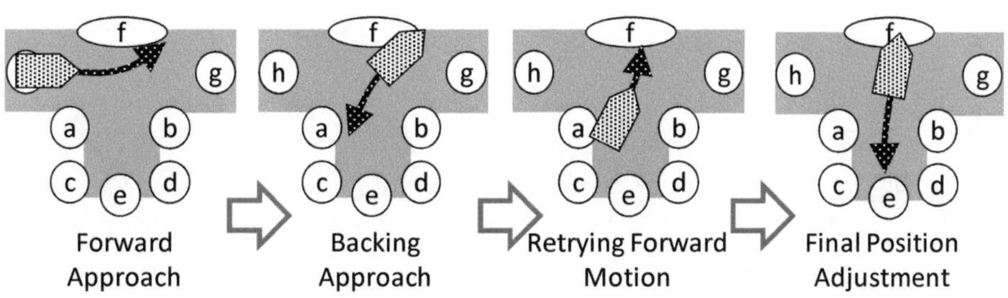

Fig. 1. Four Phases of Backward Parking Task and Obstacle Labels

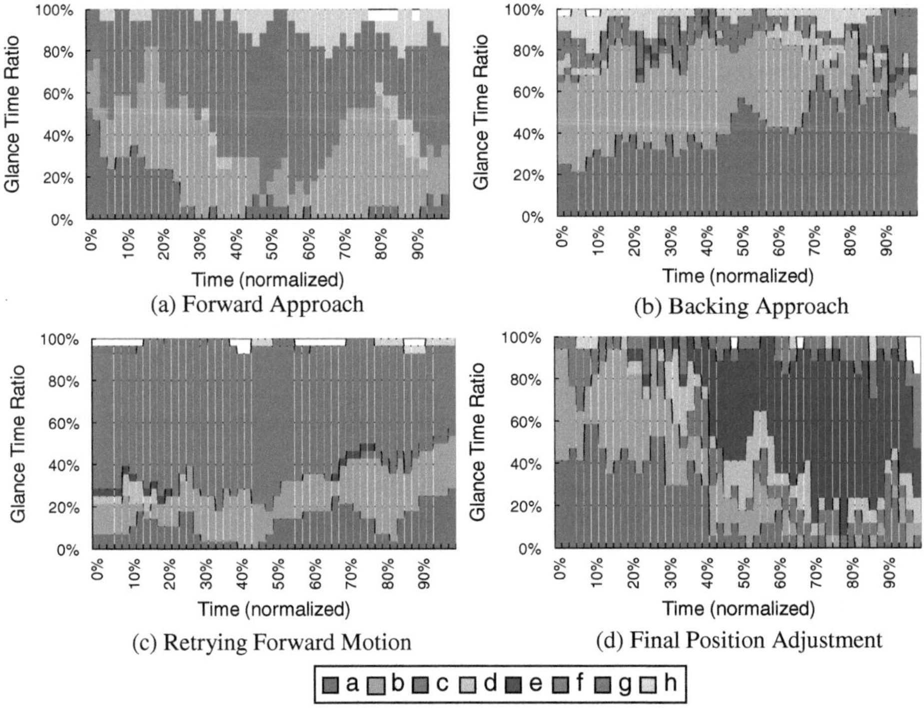

Fig. 2. Transition of Time Ratio of Staring Direction by Parking Phase

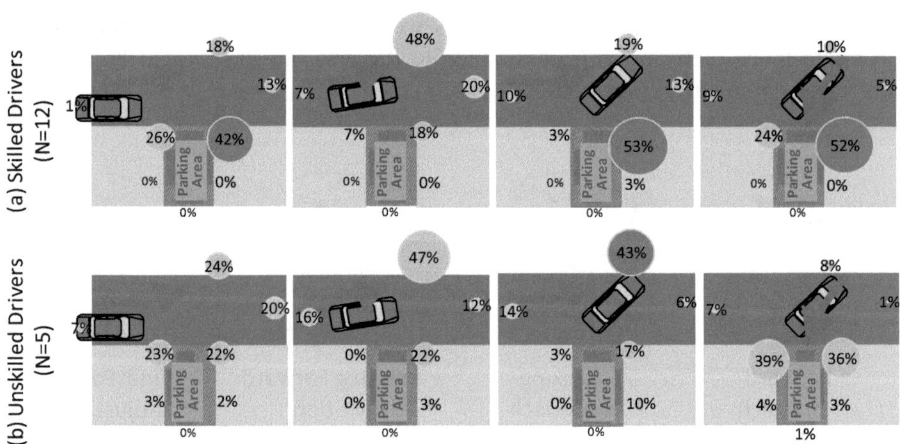

Fig. 3. Difference of Staring Direction by Parking Skill Level

Simulation for Pilot's Capability of Target-Pointing Operation

Hongjun Xue and Xiaoyan Zhang

School of Aeronautics, Northwestern Polytechnical University, Xi'an Shaanxi 710072, China
xuehj@nwpu.edu.cn, zxyliuyan@sina.com

Abstract. Target-pointing operation of the pilot is of importance for the information interaction in the cockpit, and the accuracy, rapidness and effectiveness of the operation is critical for the flight safety. The design and layout of human-machine interface in the cockpit cannot be implemented perfectly through static reach and visual zone, due to neglect the dynamic effect, such as plane vibration. In order for the optimization of layout of human-machine interface, the affect of the target-pointing operation due to multi-acceleration and vibration in cockpit is studied by manikin dynamic simulation based on both of muscle-skeleton model of LifeMOD platform and pilot motion captured data under normal condition. The results suggest that emergency operation equipment can be positioned in the area in which the acceleration and vibration has least impact to ensure that pilot can operate timely and accurately in emergency and eventually to promote flight safety.

Keywords: Cockpit, lifeMOD, target-pointing, pilot capability.

1 Introduction

Cockpit is a kind of important interface between pilot and aircraft. Pilot can respond to the information from the aircraft by control equipments. Although autopilot may reduce workload from pilots there is still much work for pilot to operate manually. Especially during takeoff or landing, or in emergency pilot would be the last decision-maker to guarantee flight safety. Usually, pilot limb's movement time, track or speed, acceleration is always used to represent the performance of nominal operation. Generally, the flight of aircraft is often affected by vibration and acceleration of engine or airflows [1, 2, 3, 4]. Sometimes, this vibration and acceleration may make the pilot's operation performance to be lower or even failure [5, 6, 7, 8]. The operation of pressing or dialing the buttons on the panel in the cockpit is defined "target-pointing". "Target-pointing" operation is also of importance for flight safety. This paper focuses on the performance of target-pointing operation from pilot muscle-skeleton model in LifeMOD. Taking experimental operation data as the basis data and the driven data, we built a manikin model to simulate various accelerations and swings influence for pilot operation. The result has given a principle of design for the man-machine interfaces in cockpit, and improvements in flight emergency to guarantee flight safety.

C. Stephanidis (Ed.): Posters, Part II, HCII 2013, CCIS 374, pp. 347–351, 2013.

2 Kinetics Model of Target-Pointing Operation

Kinetics Model of Pilot. Kinetics model in the LifeMOD includes 122 muscle units modeled by spring and damp elements and can bear and produce pull force. The forces from the muscles act on the skeleton system [9, 10, 11]. The muscle unit is originally "un-trained". During the anti-kinetics simulation, the capture data can be used to drive the manikin and the action of muscles are recorded, after once simulation, the muscle is "trained". During the later kinetics simulation, the trained muscles has now the performance as same as before.

The equation of muscle is:

$$F = \begin{cases} F_{max} & F \geq F_{max} \\ P_{gain} \cdot P_{error} + D_{gain} \cdot D_{error} & F < F_{max} \\ 0 & L_{desired} < L_{actual} \end{cases} \tag{1}$$

where, $F_{max} = p_{CSA} \cdot s_{max}$, p_{CSA} is the area of muscle transect, S_{max} is the maximum tissue stress; $P_{error} = L_{desired} - L_{actual}$, $L_{desired}$ is the force of the expected muscle motion mode, and L_{actual} is the actual force. $D_{error} = \dot{P}_{error}$. P_{gain} and D_{gain} represents scale plus coefficient and differential plus coefficient respectively. Generally speaking, D_{gain} is one tenth of P_{gain}.

Model of Pilot-Seat. Taking the ADAMS to simulate the pilot posture. In this simulation, coefficient of rigid is 10kN/m, and damp is 0.1kN · s/m[9].

3 Kinetics Simulation of Target-Pointing Operation

Operation Target. The operation target in the cockpit is the vertexes and centre of rectangle on the shield, top panel, MCD and central control panel. The optics capture system has been used to capture the motion data of pilot in the operation experiment.

Influence of Acceleration. As for civil aircraft, the direction of acceleration is always +Z, -Z, and +X (where X axis is along the fuselage and the direction of flight is +X, and Y axis directs left, Z axis directs up.). According to the CAAR 25, the range of acceleration is within +Z (0, 2.5g), -Z (-1g, 0), +X (0, 1g).

Influence of +Z-axis Acceleration. Appling +Z acceleration ranged from 0 to 2.5g to the pilot-seat model and increment is 0.1g. The movement and displacement of the finger compared with which of basis is analyzed for the four areas and shown in figure 1. The simulation result in figure 1 suggests that +Z-acceleration influences the top panel area most, central control panel least. the biggest displacement is 864mm in top panel at 2.2g acceleration.

Influence of -Z-axis Acceleration. Applying -Z acceleration ranged from -1g to 0 to the pilot-seat model and increment is 0.1g. The result is shown in figure 2 for the four areas, and suggests that -Z-acceleration influence the shield area most and central control panel least. The biggest displacement is 93mm in shield and least is 48mm in central control panel.

Influence of +X -axis Acceleration Applying +X acceleration ranged from 0 to 1g to the pilot-seat model and increment is 0.1g. The result in figure 3 suggests that when the acceleration is range from 0 to 0.5g, the function of displacement and acceleration is nearly linear in shield and top panel, but when the acceleration is bigger than 0.5, the operation can hardly finished, the biggest displacement is almost 800mm in 1g in shield, and top panel displacement is more than 600mm in 0.8g acceleration. The function is nearly linear in MCD and central control panel, and the influence is less than the other two areas.

Influence of Vibration. The vibration influences pilot operation performance through magnitude of swing and frequency. The magnitude of swing ranged from 10mm to 50mm belongs to low swing, and the frequency ranged from 5 HZ to 50 HZ belongs to low frequency too. The vibration, $S = Asin(2\pi \cdot f \cdot t)$, imposed on both Z axis and Y axis. The actual movement of right finger is not linear but oscillating around the balance position. The maximum displacement $|E|_{max}$ is used to analyze the degree of influence in vibration.

Influence of Z-axis Vibration. $|E|_{max}$ is shown in figure 4. "Throw-off" means that operation can not be carried out and vibration makes the finger uncontrollable by pilot themselves. The break points in figure 4 and figure 5 represents "Throw-off".

Under identical condition, the vibration influences shield area most, central control panel least. The maximum $|E|_{max}$ is less than 100mm. "Throw-off" has appeared in the MCD area but less influence than shield area.

Influence of Y-axis Vibration. $|E|_{max}$ of Y-axis is shown in figure 5, the contrast of $|E|_{max}$ of Y-axis vibration in four areas. Similarly the vibration influences shield and top panel more than MCD and central control panel. With Y- axis vibration the four areas all appeared "Throw-off" with different magnitude of swings.

4 Conclusions

From the pilot-seat simulation and result analysis, it seems that vibration affect the operation least when pilot operates button in the central control panel. Because the right-upper area as least affected area of pilot operation, the muscle in the model is "operational trained" better and be used to simulate pilot operation in various cockpit environments well. The result of simulation shows that cockpit vibration affects pilot's operation more than that of acceleration, and may leads to operation failure more much. The results also present the fact that the pilots are more adaptable to cockpit acceleration than vibration. The most important button for safety especially for emergency operation should be positioned in the central control panel to improve the flight safety; and other buttons can be placed in neighbor areas.

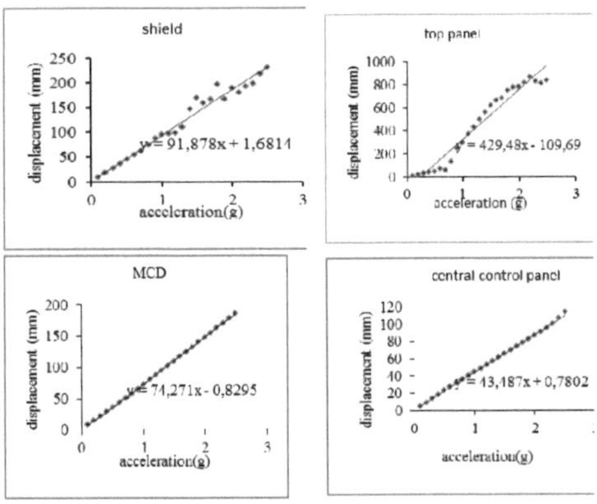

Fig. 1. Displacement with +Z acceleration

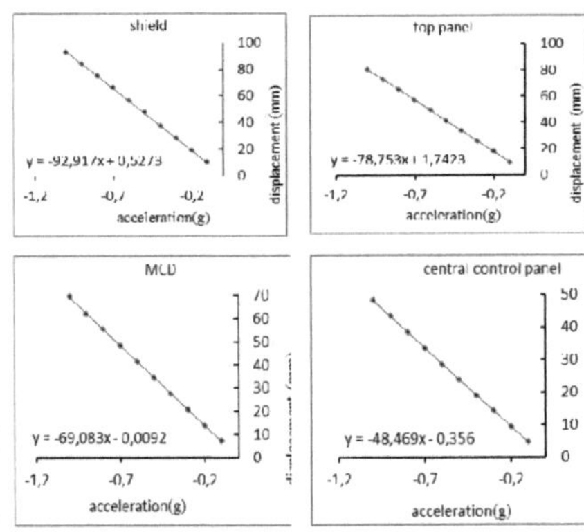

Fig. 2. Displacement with +Z acceleration

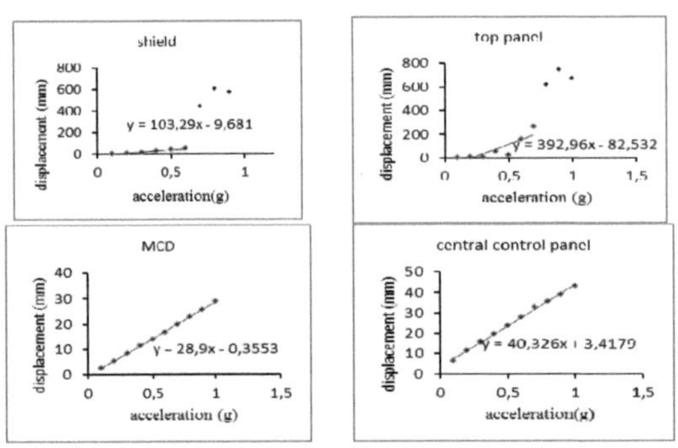

Fig. 3. Displacement with +X acceleration

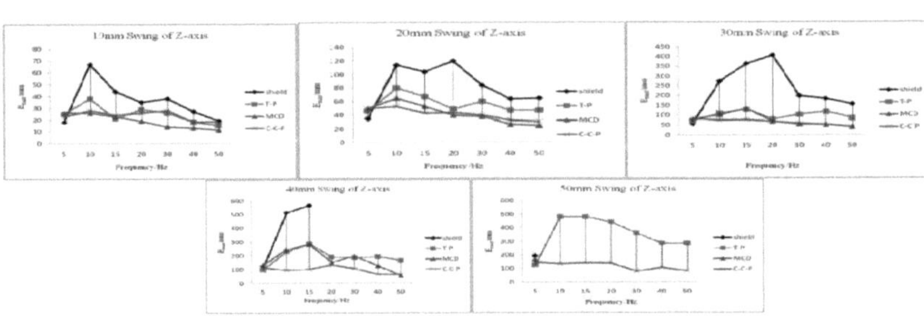

Fig. 4. Contrast of $|E|_{max}$ in four areas with Z-axis vibration

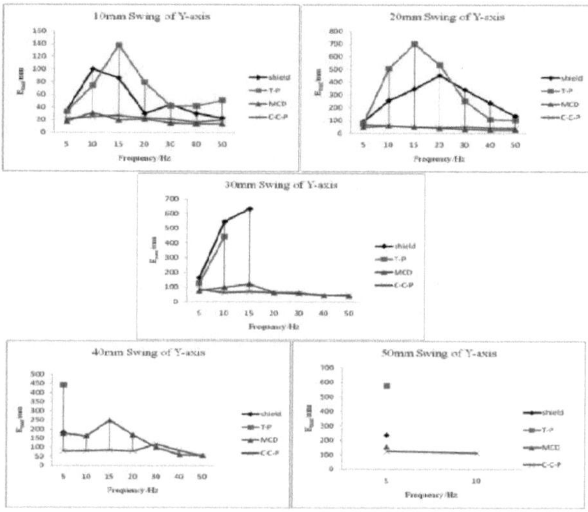

Fig. 5. Contrast of $|E|_{max}$ in four areas with Y-axis vibration

Acknowledgement. The paper is granted under National Basic Research Program of China (No.2010CB734101).

References

1. Adams, J.J.: Application of Human Transfer Functions to a Design Problem. In: Third Annual NASA – University Conference on Manual Control, NASA SP–144 (1967)
2. Long, S.Z., Chen, H.: Research on Human Fuzzy Control Model in Man-Machine-Environment Systems. In: The 33rd International Congress of Aviation and Space Medicine, pp. 138–141 (1985)
3. Yang, N.: Coordination Analysis and Parametric Description of Human Movements. TsingHua University, Beijing (2001)
4. Jiang, M., Wang, R., Jin, D.: Fitts's law for evaluating the recovery from movements of hand-held objects. Journal of TsingHua University 46(11), 1848–1850 (2006)
5. Ariff, F.H.M., Rambely, A.S.: Modeling of an Arm Via Kane's Method: An Inverse Dynamic Approach. European Journal of Scientific Research 33(2), 358–364 (2009)
6. Wang, R., Zhuang, D.: Simulation and analysis of pilots' manipulation based on SimMechanics. Journal of Beijing University of Aeronautics and Astronautics 33(7), 765–768 (2007)
7. Sun, P., Wang, S., Wang, Q.: Calculation for optimized movement trajectories of human multi-joint arm. Inese Journal of Theoretical and Applied Mechanics 42(3), 506–511 (2010)
8. Boshi, H., Fumin, C.: Research on Human Body Motion Capture and Motion Control. Computer Engineering and Applications, 60–63 (2005)
9. `http://www.lifemodeler.com`
10. Li, X., Zhang, E., Lu, C.: Driving Comfort Simulation Based on Human Biomechanics Model Under Vibration. Journal of Xi'an Jiaotong University 42(5), 556–560 (2008)
11. Shabana, A.A.: Computational Dynamics. John Wiley & Sons Ltd., United Kingdom (2010)

Part V
Web and Social Media

Increased Community Engagement via Map Based Website Modules/Plugins

Sapumal Ahangama

MillenniumIT, Malabe, Sri Lanka
sahangama@gmail.com

Abstract. This paper will look into increased community engagement in modern societies with the use of map based modules that can be integrated on common websites. The intention is to use a central system which will store crowd sourced data regarding community projects and spread the data among a variety of website users achieving highest and optimum reach.

Keywords: Community Engagement, Website Plugins, Social Media.

1 Introduction

In modern societies, inter-person engagement in real life is at a bare minimum due to the highly dynamic nature of day to day activities. The dynamic nature has made boundaries of interpersonal engagement with limitation to interaction with those only known personally [1]. As a result, even news about important community based projects in local human settlements does not spread beyond a certain level. With the development of technology, internet and social media, people nowadays tend to use electronic tools as an interaction mechanism among themselves as well as a convenient mode of spreading news. An attempt will be made to explore the possibility of using these technologies to propagate and spread information about community projects in societies, using websites, maps and social media channels. The projects vary from environmental protection, community education and to a much broader community activities such as feeding the poor, uplifting of rural health, education etc. even in distant countries.

In order to make the integration with websites based on content management systems easier, it is intended to use a plugin which can be integrated in to any website. As a measure to increase interactivity and ease of use, a map will be basically used in the plugin area to display data.

2 Goals

- All community projects should be stored in a single system accessed on demand by external systems. Cloud storage may be utilized with increase of usage. Projects should be added by the community itself with proper categorization and details.

C. Stephanidis (Ed.): Posters, Part II, HCII 2013, CCIS 374, pp. 355–358, 2013.

Easy access to the project organizers and viewing participants at events are considered as important features.

- The system should run across all platforms without limiting to a single technology. Tailor made plugins will be integrated on websites based on various content management systems capable of communicating with a common protocol.
- To reach a diverse base of web users, the plugin should be integrated into a variety of web sites in different fields exposing the system to a diverse range of users.
- The interaction with the system should be user friendly without disturbing the user experience of the main website. In the plugin map (Fig. 1), user should be provided with community projects that suit user's prime interest and should also be able to select, monitor and search community projects.

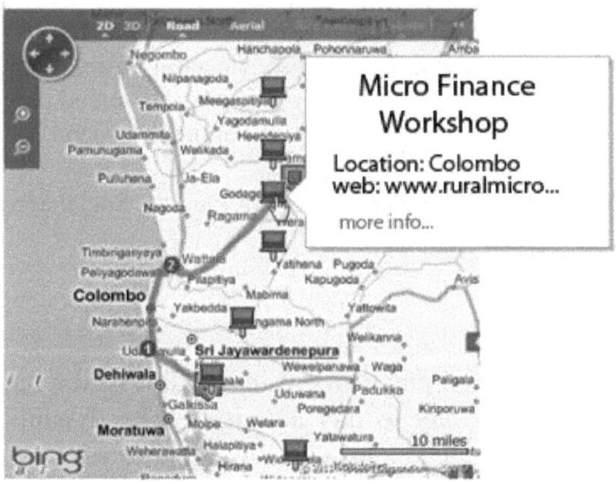

Fig. 1. Example display area of the plugin

3 Workflow of the System

Community projects organized by various organizations, civil societies etc. can be added to the central system by their project admins/organizers. These projects should be validated as genuine social projects targeting community, to avoid spam material. Use of reputation systems to fight spam will be suitable [2]. Based on seniority and past activity levels, certain participants will have the administrative power of projects added to the system.

Once a project becomes public, its information will be available to websites subscribed to the system via the installed plugins. Each project attached will include a set of basic data such as information of the project, an optional website, timelines, event admins and publicly accepted participants.

Community development projects will be most effective with increased community support and involvement. This will improve the access to local resources, building community capacity, and fostering friendship and goodwill [3]. Hence knowing other participants beforehand would enhance the success of the project. The plugin will select projects best suited and within the reach of the user to be displayed on the plugin's map. Thus the project should be in a reachable distance for the active participation of the user or the user should be able to provide assistance to the project in other ways, such as through donations even without his/her physical presence.

4 Logic for Selection of Most Suited Projects

Main criteria for selection of suitable projects for a particular user would be the distance to the project location. Html geo location capabilities of the web browser will be used to determine the user's location. Hence projects within a radius which is predefined based on reachability criteria such as distance and time of travel will be displayed on the plugin map. The user will also be able to select projects on his/her interest and search for projects of other areas too.

In an advanced logic of selection of projects, the user is required to have an account with the system. Also, it will be required to get information of user's immediate friends, as well as of the friends of friends of the user, which can be accessed from user's registered social media sites with user consent. Projects involving immediate friends will be of more interest to the user as there is a possibility of common interest and the tendency to attend an event where an immediate friend participates is highly probable.

The logic is expanded by giving further prominence to community projects participated by friends of friends too. In addition, friend suggestion algorithms using the implicit social graph as proposed by Roth et al. [4] will be helpful in identifying projects attended by possible other related parties.

5 Technical Implementation

The communication with the system for external websites will be done through the public web service made available. The web service will respond with data according to the parameters of the requests such as location of the user, optional user preferences and the unique user identification code if the user is logged with a social media platform.

The system will use a central database to store data such as details of submitted projects and users registered with the system. The project details will be those added by the project admin. Details of past projects too will be stored to track their status. The system would calculate and maintain a score associated with each project, based on user behavior such as number of views and engagement to determine its importance. Data of the registered users will be used to provide personalized user experience when community projects are displayed on the map. When a user is logged in using a social media platform's authentication method, the system will be able to access details of user's friends and friends of friends' too. As a result the system will be able to build relationships between a particular user and other members active in the system. During the project selection for a particular user, projects having participation of many connected parties of the current user will be given more weight [5] providing a better user experience with the plugin, as the projects have a high possibility of user interest.

The web service will respond with data selected by the selection logic employed by the selection engine based on the parameters. The response data will include information such as web links, contact details and tracking information of the project enabling further interaction with the project.

6 Conclusion

The aim of the proposed system would be to increase community engagement using a common map based plugin in websites. The plugin can be integrated to websites based on different technological frameworks and will fetch data from a common service. As a result, the plugin can be integrated to a variety of website types in different fields, and community projects can be exposed to a large user base. Customized user experience provided by the system using various data associated with the user will also improve the user experience with the system, thus increasing engagement in community projects.

References

1. Engaging the Community in Fort Lauderdale's Community Investment Plan, Leadership ICMA 2012 (2012)
2. Prakash, V.V., O'Donnell, A.: Fighting Spam with Reputation Systems. Queue 3(9) (November 2005)
3. Communities in Action: A Guide to Effective Project, Rotary International, http://www.rotary.org/ridocuments/en_pdf/605a_en.pdf
4. Roth, M., Ben-David, A., Deutscher, D., Flysher, G., Horn, I., Leichtberg, A., Leiser, N., Matias, Y., Merom, R.: Suggesting Friends using the Implicit Social Graph. In: Proc. KDD 2010, pp. 233–242. ACM Press (2010)
5. Gilbert, E., Karahalios, K.: Predicting tie strength with social media. In: Proceedings of the SIGCHI Conference on Human Factors in Computing Systems, Boston, MA, USA, April 04-09 (2009)

Social Networking Using Mobile Devices

Dima Kassab, Xiaojun Yuan, and Jami L. Cotler

College of Computing and Information, University at Albany,
State University of New York, Albany, NY 12222
{dkassab,xyuan,jcotler}@albany.edu

Abstract. The burgeoning domain of social media has infiltrated general populations and has achieved broad applicability [10]. This domain has been studied extensively but there is a deficiency of research in the area of social media and mobile access and use [1] [11]. This study examines not only the use of social media on mobile devices but extends the ideas of this area of research to evaluate how social media is being used on mobile devices. It reports the findings of an online survey of 73 participants recruited from different listservs in the world. The study shows that the majority of participants use social networks as consumers (e.g. read other people posts), more than producers (i.e. post status update or a photo). It also reveals some differences between the topics participants share through a mobile device and a personal computer.

Keywords: Mobile social networks, user behaviors, survey.

1 Introduction

Mobile social networking has gained the attention from academia, industry and governments during the past decade. Due to the technical advances of the WWW and mobile technologies, researchers in the field have done considerable work in promoting social communication in different ways [3][8]. But to our knowledge, few studies have investigated why (e.g. motivations) and how (e.g. when do they do social networking, and where) people do social networking using mobile devices.

Mobile devices are becoming a popular interface for accessing social networking services; when coupled with social networking these devices are allowing people to connect with family, friends, strangers and the community throughout the day, regardless of location. Mobile social networks services provide their users with instant and real-time access to their network. Based on a previous pilot study where we interviewed (12) participants from a US university regarding their information needs and search behaviors on mobile devices, we found staying connected to social networks to be one of the emergent trends that motivate users to access the mobile Internet [6]. On an attempt to further understand this new trend, we distributed an online survey to various listservs in the world. This paper reports our results of the survey data and discusses the findings and our future work.

C. Stephanidis (Ed.): Posters, Part II, HCII 2013, CCIS 374, pp. 359–364, 2013.

2 Literature Review

There is a rich set of work towards characterizing user behaviors in online social networks, however less has been done to study user behaviors in the mobile social network space. Mobile social networks could be classified into native mobile social networks and web-based social networks with mobile version. For example, Dodgeball is a mobile social networking service that allows people to broadcast their location via text messages to their networks. Dodgeball is a native mobile social network that does not have an online presence. On the other hand, Facebook, Google+ and Twitter are social networks which started online, and due to the increase in mobile devices use provide mobile access through an application.

Some of the studies on mobile social networks have focused on native mobile social networks [4] [7], while others focused on social networks that exist online and provide mobile access through an app such as Facebook, Google+ and Twitter [2] [9] [13]. Research has shown differences between the way native and web-based mobile are used.

Native mobile social networks have been used more to facilitate face-to-face interactions [4] [7]. As Köbler et al. (2011) pointed out, there has been a shift in the behavioral patterns and intentions of users of various mobile social networks towards a closer association between socializing in real life and the use of Social Network Systems. Hmphreys (2007) has focused on Dodgball. His study indicated that mobile social networks are used by people to be part of social molecularization. People use them to discover new places and alert others of the existence of such places, by checking in these places. According to him, by indirectly communicating about a place in real time, people exchange social-location information. This can result in a collective momentum of using the mobile social network system [4].

While the research reviewed above focused on native mobile social network services, this section focuses on web-based social networks. Cui & Wang (2012) conducted a diary study with 12 users in South Korea to characterize the experience of accessing social networks through mobile device. They found social connection, awareness, diversions and following notifications to be the main motivations behind this activity. "Awareness" emphasizes effortless access to information that enables people to pick it up with ease, make sense of it, and adjust their behavior accordingly. Their study reveals cross-medium alerts, especially push-messaging alert as a common trigger for mobile social networking sessions [2].

Rotman (2010) in their study of students and faculty members social networks use, reported responding to an alert is one of the major motivations to use mobile social networks. Mobile Facebook users observed in the study were continually looking for new updates, usually without a clear goal other than keeping up to date. They also observed Mobile Facebook users to check updates, but to seldom perform any active synchronous interactions with other users [9]. A more recent report (2013) by IDC Research supported by Facebook indicates that a "sense of being connected" is the strongest sentiment to use mobile social networks. It spans demographics and brands, services and applications used. In this study IDC conducted an online survey of 7,446 18-44 year old iPhone and Android smartphone owners in the U.S. over the course of one week. The study was an attempt to understand how smartphone owners use their mobile phones, with an emphasis on social media and communication. Participants in this study reports higher use of social applications during events when they are out socially interacting with others. The main reason behind this use is to instantly share experiences. Moreover, the ease of use mobile devices provide encourages sharing even more. The study has also looked at the different popularity of social networks including LinkedIn, Instagram and Twitter. In comparison to other mobile social network sites, the Facebook app dominates regarding the total time spent on social and communications activities on a smartphone [13].

Users have different concerns while using mobile social networks. Privacy is one of the main concerns regarding mobile social networking, especially for applications making use of Bluetooth sensing or applications that track users daily routines and preferences through their location [7]. Explicit, implicit, and automated sharing raise new concerns about privacy. Privacy is one of the main reasons that prevents people from sharing content online. Wiese et al. (2011) proposed creating a model of the interpersonal relationships between different people, rather than a social graph where everyone is simply a "friend" as a solution to manage information sharing in a better way. Their proposition is based on their findings that from all data they collected describing 2730 social relationships, self reported closeness was the best indicator of whether or not to share a piece of information, where common information is more likely to be shared [12].

The studies identified in this literature review did not focus on understanding any differences perceived by the users between sharing through a mobile device and a personal computer. These studies did not, as well, investigate the reasons that might discourage social networking users from accessing their networks through a mobile device. Our study is an attempt to explore these areas and to further understand mobile social networking user behaviors. In the following sections we will present our methodology, findings and future work.

3 Methodology

A survey was developed with different constructs related to social networking behaviors on mobile devices such as, frequency of usage, preferred social networks, topics shared, locations, and differences between behaviors on the mobile device and personal computer. This survey was sent to a variety of listservs including university and professional listservs. Participation on the survey was anonymous and the participants had the option of whether or not to answer specific questions in the survey. The internal validity of the survey was tested using 3 different pilots.

4 Participants

Participants (n=73) from a variety of backgrounds were involved in the study. The majority of participants (72.6%) were over 26 years old. In terms of the sex of the participants, the majority were females (60.27%). All the participants have different levels of education: 36.99% were PhD, 36.99% were masters, and 23.29% were undergraduates. Furthermore, the majority of participants (83.56%) owned a touch screen device and Most of them (82.19%) had a data plan.

5 Results

The participants in our study expressed their use of a device for social networking. This is actually the case for 68.97% of our poll. The majority of these participants (62.5%) accessed social networks on a daily basis, 12.5% participants accessed them on a weekly basis and 5% rarely accessed them. Facebook was the most visited social network website among participants. The majority of participants (65%) said they use Facebook very often, 17.5% use it often and 12.5% use it sometimes and 5% use it rarely (Figure 1). Twitter was the most frequently used social network among participants, where 17.14% of the participants use it very often, 8.57% use it often, 25.71% use it sometimes, 20% use it rarely and 28.57% had never used it. Participants had also used their mobile device to blog, where 5.71% use it very often, 8.57% use it often, 17.14 use it sometime, and 17.14% use it rarely.

Participants who access social networks through a mobile device used it mainly to read other people's updates and view photos posted by others (55% of participants). A fewer number of participants (32.5%) used these tools actively to post status updates, post pictures or comments. Only 5% of participants used the device to chat using social networks. Only 5% of participants used it to read articles.

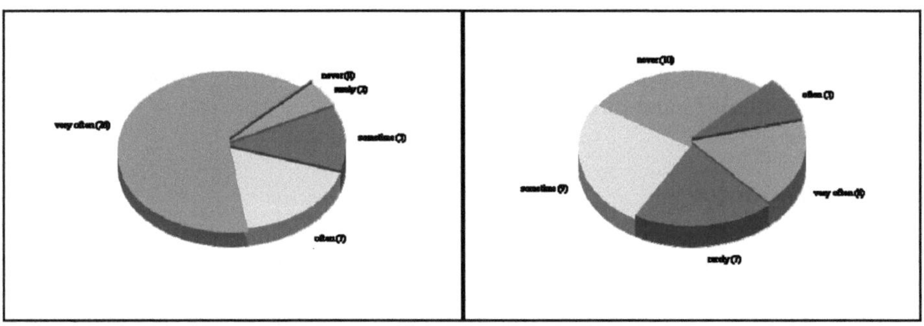

Fig. 1. Facebook usage (left) vs. Twitter usage (right)

The main reasons for participants not to use their mobile devices for social networking are: 1) Device related: "the phone is not for this purpose" or "I do not trust the app"; 2) Network related: the connection is slow or expensive; and 3) Personal preference: I am not a fan of social networks.

The majority of participants (85%) noticed minor differences between the topics they share using the mobile device and personal computers. According to participants, the topics shared through the mobile devices are more immediate, essential and pertaining to something current. One participant stated, "Topics I share through the phone are immediately pertaining to something instead of waiting to get to a computer to put up the status." These topics will be less descriptive and could be expressed with a shorter text due to the difficulty of typing on the mobile device keyboard, and as a participant pointed out "Less description because I don't like the keyboard on my phone. The phone is for quick, spontaneous thoughts or photo uploads." Topics that include links are more likely to be shared using the personal computer because of the copy-paste functionality. Pictures, on the other hand, are more likely to be shared using the mobile device instantly right after the photo is captured. The main reasons these participants prefer mobile devices to a personal computers are mobility (37.5%), convenience (37.5%) and ease of use (17.5%).

Participants access social networks through their mobile devices everywhere (27.5%), when they do not have access to a computer (15%), in bed (5%), on the go (25%), in school (10%) and at work (7.5%).

6 Conclusion and Future Work

We collected data from an online survey that asked questions regarding people's use of social networking using mobile devices. Our findings are of great interest for our area of research. It seems that Facebook and Twitter are the most popularly used social networking sites. When people do social networking, they read or write posts, and share posts and pictures with each others. They share similar topics using mobile and using personal computers. We also found that mobile devices made social networking more convenient because people can stay connected almost everywhere, whenever they want to. Privacy did not seem to prevent participants from using mobile social network. Participants in our survey did not indicate any concern regarding their privacy.

In this study, we made an effort towards a better understanding of mobile users' social networking behavior. We plan to further explore how people collaborate in the social networking environment and how they interact with each other using mobile phones. In the next phase we plan to extend our study by (1) targeting a larger number of participants; and (2) using responses from this survey to create categories for the next survey questions.

Other areas discussed in this paper are in need of more research. One of the findings indicates that the majority of activities reported by participants in our survey were more passive (consumption) than active (creation). A future research could investigate the reasons for which users prefer to be passive rather than active while using mobile social networks. The study also reports perceived differences between the topics shared using a mobile device and a personal computer. As a next step, we will emphasize more the understanding of which topics users share with others and whether or not they have any privacy concerns while sharing these topics.

Moreover, the next phase will investigate how mobile social interactions may affect social interactions with others in general. This is of great interest to the authors since it is one of the areas where mobile social networks differ from online social networks.

References

1. Chai, S., Kim, M.: A socio-technical approach to knowledge contribution behavior: An empirical investigation of social networking sites users. International Journal of Information Management 32(2), 118–126 (2012)
2. Cui, Y., Wang, L.: Motivations for accessing social networking services on mobile devices. In: Proceedings of the International Working Conference on Advanced Visual Interfaces, pp. 636–639. ACM, New York (2012)
3. González, M.C., Hidalgo, C.A., Barabási, A.-L.: Understanding individual human mobility patterns. Nature 453(7196), 779–782 (2008)
4. Hmphreys, L.: Mobile Social Networks and Social Practice: A Case Study of Dodgeball. Journal of Computer-Mediated Communication 13(1), 341–360 (2007)
5. Joinson, A.N.: Looking at, looking up or keeping up with people?: motives and use of facebook. In: Proceedings of the SIGCHI Conference on Human Factors in Computing Systems, pp. 1027–1036. ACM, New York (2008), doi:10.1145/1357054.1357213
6. Kassab, D., Yuan, X.: Understanding the information needs and search behaviours of mobile users. Information Research 17(4) (2012)
7. Köbler, F., Goswami, S., Koene, P., Leimeister, J., Krcmar, H.: NFriendConnector: Design and Evaluation of an Application for Integrating Offline and Online Social Networking. AIS Transactions on Human-Computer Interaction 3(4), 214–235 (2011)
8. Rheingold, H.: Smart Mobs: The Next Social Revolution. Perseus, Cambridge (2003)
9. Rotman, D.: Constant connectivity, selective participation: mobile-social interaction of students and faculty. In: CHI 2010 Extended Abstracts on Human Factors in Computing Systems, pp. 4333–4338. ACM, New York (2010)
10. Santos, A.C., Cardoso, J.M.P., Ferreira, D.R., Diniz, P.C., Chaínho, P.: Providing user context for mobile and social networking applications. Pervasive and Mobile Computing 6(3), 324–341 (2010)
11. Tsai, F.S., Han, W., Xu, J., Chua, H.C.: Design and development of a mobile peer-to-peer social networking application. Expert Systems with Applications 36(8), 11077–11087 (2009)
12. Wiese, J., Kelley, P.G., Cranor, L.F., Dabbish, L., Hong, J.I., Zimmerman, J.: Are you close with me? Are you nearby?: investigating social groups, closeness, and willingness to share. In: Proceedings of the 13th International Conference on Ubiquitous Computing, pp. 197–206. ACM, New York (2011)
13. Zibart, M.: IDC-Facebook Always Connected. Facebook, http://newsroom.fb.com/News/588/IDC-Study-Mobile-and-Social-Connectiveness (retrieved April 10, 2013)

When Does "Facebooking" Make Us Avoid Risks? The Effect of Social Networking Orientation on Risk Preference

Hakkyun Kim[1], Kyoungmi Lee[2], and Kiwan Park[2]

[1] School of Business, Sungkyunkwan University,
25-2 Sungkyunkwan-ro, Jongno-gu, Seoul, Korea
hakkyunkim@skku.edu
[2] Graduate School of Business, Seoul National University,
1 Gwanak-ro, Gwanak-gu, Seoul, Korea
{kiwanp,kyoungmi}@snu.ac.kr

Abstract. Will consumers' social networking orientations influence their psychological functioning on subsequent tasks in seemingly remote, unrelated domains? Prior research on social capital suggests the distinction between a bonding orientation, with which people seek to cement connectedness among exclusive and relatively homogeneous groups, and a bridging orientation, with which people focus on creating new contacts with different groups, resulting in spanning diverse social cleavages. Building on the resource depletion paradigm, we propose and find that consumers become more risk-averse after performing bridging- versus bonding-oriented activities on Facebook. We also confirm the depletion of risk-taking resources as the underlying process by showing its mediating role between social networking orientation and risk preference.

Keywords: Social media, social networking orientation, Facebook, risk perceptions.

1 Introduction

Over the past decade, social networking services have become an integral part of managing relationships with others and understanding the world. By connecting with others online and accumulating "friends," individuals can establish their social networks, thus growing their social capital. Reflecting on such a near-endemic phenomenon of living with social network services (SNS), the extant research in marketing and consumer behavior has investigated several issues regarding social network service, such as the valuation of online networks [1] or word-of-mouth communications [2]. Less is known, however, about how consumers' experiences with social networking services influence their psychological functioning, such as decision-making styles and risk preferences. By filling this gap, the present research examines downstream influences that the use of social networking sites may have on consumer decision-making, particularly on risky choices.

C. Stephanidis (Ed.): Posters, Part II, HCII 2013, CCIS 374, pp. 365–367, 2013.

We propose that an individual's primary motivational foci of social networking affect their everyday decisions associated with risk (e.g., investment-related or health-related decision-making). Building on the resource depletion paradigm that suggests that people who engage in an initial self-regulation task perform worse on a subsequent task demanding self-regulation resources [3-5], we posit that humans have a limited amount of risk-taking resources. Thus, once their risk-taking resources are drained, individuals will act more conservatively in subsequent tasks. Specifically, given that bridging- versus bonding-oriented activities are involved with a higher level of social risk, thereby depleting more resources, we hypothesize that consumers may become more risk-averse after performing bridging- versus bonding-oriented social networking activities. We conducted an experiment to examine this hypothesis.

2 Method

Sixty-five undergraduate students participated and were randomly assigned to the either bridging- or bonding-orientation condition. Participants in the bridging condition were asked to choose some people on their friend lists with whom they had not personally interacted (e.g., someone from a class or friends' friends), and visit each person's Wall. The participants were then asked to spend about 10 minutes reading their friends' recent events and leaving Wall posts. In contrast, those in the bonding condition were asked to choose some people whom they felt close to and whom they often interacted with (e.g., best friends).

After completing the task, participants were asked to indicate on seven-point scales how socially risky (1 = not risky at all; 7 =very risky) and how stressful (1 = not stressful at all; 7 = very stressful) they perceived the Facebook activities to be. We averaged the two items and used a composite index to understand underlying process. Next, as a purportedly separate study, participants were asked to engage in a task to measure their risk preferences, which required deliberation to gauge between risks and payoffs in their choices [6]. Their response to this task was used in calculation of their risk preference index.

3 Results

First, we analyzed the risk preference index to investigate whether the bridging activities made participants more risk-aversive in the subsequent task than did the bonding activities. A one-way ANOVA indicated that participants became more risk-aversive after completing the bridging versus bonding activities on the Facebook ($M_{bridging}$ = 2.81, $M_{bonding}$ = 3.73, $F(1, 56) = 7.19$, $p < .01$). Risk preference was significantly lower than the midpoint of the seven-point scale in the bridging condition ($t(31) = 5.32$, $p < .001$), whereas it was not in the bonding condition ($t(27) = 1.19$, $p > .25$).

We also confirmed that participants in the bridging versus bonding condition spent their risk-taking resources ($M_{bridging}$ = 3.55, $M_{bonding}$ = 2.59, $F(1, 56) = 6.22$, $p < .05$)

while completing the Facebook activities. Furthermore, in order to test mediation via resource depletion, we conducted a mediational analysis using bootstrapping procedures [7, 8], which demonstrated that an indirect effect via resource depletion was significant (95% CI = [–.3216, –.0053]) .

4 Discussion

These results provide evidence that when activities on social networking sites center on bonding (vs. bridging), consumers tend to make more risky decisions. Theoretically, this research can shed light on hitherto unknown influences that experiences with social networking service unwittingly exert on human decision processes, which could be explained as a result of depletion of risk seeking resources. In particular, given that the subsequent consequences of online social networking can apply to a variety of decision domains (including decisions that are not directly related to social networking sites), this research promises to advance our understanding of consumers' implicit decision-making processes, and the insights gleaned from this research can carry societal significance.

Acknowledgement. This work was supported by the National Research Foundation of Korea Grant funded by the Korean Government (NRF-2011-330-B00080).

References

1. Steele, C., Aronson, J., Spencer, S.J.: Stereotype threat. In: Baumeister, R.F., Vohs, K.D. (eds.) Encyclopedia of Social Psychology, pp. 943–944. Sage, Thousand Oaks (2007)
2. Trusov, M., Bucklin, R.E., Pauwels, K.: Effects of word-of-mouth versus traditional marketing: findings from an Internet social networking site. Journal of Marketing 73, 90–102 (2009)
3. Baumeister, R.F., Bratslavsky, E., Muraven, M., Tice, D.: Ego depletion: is the active self a limited resource? Journal of Personality and Social Psychology 74, 1252–1265 (1998)
4. Baumeister, R.F., Vohs, K.D., Tice, D.M.: The strength model of self-control. Current Directions in Psychological Science 16, 351–355 (2007)
5. Baumeister, R.F., Schmeichel, B.J., Vohs, K.D.: Self-regulation and the executive function: the self as controlling agent. In: Kruglanski, A.W., Higgins, E.T. (eds.) Social Psychology: Handbook of Basic Principles, pp. 516–539. Guilford, New York (2007)
6. Hsee, C.K., Weber, E.U.: Cross-national differences in risk preferences and lay predictions for the differences. Journal of Behavioral Decision Making 12, 165–179 (1999)
7. Preacher, K.J., Hayes, A.F.: Asymptotic and resampling strategies for assessing and comparing indirect effects in multiple mediator models. Behavior Research Methods 40, 879–891 (2008)
8. Preacher, K.J., Hayes, A.F.: SPSS and SAS procedures for estimating indirect effects in simple mediation models. Behavior Research Methods, Instruments, & Computers 36, 717–731 (2004)

Reflection on Reflection: Daily Review of Lifelog Photos and the Usability of Wearable Digital Camera

Hyowon Lee[1], Nazlena Mohamad Ali[2], and Cathal Gurrin[3]

[1] Singapore University of Technology and Design, 20 Dover Drive, Singapore 138682
[2] Institute of Visual Informatics, Universiti Kebangsaan Malaysia
[3] CLARITY: Centre for Sensor Web Technologies, Dublin City University, Ireland

Abstract. The novel activity of continuous visual lifelogging, becoming more and more affordable with small, wearable digital cameras, allows a user to visually record a day's activities in remarkable details and review or re-live later. Loaded with privacy and ethical issues but still promising so many potentially positive usage scenarios, such an extreme lifelogging has many aspects to be further explored to become a truly meaningful, usable and life quality-enhancing activity. Based on the authors' first-hand experiences of practicing visual lifelogging for a number of years, this paper describes the usability issues of wearing a typical lifelog digital camera and reviewing the photos each day.

Keywords: lifelogging, daily reflection, wearable camera.

1 Introduction

While the field of HCI is mainly concerned about improving people's lives and interaction with technologies by understanding their activities and trying to support those activities with available or developing technologies, sometimes the process takes a reverse turn whereby an available or developing technology ends up inventing a new activity that hitherto people have not practiced (thus have not voiced their wish to practice it) before. A number of novel activities as a result of such a process are expected to pour out over the coming years as the new technological advancements in terms of computational algorithms and interaction platforms are fiercely explored, experimented and exploited into end-user systems, gadgets and services. The concept of "lifelogging" is an example of such a novel activity, and is about to become a more prevalent and common practice as more convenient means to "log" one's life is becoming available and the idea of frequent tracking and recording of one's whereabouts as evidenced in the increasing membership of Quantified Self[1] is becoming more prevalent. One extreme type of lifelogging is to use a passive digital camera to visually record the details of one's life in minute details throughout the days, and such an activity is likewise becoming more and more acceptable as more compact

[1] Quantified Self: Self Knowledge through Numbers. `http://quantifiedself.com/`

C. Stephanidis (Ed.): Posters, Part II, HCII 2013, CCIS 374, pp. 368–372, 2013.

and smaller wearable photo capture devices become available in the market and as the community of avid bloggers/tweeters find the value in these capture devices to passively record their daily lives. Many novel usage scenarios of such a visual and continuous lifelogging activities are currently being investigated in different domains, including a memory aid for Alzheimer patients or memory-impaired people (Harrell 2010), discovering one's lifestyle (Doherty et al. 2011), diagnosing the heart rate irregularity among the elderly (Mohan et al. 2012) and as market research tool (Hughes et al. 2012).

Currently there are no long-term "visual lifeloggers" with photo capture devices other than a minority of dedicated researchers who actually practice the lifelogging activity in order to gain insights and obtain real data from such a practice. Awaiting more convenient wearable digital camera products and more usable and useful software applications to help organise, search, review and relive the daily amassed data, in this paper we describe the authors' experience of practicing the continuous visual lifelogging for over the past 6 years, in terms of the usability of wearing a passive capture device and in terms of reviewing the photos daily.

2 Wearability of the Passive Capture Camera

According to Heckel's Law (Derrett 2004) stating that "the quality of the user interface of an appliance is relatively unimportant in determining its adoption by users if the perceived value of the appliance is high," the enormous potential value of the lifelogging activity will likely push the prevalence of such activities in the coming years as the general public starts experimenting and finding the values in their own terms, even if the wearability, usability and other practicalities of practicing the lifelogging activity is not yet at the level where one can conveniently and effortlessly engage in today. However, as better, more convenient, lighter, smaller, more consumer-friendly wearable digital cameras are starting to be marketed and software supporting the access to the collected photos are improved, there certainly will be more uptake of the lifelogging by the general public.

Practicing a photo-based lifelogging activity today means a considerable commitment in terms of wearing the device on a continuous basis. Current form of a wearable digital camera such as SenseCam and Vicon Revue[2] is a light-weight mini black box with a strap to hang around a user's neck, so that the device itself can dangle in front of the users chest. This causes a number of inconveniences and hindrances in day-to-day activities. For example, when the user walks very fast or runs (e.g. to catch a bus, or going up the stairs quickly), the device around the neck moves like a pendulum often hitting the chest or other nearby walls/objects. When running, one ends up holding the device pressed to the chest in order to avoid such a movement. Those activities that involve the person to bend down can cause similar issues, for example, washing the face,

[2] Vicon Revue: Memories for Life: `http://viconrevue.com`

eating, shoe-lacing and picking up something from the ground. Minor inconveniences as these will be felt differently to different people due to many different factors. Other more recent wearable camera products such as Autographer[3] and Memoto[4] allow the user to clip the device on the collar or chest pocket, avoiding the dangling inconveniences of their predecessors.

Other usability issues of wearing the device worth noting include:

- Going outdoor in the winter time usually means wearing coat or jacket, in which case the user should re-adjust or re-wear the device accordingly;
- As the device is not water-proof, the user needs to take a particular care on a rainy day outdoor or in the bathroom when washing hands or face;
- Whenever the user comes to privacy/security-sensitive areas such as toilet, gym and airport security points, the device has to be taken off and turned off;
- The user needs to be always mindful about any obstacles that might block the camera lens on the device, for example, when using a seat belt in a car, care should be taken that the belt strap does not cover the device lens;

Improving the form factor of the device itself would be half the solution as some of these are outside of the issues of the product itself. Lighter and smaller hardware that will not pull down the clothes when clipped on the chest, water-proof, an easily re-clippable or re-adjustable mechanism, and appropriate privacy and ethical instruments and policies need to be developed to enhance the wearability issues felt today.

3 Daily Review and Reflection

One obvious usage scenario for lifelogging without requiring much additional infrastructure or support is a simple daily review of what happened during the day, by the camera wearer going through all the captured photos in the evening. Reviewing what happened during the day, what the wearer did, where she was, whom she met, what she ate, etc. at the end of each day can be a very beneficial and rewarding activity allowing a self-reflection similar to keeping a personal diary but in a visual and far more detailed way, and in a far more consistently-captured throughout the day than a diary-keeping could allow.

Currently the software tools that support the daily review of the photos taken by wearable digital camera are those simply presenting all the photos of the day sequentially one by one, as in a slide-show. The number of photos generated by wearing the device on a typical day is between 3,000 and 4,000 depending on the kinds of activities the wearer was engaged in throughout the day, thus going through this amount of photos everyday takes time and requires considerable effort, concentration and patience. Better photo-browsing software specifically tailored for handling and presenting a large number of photos is needed. Use of

[3] OMG Life Autographer: `http://www.autographer.com/`

[4] Memoto Lifelogging Camera: `http://memoto.com/`

computer vision and image understanding techniques to automatically index, annotate and summarise/highlight the large amount of accumulating lifelog photo collection is one of the directions the computational technology community has been exploring over the past few years. Automatically identifying people, places and other objects that appear in the photos and preparing a concise and summarised user-interface (Lee et al. 2008) will help the user more efficiently and conveniently browse the daily lifelog photos over time.

Many small and big events that happen during each day are, by the natural process of forgetfulness, completely forgotten. Furthermore, during the events that happen we focus on things that are at hand, thus unable to notice many of the other aspects of the events that unfold at the time of engagement. For example, when a person is engaged in a conversation with a colleague in the office corridor, she is usually too busy with the conversation to notice other passer-by, new signs beside the door, clothes the colleague is wearing, or any other things that happen or are around at that time. Reviewing that event later allows her to view these other aspects that might be useful or even important in the way that would have been otherwise impossible.

Extending the daily reflection, one could imagine reviewing of a whole year at the end of the year - what has she done this year, what were the important events and what other aspects of those events can she notice when she reviews? Again, facilitating for indexing, annotation and highlighting of the important activities, unusual events or memorable incidents that happened throughout a year will be a powerful end-user support tool for browsing, re-living and reflecting one's life on a longer-term basis.

4 Conclusion

Shaping future activities afforded by emerging technological possibilities is a significant and potentially high-impact effort that could transform how we work and play in a major way in the coming years, but many aspects of these shaping can be better understood only after the early adopters start practicing the activity and go through exciting but expensive, cumbersome and inefficient trial-and-error processes. Awaiting for a more prevalent use of wearable digital cameras as a personal daily reflection tool, as a memory aid for the elderly, as an educational and training tool, or as a lifestyle monitoring tool in medicine, we need to go one step ahead by actually practicing the lifelogging activity and identifying and analysing important usability issues of such a tool and suggest how we could enhance the quality of such a potentially useful activity before it happens on a massive scale in the coming years.

References

Derrett, N.: Heckel's law: conclusions from the user interface design of a music appliance - the bassoon. Personal Ubiquitous Comput. 8, 3–4 (2004)

Doherty, A., Caprani, N., O Conaire, C., Kalnikaite, V., Gurrin, C., Smeaton, A.F., O'Connor, N.: Passively recognising human activities through lifelogging. Computers in Human Behavior 27(5), 1948–1958 (2011)

Harrell, E.: Remains of the day: can a new device help amnesia patients outsource memory? Time Magazine, 46–51 (October 2010)

Hughes, M., Newman, E., O'Hare, N., Zhang, Z., Lee, H., Smeaton, A.F., O'Connor, N., Farrell, G.A.: Lifelogging approach to automated market research. In: SenseCam 2012 - 3rd Annual SenseCam Symposium, Oxford, U.K., April 3-4 (2012)

Lee, H., Smeaton, A.F., O'Connor, N., Jones, G., Blighe, M., Byrne, D., Doherty, A., Gurrin, C.: Constructing a SenseCam visual diary as a media process. Multimedia Systems Journal 14(6), 341–349 (2008)

Mohan, E.R., Lee, H., Jaichandar, K.S., Calderon, C.: LifeVision: Integrating heart rate sensing in lifelogging camera for accurate risk diagnosis for the elderly. In: The 6th Intl. Convention on Rehabilitation Eng. and Assistive Tech. (2012)

Balloting: Speeding Up the Voting Process

Pascal Lola, Wanda Eugene, Phillip Hall, and Juan E. Gilbert

Human-Centered Computing, School of Computing, Clemson University,
100 McAdams Hall, Clemson, S.C. 29634
{plola,weugene,pwhall,juan}@clemson.edu

Abstract. Long wait times at the voting polls has grown to be one of the biggest issues in the United States (U.S.) voting process. To address this issue, *Balloting* is presented as part of a solution to speed up the voting process. The *Balloting* process gives the voter an opportunity to electronically mark a ballot at his/her convenience, print the completed ballot in the form of a Quick Response (QR) code, and on Election Day, the voting machine is used to scan the voter's QR code, which brings up the voter's prior completed ballot for review and modification before officially casting the ballot. A preliminary study was conducted to measure the efficiency of *Balloting* compared to other methods of voting. As hypothesized, the study revealed that *Balloting* significantly reduced voting time, which consequently reduces long wait times at the voting polls.

Keywords: Electronic Voting Systems, Multimodal Systems, Human Computer Interaction, Evaluation.

1 Introduction

1.1 The Problem

Long wait times and lines at the voting polls have become one of the biggest issues of concern in elections across the U.S. In the 2012 November elections, voters across the U.S. faced long lines and wait times during both the early voting period and on Election Day. In Massachusetts, some voters waited 2 hours to vote [1]. In Colorado, Virginia, and Texas, voters waited in line for up to 4 hours [2, 3]. Voters in the state of Florida experienced anywhere from 5 to 8 hour [4] wait times at certain precincts. Although the recent national election's wait times set a record in states such as Florida, long lines and wait times have been an issues in the U.S. for years. Long lines and wait times discourage and prevent people from voting, as evident in the recent presidential elections, where certain precincts reported voters leaving polls without casting their ballots [4]. As many as 201,000 voters in Florida were discouraged from voting due to long wait times and lines [5]. This shows the type of voter disenfranchisement long wait times can cause and how this apparently subtle issue can affect election results, especially in close races such as the 2000 presidential election in Florida where 5,801,000 votes were cast and a 537-vote margin determined the winner [6].

C. Stephanidis (Ed.): Posters, Part II, HCII 2013, CCIS 374, pp. 373–377, 2013.

President Obama recognized the problem with long wait times at the polls in the 2012 National Elections and as a result took a pledge to form a commission to tackle this issue [7].

2 Background

2.1 Voter Preparation and Early Voting

One of the societal needs in regards to voting is facilitating the voting process in general by creating more informed voters and extending the voting period. Today, voters across the U.S. are given different options for ballot casting and voter preparation prior to Election Day. Sample ballots, early voting, and mail-in voting are some of the few employed mechanisms of engaging, preparing, and facilitating the voting process. Each of the listed approaches directly or indirectly impacts voting times and lines.

2.2 Variables That Affect Voting Times

At polling centers, many factors can influence the total voting time. According to [8] the cause of long lines are: more people or items arriving for a given transaction within a given window of time, fewer points of service, and longer transactions. The length of the ballot and ballot familiarity amongst voters also play a role in voting time. Long ballots can detain voters and can be difficult to scan in some cases, forcing the voter to use more time to vote [8]. Stewart III [8] also stated that shortening the early voting periods has an impact on voting time. The availability of polling resources can also impact the voting experience and can influence the total voting time. Examples of resources include poll workers, voting machines, etc. In November 2012, South Carolina and other states reported problems with voting machines during the Presidential election [9].

3 Approach

3.1 Balloting

Prime III is an accessible voting technology that provides universal access for ballot marking and casting using physical input (e.g. touch or voice) interchangeably [10]. In conjunction with the Prime III voting system, Balloting is a concept aimed at speeding up the voting process; but it can also be implemented on other electronic voting systems. Balloting delivers a ballot to registered voters via an online system, allowing a voter to fill out a ballot via a personal digital device (e.g. mobile device or computer) prior to officially casting a ballot on Election Day or at an early voting station. Like sample ballots, Balloting provides the voter with ballot information prior to going to the polls. In addition to delivering a ballot, Balloting, allows a voter to start the voting process early by "pre-voting" (ballot marking). Ballot marking is an important and time-consuming process in voting; hence, Balloting focuses on breaking down this process in 3 phases:

1. Conveniently and accessibly delivering the ballot to the voter.
2. Digitally capturing and storing voter selections and providing a digital and/or combined digital-analog mechanism (such as printed QR codes) to encapsulate voter selections for later access on the official voting machine.
3. Retrieving the marked ballot for review and modification before officially casting the ballot on Election Day using the voting machine.

Phase 2 of *Balloting* is implemented using a QR code, which can be printed on paper or digitally stored on a voter's mobile device and later scanned at the voting station (i.e. phase 3). In phase 3, a voter's QR code is scanned using Prime III, which then brings up the voter's prior completed ballot for review and modification before officially casting it. After the voter reviews and submits the ballot on the Prime III voting machine, it will print the official completed paper ballot, which is then cast for counting in the election.

4 Study

A preliminary study was conducted to measure the efficiency of *Balloting* compared to other methods of voting. The pilot study used a 2012 ballot from Broward County, Florida to measure the time it took each participant to vote via a (1) paper ballot, (2) electronic voting system, and (3) *Balloting*.

4.1 Methodology

A convenience sample of graduate students (n=23) participated in a within-subject experiment. All participants voted under all 3 conditions--paper, electronic voting system (Prime III), and QR (*Balloting*) ballots. The dependent variable, total voting time, was measured and automatically computed by the Prime III electronic voting system, except for the paper ballot condition, in which a timer was used instead.

4.2 Results

In summary, the study revealed that *Balloting* significantly reduced the total voting time, with an average of 48 seconds spent voting compared to 3.43 minutes and 4.46 minutes for the electronic voting system and paper ballots respectively, see table 1.

Table 1. Study results in minutes. (items in parentheses denote values with outlier included)

	Min	Max	Mean	Median	Range	St. Dev.
Paper	2.71	9.88	4.46	4.25	7.17	1.62
EVS	1.08	6.49 (13.50)	3.43 (3.87)	3.22 (3.29)	5.41 (12.42)	1.43 (2.52)
Balloting	0.13	1.42 (8.00)	0.51 (0.82)	0.44 (0.46)	1.29 (7.87)	0.36 (1.57)

4.3 Discussion and Queuing Models

As the results indicate, the hypothesis holds true that *Balloting* reduces voting time and is likely to reduce wait times. As mentioned earlier, this reduction in voting time is a result of an early ballot-marking phase of the voting process being offloaded to a voter's personal digital device and convenient time prior to casting the official ballot. To predict average wait times, queuing models were developed based on the average voting times given a total number of voters in a given time frame, available voting machines, and other variables. The results of the queuing models showed that *Balloting* would consequently reduce voting wait times

5 Conclusion

The presented preliminary study shows that *Balloting* reduces voting time and may consequently reduce wait times and improve the overall voting experience. The U.S. President has made it a cause for national concern, exposing the severity of this issue [7] and we propose that part of the answer lies with *Balloting*.

Acknowledgement. The work on *Balloting* is based upon work supported by the U.S. Election Assistance Commission (EAC). Opinions or points of view expressed in this document are those of the authors and do not necessarily reflect the official position of, or a position that is endorsed by, EAC or the Federal government. We would also like to acknowledge the graduate students of the Fall 2012 Fundamentals of Human-Centered Computing course for their participation in this preliminary study.

References

1. Earthman, M.M., Rosso, P.D., Bartlett, J., Carroll, M., Sacchetti, M.: Voters Face Long Lines and Chilly Temperatures. MetroDesk. Boston.com, Web (November 25, 2012), `http://www.boston.com/metrodesk/2012/11/06/voters-face-long-lines-and-freezing-temperatures/AxiIAXKL8efZwxIfP0anJP/story.html`

2. Bronner, E.: Long Lines, Demands for ID and Provisional Ballots Mar Voting for Some. The New York Times Politics. The New York Times, Web (November 07, 2012), `http://www.nytimes.com/2012/11/07/us/politics/long-lines-id-demands-and-provisional-ballots-mar-voting.html` (November 25, 2012)
3. Osher, C.N., Parker, R.: Metro Voters Experience Long Waits in Colorado. The Denver Post, Web (November 06, 2012), `http://www.denverpost.com/breakingnews/ci_21939411/election-day-voting-begins-swing-state-colorado` (November 25, 2012)

4. Campbell, J.: Emergency Lawsuit Filed In Florida Over Long Lines At Early Voting. Huffpost Miami. The Huffington Post, Web (November 04, 2012),

http://www.huffingtonpost.com/2012/11/04/florida-early-voting-lawsuit_n_2072435.html (November 25, 2012)
5. Johnson, L.: Florida voting lines discouraged 201,000 voters statewide: Report (January 24, 2013), http://www.huffingtonpost.com/2013/01/24/florida-voting-lines-report_n_2544373.html (retrieved)
6. Belenky, A.S., Larson, R.C.: "To Queue or Not to Queue?" Operations Research Management Science - Voting Queues. Lionheart Publishing, Inc. Web (June 2006), http://www.orms-today.org/orms-6-06/queues.html (November 25, 2012)
7. Staff, C.: Obama forms commission on long lines to vote (March 28, 2013), http://politicalticker.blogs.cnn.com/2013/03/28/obama-to-form-commission-on-long-lines-to-vote/ (retrieved)
8. Stewart III, C.: Waiting to Vote in 2012. Journal of Law and Politics, MIT Political Science Department Research Paper No. 2013-6 (April 1, 2013) (forthcoming), Available at SSRN: http://ssrn.com/abstract=2243630
9. Truitt, A., Pou, C., Werts, M., Hooks, K., Kresslein, J., Ransom, A., Riley, B.: A review of voting machines in South Carolina (March 2013), http://lac.sc.gov/LAC_Reports/2013/Documents/SEC.pdf (retrieved)
10. Gilbert, J.E., McMillian, Y., Rouse, K., Williams, P., Rogers, G., McClendon, J., Mitchell, W., Gupta, P., Mkpong-Ruffin, I., Cross, E.V.: Universal Access in e-Voting for the Blind. Universal Access in the Information Society Journal 9(4), 357–365 (2010)

Adaptive Voting Algorithms for Group and Social Recommender Systems

George Popescu

École Polytechnique Fédérale de Lausanne, Switzerland
Systemic Modeling Laboratory (LAMS), BC 167, CH-1015, Lausanne
george.popescu@epfl.ch

Abstract. Nowadays online group activities are emerging, as individuals share their preferences, collaborate, discover and interact with their friends and family. Group recommender systems (GRS) use various social resources to make recommendations of items or activities that users are most likely to consume or agree upon. Thus, aggregating preference and recommending a common set of items for a group has become a challenging topic in online systems providing group suggestions and social websites. This issue is mainly concerned with the following three subjects: eliciting individual users' preferences, suggesting the maximized overall satisfaction outcome for all users and ensuring that the aggregation mechanism is resistant to individual users' manipulation. Furthermore, both individual and group preferences change over time. In order to track all of these changes GRS need to benefit from user interaction. This paper aims to present an innovative algorithm, which adapts to individual preference dynamics for group and social recommender systems. Individuals choose their desired items with the purpose of maximizing the entire group's satisfaction.

1 General Framework

1.1 Notations

A = set of n agents (individuals, users, persons, etc.)

$$a_i \in A, \forall 1 \le i \le n \tag{1}$$

S = set of all possible items k (alternatives, e.g.: songs)

$$s_j \in S, \forall 1 \le j \le m \tag{2}$$

$score(s_j, a_i)$ = score that each agent gives to selected items

$$score(s_j, a_i) \in \{0,1,2,3,4,5\} \ \forall s_j \in l(a_i) \tag{3}$$

$u(s_j, a_i)$ = individual utility and corresponds the score given by each agent

$$u(s_j, a_i) = score(s_j, a_i) \ \forall s_j \in l(a_i), \forall a_i \in A \tag{4}$$

C. Stephanidis (Ed.): Posters, Part II, HCII 2013, CCIS 374, pp. 378–382, 2013.

$l(a_i)$ = list of items of agent a_i

$$l(a_i) = \{s_j \mid score(s_j, a_i) \neq 0\},\ \forall 1 \leq i \leq n \tag{5}$$

$N_i = N_{a_i}$ = set of neighbors of agent a_i, given a trust relationship between agents

$$N_i = \{a_j \mid \exists r \leftrightarrow (a_i, a_j)\},\ \forall 1 \leq i, j \leq n \tag{6}$$

$T_{ij} = T_{a_i a_j}$ = level of **direct** trust between agents a_i and a_j

$$T_{ij} \in N,\ \forall 1 \leq i, j \leq n \tag{7}$$

$\tilde{T}_{ij}$ = level of **indirect** trust between agents a_i and a_j

$$\tilde{T}_{ij} \in N,\ \forall 1 \leq i, j \leq n \tag{8}$$

k = length of the final list of items to be elected

$$k << \sum_{1 \leq i \leq n} l(a_i), \tag{9}$$

1.2 Computation

The motivation of this research is to find a preference elicitation and aggregation method for a group deciding on a common outcome. The method should adapt to the dynamics of the group in terms of preference change, interaction and trust. Two criteria are important for developing it: it must maximize the group satisfaction, and it must encourage users to state their preferences truthfully.

This problem is a general instance of social choice and often modeled as a voting problem. We let A be the set of all agents and S the set of all possible outcomes that can be rated. In a group music recommendation setting, the outcomes are songs s_j to be selected in a common playlist. Each individual a_i submits a numerical vote $score(s_j, a_i)$ for each song s_j. This represents the preference intensity or utility for the respective song.

$$score(s_j, a_i) = \frac{rating(s_j, a_i)}{\sum_j rating(s_j, a_i)} \tag{10}$$

Thus each person estimates self-utility and submits the respective score for each song. Votes are given as ratings, e.g.: 2 out of 5. The voting weight is chosen as a 5-steps Likert scale and represents: 1="Strongly dislike it", 5="Strongly like it". We normalize them so that the scores given by each agent sum to 1. Then, we assign a joint score to each song that is computed as the sum of the scores given by the each individual:

$$score(s_j) = \sum_{a_i \in A} score(s_i, a_j) \quad (11)$$

As such songs' scores are stored and can be listed according in a descending order, for instance. To choose the songs to be included in a playlist of length k, a deterministic method that satisfies montonicity is to choose the k songs with the highest joint rating. This is a generalized plurality rule. However, this method is not truthful.

2 Proposed Voting Algorithm

As a method for choosing a joint playlist, based on the previous discussions, we propose a method we call the probabilistic weighted sum (PWS). PWS is equivalent to the random dictator rule: we iteratively choose each of the k songs randomly:

$$p(s_j) = \frac{score(s_j)}{\sum_{s_j \in S} score(s_j)} \quad (12)$$

The algorithm will choose the playlist by selecting one song after another using this probabilistic distribution. Compared with other social choice based algorithms, PWS is incentive compatible. That is, it is to the best interest of the individual to reveal his/her preferences truthfully. It is in fact equivalent to a random dictator method, where the dictator will choose a song randomly with the probabilities given by its degree of preference – a reasonable method since nobody wants to hear the same song over and over again. The probability of a song s_j to be chosen can be written as:

$$p(s_j) = \frac{score(s_j)}{|A|} = \sum_{a_i \in A} \frac{score(s_j, a_i)}{|A|} \quad (13)$$

In other words, the probability for song s_j to be selected is the probability of choosing user a_i multiplied by the normalized score that user a_i has given to song s_j.

3 Individual Preference Elicitation

The figure below shows the steps followed by each user and the system from rating generation to recommendation. First the users choose their songs. Then they rate those songs corresponding to their utilities. The algorithm normalizes the scores into probabilities as explained above and displays a song list based on these probabilities.

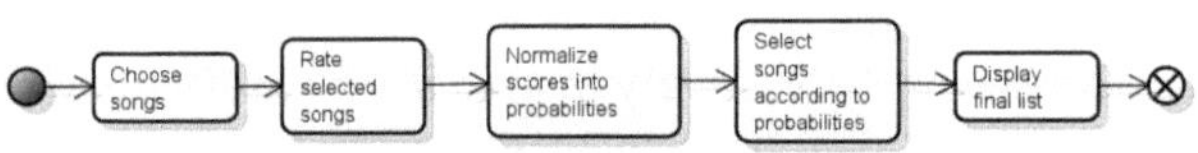

Fig. 1. The steps of the PWS algorithm

The recommendation list of songs favors diversity. Even though users will not get to have their most favorite songs selected, but with a certain probability, the more they interact with the system, the higher the chances will be to their preferences will arrive in the top k. Till this point we have considered only individual interactions with the system, i.e. individual rating. Each user gives personal scores to each of the songs, $score(s_j, a_i)$ which represent numbers from 1 to 5 (ratings).

4 Group Preference Elicitation

We now consider trust between users and define a framework for modeling trust relationships. Suppose users share their songs with other users. If one song is selected by the others then the level of direct trust T_{ij}, between the two users will increase.

For any song s_j we have the following score updating rule:

$$score(s_j) := \sum_{N_j} score(s_j, a_{N_j}) \tag{14}$$

for all neighbors who rated the same song.

$$N_i = \{a_j \mid \exists song \leftrightarrow (a_i, a_j)\}, \forall 1 \le i, j \le n \tag{15}$$

In other words, there exists at least one song rated by both users, not necessary with the same score.

$$N_i = \{a_j \mid l(a_i) \cap l(a_j) \ne \Theta\}, \forall 1 \le i, j \le n \tag{16}$$

N_i is the set of all trusted neighbors for user a_i. Until now we considered only direct trust between users.

Indirect trust can be computed by taking into account the interaction among users. We consider the case in which users critique the preferences of others. Suppose that each user has already created an individual playlist. For each songs in $k(a_i)$ the current user a_i has submitted his/her ratings. Now users can check other users' playlists and can submit their critiques in the form of "like" / "dislike".

$$critique(s_j, a_i) \in \{-1, 0, 1\} \tag{17}$$

$$score(s_j) := \sum_{N_j} score(s_j, a_{N_j}) + \sum_{N'_j} critique(s_j, a_{N'_j}) \tag{18}$$

The total direct trust for user a_i is the sum of all direct trust between all neighboring agents and the current user. We compute this as counting the number of times each other user rated same songs thus adding 1 to the overall direct trust for user a_i.

$$\sum_{j \in N_i} T_{ij} = \sum_{j \in N_j} count(score(s_j, a_i) \geq 3), \quad \forall 1 \leq i \leq n \tag{19}$$

Finally, we normalize this direct trust score to 1 allowing a comparison between the levels of direct trust among all users.

$$T_i = T_{a_i} = T(a_i) = \frac{\sum_{j \in N_j} count(score(s_j, a_i) \geq 3)}{\sum_{j \in N_j} count(score(s_j, a_i) \neq 0)}, \quad \forall 1 \leq i \leq n \tag{20}$$

We do a similar computation for indirect trust. For both direct and indirect trust we compute $trust(a_i)$ the trustworthiness score to an agent a_i, the sum between the direct and indirect trust for all neighbors.

$$trust(a_i) = T(a_i) + \tilde{T}(a_i), \ \forall 1 \leq i \leq n \tag{21}$$

Users are sorted by their trust coefficient. They are interested in proposing interesting songs and capture the direct and indirect trust of other users. In this way the GRS with the probabilistic weighted sum algorithm increases the group's welfare by giving higher probabilities to songs which "worth" being included in the final top k playlist.

5 Related Work

Addressing the problem of social choice with a general voting mechanism, Brandt and Sandholm (2005) consider the most general case of voting in which the users' rankings of alternatives are mapped to a collective ranking of alternatives by a social welfare functional. Such approach was investigated by: Hastie and Kameda (2005), Herlocker et. al (2004) and Ricci (2009). As an example, CATS is a synchronous collaborative recommender system, which helps a maximum of 4 users to reach a common ski destination using the DiamondTouch tabletop (McCarthy et. al, 2006). TV show experiments revealed important decision making consequences for the impact of scores and recommendations a recommender systems presents to its users (Adomavicius et. al, 2010).

Designing a Voting Mechanism in the GroupFun Music Recommender System

George Popescu

École Polytechnique Fédérale de Lausanne, Switzerland
georgepopescu2003@gmail.com

Abstract. In this paper we present the implementation of a truthful preference elicitation algorithm that favors item diversity in our group music recommender system, GroupFun. First, we discuss our methodology and relate to other group decision mechanisms already implemented in state of the art group recommender systems. Then, we formalize the implementation of the probabilistic weighted sum algorithmic in GroupFun. In addition to this we discuss user strategies and incentives for submitting ratings and show how PWS favors music diversity maximizing the group's overall satisfaction. Due to space constraints in the following we highlight only the main characteristics of our system presenting its design, interfaces and user actions.

1 "Home" Page in GroupFun

GroupFun is a Facebook application available at the address and hosted at EPFL. The "Home" page contains the visual identify of the GroupFun and three playlists: Top 8 GroupFun, Christmas and Lausanne Party. Three entities are samples of what GroupFun can have as output, as shown below.

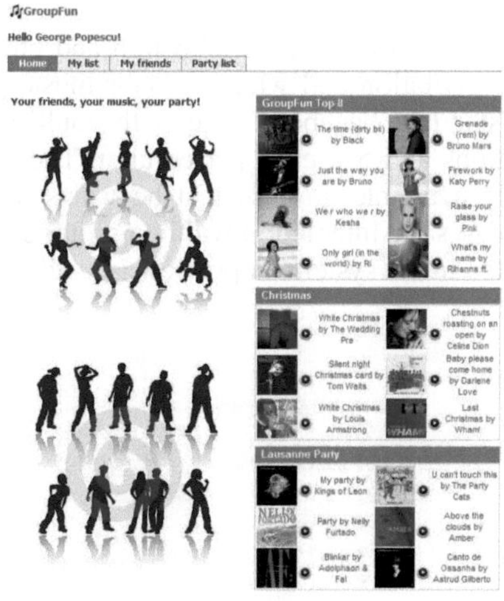

Fig. 1. "Home" tab

C. Stephanidis (Ed.): Posters, Part II, HCII 2013, CCIS 374, pp. 383–386, 2013.

2 My List

Users can create their own playlist from a number of about 10,000 songs. After the playlist is created, the user can rate the songs, as in the Figure 2. The music player, soundmanager, can help the user to take the right decisions. The user can edit his/her playlist and add/remove songs from the playlist.

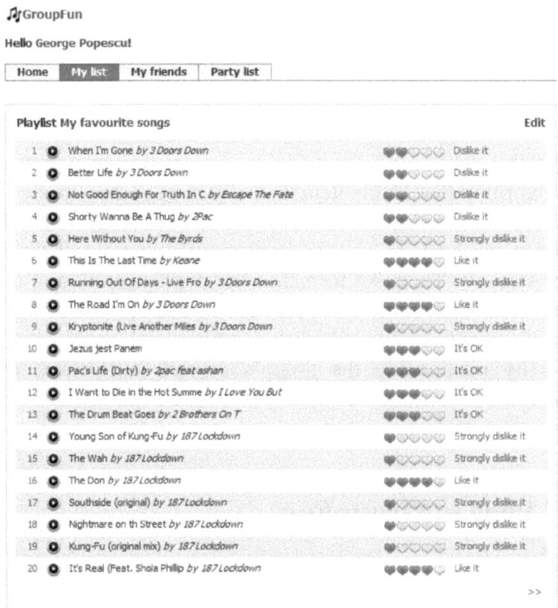

Fig. 2. "My list" tab

3 My Friends

The user can invite his friends to use the application and check their activity: whether they accepted or not the invitation and what are their music preferences. In the implementation, we used the standard Facebook request fb: multi-friend-selector, customized with 6 maximum invitations and 5 friends per column. The activity of user's friends in GroupFun is additionally available, in case that he wants to check their music preferences. This feature increases the interaction within a group of friends, as some users can rate the songs already rated in the system. A preview is available in the figures below.

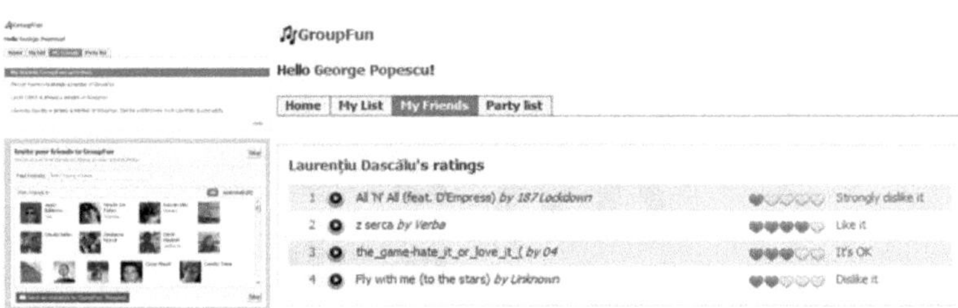

Fig. 3. "My friends" tab

4 My Scrobbler

Using the Last.fm music recommender system called "Audioscrobbler", we imported users data into GroupFun by taking advantage of the profile of each user's musical taste after recording details of the songs the user listens to, either from Internet radio stations, or the user's computer or many portable music devices. This information is transferred to Last.fm's database ("scrobbled") and then scrobbled again into GroupFun. The profile data is then displayed on the user's profile page.

5 Discussion

The total number of users, n, we currently have logged into our system is between 200 and 300 users. This is not a strict limitation since a virtually infinite number of Facebook friends can access the shared space of GroupFun in the same time. Some users may be friends with one-another. In this regards they may be strongly (or weakly) influenced by other friends' (or strangers') choices.

GroupFun offers unbounded preference elicitation all users: they can choose which and how many songs as desired in constructing their individual playlist. Songs can be extracted from a list of popular songs (like billboards) or can be searched within a shared database: the filtering can be set upon artists' names, song name, album, genre, etc. Users also may directly recommend music to other users or (sub) groups of users (eventually friends but not necessary) – they can send e-mail notifications to other user profiles using the same platform or they can interact verbally being in the same place.

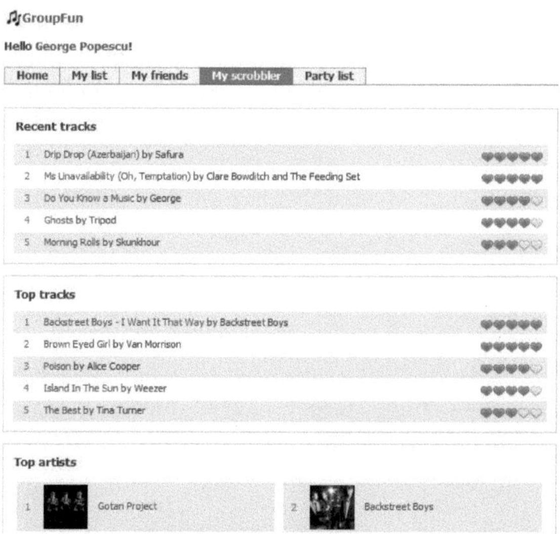

Fig. 4. "My scrobbler" tab

With respect to information overload, computational limitations and users' ratings we include an incomplete ranking of all items: users do not need to know all songs because they only vote for the songs they are interested in – giving their vote to songs which are relevant for them. The amount of user interaction through GroupFun is user-depended: individuals rate either the available songs in GroupFun or the displayed ones. Rating all group songs would be very time consuming considering users' time and interest in doing so. Here we rely on recent research that has provided design guidelines for reducing users' effort by focusing on preference dynamics.

In terms of the length of the common playlist, it can virtually be infinite. However, this case does not represent an interest research case since songs will only need to be ordered by their final group score and users will get to see all songs (e.g. 300 friends composing a list of 1,000 songs). Since they will not be able to listen or visualize them all we aim at recommending top k songs based on the probabilistic weighted sum algorithm, where k is group-specified (the group agrees on a common value for k for a specific event, e.g. Birthday party).

6 User Feedback

We used GroupFun in a series of pilot tests and targeted user experiments. The general feedback we received was positive, users emphasizing the need to "discover other people's tastes" that "match their own". From an interaction point of view our users mentioned the fact that they would prefer a system that is easy to use and intuitive, and would allow all members to have the same importance in choosing the common music playlist. The system's algorithm would then benefit the group by suggesting a list of songs that would favor everyone. Individuals also expressed their interest in using the predefined playlists, which would include recent songs, or are event-specific. Furthermore, our test users suggested that since both the music itself and the people forming the groups are equally important, it could be interesting to implement an algorithmic mechanism that would allow groups to compete among them-selves with respect to their music preferences, ratings, listening times, interaction, etc.

Design of a Web-Based Voting Application

Jerry Ray, Linda Harley, Keith Kline, Carrie Bell, Andrew Baranak, Chandler Price, Matthew Hung, and Brad Fain

Georgia Tech Research Institute, Atlanta, GA, USA
{jerry.ray,linda.harley,keith.kline,carrie.bell, andrew.baranak,chandler.price,matthew.hung, brad.fain}@gtri.gatech.edu

Abstract. According to the U.S. Department of Defense, over 50,000 U.S. troops have been wounded during the recent and current conflicts in Iraq and Afghanistan, many returning home with a range of conditions including traumatic brain injury, post-traumatic stress disorder, and polytrauma. These conditions can lead to impairments that cause difficulty with the voting process. Researchers at the Georgia Tech Research Institute have developed an accessible voting web application to serve as an exemplar of an accessible voting interface and to serve as a testbed to support research into ways to improve voting accessibility.

Keywords: voting system, ballot marking, disability, accessibility, human factors engineering, web application.

1 Introduction

According to statistics compiled by the U.S. Department of Defense, as of April 5, 2013, over 50,000 U.S. troops have been wounded in the recent and current conflicts in Iraq and Afghanistan [1]. Many of these service members have returned home with a range of conditions including traumatic brain injury, post-traumatic stress disorder, and polytrauma (defined as "concurrent injury to the brain and several body areas or organ systems that results in physical, cognitive, and psychosocial impairments" [2]). The resulting impairments, including physical impairments (loss of limbs, loss of fine motor control, or reduced endurance), sensory impairments (loss of sight or hearing), cognitive impairments (memory problems or difficulty concentrating), and emotional issues (frustration, loss of motivation, or aversion to crowds), can cause difficulties with the voting process.

Because these service members became disabled relatively recently, many of them have not had time to adapt to their new situation, for instance by learning to use assistive technologies. Furthermore, many wounded service members spend extensive periods of time away from their homes in rehabilitation facilities. This requires them to cast absentee ballots, which are often simple pencil-and-paper ballots with little or no support for accessibility. A more accessible method for filling out absentee ballots is needed.

C. Stephanidis (Ed.): Posters, Part II, HCII 2013, CCIS 374, pp. 387–391, 2013.

To meet this need, researchers at the Georgia Tech Research Institute (GTRI) developed an accessible voting web application ("Voting App") to support marking absentee ballots. The purpose of the Voting App is twofold. First, the Voting App is intended to serve as an exemplar of an accessible voting interface to demonstrate ways in which technology can assist in the voting process. Second, the Voting App is designed as a testbed to support research into various technologies and methods of presenting information to improve voting accessibility. Although the Voting App was developed to address the needs of wounded service members, the design principles it embodies can improve voting accessibility for all users with disabilities.

The Voting App is a web-based application developed with jQuery Mobile, a cross-platform user interface system for mobile devices based on HTML5, supplemented with JavaScript and Ajax. CSS3 style properties control the appearance of the interface. The Voting App is viewable on any web-enabled device, including personal computers, tablets, and smartphones. It was designed to be compatible with a variety of assistive technologies, in order to accommodate users with different abilities without requiring changes to the appearance of the user interface.

2 Design Features of the Voting App

The voting difficulties and accessibility needs of recently-disabled service members were identified through interviews, literature reviews, and other methods. Hardware and software considerations for an accessible voting system were identified, and a user interface was designed with features to address accessibility needs. Figure 1 shows a typical user interface screen of the Voting App, and the following sections describe the features of the user interface in more detail.

2.1 Ballot Design

Many of the software considerations for an accessible voting interface are in the area of ballot design – the visual appearance and spatial layout of the information in the ballot. The major ballot design features are described below.

- *Sparse layout.* Only essential information is displayed on ballot pages, to reduce clutter and focus attention on the most important elements on the page.
- *Large controls.* Active areas of controls are large to facilitate touchscreen use and to reduce selection errors for users with dexterity and fine motor control issues.
- *Large fonts.* The smallest font used in the interface is 14 point, with larger fonts used for critical information such as contest titles and candidate names. The sparse design of the interface allows the use of larger fonts without the display becoming cluttered. The font size is adjustable by the user.

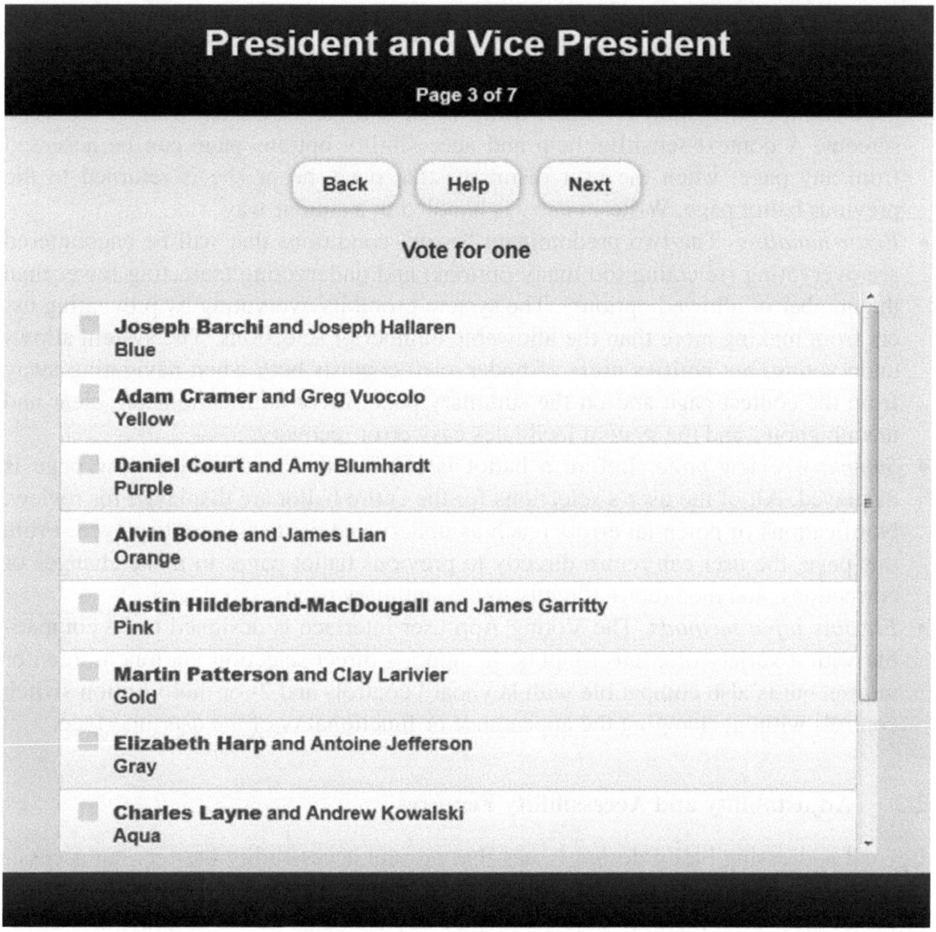

Fig. 1. Sample Voting App Screen

- *Mixed case.* All of the text in the interface is presented in mixed case for improved readability. Varying font sizes and weights and other techniques are used to distinguish headers and other information.
- *Plain language.* User instructions are presented in plain language to ensure that they are easy to read and understand.
- *High contrast.* The basic presentation of the ballot provides high contrast between the background and the foreground. Color is used sparingly for high priority elements like user selections and error notifications. Users will be able to select from an assortment of color schemes providing a range of contrast levels.
- *Consistent layout.* Key elements of the ballot appear in the same location across all pages. The page title or contest name appears in a title bar at the top of each page, along with a progress indicator. A navigation and control bar appears directly below the title bar, followed by contest instructions. Contest-specific information appears in a scrollable area that occupies the bulk of the page.

- *Simple, linear presentation.* Initial screens present basic instructions to users and allow them to configure accessibility options (or have them configured by someone else) before entering the ballot. The ballot is organized to present one contest per page. Ballot navigation is linear, using Back and Next buttons to move between screens. A context-sensitive help and accessibility options page can be accessed from any page; when the user dismisses that page, he or she is returned to the previous ballot page. Write-in entry is handled in a similar way.
- *Error handling.* The two predominant "error" conditions that will be encountered are overvoting (selecting too many options) and undervoting (selecting fewer than the number of allowed options). The system prohibits overvoting by preventing users from making more than the allowable number of selections. The system allows undervoting, but notifies users of undervoted contests both when navigating away from the contest page and on the summary page. Error notifications are clear and unambiguous, and the system facilitates easy error recovery.
- *Summary/review page.* Before a ballot is submitted, a summary/review page is displayed. All of the user's selections for the entire ballot are displayed for review. Notifications of potential errors (such as undervoted contests) are displayed. From this page, the user can return directly to previous ballot pages to make changes or corrections, and then return directly to the summary page.
- *Flexible input methods.* The Voting App user interface is designed to be compatible with a variety of control inputs. It supports direct selection via touchscreen or mouse, but is also compatible with keyboard controls and 2- or multi-button switch controls without changing the appearance or functionality of the user interface.

2.2 Adjustability and Accessibility Features

Beyond addressing ballot design issues that present accessibility barriers, an accessible voting interface must also provide assistive features to support users with a variety of disabilities. This includes adjustability of key elements of the display, as well as features designed to provide accessibility for specific types of disabilities.

- *Adjustable font size.* Users can adjust the display to increase (or decrease, if desired) the size of all fonts used in the system. The screen layout automatically reflows to accommodate changes to font size while preserving the overall layout.
- *Adjustable contrast.* Users will be able to select from display schemes that provide a variety of contrast options, including light text on a dark background, dark text on a light background, and an overall dim presentation for users who are sensitive to light.
- *Context-sensitive help.* A context-sensitive help system is available to users via a Help button on the control bar at the top of each page. Help content relevant to the current page type is displayed, and users can also access controls for adjustments and accessibility features through the help system. When the user exits the help system, the interface returns to the screen that was previously displayed.
- *Voice output.* The Voting App will provide a simple, integrated voice output system. Only basic adjustments will be available (voice output on or off, volume

adjustment, and possibly speed adjustment), and the ability to pause, resume, and repeat audio output will be provided where necessary. The voice output system will be simple and easy to operate for a novice user.
- *Save and resume.* Concentration and fatigue issues are considerations for some users. Because ballots can be long and can take an extended period of time to complete (especially when using assistive technologies), the system will provide the ability for users to save an in-progress ballot and return to it after a period of rest.

2.3 Hardware Features

The Voting App has been designed to be accessed from a variety of hardware platforms. As part of the current research, desirable hardware features for a device running the Voting App were identified.

- *Headphone jack.* The hardware platform should provide a standard headphone jack so that the Voting App can be used privately with speech output.
- *Accessible touchscreen.* The touchscreen of the hardware platform should be compatible with materials other than skin, such as prosthetic devices.
- *Interface with external controls.* The hardware platform should be capable of interfacing with a variety of external controls, such as keyboard, mouse, or button panels and switches. Wireless interface with those devices is preferred where possible.

3 Conclusion

Research and development of the Voting App is ongoing. An initial round of user testing was conducted to assess differences in user performance when two factors were varied: information density of the interface and input device type [3]. The findings of that testing were used to refine the Voting App interface design, and additional user testing activities are planned to investigate other user interface considerations.

References

1. U.S. Casualty Status for OIF, OND, and OEF, `http://www.defense.gov/news/casualty.pdf`
2. Lew, H.J., Poole, J.H., Vanderploeg, R.D., Goodrich, G.L., Dekelboum, S., Guillory, S.B., . . . Cifu, D.X.: Program development and defining characteristics of returning military in a VA Polytrauma Network Site. Journal of Rehabilitation Research & Development 44(7), 1027–1034 (2007)
3. Harley, L., Kline, K., Ray, J., Bell, C., Baranak, A., Price, C., Hung, M., Fain, B.: The Evaluation of a Voting Web Based Application. In: Kurosu, M. (ed.) Human-Computer Interaction, Part III, HCII 2013. LNCS, vol. 8006, pp. 285–294. Springer, Heidelberg (2013)

Network Propagation – Chance or Design?

Why Do People Share Online Content?

Johanna Schacht and Margeret Hall

Karlsruhe Service Research Institute, Karlsruhe Institute of Technology, Germany
johanna@sch-8.de, hall@kit.edu

Keywords: Network propagation, online social media, viral marketing.

1 Introduction

New media offer new opportunities. Does this also provide stronger influence over potential customers? With the possibility of ad block, the forward goal must be to develop consumer's desire to consume advertising. Having consumers' attention immensely increases likelihood them to remember content. (Cowan, 1995) This drives researchers to investigate the reasons artifacts become viral on the internet. What factors need to be in place to guarantee virality? Can there be a 'how-to' instruction guide? What needs to be considered when creating ads in order for this new advertising mechanism to be successful? In what way does the content of ads predict viral potential?

Placing an artifact online and achieving organic distribution through potential customers is the high point a company can hope for in adverting; it is cheap, easy and possibly fast, depending whether the artifact is being distributed quickly by the prospective users, is placed well on the internet, and reaches a lot of potential forwarders in the social graph. How can it be determined if the forwarding process works or fails? Is it possible to design a viral marketing campaign, or is success in these cases only by chance? Does the sending person make a difference?

This research investigates the design of viral marketing campaigns to evaluate the occurrence of virality. Section 2 proposes a virality research model. Using fifteen preselected YouTube video clips, we extend the model and review virality factors in Section 3, such as reach and activation, which enable artifacts to 'go viral.' Also under consideration are the needed attributes of artifacts in order to sponsor virality – the chance or design of virality. Section 4 finds and discusses that video clips 1 through 10 are successful in both spread and design, while the other five unsuccessful. The discussed results and future research of Section 5 reveal design implications for the marketing and social network analysis communities.

2 Related Literature: Milkman and Berger

Berger and Milkman (2012) looked into the '25 Most E-mailed List' of the New York Times to explore why certain articles became viral using a logistic regression model

C. Stephanidis (Ed.): Posters, Part II, HCII 2013, CCIS 374, pp. 392–396, 2013.

to predict whether an article makes the '25 Most Emailed List.' By testing the impact of the consumers' emotions when reading an article, and the benefit and reasoning from forwarding it, their conclusion argues that in order for forwarding to happen people need to feel some kind of activation and motivation. Their study shows that activation is highly correlated to the consumers' emotional state. In increasing order, the viral potential emotions they explored are disgust, sadness, anger, surprise, anxiety, amusement and awe. Also other categories like practical utility help virality. Milkman and Berger's results can be used for predicting whether or not a viral marketing campaign will be successful, but in order to determine range of success, more criteria will be necessary. Looking into the compilation data it is obvious that activation is very important in order to make a viral marketing campaign successful, according to the fact, that the most successful marketing campaigns were interesting and awe-inspiring or surprising and that the unsuccessful viral marketing campaigns often did not inspire a specific emotion.

3 Viral Marketing on YouTube

Like in the paper of Milkman and Berger the artifacts used in this research cover a wide range of different target audiences. Since this paper not only looks at whether or not something is successfully viral, but also at the success rate, a standard logistic regression as used by Milkman and Berger is inappropriate. The authors thus extended the formula to prominently calculate the even more important existence of emotionality and positivity, which leads to the quantifier as shown in the formula 'forecasted successes'.

$$\text{Forecasted Successes} = \frac{1}{a} + \frac{8}{36} * \text{emotionality} + \frac{7}{36} * \text{positivity} + \text{evoked emotion} + \text{interest} + \text{practical utility} \tag{1}$$

The variable a (average liked), measured via a convenience survey (n=27), a 5-point questionnaire where 4 is 'like the video extremely' and 0 is 'do not like the video at all', is the average of the answers of this survey for each video.

$$\text{Positivity} = \frac{\frac{\text{positive play time}*100}{\text{Total play time}} + \frac{\text{Amount of positive words}*100}{\text{Total amount of spoken words}}}{2} \tag{2}$$

$$\text{Emotionality} = \frac{\frac{\text{Emotional play time}*100}{\text{Total play time}} + \frac{\text{Amount of emotional words}*100}{\text{total amount of spoken words}}}{2} \tag{3}$$

Positivity is the amount of time, where the video shows positive content and emotionality is the time the video shows emotional content (including positive emotions).

$$\text{Evoked emotion: Awe} = \frac{6}{36}, \text{ Amusement} = \frac{5}{36}, \text{ Surprise} = \frac{4}{36}, \text{ Anger} = \frac{3}{36}, \text{ Anxiety} = \frac{2}{36}, \text{ Sadness} = \frac{1}{36}, \text{ Disgust} = \frac{0}{36} \tag{4}$$

The specific emotions, like awe, amusement, anger, sadness, disgust, surprise and anxiety, where determined through the convenience survey, by asking about the emotion(s) evoked.

$$\text{Interest: if yes} = 0{,}05, \text{else } 0; \text{ Practical Utility: if yes} = 0{,}05, \text{else } 0 \tag{5}$$

Additionally, the questionnaire asked whether or not an article is practically useful and interesting. The video is considered emotional when one of the emotions is shown or said in words. This calculation serves both to make the success rate results more comparable and to prove the correctness of the classification above, as shown in Figure 1. It is formed by the division of YouTube clicks and potential customers of the company or the people that are supposed to be reached.[1] Using this division the campaigns are more comparable to each other.

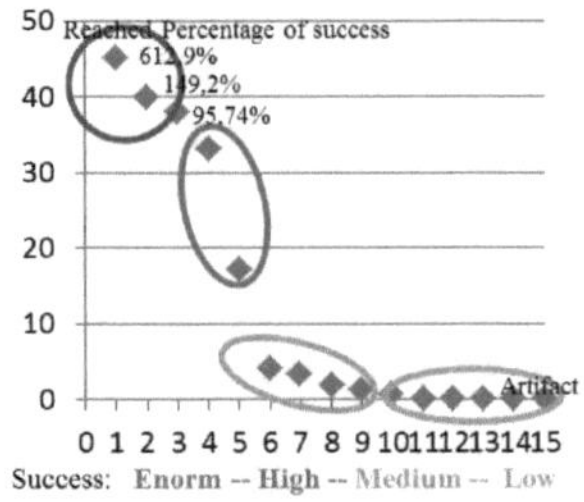

Fig. 1. Percentage of possible consumer reached per video clip (n=15)

The number of reached potential customers is only an approximation and not an exact number. The reasons for this fuzziness are numerous: It is currently not possible to know how often one person watched a video, nor how many people watched it at a time. Also while YouTube is a worldwide platform, not every video are accessible worldwide. Finally, this research does not consider how many consumers have internet access in the countries which companies distribute.

3.1 Context Specificity

Watching the videos one notices that the most viral videos do not seem to have a lot in common with the product they promote. The second question the authors explore measures the strength of connection between the artifact's content and the actual product the online content is promoting by calculating the length of the video compared to the time the promoted product is seen in the video (Formula 6).

$$\text{Percentage of time product was shown} = \frac{\text{Time promoted product is in video} * 100}{\text{Total play time}} \tag{6}$$

Also the total amount of words that are spoken in the video are compared to the total of words that mention the promoted product, Formula 7.

$$\text{Percentage of words that broach the product} = \frac{\text{Amount of words broach the promoted product}*100}{\text{Total amount of spoken words}} \tag{7}$$

[1] The number of potential customers is the sum of people living in the countries where the company is distributing (according to each company's website). 1,705,670,000 is the predicted calculation of how many people have internet access in 2012.

Again the average of these two, as shown in Formula 8, is a useful measure, because, as mentioned earlier, watching a video two senses are addressed – sight and hearing. The total play time is taken from the YouTube video and total play time that broached the video is measured and the time is added up. The total amount of word is counted as well the amount of words that broach the product.

$$\text{Average} = \frac{\text{\% of time product was shown} + \text{\% of words that broach the promoted product}}{2} \quad (8)$$

Figure 2 shows the correlation between forecasted success and the success rate of all fifteen viral marketing campaigns. They have a moderately strong positive correlation, meaning that success can be forecasted using the given criteria. Considering the correlation strength and samples of this initial study of viral marketing examples, probability of success cannot yet be determined or interpreted. It does however show a trend that using the above criteria increases the chance of virality.

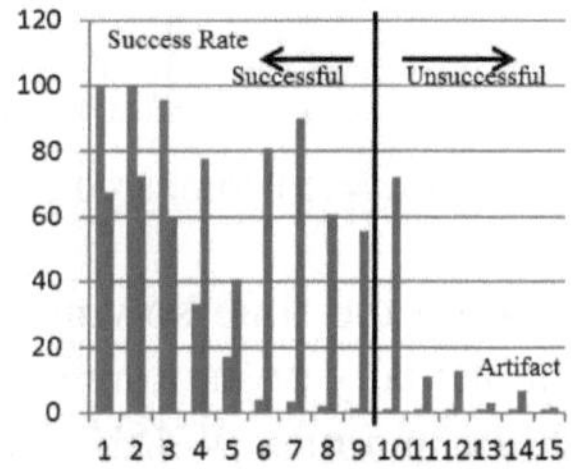

Fig. 2. Success rate decreasing (blue) and forecasted Success (red)

The connection between the total play time and time that is spent actually telling about the product to be promoted (Figure 3) is proved through a linear regression model: $f(x) = -4{,}69 + 5{,}77x$. When a company increases the percentage of time showing their product in the video, the chances for their campaign to go viral decreases. The unsuccessful viral marketing campaigns mainly reside to the right in Figure 3, where the percentage of the time spent showing the product to be promoted is high. Successful viral marketing campaigns mainly reside in the left side, where the percentage of time spent showing the product to be promoted is rather low.

The connection between the word total and amount that is spent actually on the product is proven through linear regression: $f(x) = -16{,}48 + 6{,}99x$ (Figure 4).

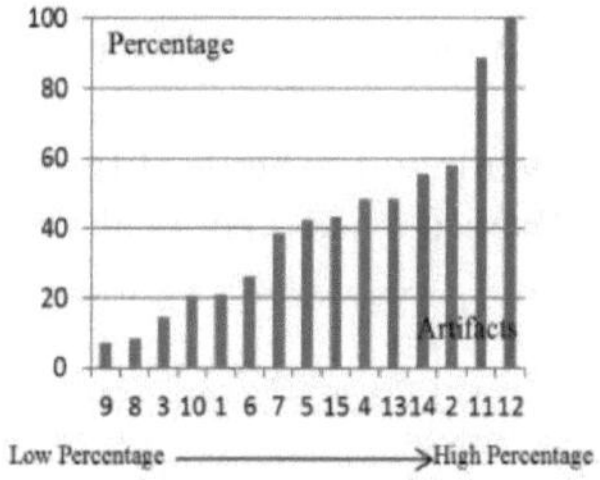

Fig. 3. Percentage of time referencing Product

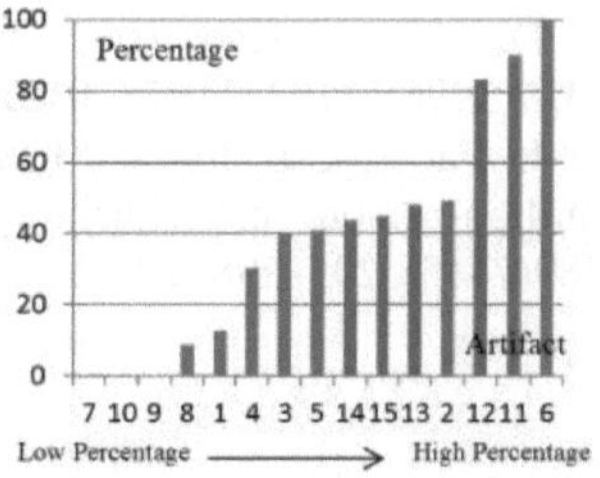

Fig. 4. Percentage of words promoting product

4 Evaluation and Future Work

Similar to the above findings, when a company increases the percentage of time mentioning their product in the video, they decrease the change for their campaign to go viral. In Figure 5 the correlation between the averages of the results of Figure 3 and Figure 4 and the success rate of all fifteen viral marketing campaigns displayed, with a correlation coefficient of−0,060.

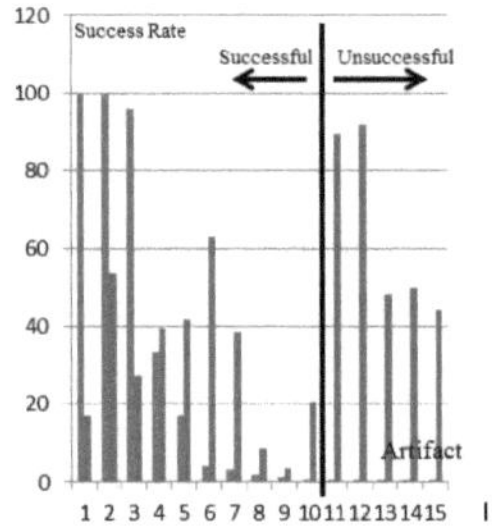

Fig. 5. success rate of videos (n=15) compared to product promotion time

In summary, it is useful to keep the time sowing promoted product between 5% and 40%. In addition word total actually promoting the product and the time the product appears in the video should be at a max of 45%. This creates the recommendation that in order for higher return on investment when attempting to start a viral marketing campaign, keep the average between promotion time and words low.Looking at the results of this paper, it becomes obvious that it still is a long way to reach a functional instruction series on making content viral. But what is for sure it is not only chance. One further research need is an impact assessment of where an artifact is published. Another area is linking virality assessments to social network analysis, and node placement. Finally, content appearance needs to be carefully researched.

References

1. Berger, J., Milkman, K.: Social transmission, emotion, and the virality of online content. Wharton Research Paper (2010)
2. Cowan, N.: Attention and memory: An integrated framework, vol. 26. Oxford University Press on Demand (1995)
3. Centola, D.: The spread of behavior in an online social network experiment. Science 329(5996), 1194–1197 (2010)
4. Bond, R.M., Fariss, C.J., Jones, J.J., Kramer, A.D., Marlow, C., Settle, J.E., Fowler, J.H.: A 61-million-person experiment in social influence and political mobilization. Nature 489(7415), 295–298 (2012)

Applying Facebook as a Management Method for the Teaching Platform to Develop Product Design

Chien-Kuo Teng[1] and Buo-Han Lin[1,2]

[1] Department of Industrial Design, Shih Chien University
[2] Graduate Institute of Design, National Taipei University of Technology
teng@mail.usc.edu.tw

Abstract. This empirical study investigated how to form a club with Facebook (FB) as an assisted instruction platform for design courses to observe the actual performance of a design agendum combining three design projects over three months. The research contents included (1) change of classroom curriculum design by proposing a design procedure for developing a FB-based design discussion platform. (2) Provider a concept for a visualization of dynamically exposed contents by developing a format with horizontal timeline that right-to-left based on the administration process of the three design projects. A feedback distribution map was produced based on two types of information, "Like" clicks and comment frequency, corresponding to the timeline. Lastly, suggestions for enhancing learning motivation by incorporating group activities, demonstrating fun and showing off characteristics were made in the conclusion.

Keywords: online education, design, social network, visualize.

1 Introduction

In product design, we need to consider multicultural characteristics and universal design concepts. After globalization, how to discover the localized value of tourism and cultural characteristics in cultural and creative product development has become a new issue to product designers. To the internet generation in the 21st century, the applications of social networks are thriving. It is an important trend that internet social networks with a prominent function in human communication that was arisen as powerful tools where people exchange knowledge [1; 2; 5]. In addition, it was the resources for the learning, problem solving, and self- improvement. According to Lewin [4], the new term "SoLoMo" appeared at the end of 2011 and originates from the social, local, and the mobile instant messaging experience, allowing us to more dynamically capture the 5w's (who, what, when, where, and what) of our friends. Lewin [4] described that" the online education company Coursera, its free college courses had drawn a million user, a faster launching than either Facebook(FB) or Twitter. Universities across the United States are increasing their online offerings, hoping to attract students around the world". This trend was also invokes gigantic marketing and advertising opportunities. As users can now "instantly" share information over mobile networks, instant messaging has become the part of daily life of the majority

C. Stephanidis (Ed.): Posters, Part II, HCII 2013, CCIS 374, pp. 397–401, 2013.

university students in Taiwan. Besides a social networking platform for searching friends and communicating via graphics and text, famous social networking website Facebook influences the gustatory, visual, and spatial experiences of users through the instant sharing of gourmet foods, designs, and videos. By uploading different images, users can share their world with friends and relatives. However, if FB has so many advantages, apart from sharing the bits and pieces in daily life, what other functions can it demonstrates in design learning? This study will apply a case study that investigates how to arouse the learning interest of students with the affective sharing of FB.

2 Out of Classroom Curriculum Scheme

When a course asks designers to associate product design with daily life, and the product must be presented the characteristics of a specific environment, event, or urban landscape. Then, designers will need to walk in such an environment to observe the characteristics within it. In practice, designers need to properly combine the environment, scenario, aesthetics, and functions. Did it still need concern during at online social networking? According to the series relevant researches [2, 6] that defines online social networking sites are "free online services that facilitate communication through an interactive network that includes the following: user profiles, photos, groups, email, blogs, surveys, chat room, wikis, social bookmarking, document management, instant messaging music and other media". Din & Haron [2] findings showed online social networking culture is related to knowledge sharing as a way of life. Cuéllar, et al. [1] suggest a purpose for personalized social network is extracted from the ontology, that a Learning Management Systems(LMS) could be a challenge to make further studies about learners, teachers and learning resources to obtain a better understanding of their social structure, and therefore to make or improve decisions about the learning process. Marques, et al. [5] was defined an investigation on the structure of messages on blogs and microblogs, two different categories of social networks. That "blogs are author-based (also called content-based or push-based) social networks while microblogs are reader-based (also called contact-based or pull-based) social networks. They was categorization of social networks is explained and some characteristics of messages' structuring messages in blogs were comment, reply and quote. At this moment, the alternative website of most people knows: FB has become an effective platform for designers to instantly share their experiences with friends through photographs and thus this study formed a group of 18 members with FB. In order to expand the space of design learning, we have designed three design projects for this course. Project 1 set an off-campus environment as the target for observers to experience the more real behavior away from the campus or the unmodified natural scenery in that environment. Designers were requested to capture the elements in that environment based on each group in order to design an installation with these elements. Although the characteristics of an environment are an open case, we can share, discuss and analyze the drawings with each member. As an extension of this study of Project 1, Project 2 requested each designer to design a single-function product. Project 3 will ask each designer to design a special product based on the emotions evoked by fairytales, sci-fi or action films. There was some point for the acts of process of communication were noted as below.

Differences between Virtual Group and Classroom Instruction. The aim of this study is to design and establish a brain- storming and creative platform for combing classroom instruction and sharing of the bits and pieces in daily life. With this platform, students can post or share their designs ubiquitously in the virtual space. Also, this platform will act as a reminder, such as the class summary and notes for handing out assignments. The design course in this study included three design projects; Project 1 is the group observation (two students in one group) to reduce the number of discussion groups to eight groups. Projects 2 and 3 will request each student to hand out work. This will facilitate the observation of the difference between group and individual work.

Observation of Graphic Records. Based on the outcomes from the class discussions and the instructor's notes, we can further share the project concept framework via this platform. Apart from a reminder, this brings more opportunities for brain-storming. In terms of sketch sharing, designers usually communicate with themselves with sketches but due to reasons of privacy, designers are usually reluctant to disclose their sketches. Also, whether or not the sketches uploaded are the ideal outcomes is an interesting question for designers might have doubts about their sketches and need their friends to approve them (by clicking "Like"). Therefore, the platform is another way to give designers positive reinforcement. The operating process of the FB-based design discussion platform is illustrated as figure 1.

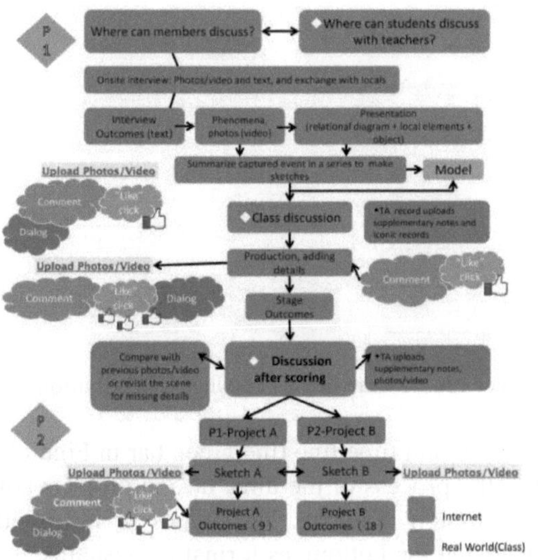

Fig. 1. Operating Process of the FB-Based Design Discussion Platform

Sharing of Personal Thoughts. Uploading student's concepts, sketches, and photos to the platform for group discussions may be not a perfect solution, but teamwork is always far more effective and efficient than working all alone. For fear of being embarrassed, some choose not to share with others when their work is not as good as that of others. This is not the intention of this study. Feedback (either comments or "like" clicks) is another factor affecting the students' intention to share. A "like" click suggests approval and positive reinforcement, and comments can be criticisms or suggestions. If there is no feedback to some ideas, students will be unwilling to share their work again. Therefore, deeper considerations are needed before implementation.

3 Visualization of Dynamically Exposed Contents

FB is an important tool demonstrating interpersonal soft power, and the dynamic exposure featuring the EdgeRank is the most interesting element. According to Kabasawa [3], the higher the EdgeRank score, the higher the exposure of a work will be. All stories are called objects, and an edge forms when there are users feeding back to a story (clicking "Like", commenting, or bookmarking). There are three elements in an edge: affinity score, weight, and time decay factor. After multiplying these three elements and the edge score of the object, the EdgeRank is calculated. Although users are unable to check the score, they can visualize the dynamically exposed contents as the reference for assessment.

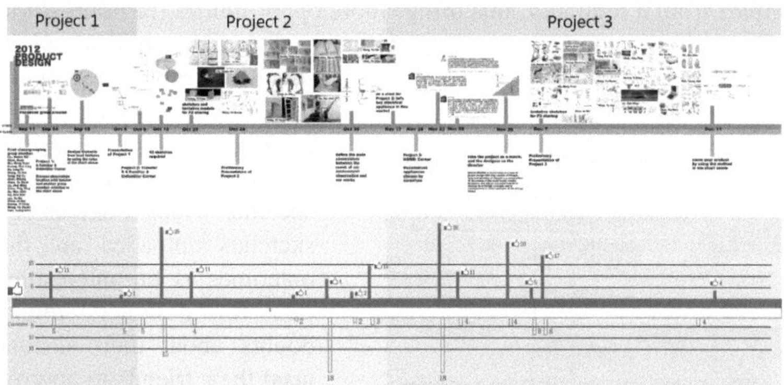

Fig. 2. A format for visualize of Project Club's Timeline as Feedback Distribution

This study produced a right-to-left horizontal time line (the green bar in Figure 2, a total of three months) corresponding to the process of the three design projects administered over the FB-based design discussion platform. Two types of information corresponding to the timeline are indicated at the bottom, as format for visualize show in Figure 2. The line will be integrating two parallel information with "Like" clicks (grey bar chart, minimum 0 click and maximum 26 clicks) and comment frequency (white bar chart with orange frame, minimum 0 comment and maximum 18 comments). Member response was low in the early stages after the formation of the club, but after sharing some course notes over the platform in the middle of Project 1, the first peak of feedback appeared. From then on, nearly all feedback peaks are associated with course notes sharing. From the review and discussion after Project 1 to Projects 2 and 3, we found that members were getting more familiar with the progress of the class and the club, as witnessed by the escalation of feedback frequency. The intensity also doubled (the peak appeared on Project 2 and P 3 began). These results as bar chart could show the formation of a club by emotional arousal by each month or end of one project. That would offer a visual massage to manage his education topic for leading its group to encourage or discuss and share other information for his members. This also affirms that design requires discussion.

4 Conclusion

The conclusions of the administration of this design issue include:

Enhancing Learning Motivation by Incorporating Group Activities. In terms of grouping members, when there are two students in each group, "group pressure" will be a motor to push members to work harder in order not to burden his/her partner. This is also a way to promote mutual encouragement. If we consider learning as a dynamic line, we can link up the observation and sharing experiences made at different times into a new pathway of the individual's special memories. By sharing the exploration outcomes of a specific environment on FB, groups can resourcefully update their contents. When someone clicks "Like", this brings positive reinforcement to the effort that the uploader has put in for this topic. This research also proposed a format that visualize for project club's timeline and feedback distribution. It would give administer an image to offer some hints more easily.

Demonstrating the Fun and Showing off Characteristics. In terms of design observation, analyzing a selected target may be a standard and boring procedure, and conceptualization may be narrowed due to prior experience. Human beings love fun and learn from fun. If sharing is a fun experience, this will be easier to learn new things. A boring thing becomes interesting when one sees it from a different angle. If we can share our discoveries with other people, observation may become more interesting, and the motivation to explore curiosity will increase. Requesting students to share after recording will increase the expectation of sharing.

Issues Concerning Members in the Virtual Group. Compared the virtual FB club and the physical class, the disadvantages was included that members without a FB account would be unable to participate in discussions. It would also be necessary to consider the privacy of members after joining the FB club and the limitations that the FB club brings. The picture right and right of privacy was other issue necessary to consider by the platform within on-line or internet.

References

1. Cuéllar, M., Delgado, M., Pegalajar, M.: Improving learning management through semantic web and social networks in e-learning environments. Expert Systems with Applications 38(4), 4181–4189 (2011)
2. Din, N., Haron, S.: Knowledge Sharing as a Culture among Malaysian Online Social Networking Users. Procedia - Social and Behavioral Sciences 50, 1043–1050 (2012)
3. Kabasawa, Z.: TWITTER NO CHO-PRO GA OSHIERU Facebook SHIGOTO-JYUTSU. Sunmark Publishing, Tokyo (2011)
4. Lewin, T.: Web classes grow, but profits trail. The New York Times International Weekly, by United Daily News (2013)
5. Marques, A., Krejci, R., Siqueira, S., Pimentel, P., Braz, M.: Structuring the discourse on social networks for learning: Case studies on blogs and microblogs. Computers in Human Behavior 29, 395–400 (2013)
6. Miller, E.M.: Phenomenological Exploration of Residential Students' Use of OSN Sites. Unpublished master's thesis, California Stste University, Long Beach (2007)

Film as the Future Information System

Katrin Vodrážková

Information Science and Librarianship, Charles University, Prague, Czech Republic
vodrazkova.katrin@gmail.com

Abstract. The poster will show the medium of film as the future information system, what are the future trends of imaging techniques, on what philosophical background we could analyze them, and how we could predict the future evolution of the film media. The film itself is not only the imaging, cultural, and artistic technology, but also a specific information system, which have an important impact on the changes of media thinking in our information society. In this system all the essential features from the photographic medium are reproduced, and are further enhanced by the movement dynamics, time, depth of space, and interaction. Film and photography are being based on binary coding and difference between the internal Self-reference of system and external Other-reference of environment. The poster shows the film medium as social system, which have influence on the model of reality in the information society and culture of electronic pictures.

Keywords: media of film and photography, media thinking, models of reality, formation of a form in context of information, communication, society, culture and new media.

The topic of the poster focuses on the film medium as a future information system. This idea for the term future information system should explain how the film medium can influence society, culture, new media, art and perception of each person in the information society and culture of electronic pictures, and the design of the information apparatus as a dynamic medium. The background of the whole topic is connected on the one hand with the area and theory of information science, media theory and communication, and on the other hand with the dissertation called Phenomenon Of Film - Information - Society.

The film medium is the form of new imaging techniques and will show how the form could be formed and how many classes and parts the system of the film really has. The film will be described as the special information and imaging system, better to say as the system of new display techniques, but the film is also held as a cultural, artistic and communication system. It is the unique combination of new technology and model of reality, which should differentiate the film reality and actual reality; in other words to the actual reality and virtual reality (Deleuze 1989: 84). Therefore the topic also speaks about the problem of time and space, motion and depth, interface and new imaging design of the systems.

Because the film is a medium set mainly on motion pictures, so the film as the imaging and sound system, this poster and also the dissertation is analyzing the medium

C. Stephanidis (Ed.): Posters, Part II, HCII 2013, CCIS 374, pp. 402–406, 2013.

of photography at first. The film resulted from the sequential photography and brought motion as the new and the most important element to the system of media. The film medium is reflexive and characterized as a self-reference medium (Luhmann 1996: 16). So the medium itself gives evidence about itself, can inform us and show us how the form and model of reality is forming and working.

The topic of the poster and also the doctoral thesis are based mainly on the system theory of Niklas Luhmann, who described the social systems, what produce the communication. The main thesis of the Luhmann´s system theory says, that the system can communicate (Luhmann 1996: 207), and each person should de-code how the system works, what are specific attributes of the environment of the system, what is the background of the whole interface of the media system. Other important authors who also present the discursive and semiotics methods are especially Flusser and his theory of apparatus and media thinking; Lotman and his semiotics of the film medium; Eco and his semiotics diagrams; Hofstadter and his theory of systems, structure and construction of figures; Deleuze and his theory of motion, time and space; Floridi with information and binary coding.

As the method the discursive analysis with semiotics elements has been chosen. That is the best method regarding the information science, media theory and communication sphere. The conception of the discursiveness itself means form, what can create other and new types of form and concepts. This topic and method will draw a comparison between the coding, symbols and elements of film, which are the special cases of new imaging techniques forming in the information society and culture of electronic media and electronic pictures. The discursive and semiotics analysis can also explain the differences between the inside and outside of the social system, or between the real reality and the film reality, what should be separated in our information society and type of culture based on the electronic pictures and especially electronic media in comparison to classic media, such a book or system of writing. These differences could clarify, how are special and new forms of the conceptual thinking (pictures, electronic images, electronic media, information systems) in comparison to the linear thinking (traditional pictures, script, writing). In our information society are people situated in the system of technical images like medium of film and medium of photography that means the third level of media thinking.

The main difference is that the medium of photography is static, whereas the structure of the film medium content is always motion. The medium of film is like motion in motion, because only the film medium has possibility to move forward and back in time. Photography shows us only one event at one moment, which is always happening in present or concrete time. The film medium can imagine and show sequences of many events and keep digressing from present to future or past. But the images based on these imaging techniques are everywhere - books, posters, information screens in shopping centers, shop windows, clothes, shopping bags, CD, DVD or Blu-ray disc. And the human being should recognize how the technique works and what is behind this, not only see inputs and outputs, so the man should scan every image to the depth, de-code each of those images and learn how to read (de-code) and understand them.

The point and goal is that everyone should understand the deep meaning of images and form the abstract thinking in the electronic culture and information society. Then the system of the society as such and people can communicate and they will understand the concrete message and also each other. Communication within a system operates by selecting only a limited amount of all information available outside (Luhmann 1996: 28). For the system of communication, imagination and information systems at all is the operation hold as the most important activity. Therefore the system theory is talking about social and information systems which are operative and have recursive structure. The motion which is still forming too could be also seen there.

The dissertation will show different and other forms of imaging and thinking which are inside the system and based on media thinking. The important element and other side of the media references regarding Luhmann´s social system theory is not the recursive Self-reference - formula, which refers to itself and which occurs in reflection in information and computer science, but the Other-reference, which influence the media thinking and relate to the thinking per se from the outside - from the external side, that means from the environment (Luhmann 1996: 24). The Other-reference is the most important concept of the research, because it can answer the question of the model of reality and film thinking, if it is the technique and apparatus or the thinking, what has the biggest influence and important effects on the media thinking and related back to the human thinking. In all cases the film has the biggest power as dynamic and future information, imaging, culture and social system.

The system will show the internal side with binary coding of media (Hofstadter 1999: 152), which are in the system inside, whereas the environment represents the external side. The binary coding is being based on the code "yes", or "no" (Floridi 2010: 28). For the economic system for example, we have money as the medium with coding based on "I pay", or "I will not pay" (Luhmann 1996: 42). So there should be always something on the one side which communicates with the other side. The "reality" can therefore only be, as Luhmann said, an internal correlate of the system´s operations (Luhmann 1996: 6). That means, the reality is an indicator of successful tests for consistency in the social and information system. Thanks the forming and models of reality and constructions of systems could a specific sense of communicative paradoxes be implemented to the information system and today´s electronic culture.

The poster and doctoral thesis will show the future trends in media thinking and use of apparatus with important consequences for the information society, mass production and communication processes at all. The main work and effective elements come from James Cameron´s first part of the movie "Avatar", who is also working and testing following imaging techniques and new forms for the second part of the film "Avatar": motion capture, fusion camera, HFR 3D, computer-generated imagery and other new technologies (Fitzpatrick 2010: 243). Also Peter Jackson will show in the second part of the movie "Hobbit" new combination of the imaging techniques. In the first part of "Hobbit" there could be seen the essential combination of 3D HFR for image and 3D sound together, what has influence not only on the people sitting in the cinema and watching the film reality in comparison to real reality in our daily life.

The form of motion capturing is also being used for computer games, what show us the second life. But the motion capture in the motion picture will especially imagine the motion from one point to another point in the film and virtual reality that means the real reality for the film medium, the motion which is permanently moving. This effect is typical for the fusion camera (Fitzpatrick 2010: 255), which connect the environment, time, motion and objects or one point with the depth of space and with the whole system of the film medium. In all cases the human being should be the essential article and the special 3D camera for stereoscopic pictures will scan concrete points on the face and body of the concrete character, who is implementing into the computer system for final editing. The apparatus of the motion capture and fusion camera technology create form, which has big influence on the media thinking in a relation to the thinking of the human being, and change the attributes of thinking while creating new forms and conceptions of imaging techniques.

This forming of reality construction results into the new forms of depth of space, new formation of thinking and seeing. The principal medium which can determine and move the media thinking into the deepness is human eye. Also Cameron and others will show how can eyes influence and change the media thinking in relation to the thinking of human being in the system of film or photography. Medium of eye is presented as model which determine the motion between the inside and outside in the system of imagination and communication. Medium of eye bring special types of information which is coming from outside, but every man should set his or her thinking in that form, that each person will de-code and understand the information via eye medium from the internal side. Eye medium as a complicated apparatus shows types of reality forming in the system of media. The eye is the important element using in the dissertation which connect our real reality with the film reality based on medium of photography, and will be having big impact on the thinking in the social and future information systems.

The current information system and forming of imaging and communication in our society force each person to think in a different way and first of all to de-code the sense and symbolic and deep meaning of the images, because every image is encoded, but could and should be decompose. For the current electronic culture are mainly the dynamic, speed and abstraction as characteristic feature. And the amount of information is a correlative of amount of times. Therefore is the medium of film, but also the medium itself hold as active medium in general, as it would be a perceiving and thinking organism.

Important in the social systems and for the information society is, that the human being is understand as observer. Observing is a special form of watching and make together with operate basic and principal activities of the system in a relation to the environment (Luhmann 1996: 162). What is interesting is that two levels of the observing activity are there. Firstly the observer is observing some object. In the second case should be resolved, how the observer are observing, so this is the level of observing of the observers, understand as the Other-reference. So the form of this operative activity should be found and recognized. The system is the society, as Luhmann said in his theory of social systems (Luhmann 1996: 173). And everything we know, all information, we know from the media system and film medium as cognitive system.

References

1. Deleuze, G.: Cinema 2. The Time – image. University of Minnesota Press, Minneapolis (1989)
2. Floridi, L.: Information. Oxford University Press, Oxford (2010)
3. Fitzpatrick, L.: The Film – Making of AVATAR. Knesebeck Von Dem GmbH, Munich (2010)
4. Hofstadter, D.: Gödel, Escher, Bach: An Eternal Golden Braid, 20th anniversary edn. Basic Books, New York (1999)
5. Luhmann, N.: The reality of Massmedia. Stanford University Press, Stanford (1996)
6. Avatar (film). Directed by Cameron, J. Twentieth Century Fox, USA (2009)
7. Hobbit: Unexpected Journey (film) Directed by Jackson, P. Warner Bros, USA (2012)

Multi-dimensional Aesthetics Mining for Social Photo Recommendation

Zhanwei Wu, ZhenYu Gu, and Zhanxun Dong

Department of Media and Design, Shanghai Jiaotong University
{Zhanwei_wu,zygu,dongzx}@sjtu.edu.cn

Abstract. The success of a social photo recommendation system mainly depends on its ability to provide high quality photos, which also means the recommended photos will have a greater chance to meet the interests of the users. We believe the quality of photos may originate from three dimensions. Two experiments was conducted to validate the relation of various features from these dimensions and the attractiveness of social photos. Result show, by integrated use of three dimensions, classifiers could be constructed effectively with fewer features.

Keywords: social photo, aesthetics, user study.

1 Introduction

Photo recommendation plays an important role in how people browse large photo collections on social network sites. To find visually appealing photos, many methods have been proposed from the perspective of visual aesthetics. The typical approach is to extract features and model it as a machine learning problem. Then, photos will be labeled or rated using classifiers and regression models constructed by those features. Most methods use low level characteristics [1][2][3][4], such as: HSV, contrast, level, histogram, etc. However, there exits too many low level features in photograph. It's hard to explain why some features should be selected, while others not. Recently, many high level attributes (which means more human centered) were proposed to address this problem [5][6][7]. However, most features are borrowed directly from photography theories without convincible reasons, rather than by studying user behaviors.

In this paper, three dimensions of aesthetic features are extracted and evaluated in a more intuitive way, by conducting user-centered studies. We believe, by integrating features that describe all the dimensions of the photography aesthetics, a more complete model could be constructed to achieve better performance. Moreover, not only image characteristics, but different types of data related to those photos should also be taken into consideration. For example, remarks may provide information that whether subject in the photo is attractive or not, mining EXIF data may reveal the quality of photography equipment.

C. Stephanidis (Ed.): Posters, Part II, HCII 2013, CCIS 374, pp. 407–412, 2013.

2 Experiment and Method

2.1 User Observation

First, a user observation experiment was conducted to learn what kind of key factors would affect user's social photo aesthetics evaluation. Take the fact into consideration that normal users lack of specific photography knowledge and could not describe their feeling precisely, we specially invited users with professional background as a complementation.

There are 10 normal users(non-design-majored students without professional photography training) and 10 professional users(design-majored students with professional photography training) taking part in our study. We requested the normal users, first, to randomly browse and then point out those they specifically interested in among all the social photos. By analyzing the observation result, we found that there were usually two stages of user behavior during the process of browsing pictures: the first stage was rapidly scanning the thumbnails in order to target the albums they may be interested in; while in the second stage, users would browse the pictures in sequence or view them in detail within the selected album.

The eye-tracking record showed that the average time cost in the first stage was relatively shorter than 0.7 second per picture. Moreover, most of the users' attentions were focused on the photo subjects. However, the average time spent on the second stage was significantly longer than on the first stage and the user behavior mode varied intensively according to user differences: some users scanned the whole album orderly, while the other skimmed or jumped over some pictures by "click and return". Still when viewing closely, users paid more attention to the subject.

Later we paired each nonprofessional user with one professional user and asked them to browse the social photos again. Under the assistance of professional users, nonprofessional users were supposed to pick up technical terms and describe the factors affecting their choices upon pictures in an accurate way. We concluded those factors into 3 dimensions: Attractiveness of subject (cute face, good body shape, graceful body curve and elegant pose), skill of photographer (subject size, angle, position, background simplicity, narrow DOF, accurate focus, light scheme) and quality of camera (aperture, shutter speed, noise, accurate color reproduction, sharpness, white balance accuracy).

2.2 Evaluation and Experiment Design

Though intuitive relationship could be found between visual quality and 3 dimensions mentioned above, to evaluate this relationship more objectively, experiments was proposed as follows:

Pre-processing of Photos

The main purpose of pre-processing was to filter out unsuitable photos, including three aspects:

- First, we found most pictures were screened out in the first phase of rapid scanning, without actual visiting, which consequently led to a lower click rate compared to the average level of the whole album. The user interview suggested that by simulating this kind of user behavior we may be able to filter out low quality pictures effectively. Therefore we deleted all the photos under average click rate.

- Second, the object of our study was limited to portrait photography, so we deleted other photos by using face recognition.
- Last, since the object of our study was pictures taken and uploaded by users themselves, we simply deleted those photos without EXIF information.

The Evaluation about Attractiveness of Subject

According to survey, the attractiveness of subject included various aspects such as: face, body shape, body gestures, and etc. The aesthetic evaluation of these features is too complicated for computer vision to handle with. Considering the fact that social photos contain various social information which could be used for aesthetic evaluation, like: the click rate of photos, the total amount of replies, contents of replies and etc. We premised that:

H1.1 Good-looking subjects will induce more clicks in the rapid scanning stage.

H1.2 Good-looking subjects will make viewers more willing to comment and thus get more replies.

H1.3 Good-looking subjects will give viewers positive arousals and thus generate positive comments.

If the hypothesis above can be proved, we then be able to use these social features to construct a classifier. So we designed experiment 1-(1) to test and verify what we had proposed.

In Exp. 1-1, we asked a user to randomly browse social pictures and recorded his browsing history. All the browsed photos were sent to another 10 users for rating, and we used five point grade scale: -2(ugly), -1(bad looking), 0(so so), +1(good looking), +2(beautiful). The average rating from these 10 users was regarded as the final aesthetic rating and put into correlation test together with click rate, numbers of replies and positive comments. To notice that when we talk about positive replies, it meant that comments containing emotional remarks about affinity, admiration and praises. Instead of semantic analysis, we actually adopted the method of detecting the corresponding emoticons.

The Evaluation about Skill of Photographer and Quality of Camera

In recent studies, photography rules, for instance rule of thirds, have already been widely used in photo aesthetics evaluation. However, there is no evidence that using rules is always better. The fact is, many photographers believe that sometimes breaking the rule equals to breaking new ground. We argue that it's the photographer's experience and skills behind these rules makes photos more attractive, rather than a single rule. Thus, hypothesis were proposed as follows:

- H2.1 Photos meet the rule of thirds rank higher than those not.
- H2.2 Photos of which subject size can meet portrait photograph requirement rank higher than those not.
- H2.3 Photos with narrow DOF rank higher than those with wide DOF.
- H2.4 Photos with clear subjects rank higher than those with dim ones.
- H2.5 The more photography rules satisfied, the higher ranking photo will get.

Besides, we also took equipment evaluation into consideration at the same time because: First, some of photography rules request for equipment support. For instance, big aperture is usually necessary to narrow DOF, known as "selective focus". Technologically, it is unable to separate techniques from equipment. Second, veteran photographers tend to use professional cameras according to the survey. It is unnecessary to separate them apart either. As a result, we verified another hypothesis in the same experiment:

– H3 Social photos taken by professional camera are more aesthetic.

In order to verify hypothesis above, we designed Exp. 1-2:We collected 50 photos of one subject and asked 10 normal social network users and 10 professional users to make a rating. Still the average rating was regarded as the final result.
Then we tested photography rules on whether it was related to the result or not:

- Rule of thirds was measured using midpoint between two eyes. Eye recognition algorithm in OpenCV was used for targeting the eye positions. We used midpoint because it was the visual focus from most photographers' opinion. Eye midpoint ranging from 0.33±0.1 of the entire frame were regarded to satisfy the rule, otherwise not.
- Rule of subject size was measured using face size of subject, which decided by the face recognition algorithm in OpenCV. If the proportion of the face area in the whole frame reached the requirements listed below: 0.5%-5% as Full length photo; 5%-12.5% as Half length photo; 12.5%-50% as Close-up. Then we defined it to satisfy the rule. Otherwise not.
- Rule of DOF was measured by manual judgment (on whether background is blurred or not.), because image-sharpness calculating functions proposed in previous studies could not give a satisfactory accuracy.
- Rule of focus is measured by manual judgment for the same reason.

Quality of camera was measured using EXIF data and divided into 5 categories: 1. Cellphone Camera, 2. Normal Consumer Camera, 3. High-Quality Consumer Camera, 4. Professional Camera, 5. High-Quality Professional Camera. Camera model library was also built manually.

Photo Recommendation Using Multi-dimensional Features
Exp.1-1 and Exp.1-2 explored how the features from 3 dimensions affected viewers' aesthetic evaluations respectively. In order to combine all the three dimensions and evaluate its comprehensive effects upon practical photo recommendation, we chose part of the parameters in exp.1-1 to construct a classifier and used training set to train it in Experiment 2. Later, 10 users' social friends albums were randomly selected as testing set. We recommended photos that classifier evaluated as above "good looking" to another 10 users and collected actual feedbacks as a comparison.

3 Result and Discussion

H1.1: negative; H1.2: negative; H1.3: positive;
Both H1.1 and H1.2 were not supported by correlation test, though click rate and the total amount of replies are widely used in many photo recommendation system. After investigation, we found most social photo browse came from friends which suggest

browse and replies have significant relation with active friends. Moreover, users browse and comment a social photo for many reasons, including but not limited to aesthetics experience. However, H1.3 were supported. Feedback shows, emoticons are only used when users experienced strong emotional arousal, some are mostly related to aesthetics experience.

H2.1 negative; H2.2 negative; H2.3 negative; H2.4 negative; H2.5 negative; H2.1 to H2.4 are hypothesis regarding single photography rule. All four hypothesis are rejected by t-test with 95% confidence level, though photos satisfy certain rule usually have better score than photos satisfy none. Among them, the effect of subject sharpness (H2.4) is the least significant because users rarely upload photos that are seriously out of focus. The most significant one is DOF (H2.3). This hypothesis could be accepted if confidence level is 90%. Subject size (H2.2) is an interesting feature. Out of size photos and full length photos have almost the same score, but are significantly less than half length and close-up photos. The possible reason is, taking a good full length photo requires much more skills than half length or close-up, which is

H2.5 is rejected by correlation test with 95% confidence level. However, photos satisfy all rules have significantly higher mean rating than photos satisfy none. Since rules studied in this paper are just a small part of photography aesthetics, a more considerable effect should be observed if we take more rules into account.

H3 positive.H3 is accepted. Photos taken by professional camera (4, 5) have significant higher mean ratings than photos taken by consumer camera (1, 2, 3). Survey after experiment also shown photographer using professional camera have more photography knowledge and are more skillful.

After studying the results of experiment 1, several features were selected to construct a classifier, include: emoticon number and click rate (from dimension 1), subject size, DOF and usage of photograph rules (from dimension 2), camera type (from dimension 3). 100 photos were randomly chosen from 10 album and used as training set. Another 100 photos were used as test set. After classification, 14 photos from test set were labeled as good-looking or above. These 14 photos were recommended to 10 users for validation. Feedback shown, 10 of 14 were rated above good-looking by users.

4 Conclusion

Social photo recommendation is a challenging task. In this paper, a model consists of three dimensions was used to explain user's aesthetics preference. Integrated use of aesthetic features from those dimensions could help to address photo recommendation problem. However, additional studies should be carried out to verify the feasibility of this model. Future studies could determine whether this model hold true for different types of photo aesthetics and for various kind of users.

Moreover, there are considerable features from dimensions mentioned above. Some have not been discussed in this paper yet, especially many photography rules. Additional studies could focus on validation of these rules and take good use of photographer's experiences.

One classifier evaluated by participants in this study, using features mentioned above, proved to be effective for photo recommendation. However, several features are decided by manual judgment instead of computer processing, though some calculating functions have already been proposed in previous studies. The main reason is to ensure accuracy. Thus, to improve the accuracy of these functions might be the basis for the future studies.

References

1. Datta, R., Joshi, D., Li, J., Wang, J.Z.: Studying aesthetics in photographic images using a computational approach. In: Leonardis, A., Bischof, H., Pinz, A. (eds.) ECCV 2006, Part III. LNCS, vol. 3953, pp. 288–301. Springer, Heidelberg (2006)
2. Luo, Y., Tang, X.: Photo and video quality evaluation: Focusing on the subject. In: Forsyth, D., Torr, P., Zisserman, A. (eds.) ECCV 2008, Part III. LNCS, vol. 5304, pp. 386–399. Springer, Heidelberg (2008)
3. Dalal, N., Triggs, B.: Histograms of oriented gradients for human detection. In: CVPR (1), pp. 886–893. IEEE Computer Society (2005)
4. Li, C., Chen, T.: Aesthetic visual quality assessment of paintings. IEEE Journal of Selected Topics in Signal Processing 3(2), 236–252 (2009)
5. Cerosaletti, C.D., Loui, A.C.: Measuring the perceived aesthetic quality of photographic images. In: First International Workshop on Quality of Multimedia Experience, QoMEX, pp. 47–52 (2009)
6. Jiang, W., Loui, A.C., Cerosaletti, C.D.: Automatic aesthetic value assessment in photographic images. In: ICME, pp. 920–925. IEEE (2010)
7. Dhar, S., Ordonez, V., Berg, T.L.: High level describable attributes for predicting aesthetics and interestingness. In: CVPR, pp. 1657–1664 (2011)

Aisthésis of Communication Visualization through Twitter

Miohk Yoo and Kyoungju Park

GSAIM, Chung-Ang University, Korea
vogue901@naver.com, kjpark@cau.ac.kr

Abstract. As technology develops, the communication methods are diversified, and, among them, the social network service (SNS) becomes popular by spreading intuitive and instant messages in cyber-physical space. Due to its unique features, this SNS-based communication inspires many media artists, who produced the visualized artworks after analyzing and extracting text messages on the SNS. We produce a prototype for interactive art installations, which involves audiences, analyzes the Twitter messages between audiences and many others, and visualizes the data on the screen in 3D, so that the audiences can experience and enjoy sensual Aisthésis of their communications. The works are made as follows. Once the Twitter messages are sent to the randomly designated accounts, they are animated by varying properties, such as the translation, rotation, font size, and color, and then the animated messages overlay with thc existing messages that other audiences already sent. The animation follows either predefined shapes or paths, changes the velocity of message, and swings the individual letters of messages randomly. (To better express the process of mutual communications through twitter messages,) We also visualize the animated messages in 3D space that allows changing camera viewing and lighting, and divide messages into letter by letter so that each letter are able to be animated as a single object.

Keywords: Twitter, SNS, Aisthésis, Information Visualization, Media Art.

1 Introduction

With the high penetration of smart mobile phones and the constant development of ubiquitous environment and its relevant technologies and ideas, the public has easily faced and experienced such environment. Besides, social networking service (SNS) in which smooth communication among multiple people is made possible has been on the rise [1]. SNS is a sort of networking service that has the advantage of the temporal and spatial flexibility to send simple messages and experience mutual communication through direct and indirect communication structures [2]. With diversification of the types and methods of mutual communication participation, the interactive artworks that focus on multiple-communication are very interesting. As a feature of SNS, the smooth multiple-communication way can be used to present the interactive art that has the linear and spatial restriction shape in diversified ways.

In this paper proposes the diversified presentation methods and possibility of interactive art on the basis of the SNS feature described earlier. It gives both spectators

C. Stephanidis (Ed.): Posters, Part II, HCII 2013, CCIS 374, pp. 413–417, 2013.

and others in a different space an opportunity to provide a variety of experiential factors of media art by combining SNS with interactive art. By combining the mutual communication networking of SNS with the media art leading aisthésis, this work produces a system through which spectators who look at artworks in an exhibition space share aisthésis with SNS users in a different space, and telepresent about mutual communication between users, and thereby tests the environment where aisthésis is delivered through "HOSHI" and "KKAMUU".

2 Aisthésis of Interactive Art

Aisthésis appears in the cognitive processes of a genuine existence through human sensible perception. Also, people understand and experience this, realizing essential and genuine meaning through experience of sensitivity, sense and perception [3]. Interactive Art is a part in Art that chances audience can experience personally are occurred frequently [4]. For audience, art formation such as movement change and finishing work with their experience through audience's intervention is very interested. Also, work of Interactive Art that can make a work of art with human various and sensible components using five senses, has sensible experience with interaction of various approach in contrast to earlier approaches. This is used as possibility that when audience encounter works, they experience this directly, and audience's experience at accepting sensuously experiences things artist wants to express sensuously through subjective reinterpretation.

3 Related Works

Interactive art is a form of art that involves spectators in a way that they interact with artworks, offering multiple spectators experiential experiences [5]. The art form that uses interactive art and the temporal and spatial mutual communication way of SNS plays a role to offer spectators direct and indirect experiential factors and drawing the empathy and communication between spectators and users. For example, Jon Montengro's 'happyrain' in 2011 used social media information in twitter. Twitter messages are information of designated time, and are comprised of sensitivity messages involved happiness [6]. Also, independent messages are personified with shape like rain, so message color is expressed variously. Lee Jun's 'A dream of tree' [7] is an installation work impacted a meaning that vitality of dead branches is recovered; with using twitter messages involved a city [Fig.1].

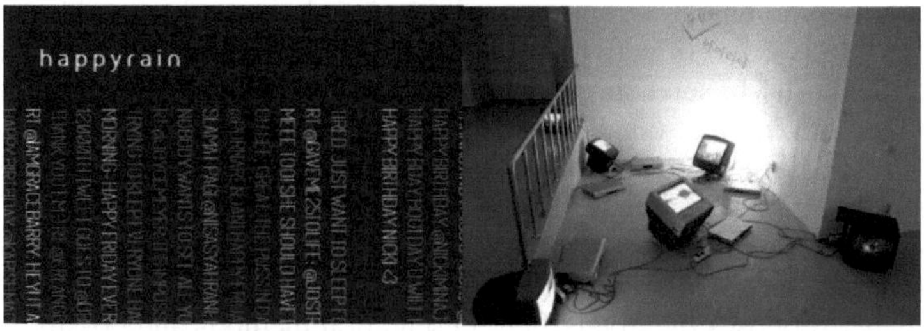

Fig. 1. "happyrain" and "Dream of Tree"

4 Concept of Artwork "HOSHI" and "KKAMUU"

To reflect to concept based on above-suggested SNS characteristic and aesthesis of Interactive Art, basic components are twitter and typography design, so with borrowing these, work is formed. Therefore, system structure, aesthesis, multilateral communication and sharing telepresent, is made through messages from audience seeing exhibition. Both artworks have been installed in exhibitions by visualizing the communication between audiences and random other people, and by providing the sensual experience of the communications in cyber-physical space.

4.1 "HOSHI"

"HOSHI" [8], in which there are existing messages in 3D space, new messages are generated and are harmonized with the existing messages after undergoing the camera viewing and text color change. New message color is changed, so camera is zoomed in. Therefore, audience can enjoy messages they send, in real time. These messages not create once thence become extinct, but coexist with as-found text as optical typography with new messages in 3D space.

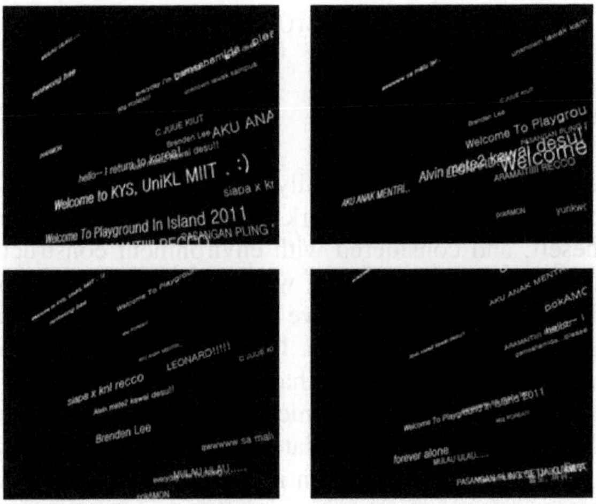

Fig. 2. "HOSHI" Artwork Screen image

4.2 "KKAMUU"

"KKAMUU", in which the new messages are divided into each letter, the letter is animated following the shape of the designated 2D image texture, and is gathered together on the bottom of the image in the end. Messages received form twitter are exposed to the top of tail of cat texture fixed in 2D, so legibility and meaning of messages appearance are given by audience. And then, after about 2 seconds, each independent shaped text is animated and is accumulated so is piled up among texts. Texts which are stored before are located under cat texture, and visualize like Figure.3 in limited texture space.

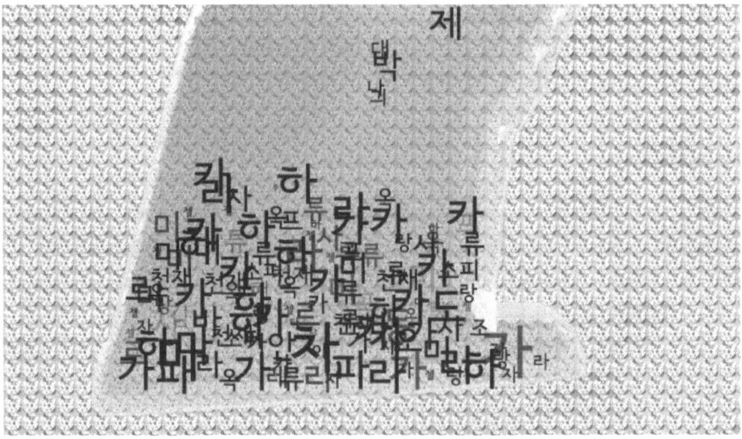

Fig. 3. "KKAMUU" Screen image

5 Conclusion

The thesis made Media Art experimentally with SNS characteristic, delivered a telepresent differentiated from as-found work with suggesting connected passageway to communicate oneself, and considered with environment construction that people do aisthésis of mutual communication, and work producing. Also, the thesis suggested the possibility that aisthésis of Interactive Art is amalgamated, based on characteristics such as free mutual communication, liquidity of time and space, and delivering telepresent among active parts that SNS has, so telepresent is delivered, is shared and is communicated with network communication between audience in exhibition and non-exhibition, so communion of multilateral aisthésis is maximized. SNS can supplement the limitation of exhibition form in interactive art with freedom of time and space. In the future works, if people use not only text but also various media such as image, video and sound, it will be possible to make production environment of various Interactive Art rather than aisthésis in as-found.

References

1. Sung, J.-S.: A Study of Contents Secure in Smart Phone, Security Engineering Research Support Center. Journal of Security Engineering 8, 665–672 (2011)
2. Boyd, D.M., Ellison, N.B.: Social Network Sites: Definition, History, and Scholarship. Journal of Computer-Mediated Communication 13(1), 210–230 (2007)
3. Ranciere, J.: Thinking between disciplines: an aesthetics of knowledge. Parrhesia 1 (2006)

4. Lee, S.J.: Die Kunstlehre bei M. Heidegger. Heidegger-Gesellschaft in Korea, 7, 209–243 (2002)
5. Jung, H.H.: A study on the Aesthetic Characteristics of Digital Art. Korea Digital Design Council 33, 203–212 (2012)
6. http://www.variousways.com/blog/2011/03/happyrain-twitter-art/
7. Korean Cultural Service New York, http://www.koreanculture.org/?document_srl=28834&mid=cr_exhibitions
8. Hoshi, Digital Playground in Island, in Malaysia, International Exhibition, Total Museum (2012)

A Study on Intention Network Modeling Based on User's Interest Web-Page

Taebok Yoon[1] and Jee-Hyong Lee[2]

[1] Department of Computer Software, Seoil University, Seoul, Korea
[2] Department of Computer Engineering, Sungkyunkwan University, Suwon, Korea
tbyoon@seoil.ac.kr

Abstract. There are various studies to try to provide useful information to users in the Web. Web usage mining is a method to extract meaningful patterns based on web users' log data. Most of existing approaches of web usage mining, however, had not considered users' diverse intention but created general models. Web users' search keywords can have various meaning upon their preference and context. This study is for generating the User Intent Network Model (UIN-Model) after collecting and analyzing web usage information corresponding to keywords. UIN-Model can supply web page navigation networks reflecting users' various intention information. It can also be used to recommend most proper web pages and it has been confirmed that the suggested method was useful enough.

Keywords: UIN-Model, Web Mining, User Preference.

1 Introduction

Upon development of Information Technology, information on websites are rapidly increasing so that people should spend more time and make more effort to get right information that they want. Therefore, there are various studies to attempt to reduce the burdens. The studies can be sorted into two parts: a study to understand contents and structure of web pages [1] and a study to analyze a web-user's choice on web pages [2]. The contents and structure of web pages can be understood by analyzing images, texts or video in the pages, or by analyzing the stratified structure and linking structure of websites. To analyze a web-user's choice on web pages, the web user's activity, such as visiting pages and choosing menus, are logged. There are also several researches to analyze a user's visited web pages by observing mouse drags and clicks, or keyboard typing. However, the existing analysis and estimation on web pages is limited so that it is hard to offer services that consider various users' intention. For example, let us assume there is a keyword of "soccer". What comes across in your mind first? It reminds someone soccer games like World-cup or Champion's leagues, famous soccer players like “Pelé”, “Maradona” or “Ji-Sung Park”, or soccer supplies like soccer balls, shoes or uniforms. A keyword, thus, can have diverse meanings for users upon their preference, context and current status. It may not be said as an

C. Stephanidis (Ed.): Posters, Part II, HCII 2013, CCIS 374, pp. 418–421, 2013.

intelligent and applicable service if users have common results on their interest keywords in spite of their diverse intention. The User Intent Network Model (UIN-Model) is a navigation network that can reflect users various search intention, generated by reviewing web pages that users hit on keywords. Also, we collect the web users' web page visiting information with a keyword and create the UIN-Model as a model of navigation patterns according to search intention. The UIN-Model is useful for recommending web pages, advertisements upon keywords and grasping the meaning that a user intended to represent.

2 Related Works

Researches related to recommending web pages to supply meaningful information related to users' interest keywords are very diverse. Joh et al. [3] and Hay et al. [4] illustrated sequence alignments of web-users activities and compared the similarities among them, and Sufyan and ahmad[5] studied web search enhancement by mining users' actions to analyze their website visiting information. Also, Ahmed et al. [6] was introduced the methods to know the user's interest using Web log.

These existing researches collect and analyze web-users log information, find out patterns and model their web using information. Those models utilize standard technology to perform services like automation, intelligence and personalization types etc. Those, however, have limited features for their extent of usage due to their models which did not regard various users' intention. It is necessary to analyze various users' intention and research to reflect them to create models.

3 Design of UIN-Model

On web environment, users can access any website to get information that they wanted through various searching engines like Google, Yahoo, Naver etc. If a user searches with a keyword and reviewed a website carefully, the information can be used as useful information to recommend web-searching.

The user's interest keyword, user ID and user's activity information on the website can be tools to measure how visited web page was meaningful for the user. There is many users' activity information on visited web pages: user ID to distinguish users, browsed website URL by using interest keywords, starting and ending time of web pages, activities of download, copy and paste and bookmark, contents size of web pages etc. Web-page scoring must be used to value a website in number. We need to consider how each of elements affects each other for scoring. Each element can decide importance by using weight value. The numerical formula as below has been used to measure how important a web-page for a user regarding weight of each element.

$$PageWeight_j = 1 - \left[\frac{1}{\sum_{i=0}^{n} (C_i \bullet Attribute_i)} \right] \tag{1}$$

PageWeight$_j$ means the weight of web-page ***j*** among various referred pages based on some keyword, and ***n*** means number of elements (web-users' activities like duration, book-marking etc.) used for assessing web-pages. ***Attribute$_i$*** means element ***i*** and ***C$_i$*** means weight (constant) of element ***i***.

If ***n*** of users' information had been collected, cost for managing and calculating network will increased by having ***n*** branches. It will be helpful to understand created network if groups of web-pages referred by users based on interest keywords are not simply listed but can be implied expression of users referred to similar web-pages. We can call it intentions, collected personal web-page browsing information by keywords. For more important expression of network, similarities of intentions and relationship of inclusion are compared and unified. Unification of intentions are assorted to Unity type, Inclusion type and Partly-unity type. Partly-unity type can be decided their similarity by using formula below and possibility of unification by status of similarity.

$$Sim(X,Y) = w_S S - w_u U \tag{2}$$

From ***Sim(X, Y), S*** means the number of web-pages that two sets include commonly and ***U*** means the number of web pages that two sets didn't. ***w$_u$*** is weight on web-pages that two sets have commonly and ***w$_u$*** is weight on web pages that two sets don't. If threshold is more than two group's similarity, they must be unified and weight of web-page should be unified and become one weight. Combining method by analyzing web-page similarities measured similarity of two groups by multiplying number of repeated pages and weight of number of not repeated pages.

4 Experiment

The experiment used twenty keywords except games or specific searching engine among top 30 popular keywords in 2010 and 2011 on Google, Yahoo and Naver. In case of keywords to access specific sites like the lottery site, National Tax Service or games like Sudden Attack or Dungeon fighter, one-click on searching results leads

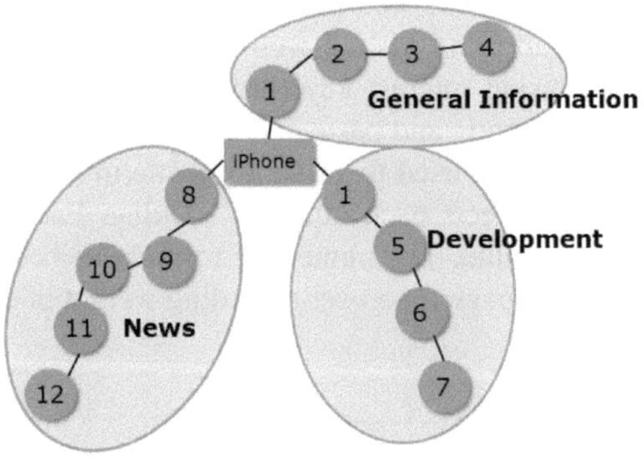

Fig. 1. UIN-Model of keyword "iPhone"

you to the right sites for a user's want. If there is only one absolute website for all users' want on some keywords, recommendation has no meaning.

Seven staffs have been selected for this experiment. They visited 823 web pages and 451 of collected data have been used for UIN-Model creation after deleting meaningless web pages. 141 groups also have been combined to 83 groups through UIN-Model. Figure 7 illustrated a keyword of iPhone network by using UIN-Model. The group with web pages 1, 2, 3 and 4 were about general information of iPhone, web pages 1, 5, 6 and 7, news of iPhone and web pages 8, 9, 10, 11 and 12, development for iPhone.

5 Conclusion

This study suggested UIN-Model as a method to include diverse propensity information on web-users' searching. It created network of web pages based on web-users' using information through keywords, measured and united similarity among users' intentions and made more meaningful network. Generated UIN-Model can be utilized for web pages recommending service and basic technology to compare, analyze and decide similarities among keywords on networks. UIN-Model based on keywords created from experiment was describing information on users' searching activities carefully so that they can be useful for recommendation service.

References

1. Eirinaki, M., Vazirgiannis, M.: Web Mining for Web Personalization. ACM Transactions on Internet Technology 3(1), 1–27 (2003)
2. Srivastava, J., Cooley, R., Deshpande, M., Tan, P.-N.: Web Usage Mining: Discovery and Applications of Usage Patterns from Web Data. SIGKDD Explorations 1(2), 12–23 (2000)
3. Joh, C.H., Arentze, T.A., Timmermans, H.J.P.: A position-sensitive sequence alignment method illustrated for space-time activity-diary data. Environment and Planning A 2001 33, 313–338 (2001)
4. Hay, B., Wets, G., Vanhoof, K.: Clustering Navigation Patterns on a Website using a Sequence Alignment Method. In: Proc. Intelligent Techniques for Web Personalization: 17th Int. Joint Conf. Artificial Intelligence (2000)
5. Sufyan Beg, M.M., Ahmad, N.: Web Search Enhancement by Mining User Actions. Information Sciences 177, 5203–5218 (2007)
6. Ahmed, A., Low, Y., Aly, M., Josifovski, V., Smola, A.J.: Scalable Distributed Inference of Dynamic User Interests for Behavioral Targeting. In: The 17th ACM SIGKDD Conference on Knowledge Discovery and Data Mining 2011, KDD 2011 (2011)

Part VI
Information Search and Retrieval

A HCI-AI Tool for Astronomy

Jerry D. Cavin

Bridge360, 10415 Morado Cir #350 Austin, TX 78759
Jerry_Cavin@bridge360.com

Abstract. The historical use of Artificial Intelligence (AI) combined with Human Computer Interaction (HCI) has raised many philosophical and psychological questions about whether this merger is appropriate. While this debate continues to rage on there is a world of people waiting to be relieved of time consuming and tedious tasks. The current state of machine learning has proven that interaction between humans and computers is capable of supporting people performing scientific investigations.

This paper proposes a HCI-AI application for such a scientific investigation. The Lowell Amateur Research Initiative (LARI) program for the Lowell Observatory provides the opportunity to assess the viability of such an application. The LARI program offers amateur astronomers access to large photometry data sets to search for patterns of exoplanet transits, orbiting binary stars, and variable stars. These data sets contain measurements over a standard R (red) wavelength passband taken from 6x6 degree areas of the sky and contain tens of thousands of stars.

The key to the success of this HCI-AI application is the speed of processing large data sets and the ability of the HCI-AI application to interact with the amateur astronomer assisting in the identification of objects exhibiting known patterns.

1 Introduction

Photometry is a technique to measure the intensity of an objects emission of electromagnetic radiation. Differential photometry is the measurement of the changes in the intensity of the emission compared to nearby stars without regard to a standard absolute magnitude scale. The changes in the intensity of the emission are compiled into light curves. The light curves are analyzed for patterns that may indicate the presence of astronomical events and objects such as exoplanet transits, orbiting binary stars, or variable stars.

The Lowell Amateur Research Initiative (LARI) Program provides the amateur astronomer with the data to search for patterns that may indicate the presence of one of these objects. The data used by the LARI Program is from the Transatlantic Exoplanet Survey (TrES). TrES Program was developed by teams of scientists from the Lowell Observatory, National Center for Atmospheric Research and the Harvard Smithsonian Center for Astrophysics. TrES consists of a worldwide network of inexpensive telescopes gathering data on stars since 2003. The TrES catalog currently contains

C. Stephanidis (Ed.): Posters, Part II, HCII 2013, CCIS 374, pp. 425–429, 2013.

photometry data on thousands of stars in the constellations of Lyra, Draco, Hercules, Cygnus, and Andromeda.

A HCI-AI framework is proposed to support LARI members' analysis of the vast amounts of photometry data available. To achieve this goal the framework must provide continuous learning for the amateur astronomer and adapt to change in a collaborative environment. For the purpose of this paper the HCI-AI framework proposed will be called the DataExplorer application. The components of the DataExplorer application discussed in this paper are illustrated in Figure 1.

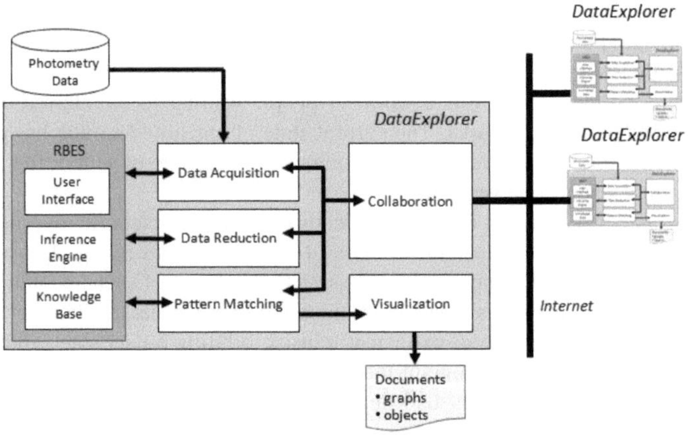

Fig. 1. The proposed components of the DataExplorer application (Source: author)

2 The Data Acquisition Stage

The first stage of the DataExplorer will be a Data Acquisition Component (DAC) to process incoming data files. The raw data files may contain extraneous data elements that need to be removed before they are introduced to the analysis stage. The raw data is presented to DAC component in an assortment of formats. DAC uses a Rule-Based Expert System (RBES) to process the raw data file according to a set of predefined rules. If the raw data file contains an unknown element, the expert system will collaborate with the user to learn how to parse the raw data file. The RBES will collaborate with the user by using a visual interactive display to parse the raw data file. In DataExplorer, the knowledge (rules) will be constructed by the expert system from the user actions in the visual display. The interactive portion of DAC will consist of a main window with a raw data file parsing display and a set of icons representing actions to perform on the data displays. The user interaction performed in the data file identification window is used for the conditional part of the rule. The user actions performed in the raw data file parsing window is used in the action portion of the rule. When the Rule-Based Expert System has been trained to process a raw data file of a particular format, other data files of the same format can be automatically processed without the need for user interaction. After the processing has completed, the processed data is stored in the DataExplorer internal data set.

3 The Data Reduction Stage

In the second stage the Data Reduction Component (DRC) will perform reduction and transformations on the data set based on rules in the Rule-Based Expert System. These rules provide the action to be taken depending on the type of data present in the TrES data file, and the type of object selected for the search. The data reduction techniques used for exoplanets is similar to the techniques used for variable stars.

The Rule-Based Expert System will reduce data by executing rules to carry out tasks for each type of search object. It may also perform tasks such as removing data with excessive uncertainty, dividing the data set it into smaller time specific data sets. Other data characteristics will execute rules to make transformations of the data. The data set might exhibit a 'large' variability over days or weeks. If the user selected to investigate the presence of exoplanet transits in a data set with large variability, the variability must be subtracted to reveal the smaller subtle changes. The pattern of an exoplanet transit event changes the magnitude of the star it orbits by one percent.

As detection techniques improve, editing the rules of the expert system will allow the user to add and redefine the data reduction techniques. Once the new data reduction rules have been established the user will make use of the DataExplorer's collaboration feature to exchange the new and modified data reduction techniques with other users.

4 The Pattern Matching Stage

The Pattern Matching Component (PMC) would use the expert system whose rules would apply a variety of statistical methods to analyze and classify objects of interest. A similar automated form of classification has been used to classify 1700 variable stars in the All-Sky Automated Survey. (Blake, 2005) For the variable stars the data must be folded. If the measurement of a star is not taken on a continuous basis statistical techniques must be used to merge the data or fold it to see if a period can be found in the data. One statistical method with this capability is Phase Dispersion Minimization. (Schwarzenberg-Czerny, 1997) Another statistical method that creates a power spectrum like Fourier analysis that works with irregularly spaced data is the Lomb-Scargle Periodogram (Kürster, 2009). Methods such as these are used to identify patterns of eclipsing binaries (Fig 2) and variable stars (Fig 3). The statistical method used to search for exoplanet transits is the Box Least Square (G. Kovács, 2002). This technique has been proven to be very fast due to its finer grid search. (A. Collier Cameron, 2006) Once this stage completes the positive hits would be stored for later analysis, visualization and sharing with colleagues through the collaboration feature.

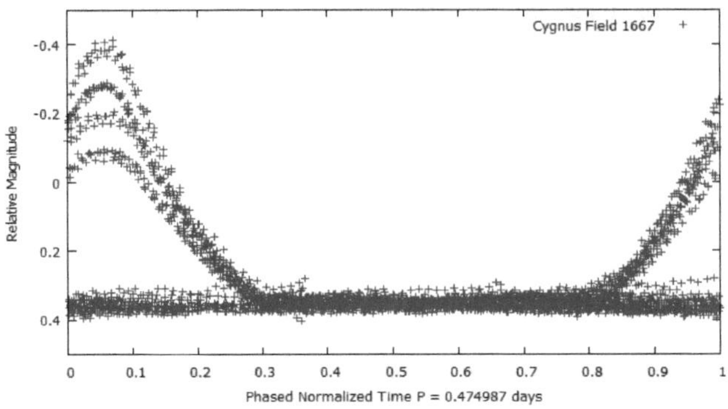

Fig. 2. TrES Cygnus 1667 – Light curve pattern of an eclipsing binary star found by an amateur astronomer in the LARI program (Source: Lowell Observatory LARI Program, with permission of Bruce Koehn, Lowell Observatory)

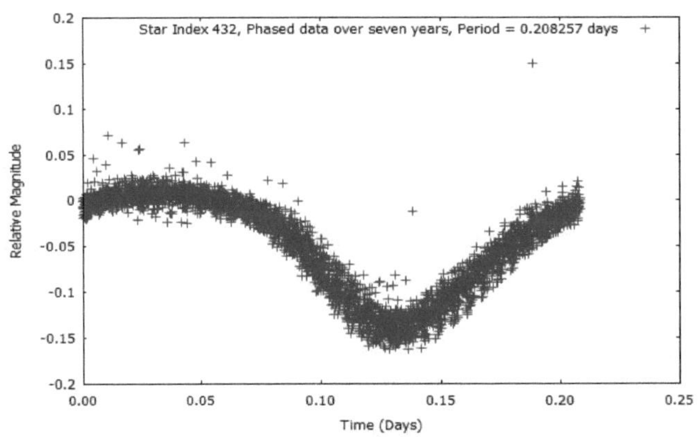

Fig. 3. TrES Cygnus 432 – Light curve pattern of a variable star found by an amateur astronomer in the LARI program (Source: Lowell Observatory LARI Program, with permission of Bruce Koehn, Lowell Observatory)

5 The Visualization Feature

Visualization of an object of interest can be performed by the end-user after the Pattern Matching Stage has been performed. The end-user is presented a list of possible objects to select. Once selected the object is visualized in a standard graph. The end-user can add additional documentation to the graph, classify the object, store and retrieve it, print it, and share the graph with other users through the Collaboration Feature.

6 The Collaboration Feature

There are many benefits to collaboration in this environment. Some problems are too complex for an amateur astronomer to handle alone. Through collaboration every astronomer may gain new skills and knowledge, and bring credibility to their work. Collaboration can also reduce duplication of effort in the analysis of massive amounts of information.

In astronomy, the set of analysis techniques are continually updated and replaced to gather more accurate results. DataExplorer must allow for interaction and exchange of rules, statistical methods, and results among amateur astronomers. By working together as a team LARI will be able to reach goals that could not be reached by individuals working alone.

7 Conclusion

The number of objects discovered in the data of the TrES catalog has been prolific. At least 773 eclipsing binary stars have been found, 34 of these are binaries with eccentric orbits, and 20 binaries have abnormal light curves. (Jonathan Devor, 2007) Six candidate exoplanet transits have been discovered in the TrES catalog (Francis T. O'Donovan, 2007). Each new discovery has led to new constraints on current astronomical models and theories. This paper has described the techniques and technology required to identify astronomical objects within massive amounts of raw data. With the DataExplorer application proposed in this paper, and with the aide of amateur astronomers collaborating around the world, the number of new discoveries can increase dramatically.

References

1. Collier Cameron, A., Pollacco, D.: A fast hybrid algorithm for exoplanetary transit searches. Mon. Not. R. Astron. Soc. 373, 799–810 (2006)
2. Blake, Eyer, L.: Automated classification of variable stars for All-Sky Automated. Mon. Not. R. Astron. Soc. 358, 30–38 (2005)
3. O'Donovan, F.T., Charbonneau, D.: Outcome of Six Candidate Transiting Planets from a TrES Field in Andromeda. arXiv:astro-ph/0610603, 658–668 (2007)
4. Kovács, G., Zucker, S.: A box-fitting algorithm in the search for periodic transits. A&A 391(1), 369–377 (2002)
5. Devor, J., Charbonneau, D.: Identification, Classifications, and Absolute Properties of 773 Eclipsing Binaries Found in the TrES Survey. arXiv:0712.0839v1 [astro-ph] (2007)
6. Kürster, Zechmeister, M.: The generalised Lomb-Scargle periodogram. A&A, 577–584 (2009)
7. Schwarzenberg-Czerny, A.: The Correct Probability Distribution for the Phase Dispersion Minimization Periodogram. ApJ 489, 941 (1997)

The Importance of Choice Design for Low Literate User Experience

Lisa Harper, Melissa McMacken, Lianne Appelt, and Kathryn Summers

University of Baltimore
Baltimore MD, 21201
{lisa.harper,melissa.mcmacken,lianne.appelt,ksummers}@ubalt.edu

Abstract. This research addresses a significant gap in our understanding of low literate behavior in online search. We explore how both low- and high-literate online consumers make decisions at the point of purchase in an online shopping task. We measured percentage fixation duration of AOIs during decision-making on four search engine results page (SERP) tasks. Qualitative and quantitative results combined suggest that tabular SERP may contribute to the success of low literate consumers making sophisticated trade-off decisions. Furthermore, we propose that tabular SERP choice design may improve low literate user experience for more general SERP choice design.

1 Introduction

Literacy involves a range of cognitive skill including discourse understanding, inferential reasoning, and numerical calculation. Low literacy may also negatively impact memory processes [1] and be associated with reduced working memory. The 2003 National Assessment of Adult Literacy (NAAL) indicates that 14% of adult Americans have no more than the most basic and concrete literacy (below basic), while an additional 29% can perform only basic every day literacy activities.[1]

Viswanathan, Rosa, and Harris [2] find that functionally illiterate consumers exhibit cognitive challenges and coping behaviors that differ markedly from literate consumers. Low literate consumers tend toward **concrete reasoning**, basing decisions on the concrete meaning of single pieces of information without regard to other product attributes or information [2]. This manifests during decision-making and analysis of trade-offs. Low literate consumers may focus exclusively on one dimension — such as price — without regard to size, number, quality, or other attributes.

Another common tendency is toward **pictographic thinking**. Low literate consumers may visualize verbal information in a scene (such as brand, price, store sign, etc.) as an image rather than actual text [2]. Low literate consumers may also make trade-offs between price and size using physical package size rather than unit or volume price information [2].

[1] `http://nces.ed.gov/naal/kf_demographics.asp`

C. Stephanidis (Ed.): Posters, Part II, HCII 2013, CCIS 374, pp. 430–434, 2013.

Finally, Jae and Delveccio [3] find that low literate consumers may be influenced by **peripheral cues** such as stylistic attributes of packaging over more central information such as written attributes. They suggest that visual decision aids may help low-literacy consumers reach more normative decisions: for example, by depicting a count attribute visually rather than textually.

While Russo and Leclerc [4] studied consumer behavior in eye fixations in a laboratory simulation of supermarket shelves, to our knowledge there exist no comparable studies of low literate consumer behavior in an online shopping environment.

2 Procedure and Measures

This experiment required two groups of native English (low and high literate) subjects to interact with search engine results pages (SERP) from Walmart.com (fig 1). 30 low and 15 high literate participants were recruited in the Baltimore, MD area. They were screened using the Rapid Estimate of Adult Literacy in Medicine (REALM) test. Potential low literate subjects were recruited only if they scored 60 or less on the REALM test and also self-reported as having basic computer skills (use of a mouse, typing, scrolling, navigating to a web page, and click on a link).

Eye-tracking was accomplished using the Tobii T60 eye-tracker on a 17" TFT monitor set at a resolution of 1024x768 sampling at the rate of 60 Hz. We used the I-VT Fixation filter from which fixations of less than 60 ms were discarded. By marking search results with rectangular areas of interest (AOIs), we were able to examine behavior such as fixation counts and duration in AOIs.

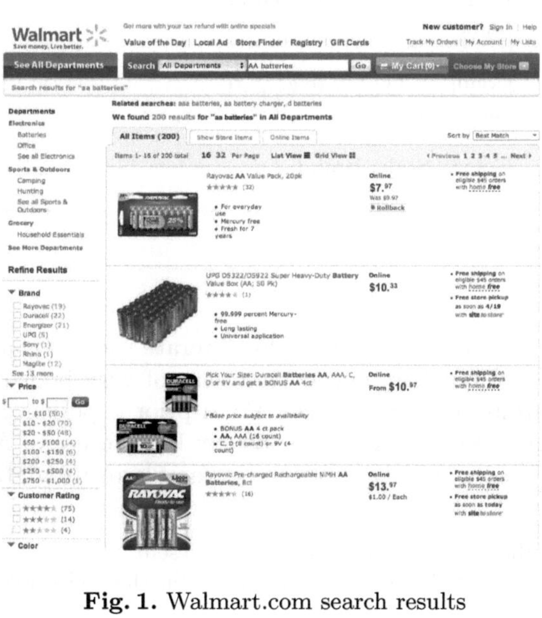

Fig. 1. Walmart.com search results

At the start of each session, the eye tracker was calibrated. Each subject was given the same set of four tasks in the same order (table 1). Subjects were directed to search for a particular item using the search bar. In order to make SERP comparable across participants, we generated a static SERP for each search query. Participants were later asked questions about the tasks presented.

Table 1 illustrates information available to the user per column (AOI).[2] Though the columnar format provides the means to organize comparable data, some fields contain more than one piece of information. For example, users can see count and type information for AA batteries both visually (in the image column) and textually (in the description column). This made the use of post-task questions that much more important for understanding what subjects were thinking.

For our analysis, we were concerned with difference in choice behavior between high literate and low literate subjects in terms of percentage fixation duration for an AOI relative to all four AOIs. We did not have time to complete a scan path analysis, which might have revealed patterns such as co-variance between specific columns as well as phases of behavior such as orientation, evaluation, and verification [4].

Table 1. User choice tasks

Item	Image	Description	Price	Shipping
Broom	Style, Options (e.g., dust-pan)	x	x	x
Laundry Soap	Brand, Type (e.g., cubes, liquid)	x	x	x
AA Batteries	Count, Type (e.g., re-chargeable)	x	x	x
Walking Shoes	Colors, Style, Brand	x	x	x

3 Results

Collecting quality eye-tracking data for low literate users is challenging. A substantial proportion of our low literate data was of very poor quality: we were able to use data from only 11 subjects. From prior experience, we find this is not uncommon for eye-tracking studies of low literate users. And, though the high literate data was generally good, we were able to use data from only five subjects.[3]

[2] An "x" simply indicates that the element was present.

[3] 7 sessions were eliminated due to a discrepancy in the collection procedure and 3 were of poor quality.

Though video, gaze plots, and questionnaire results were informative, fixation data was particularly helpful for comparing low and high literate behavior within and across trials. It is difficult for researchers to visually gauge behavioral changes that occur on the scale of milliseconds. The graphs below illustrate percentage of fixations across the four AOIs for each trial. Blue bars represent low literate subjects, while pink bars represent high literate subjects. Vertical black lines within blue and pink bars indicate standard deviation at 95% confidence. The sample size was too small to draw conclusions from eye-tracking data alone.

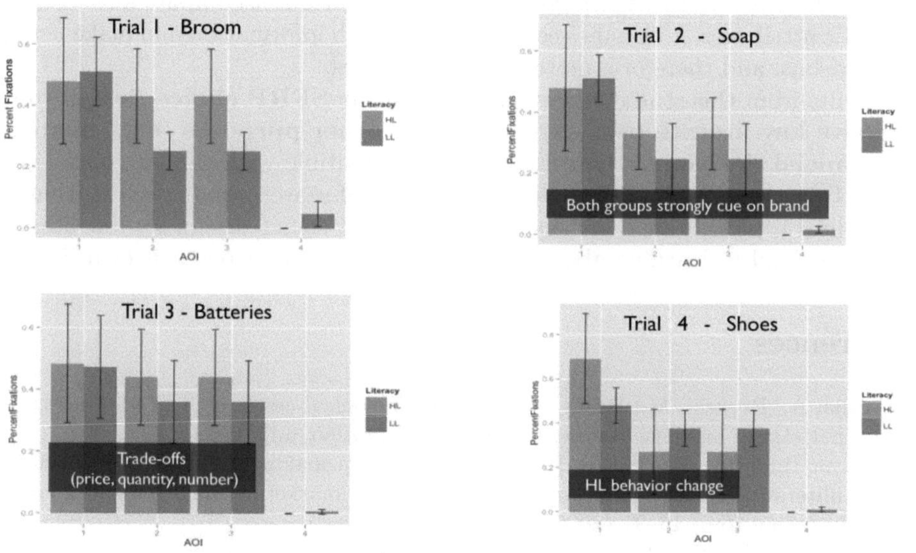

Fig. 2. Percent fixation duration for each task

However, we observed in task 3 (batteries), low literate behavior very closely resembles high literate behavior. **For the AA battery condition, low literate subjects were able to make decisions of comparable complexity and sophistication to high literate users**. Even in post-task questions, both populations indicated very similar choice decisions based on trade-offs of price, quantity, and number of batteries. In task 2 (laundry soap), both groups strongly identified with a brand choice. Considering both eye fixation duration and answers to post-task questions, it seems high and low literate subjects both cue strongly on brand. Finally, in task 4 (shoes), we observed that high literate subjects more strongly cued on visual attributes than they had in previous tasks.

4 Discussion and Conclusion

In a study of low literate consumer behavior in an online shopping point-of-purchase task, we did not see the sorts of behaviors described by Viswanathan,

Rosa, and Harris [2]. We found that **low literate users were able to make successful complex trade-off decisions**. Though some high literate subjects seemed bored with the task, low literate subjects were engaged and reportedly enjoyed the tasks. Most had never done online shopping before and left feeling confident and interested in trying this on their own. We believe this is largely attributable to the information organization of the columnar SERP product data that made it easier to make choice comparisons across a range of product attributes.

Our pilot study supports Thaler, Sunstein, and Balz [5]: a good choice architecture helps people improve their ability to map and therefore select better options. In other words, when complex information is teased apart into distinct semantic attributes, it becomes easier to distinguish information and make better comparisons, and therefore, more informed choices.

Results from this study suggest that a **tabular SERP choice design may improve low literate user experience for other purposes (e.g., medical or financial decisions)**. Our findings are compatible with similar conclusions drawn by Kammerer and Gerjets [6] in a study of search result trustworthiness on medical topics. In fact, we suspect that a good choice design for low literate users may lead to learning about how make better choices on their own [5].

References

1. Ardila, A., Rosselli, M., Rosas, P.: Neuropsychological assessment in illiterates: Visuospatial and memory abilities. Brain and Cognition, 147–166 (1989)
2. Viswanathan, M., Rosa, J.A., Harris, J.E.: Decision making and coping of functionally illiterate consumers and some implications for marketing management. Journal of Marketing (69), 15–31 (2005)
3. Jae, H., DelVecchio, D.: Decision making by low-literacy consumers in the presence of point-of-purchase information. Journal of Cosumer Affairs 38(2), 324–354 (2004)
4. Russo, J.E., Leclerc, F.: An eye-fixation analysis of choice processes for consumer nondurables. Journal of Consumer Research 21(2), 274–290 (1994)
5. Thaler, R., Sunstein, C., Balz, J.: Choice architecture. Available at SSRN 1583509 (2010)
6. Kammerer, Y., Gerjets, P.: The impact of discrepancies across web pages on high-school students' trustworthiness evaluations. Behavior and Information Technology (31), 83–97 (2012)

Performance Analysis of Naïve Bayesian Methods for Paragraph Level Text Classification in the Kannada Language

R. Jayashree[1], K. Srikanta Murthy[2], and Basavaraj S. Anami[3]

[1] Department of Computer Science, PES Institute of Technology, Bangalore, India
[2] Department of Computer Science, PES School of Engineering, Bangalore, India
[3] Department of Computer Science, KLE Institute of Technology, Hubli, India
{jayashree,srikantamurthy}@pes.edu, anami_basu@hotmail.com

Abstract. Text Categorization plays a predominant role in Natural Language Processing (NLP) and Information Retrieval (IR) applications. This work highlights the performance of different Naïve Bayesian methods for paragraph level Text Classification in the Kannada language. The dimensionality reduction technique is achieved using minimum term frequency, stop word identification and removal methods.

Keywords: performance, classifier, paragraph level classification, Kannada text classification, Naïve Bayesian, Multinomial, naïve Bayesian upbeat able, Bayesnet.

1 Introduction

When we browse information present on the internet, the point worth noting is that information is mostly present as documents, paragraphs and sentences. Another important point to be noted is the way in which the information gets updated. Whenever the information updation needs to be done, the problem of finding the correct location to update information in a document is challenging.

This work looks at the possibility of paragraph classification in the Kannada language which helps in information updation online.

The rest of the paper is organized as follows. Section-II highlights the literature about paragraph level text classification in particular, Text categorization and Research on Naïve Bayesian models in general. Section-III describes how the corpus was prepared for use in this work. Section-IV discusses the methodology of our work. Section –V is about Results and Discussion.

2 Literature Survey

Jayashree.R Et.al, have investigated two classical approaches such as Naïve Bayesian and Bag of Words to Sentence Level Text Classification in the Kannada Language

C. Stephanidis (Ed.): Posters, Part II, HCII 2013, CCIS 374, pp. 435–439, 2013.

and looked at the possibility of extending sentence level classification task to Paragraph Level Text Classification in their future work [1].

Erdong Chen Et.al [2] in their work on 'Incremental Text structuring with on line hierarchical ranking' present an online ranking model which exploits the hierarchical structure of a given document.

The importance of paragraph segmentation is highlighted by Alex Smola Et.al [3], the application is speech to text conversion, wherein there is necessity to identify punctuations, paragraphs etc.

Isaac Persing Et.al [4] have worked on' modeling organization in student Essays', wherein the organization could be treated as collection of paragraphs with respect to the structure of the Essay.

'Genre Based Paragraph for Sentiment Analysis' is an interesting work carried out by Maite Taboada Et.al [6]. They present a classification system for representing different paragraphs within movie reviews.

Work by Andrew Mccallum Et.al[7] makes an attempt to clarify the confusion between Naïve Bayesian models; Multi variant Bernoulli model and multinomial model. They claim that multinomial model is better than the multi variant Bernoulli model.

ABOUT The Corpus

The TDIL(Technology for Development of Indian Languages) corpus developed by Central Institute of Indian Languages(CIIL) is considered for use in this work. TDIL corpus contains pre categorized documents.

Table 1. Class wise Distribution of paragraphs in TDIL corpus

Category	No. of Paragraphs
Commerce	476
Social	413
Natural	475
Aesthetics	427

3 Methodology

Dimensionality Reduction:
In this work, we have achieved dimensionality reduction technique using two methods:

1. Stop word identification and removal
2. Using a restriction based on the word occurrence.

3.1 Naïve Bayes

The Naïve Bayesian is a probabilistic classifier. The dimensions in the vector indicate the presence of the word and no special weight age parameter was used in the classification process.

3.2 Naïve Bayesian Multinomial

According to Naïve Bayesian methods, a document is to be treated as bag of words wherein multiple occurring words appear multiple times. Hence we have used a modified form of Naïve Bayes which is Naïve Bayes Multinomial.

3.3 Naïve Bayes Multinomial Upbeatable

Bayes net is a probabilistic graphical model that represents a set of random variables.

3.4 Bayes Net

Is an incremental version that processes one instance at a time.

4 Results and Discussion

K-fold Cross Validation is used in this work for evaluation of the classifier performance, which is needed to ensure that each partition is used as a test set only once.

A classifier's performance can be measured by using parameters: Precision (P), Recall (R) (also called as TP rate) and F-Score (F). The definitions of the parameters are as shown:

$$\text{Precision} = \frac{\text{Proportion of the examples which truly have class x}}{\text{Total classified as class x}} \quad (1)$$

$$\text{TP rate/True Positive(TP)} = \frac{\text{Proportion classified as class x}}{\text{Actual total of class x}} \quad (2)$$

$$\text{False Positive (FP)} = \frac{\text{Proportion incorrectly classified as class x}}{\text{Actual total of all classes, except x}} \quad (3)$$

$$\text{F} - \text{measure} = \frac{2 \times \text{Precison} \times \text{Recall}}{(\text{Precision} + \text{Recall})} \quad (4)$$

4.1 Naive Bayes

with decreasing 'm', which is minimum term frequency, the evaluation parameters showed a significant rise, hence, we need to consider such words and their impact on classification. Taking m=2, the class-wise break up for the classification results by taking into consideration stop word removal, is as shown.

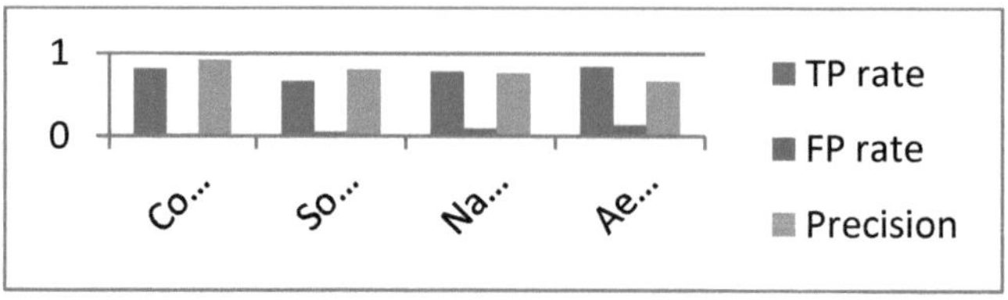

Fig. 1. Classification Results

4.2 Naïve Bayesian Multinomial

Taking M=2, the class-wise breakup for the classification results using Naïve Bayes multinomial is as shown:

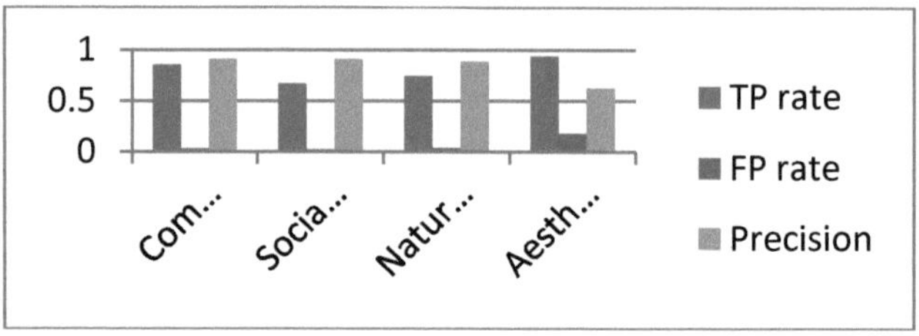

Fig. 2. Classification results for BayesNet

4.3 Bayesnet

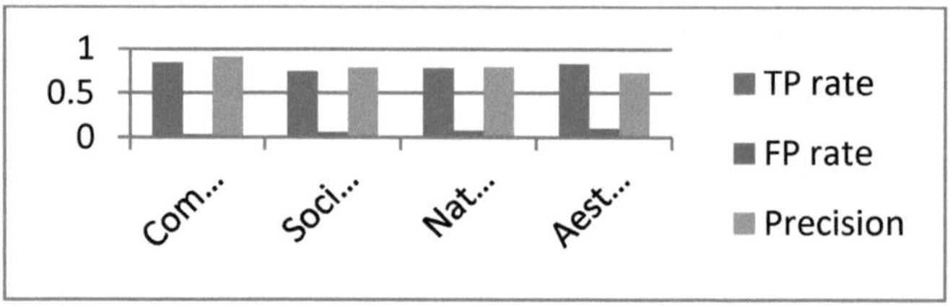

Fig. 3. Classification results

4.4 Naïve Bayes Multinomial Upbeatable

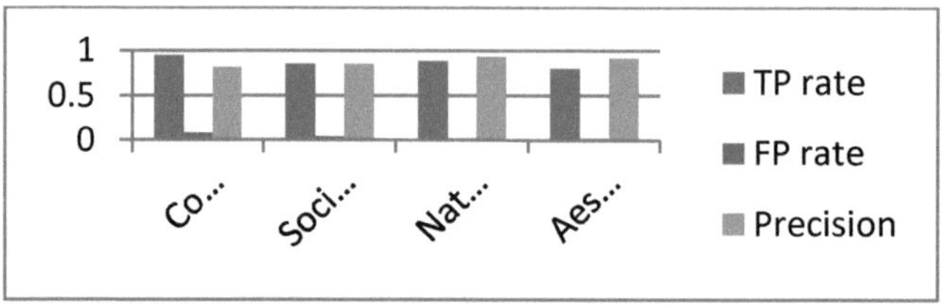

Fig. 4. Classification results

5 Conclusion

The distribution of the Minimum term frequency across categories varies in our experiments. Manual error analysis has shown that there is a significant possibility of paragraphs belonging to multiple classes. In some cases, paragraphs might not have sufficient information which indicate category and hence might use neighboring paragraphs to convey the class information.

References

1. Jayashree, R., Srikantamurthy, K.: Analysis of Sentence Level Text Cassification in the Kannada Language. In: Proceedings of the 2011 International Conference on Soft Computing and Pattern Recognition (SOCPAR 2011), Dalian, China, pp. 147–151 (October 2011)
2. Chen, E., Snyder, B., Barzilay, R.: Incremental Text Structuring with Online Hierarchical Ranking. In: Proceedings of the 2007 Joint Conference on Empirical Methods in Natural Language Processing and Computational Linguistics, Prague, pp. 83–91 (June 2007)
3. Shi, Q., Altun, Y., Smola, A., Vishwanathan, S.V.N.: Semi-Markov Models for Sequence Segmentation. In: Proceedings of the 2007 Joint Conference on Empirical Methods in Natural Language Processing and Computational Linguistics, Prague, pp. 640–648 (June 2007)
4. Persing, I., Davis, A., Ng, V.: Modeling Organization in Student Essays. In: Proceedings of the 2010 Conference on Empirical Methods in Natural Language Processing, October 9-11, pp. 229–239. MIT, Massachusetts (2010)
5. Hearst, M.A.: TextTiling: Segmenting Text into Multi-paragraph Subtopic Passages. Association for Computational Linguistics (1997)
6. Taboada, M., Brooke, J., Stede, M.: Genre-Based Paragraph Classification for Sentiment Analysis. In: Proceedings of SIGDIAL 2009: The 10th Annual Meeting of the Special Interest Group in Discourse and Dialogue, Queen Mary University of London, pp. 62–70 (September 2009)
7. McCallumzy, A., Nigamy, K.: A Comparison of Event Models for Naive Bayes Text Classication. In: AAAI 1998, Workshop on Learning for Text Categorization (1998)

Making It Everyone's Finna – Cross-Sector Collaboration and User Experience Design in a Digital Library

Heli Kautonen[1,2]

[1] The National Library of Finland, Helsinki, Finland
heli.kautonen@helsinki.fi
[2] Aalto University, Helsinki, Finland
heli.kautonen@aalto.fi

Abstract. This is a report on ongoing work on a digital library service focusing on user experience design. The service examined is the Finnish Digital Library, also called Finna. The service is being developed in collaboration between Finnish libraries, archives, and museums, which brings challenges and opportunities to the design of user experience. The report describes the current organizational settings of the design process by listing its actors, activities, and aims.

Keywords: User experience design, collaboration, digital libraries.

1 Introduction

More sophisticated information retrieval systems are needed for utilizing the material collected on the – increasingly virtual – shelves of libraries, archives, and museums (LAM). Projects carried out worldwide aim at uniting cultural heritage repositories by using different digital tools and technologies. Some of these projects reach beyond the boundaries of organization types, such as the Digital Public Library of America (DPLA), or even countries and languages, such as Europeana.[1]

Cross-sector digital library initiatives are usually launched because of the needs for economic efficiency and better end-user services. LAM organizations must have a strong motivation to join a deep and long-term collaboration project.

This is a report on the ongoing work on a digital library service focusing on user experience design. The report is part of an intensive case study investigating the strategic usability of a digital library service.

The service described here, namely the Finnish Digital Library, also called Finna, is exceptional in many respects. The current developments in open source software (OSS) and the agile development method alone are new to many libraries, archives, and museums in Finland. Furthermore, the development of Finna has brought the expertise of LAM sectors together in a way that no previous collaboration project has

[1] More information available online at dp.la and europeana.eu.

C. Stephanidis (Ed.): Posters, Part II, HCII 2013, CCIS 374, pp. 440–444, 2013.

been able to achieve. The collaboration also covers the design and evaluation of user experience.

The idea of Finna is to serve as a national infrastructure for various types of LAM organizations in need of a user interface for their online services. In time, Finna will replace several existing interfaces. The project and the maintenance of the service are financed by the Finnish Ministry of Education and Culture. The National Library of Finland is in charge of the development of the Finna service and the OSS production, and it hosts the Finna Office.

The Finna service is based on open source software modules constituting a range of end-user interface services. The same software can be used for tailoring an interface for an individual organization's needs, but it is also the core of the national view, i.e., the basic Finna.[2] At the same time, the name Finna refers to the project developing the service and uniting the Finnish LAM community in the collaboration. In this report we refer to all these various aspects of Finna.

2 Digital Libraries and User Studies

In the context of digital libraries, usability and user studies have been a significant area of research in the past few years. While the definition of a digital library has developed from a simple extension of the physical library into a heterogeneous set of information facilitation concepts that "cannot be captured by a simple definition" [1], the core interest in the user's preferences has remained the same.

A substantial part of research focuses on user studies: who are the users of a digital library, and what do they need from their digital service? Changes in the information environment and the consequentially evolving user needs are a challenge for digital library developers [2–4].There is also a call for stronger user involvement in design [5].

The debate on the most appropriate usability evaluation methods and usability indicators for digital libraries continues. Some researchers strongly favor the mixing of methods [6–7]. There is still a strong demand for universal instruments for this domain and attempts to develop them, e.g., [8].

Rarely do these studies on digital libraries and usability describe the organizational settings of design. It seems that practitioners and their role gain attention only if the circumstances have affected some of the challenges or solutions, e.g., [5] and [6]. Yet user experience design requires collective problem solving, as is argued by Buxton [9]. Therefore, the process and actors can be considered to be influential to the quality of the outcome, and more so when the digital library is built in collaboration.

3 Uncovering the Activity Framework

The organizational structure in which Finna's user experience design takes place has already changed. However, documenting its current status is important for further studies and interesting for other user experience practitioners.

---

[2] Available online at `finna.fi`.

Finna's organizational structure can be better understood through the question: *Which activity elements constitute the collaborative design of the user experience of Finna?* We took an emic action research approach and carried out a thematic analysis of Finna's design process using cultural historical activity theory as a guiding framework. Activity theory has proven useful for tracking collective activities in the context of human-computer interaction and consequentially for identifying the strengths and weaknesses in a design activity [10].

The core of this report is an account of three activity components: the *Actors*, who currently contribute to the user experience design of Finna; the *Activities* conducted by the actors; and, finally, the *Aims*, which are either tangible or more conceptual objectives of Finna's user experience design. The account is based on proactive participant observation, i.e., our experience in working with Finna, but can also be assembled from the project documentation available on the Internet.[3]

3.1 The Actors of Finna's User Experience Design

- *The in-house team at the Finna Office.* The team is the central task force for conducting the usability work. It consists of interaction designers, front-end programmers, and coordinators.
- *The partner organizations' implementation teams.* Their role is to communicate their organization's requirements to the Finna team, and vice versa.
- *The Usability Working Group.* The group consists of usability experts or customer service personnel from participating organizations. The group's role is to steer the operative work, establish guidelines, and estimate future demands.
- *Commercial service providers.* Thus far, Finna has consulted one international and a few Finnish partners for concept analyses and visual user interface design.
- *Students and researchers.* Several universities in Finland have degree programs and graduate schools that focus on usability, user interaction, and user experience. Their students and researchers have made case studies of Finna.
- *The OSS community.* The communities that actively develop the software inevitably influence the user experience.

3.2 The Activities of Finna's User Experience Design

- *Planning.* The first task of the Usability Working Group was to make a master plan for usability work. The updated version of the Usability Plan now serves as a framework for current and future activities.
- *Design and implementation.* Most of the in-house team's manpower is put into design and implementation activities.
- *Usability evaluation.* Proper usability tests with prospective users as well as rapid user tests following the pace of agile development have been conducted.
- *Tracking and analyzing actual use.* Actual use is currently monitored only with one software module, which stores and analyzes the data on site traffic and visitors. Plans for qualitative surveys and usage analyses have been made.

[3] In English at `kdk.fi/eng` and in Finnish at `www.kiwi.fi/display/finna`.

- *Coordination and management.* The Finna Office has been responsible for coordinating the collaboration and managing most of the activities.
- *Dissemination.* We have made the usability work known to the collaboration community, stakeholders, and wider audience in various presentations and publications.

3.3 The Aims of Finna's User Experience Design

- *User interface and interaction.* Although Finna utilizes OSS modules that have ready-made user interfaces and functionalities, we have modified the final end-user interfaces for our needs. The visual appearance, the layout, and the interaction elements have been and will be further redesigned.
- *Integrated services.* Each new integrated service alters the overall user experience and thus requires some designing or redesigning.
- *Service concept.* Each new partner joining Finna brings along new users and contexts of use, and therefore the service concept has to be frequently reviewed.
- *End-users.* With the beta version, there has been no actual use, but we have invited potential end-users to participate in testing via the contacts of the Usability Working Group and participating organizations.

4 Challenges and Opportunities of Collaborative User Experience Design

The analysis of Finna's current activity framework in itself cannot bring about transformation. However, reviewing it against the literature revealed some challenges and opportunities.

Examining the list of actors reveals that there is at least one potential resource that we have not involved in the design process, namely our end-users. In the context of public services, users can prove to be valuable co-designers [11]. In order to utilize the full potential of the collaboration network, the OSS community, and end-users, we should develop a strategy for how design activities can be distributed and led.

An examination of the activities indicates that our approach is still too narrow. Our current activities do not consider the flexibility or the power of open networks. The methods should also be reviewed. For example, the combination of agile software development and user experience design requires methodological awareness [12]. In the coming years of service development, we should engage in more reflection on our methods and approaches.

Reviewing the aims shows that the central element influencing the end-user experience of the service, namely the content and its representations, lacks explicit attention to its design. When partners join the project gradually over time, the process cannot be controlled as optimally as, e.g., Garrett suggests [13]. Nevertheless, Finna's contents will require design thinking.

The fact that Finna is being developed within a cross-sector community will inevitably change the mindset behind its design. All actors have to keep in mind that their design solutions will be influencing the experience of users throughout the collaboration network. The service will bring new users to the old services, and designers will have to consider new solutions, e.g., for ensuring accessibility.

The development phase will continue until the year 2016, but we already foresee that the user experience will require redesign as long as the service is in use. By strategically balancing the different activity components of user experience design, we aim ultimately to make Finna usable for everyone.

References

1. Candela, L. (ed.): The Digital Library Reference Model. DL.org Project Deliverable (2010)
2. Agosti, M., Crivellari, F., Di Nunzio, G.M., Gabrielli, S.: Understanding user requirements and preferences for a digital library Web portal. IJDL 11(4), 225–238 (2010)
3. Dobreva, M., Chowdhury, S.: A User-Centric Evaluation of the Europeana Digital Library. In: Chowdhury, G., Koo, C., Hunter, J. (eds.) ICADL 2010. LNCS, vol. 6102, pp. 148–157. Springer, Heidelberg (2010)
4. Khoo, M., Hall, C.: What Would 'Google' Do? Users' Mental Models of a Digital Library Search Engine. In: Zaphiris, P., Buchanan, G., Rasmussen, E., Loizides, F. (eds.) TPDL 2012. LNCS, vol. 7489, pp. 1–12. Springer, Heidelberg (2012)
5. Somerville, M., Brar, N.: A user-centered and evidence-based approach for digital library projects. The Electronic Library 27(3), 409–425 (2009)
6. Buttenfield, B.: Usability Evaluation of Digital Libraries. Science & Technology Libraries 17(3-4), 39–59 (1999)
7. Agosti, M., Crivellari, F., Di Nunzio, G.M.: Evaluation of Digital Library Services Using Complementary Logs. In: SIGIR 2009. ACM (2009)
8. Joo, S., Lee, J.Y.: Measuring the usability of academic digital libraries: Instrument development and validation. The Electronic Library 29(4), 523–537 (2011)
9. Buxton, B.: Interactive Technologies: Sketching User Experiences. Getting the Design Right and the Right Design. Morgan Kaufmann, Burlington (2007)
10. Kaptelinin, V., Nardi, B.A.: Acting with Technology: Activity Theory and Interaction Design. MIT Press, Cambridge (2006)
11. Szebeko, D.: Case study 01: Co-Designing Services in the Public Sector. In: Meroni, A., Sangiori, D. (eds.) Design for Services, pp. 131–138. Gower Publishing, Surrey (2011)
12. Ferreira, J., Sharp, H., Robinson, H.: Agile Development and User Experience Design Integration as an Ongoing Achievement in Practice. In: Agile Conference, pp. 11–12 (2012)
13. Garrett, J.J.: The Elements of User Experience: User Centered Design for the Web. New Riders, Indianapolis (2003)

Exploring Technical Documents: A Prototype Study

Marcus Nitsche, Stefan Haun, and Andreas Nürnberger

Otto-von-Guericke-University Magdeburg, 39106 Magdeburg, Germany
{marcus.nitsche,stefan.haun,andreas.nuernberger}@ovgu.de

Abstract. Finding information in unknown, large data sets is not an easy task, especially if they consist of documents in an unfamiliar domain. A collection of several hundred technical reports has been analyzed in order to organize it for efficient and fluent searching, browsing, navigation and even exploration. We describe a user study on an interactive system – the *EFB-Explorer* – that visualizes the data set by different attributes to reflect the specific relevance of a retrieved document to a user's query and offers easy-to-use zooming interaction as well as semantic zooming.

1 Introduction

While fact queries, like an ad-hoc Web search, are well covered by search engines, e.g. Google, finding relevant parts of large documents in a data set is not an easy task; especially when the collection is unknown to the user or the correct query itself must yet be ascertained. The EFB-Explorer has been developed to address the problem of finding relevant pages in large (ca. 300 pages) technical reports and to decide whether a complete copy of the report is relevant and therefore should be bought. We conducted a user study which showed the usefulness of the explorer. The results will be presented in this paper, after a short introduction into exploratory search and zoomable user interfaces.

2 State-of-the-Art

Tominski [16] writes about *visual exploration*:

> The aim pursued with visual exploration is to give an overview of the data and to allow users to interactively browse through different portions of the data. In this scenario, users have no or only vague hypotheses about the data; their aim is to find some. In this sense,visual exploration can be understood as an undirected search for relevant information within the data. To support users in the search process, a high degree of interactivity must be a key feature of visual exploration techniques.

C. Stephanidis (Ed.): Posters, Part II, HCII 2013, CCIS 374, pp. 445–449, 2013.

Interaction is eased by structuring elements, leading to a multitude of representations from classic list representations up to multi-dimensional structures in space. A possible technique for representation are graph-based layouts [2]. Graphs can reflect explicit connections between documents, which is is important for a directed exploration. In "CET: A Tool for Creative Exploration of Graphs" [9] a graph representation is used to represent similar topics and enable the user to view large data spaces by selecting a directly connected document set based on the visible sub-graph.

A static variant of a layout representation is shown in "ERIS – Ein Thesaurus-basiertes Bildsuchsystem" [6]. Here, the data is not discovered by expanding graphs but displayed as a radial layout [8], i.e. a tree, generating an overview for the results. Zoomable User Interfaces (ZUI) can support navigation in these overviews. A further method is interaction through Fisheye lenses [15]. A mouse-focused area is distorted and gradually enlarged, so that the user has a much more detailed view on the data at hand, yet can still see the context of the focus. In contrast, ZUIs have the advantage that they are able to focus on a local exploration. The space is not represented completely as it would be in Fisheye visualizations. Users can zoom into specific areas of interest, discarding the information about context and thus switch the frame of reference during an exploration process.

Kerren und Ebert [10] provide a more general overview in "Human-Centered Visualization Environments":

> Zoomable interfaces allow users access information by panning and zooming [13]. Space and scale are the fundamental means of organizing the information [3,13]. The most common appearance of elements is geometric zoom, but there exist more complex ones as semantic zooming [1,4,13], constant density zooming [19], or non-linear panning and zooming [5]. Also, smoothness in zooming transitions have been studied: smooth zooms [1,7,17] and non-smooth zooms [13,14].

3 Concept and Implementation of the Explorer System

We developed the *EFB-Explorer*, an interactive system to visualizes a collection of documents (in this case: technical reports) by different attributes and reflect the specific relevance of a retrieved document regarding the query. The tool offers easy-to-use zooming interaction as well as support for semantic zooming (see also [18] for the basic idea of the applied exploratory search paradigm). Results set can be views either in a classic list visualization or in a spatial arrangement (Fig. 1). We suppose that this spatial arrangement enables users to follow visual shortcuts as it supports a user in changing perspective [12], which is of benefit in exploratory search tasks [11]. Relevance is not coded by a high position, as it would be in a list representation, but by size, a more central position, depth of detail information, color and saturation.

In order to start an exploration, the user provides one or more keywords, which are used to generate a basic document set. During search, the documents are

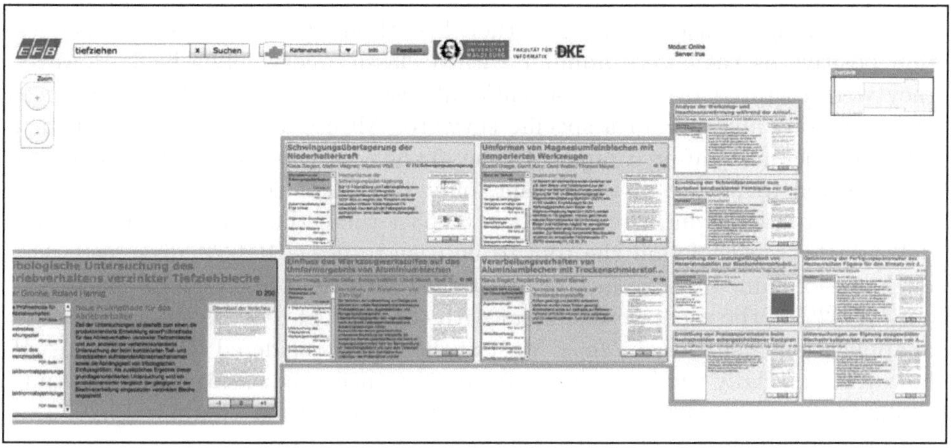

Fig. 1. EFB-Explorer – Spatial arrangement of search results, providing an alternative starting point for exploration in unfamiliar documents

regarded by their paragraphs, leading to a list of relevant text snippets which are merged back into documents for the visualization. Using smaller portions allows a more fine-grained search in parts of the documents. Based on the relevance towards the query the paragraphs, merged back to documents, are spatially arranged starting with the most relevant document on the left and leading to less relevant documents on the right side. The size of each document item is scaled to reflect the relevance value. As a result, more relevant documents take up more screen estate and are more likely to gain the user's attention. On zooming into the document set previously hidden information on less relevant documents are revealed. This allows for a clean visualization of many documents and yet enables the user to display each detail if desired. When an interesting document is found, the relevant pages can be viewed or distinct snippets can be marked for further reference. This feature, however, was not part of the study. The system was implemented as a Rich Internet Application (RIA) using the *Adobe Flex* framework and is currently being re-implemented and improved using the *HTML 5* web standard.

4 Evaluation and Results

We conducted a user study with 19 expert users that were familiar with the domain, but not familiar with specific documents of the underlying collection. The qualitative usability of the tool has been tested using different search tasks. On a two-day conference meeting of experts we exposed a test system to 19 users and asked for their opinion. Our test users had an average age of 40.3 years, 16.7% were female with an average computer usage experience of 17.6 years and 13.3 years experience in using the WWW. 44.4% were familiar with documents contained in our test collection, 61.11% were familiar with the interaction concept of a zoomable user interface (ZUI).

The users were asked to describe their first thoughts and answered this question positive as they were familiar with a classic query input field. However, they were irritated by the unconventional result visualization that they faced after releasing a search for a specific keyword. All users were able to find the a relevant document after 5 minutes time; 53.63% of them found the document we expected to be the most relevant; only 15.79% of them identified another document to be the most relevant one. 52.63% think the tool is useful for their daily work; 57.89% found the tool to be easy-to-use – 10.53% disagreed. This might be explained by the lack of experience with the presented UI concept, as only 26.32% of the users were familiar with the concept of ZUIs – partly because of applications like *Google Maps*. Most of the users considered UI to be unusual, however, especially the interaction concept was accepted: 73.68% liked the possibility to zoom in and out of documents to explore their content; 15.79% did not answer the question; 10.53% did not like this feature.

The *results* of this user study revealed a positive outcome, since 74% of the test users liked the opportunity to explore the document set using a semantic zooming technique, 79% could imagine to use the exploration tool on a daily basis and with an overall rating of 5.24 on a 7-point-Likert-Scale the tool's usefulness was rated good.

5 Conclusion and Outlook

As the study has shown, the general ZUI concept was accepted and should be further supported. However, the alignment of single documents should be revised. on the one hand to support user's understanding of the logic in the result representation, on the other hand to reduce the flood of data. Several times users complained that to many details were revealed by the system, so a more sensitive semantic zooming could be of advantage. Additionally, a relevance ranking and numbering of retrieved documents was wished by the users. The alignment of result surrogates could be more flexible and use overlapping, leading to a reduced map size. Finally, users could place elements by their own to give relevance feedback. The system will be improved and transferred in a platform-independent web-based solution using HTML5.

Acknowledgement. Part of the work is funded by the German Ministry of Education and Science (BMBF) within the ViERforES II project (no. 01IM10002B). We thank Rene Müller for developing and testing a predecessor version of the proposed concept in his Bachelor's Thesis.

References

1. Bederson, B.B., Meyer, J., Good, L.: Jazz: an extensible zoomable user interface graphics toolkit in Java. In: Proceedings of the 13th Annual ACM Symposium on User Interface Software and Technology, pp. 171–180 (2000)

2. Cui, W.: A Survey on Graph Visualization (2007)
3. Furnas, G.W., Bederson, B.B.: Space-scale diagrams: understanding multiscale interfaces. In: CHI 1995: Proceedings of the SIGCHI Conference on Human Factors in Computing Systems, pp. 234–241 (1995)
4. Frank, A.U., Timpf, S.: Multiple representations for cartographic objects in a multiscale tree – An intelligent graphical zoom. Computers & Graphics 18, 823–829 (1994)
5. Furnas, G.W., Zhang, X.: MuSE: a multiscale editor. In: Proceedings of the 11th Annual ACM Symposium on User Interface Software and Technology, pp. 107–116 (1998)
6. Gundelsweiler, F., Öttl, S.: ERIS - Ein thesaurusbasiertes Bildretrievalsystem mittels Zoomable User Interface. In: Informationskonzepte für die Zukunft: ODOK 2007, pp. 47–60. Neugebauer Verlag (2008)
7. Guo, H., Zhang, V., Wu, J.: The Effect of Zooming Speed in a Zoomable User Interface. In: Student CHI Online Research Experiments, SHORE (2000)
8. Herman, I., Melancon, G., Marshall, M.S.: Graph Visualization and Navigation in Information Visualization: A Survey. IEEE Transactions on Visualization and Computer Graphics 6, 24–43 (2000)
9. Haun, S., Nürnberger, A., Kötter, T., Thiel, K., Berthold, M.R.: CET: A Tool for Creative Exploration of Graphs. In: Balcázar, J.L., Bonchi, F., Gionis, A., Sebag, M. (eds.) ECML PKDD 2010, Part III. LNCS, vol. 6323, pp. 587–590. Springer, Heidelberg (2010)
10. Kerren, A., Ebert, A., Meyer, J. (eds.): Human-Centered Visualization Environments 2006. LNCS, vol. 4417. Springer, Heidelberg (2007)
11. Marchionini, G.: Exploratory Search: From Finding to Understanding. Communications of the ACM 49(4), 41–46 (2006)
12. Noël, L., Carloni, O., Moreau, N., Weiser, S.: Designing a knowledge-based tourism information system. International Journal of Digital Culture and Electronic Tourism 1(1), 1–17 (2008)
13. Perlin, K., Fox, D.: Pad - An Alternative Approach to the Computer Interface. In: Proc. of ACM SIGGRAPH, pp. 57–64 (1993)
14. Schaffer, D., Zuo, Z., Greenberg, S., Bartram, L., Dill, J., Dubs, S., Roseman, M.: Navigating hierarchically clustered networks through fisheye and full-zoom methods. ACM Trans. Comput.-Hum. Interact. 3, 162–188 (1996)
15. Tatemura, J.: Dynamic label sampling on fisheye maps for information exploration. In: Proceedings of the Working Conference on Advanced Visual Interfaces (AVI 2000), pp. 238–241 (2000)
16. Tominski, C.: Event-Based Visualization for User-Centered Visual Analysis. Rostock, Germany, University of Rostock, Diss. (2006)
17. Van Wijk, J.J., Nuij, W.A.A.: Smooth and efficient zooming and panning. In: Proceedings of the 9th Annual IEEE Conference on Information Visualization, pp. 15–22 (2003)
18. White, R.W., Roth, R.A.: Exploratory search: Beyond the Query-Response paradigm. In: Marchionini, G. (ed.) Synthesis Lectures on Information Concepts, Retrieval, and Services. Morgan & Claypool Publishers (2009)
19. Woodruff, A., Landay, J., Stonebraker, M.: Constant information density in zoomable interfaces. In: Proceedings of the Working Conference on Advanced Visual Interfaces, pp. 57–65 (1998)

Improved Keyword Extraction by Separation into Multiple Document Sets According to Time Series

Ryosuke Saga and Hiroshi Tsuji

Osaka Prefecture University, 1-1, Gakuen-cho, Naka-ku, Sakai-shi, Osaka, Japan
{saga,tsuji}@cs.osakafu-u.ac.jp

Abstract. This study proposes a method of extracting keywords including those that appear locally. Useful keyword extraction methods are available for text mining, such as TF-IDF and support vector machine. However, when keywords are extracted on the basis of time series, the local keywords are not often extracted. We propose a method of extracting the local keywords by separating a document set, which we call the document separation approach. The approach splits a document set into multiple sets according to time series, extracts the keywords for each document set, and integrates them. Using 1812 newspaper articles, we experimentally demonstrate that we can extract the local feature keywords using the document separation approach.

Keywords: keyword extraction, document set, text mining.

1 Introduction

Many computerized documents continue to be generated as information technology progresses. In addition to newspaper and magazine articles from publishers, blogs and tweets in social media are generated daily by users, and a document set consisting of these documents can include several topics over several genres.

Keyword extraction is an essential technique because the extracted keywords of-ten express the topics covered, and we can analyze the topics using them. The extracted keywords are used not only for identifying the topics but also for query generation for a document set (often called a corpus). Thus, the extraction method is important when treating a document set [1].

Many methods are used to extract keywords from document sets. These methods are categorized as supervised or unsupervised. As an example of the former category, support vector machine [2] has been used to extract keywords from answer sets. In the latter category, term frequency–inverse document frequency (TF–IDF) [3] is a representative method that uses the word frequency in documents. Extraction methods for the latter category in particular depend on word frequency, document frequency, and the relationships between keywords. In fact, the relationships also depend on word frequency and document frequency, and so the term frequency and document frequency play important roles in keyword extraction. However, this method cannot extract keywords that appear locally (defined as local keywords) in time series. Such

C. Stephanidis (Ed.): Posters, Part II, HCII 2013, CCIS 374, pp. 450–453, 2013.

keywords are also important, but their frequencies are lower than those of global keywords. As a result, these keywords are regarded as unimportant.

In this study, we propose a method of extracting keywords including local keywords by splitting a document set into multiple sets according to time series. This method is called the document separation approach in this study.

2 Keyword Extraction by Document Separating Approach

The document separation approach is used to extract local keywords. The basic concept is that importance is attached to not global but local keywords, and that most local keywords are as useful as global keywords. The approach consists of three steps: splitting a document set into multiple sets according to time series, extracting keywords from each document set, and integrating and identifying the keywords.

1. Separation into multiple document sets

This step generates document sets from which keywords will be extracted. Several approaches can be used to separate a document set. For example, the equal-width approach separates a document set according to time series. The equal-frequency approach separates a document set by counting documents.

2. Keyword extraction for each document set

This step extracts the keywords. Many methods are available for extracting keywords. This study uses the TF–IDF method, which calculates an importance score. We can regard high-scoring terms as keywords when using this method. If there are N documents in a document set, a term i appears TF_i times in a document set, and the term appears in N_i documents. The TF–IDF approach is given by the formula

$$w_{i,j} = \mathrm{TF}_i \times \mathrm{IDF}_i, \tag{1}$$

where wi,j is the importance score of keyword i, and IDF_i = log (Ni /N). By splitting the document set, we can consider that local keywords can be well calculated. The top k high-scoring keywords are extracted as temporary keywords.

3. Keyword integration and identification

This step integrates the temporary keywords for each document set and identifies the keywords. To integrate the temporary keywords, we perform the set operation of union. Here when the same keywords appear in multiple document sets, we choose the higher scores and regard the score as the weight of the keyword. Finally, the top k high-scoring keywords are chosen and identified as keywords for the entire document set.

3 Experiments

We performed an experiment to validate the document separation approach. In this experiment, we used 1812 Mainichi newspaper articles published in Japan between January 1, 2006 and June 30, 2006 as a time series document set. We used the equal-width approach to separate the set into multiple document sets. Further, we extracted 50 keywords (that is, k = 50) and split the set into one (original), two, or six sets.

Part of the extraction results are shown in Table 1. This table shows pairs consisting of the top 30 keywords and TF–IDF scores for each type of split. These keywords seemed to be generic keywords, and the keyword sets were very similar for each case. However, the keywords "mail," "election," and "secretary-general" were ranked 20, 21, and 28, respectively, when the number of set was six. This keyword indicates the incident called the Horie mail problem, in which a councilor made a perjured statement that there was mistrust between a business person and a secretary-general about the Lower House election. This incident occurred suddenly in February 2006 and came to an end on March 31, 2006 (that is, the end of the incident was reported on April 1, 2006). As shown in Figure 1, the keyword "mail" is one of the local keywords; thus, by using the document separation approach, we could extract the local keywords.

Table 1. Result of extracted keyword (Top 30)

# of sets	1		2		6	
Rank	keyword	TFIDF	keyword	TFIDF	keyword	TFIDF
1	Prime Minister	1695.89	Prime Minister	976.54	Leader	273.47
2	Japan	1521.69	Japan	726.72	Prime Minister	256.52
3	government	1357.20	government	650.35	Japan	236.57
4	China	1314.22	Koizumi	585.81	China	208.63
5	problem	1259.09	problem	570.13	confer	208.20
6	Koizumi	1135.75	Devolution	565.99	government	207.79
7	confer	1079.98	China	562.26	Koizumi	196.96
8	Devolution	1012.85	Leader	543.50	Democratic Liberal Party	195.33
9	Democratic Party	1011.00	Democratic Liberal Party	525.82	Democratic Party	186.03
10	Democratic Liberal Party	1008.73	Democratic Party	492.89	Devolution	176.52
11	Leader	946.74	confer	474.64	talks	172.83
12	investigation	944.06	talks	468.82	problem	171.63
13	USA	928.25	society	460.91	councillor	157.73
14	relationship	899.65	governing party	448.38	committee	157.55
15	councillor	881.20	relationship	447.13	Tokyo	156.42
16	committee	878.46	Director-General	436.34	investigation	148.42
17	society	860.03	investigation	433.41	congress	146.27
18	talks	859.20	economy	432.38	economy	142.66
19	economy	837.82	councillor	425.53	politics	142.06
20	Diet	837.45	committee	423.96	**election**	141.64
21	Tokyo	807.48	Diet	418.50	**mail**	141.44
22	Director-General	793.87	USA	407.20	Director-General	134.39
23	governing party	756.02	Tokyo	403.60	USA	128.91
24	board chairman	712.68	board chairman	375.54	Diet	128.65
25	citizen	709.66	policy	366.72	relationship	112.33
26	policy	708.14	citizen	358.14	citizen	111.16
27	last year	707.23	congress	357.38	Mayor	110.24
28	politics	668.28	politics	348.08	**secretary-general**	109.66
29	congress	664.62	discussion	338.74	governing party	106.61
30	discussion	656.87	system	335.47	explanation	104.73

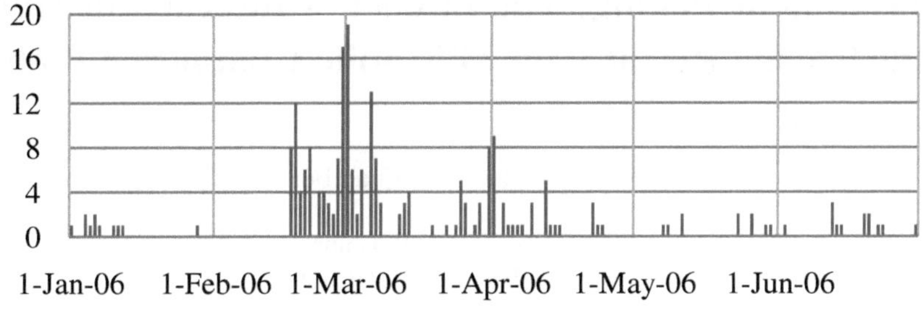

Fig. 1. Frequency movement of "mail" between January and June in 2006

4 Conclusion and Future Works

This study proposed a document separation approach for extracting keywords, including local keywords. The approach splits a document set into multiple sets ac-cording to time series, extracts the keywords from each document set, and integrates them. We showed experimentally that this approach can extract local keywords as well as global keywords.

This approach worked well for newspaper articles by separating them as per months. In addition, this method can be used for several applications such as FACT-Graph [4]. However, we could not observe local keywords when the document set was divided in half. Therefore, we have to identify effective separation points as a future work.

Acknowledgement. This research was supported by The Ministry of Education, Culture, Sports, Science and Technology (MEXT), Japan Society for the Promotion of Science(JSPS), Grant-in-Aid for Young Scientists (B), 23760358, 2011.4-2014.3

References

1. Manning, C.D., Raghavan, P., Schütze, H.: Introduction to Information Retrieval. Cambridge University Press, New York (2008)
2. Zhang, K., Xu, H., Tang, J., Li, J.: Keyword extraction using support vector machine. In: Yu, J.X., Kitsuregawa, M., Leong, H.-V. (eds.) WAIM 2006. LNCS, vol. 4016, pp. 85–96. Springer, Heidelberg (2006)
3. Salton, G.: Automatic Text Processing: The Transformation Analysis and Retrieval of Information by Computer. Addison-Wesley Publisher (1988)
4. Saga, R., Terachi, M., Tsuji, H.: FACT-Graph: Trend visualization by frequency and co-occurrence. Electronics and Communications in Japan 95, 50–58 (2012)

Scrolling or Paging: The Impact of Interaction Style on the Search Result Page of Mobile Commerce Website

Pingfei Wang[1] and Qian Fei[2]

[1] UX.etao.com, P.R. China
[2] www.taobao.com, P.R. China
qinfeng.wpf@taobao.com, fairyqq878188@gmail.com

Abstract. Increasingly, users are accessing the e-commerce website by mobile device. Users are performing complicated tasks when they are shopping on line, like searching, comparing and adding products to cart. Due to the vast application on PC and limited size of the screen of the mobile device, it is common to present web page in scrolling format, especially on the SRP (Search Result Page) of mobile Commerce Site. Although a large body of work have done to investigate the impact of the scrolling and paging on the words reading, comprehension and even recall, the results of these studies have few implications for the SRP of e-commerce web site. The purpose of this study was to investigate the impact of interaction style (paging or scrolling) on the SRP of mobile commerce web site. We examine execution times for within SRP searching tasks varying interaction styles (scrolling and pagination). Meanwhile, error rate of recall task was recorded to indicate the influence of interaction style on the working memory.

Keywords: paging, scrolling, SRP, working memory, mobile device.

1 Introduction

Increasingly, users are accessing the e-commerce website by mobile device, Including smart phones and tablets. Users are performing complicated tasks when they are shopping on line, like searching, comparing and adding products to cart. Due to the vast application on PC and limited size of the screen of the mobile device, it is common to present web page in scrolling format, especially on the SRP (Search Result Page) of mobile e-commerce site.

Some Researchers have found that scrolling can enhance the efficiency of skimming or scanning behaviors on visual search tasks (Bernard, Baker, & Fernandez, 2002; Madathil, Koikkara,Gramopadhye , 2011), but another study indicated that a scrolling format reduced understanding of complex topics from Web pages, especially for readers who were lower in working memory capacity(Sanchez and Wiley, 2009) .Although a large body of work have done to investigate the impact of the scrolling and paging on the words reading , comprehension and even recall, the results of these studies have few implications for the SRP of e-commerce web site that present information in the scrolling format. There are 2 main reasons limit the implications. First,

C. Stephanidis (Ed.): Posters, Part II, HCII 2013, CCIS 374, pp. 454–457, 2013.

the materials used in prior research were texts, it is not the same as the SRP which including pictures and texts. Second, the tasks in previous study are visual search or reading, but when users visit the SRP, they scan and then decide which products they like or not, during this progress, more complicated mental activities are required.

The purpose of this study was to investigate the impact of interaction style (paging or scrolling) on the SRP of mobile commerce web site. Our experiment including 2 tasks. In task 1,we discuss the influence of the interaction style on the perception of the products information presented o the SRP; In task 2, we examine the efficiency by the search task on the paging or the scrolling SRP.

2 Method

2.1 Participants

9 participants were employed in our study, all of them were retained in the final analyses. Participants were compensated with a gift.

2.2 Material

The materials in the study are 3 difference kinds of search result pages(see Figure 1). Material A is a traditional paging SRP , participants navigated between pages using "Next" and "Back" links embedded at the bottom of each page. Material B is a scrolling SRP without any location information (e.g., page number), so participants do not know their "place on the page". Material C is a mixed SRP in scrolling and paging style, participants scrolling first and at the end of certain length of scrolling page there are "Next" and "Back" links embedded at the bottom. 100 products were presented on each material page.

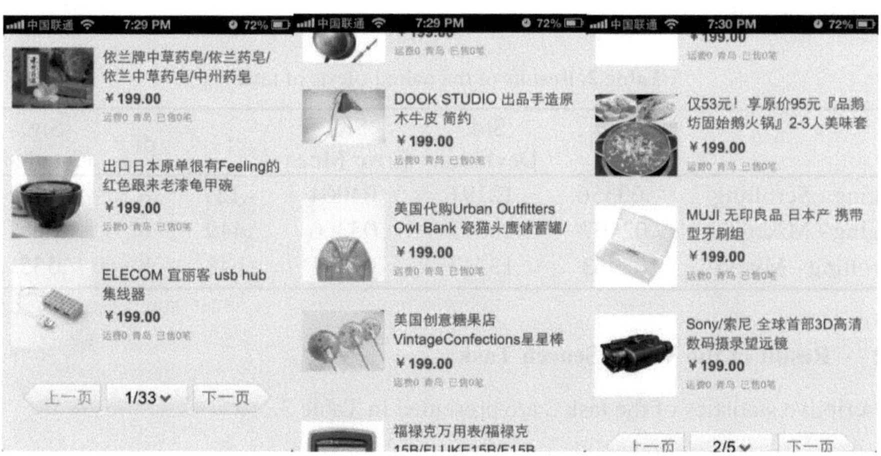

Fig. 1. The 3 demo search resulted page in the study

2.3 Tasks

There are 2 main tasks in this study. During the task 1, participants are asked to scanning all 100 products listed on material pages and then complete a recall test. In task 2, participants are asked to find the specified products by searching the material page. Tasks are going to performed by participants using an Apple Iphone 4s. Each participant completes tasks with 3 different kinds of pages (A, B, C). Error rate in the task 1 and time to complete the task 2 are recorded as the quantitative measure.

This study is within subject design, to prevent sequence effects and practice effects, the materials are well balanced.

3 Results

3.1 Result of the Recall Test

Descriptive statistics of the task 1 are presented in Table 1.

Table 1. Descriptive statistics of the error rate in the task 1

Interaction style	Mean	N	Std. Deviation	Std. Error Mean
Paging	.8037	9	.12904	.04301
Scrolling	.8093	9	.12967	.04322
Mixed	.7796	9	.14428	.04809

Paired t-tests were performed to investigate the effects of the interaction style on the perception of the SRP (see table 2). There was no significant difference on the error rate between the paging and scrolling SRP($t=-.137, p>.05$). It is the same between the paging and mixed style page ($.449$, $p>.05$), scrolling and the mixed style page($.648$, $p>.05$).

Table 2. Results of the paired t-tests of task 1

	Mean	Std. Deviation	Std. Error Mean	t	df	Sig. (2-tailed)
Paging - Scrolling	-.00556	.12191	.04064	-.137	8	.895
Paging - Mixed	.02407	.16097	.05366	.449	8	.666
Scrolling - Mixed	.02963	.13713	.04571	.648	8	.535

3.2 Result of the Visual Search Task

Descriptive statistics of the task 2 are presented in Table 3.

Table 3. Descriptive statistics of the execution time in the task 2.

Interaction style	Mean	N	Std. Deviation	Std. Error Mean
Paging	34.3333	9	5.50000	1.83333
Scrolling	38.4444	9	10.73675	3.57892
Mixed	36.1111	9	4.31406	1.43802

Paired t-tests were performed to investigate the effects of the interaction style on the visual search execution time in task 2 (see table 4). There was no significant difference on the visual search execution time between the paging and scrolling SRP($t=-.968, p>.05$). It is the same between the paging and mixed style page (1.042, $p>.05$), scrolling and the mixed style page (.624, $p>.05$).

Table 4. T-test results of task 2

	Mean	Std. Deviation	Std. Error Mean	t	df	Sig. (2-tailed)
Paging - Scrolling	-4.11111	12.74210	4.24737	-.968	8	.361
Paging - Mixed	-1.77778	5.11805	1.70602	-1.042	8	.328
Scrolling - Mixed	2.33333	11.22497	3.74166	.624	8	.550

4 Conclusion

In our study, we found that when comes to the SRP of the mobile e-commerce site, the interaction style has no impact on the perception of the products listed on the page .Meanwhile, searching task result indicates that the scrolling or paging cannot affect the efficiency on the SRP of the mobile e-commerce site.

References

1. Bernard, M., Baker, R., et al.: Paging vs. scrolling: Looking for the best way to present search results. Usability News 4(1) (2002)
2. Sanchez, C.A., Wiley, J.: To Scroll or Not to Scroll: Scrolling, Working Memory Capacity, and Comprehending Complex Texts. Human Factors: The Journal of the Human Factors and Ergonomics Society 51(5), 730–738 (2009)
3. Marcial, L., Hemminger, B.: Scrolling and pagination for within document searching: The impact of screen size and interaction style. Proceedings of the American Society for Information Science and Technology 48(1), 1–4 (2011)
4. Chalil Madathil, K., Koikkara, R., et al.: An Empirical Study of the Usability of Consenting Systems. SAGE Publications (2011)

A Personal Document Network Building System for Digital Document Searches

Masahiro Yoshikoshi, Kenji Matsunaga, and Kyoko Yoshida

School of Network and Information, Senshu University, Kanagawa, Japan
m.yoshikoshi106@gmail.com,
{matunaga,k-yoshida}@isc.senshu-u.ac.jp

Abstract. The popularity of eBooks has spread in recent years with the launch of eBook readers and more contents. Managing purchased eBooks is becoming problematic with the spread of eBooks which allows individuals to possess many books as digital documents. The volume of eBooks as well as digital documents owned by individuals is also increasing, necessitating the development of a method to search and browse them. This study led to the development of a Private Library Surfing (PLS) system as a browsing system for digital documents typified by eBooks, etc. in order to resolve this problem.

Keywords: eBooks, Digital Document.

1 Introduction

The popularity of eBooks has spread in recent years with the launch of eBook readers and more contents. Managing purchased eBooks is becoming problematic with the spread of eBooks which allows individuals to possess many books as digital documents. The volume of eBooks as well as digital documents owned by individuals is also increasing, necessitating the development of a method to search and browse them.

This study led to the development of a Private Library Surfing (PLS) system as a browsing system for digital documents typified by eBooks, etc. in order to resolve the problem described above. The PLS system targets the effective use of many digital documents possessed by individuals. This system allows users to search across multiple digital documents, summarize them as a new document using the link function based on the search results to browse this book. This linked and newly summarized one arranges documents the individual has into a network form, and we believe it to be a format that is easy to use.

2 Background

eBooks have the advantage of being able to transport a massive number of books with the eBook reader. Yet the search method for paper books still has many more superb

C. Stephanidis (Ed.): Posters, Part II, HCII 2013, CCIS 374, pp. 458–461, 2013.

features. Multiple related books can be compared on the tabletop while reading to conduct a search using paper books for example, perfect for a fuller understanding. Nevertheless, current eBook readers have insufficient functions for reading and comparing multiple books in series, and searching target items from multiple books. Digital documents individuals possess also have similar problems like eBooks in that it is time-consuming to search their contents.

The Internet at present allows for gathering webpage information on the dispersed server easily. Relevant webpages can be browsed by entering a keyword into the browser, and you can move through successive pages linked from this webpage.

If there is a system which allows for searching and browsing using a similar method for personal digital documents, and make it easy to reuse them, it will be useful for users.

3 PLS System

The PLS system was created to search, browse and reuse digital documents, typified by eBooks, efficiently. It is a useful system for searching if there are any interrelated items, or to compare and reuse related items in multiple digital documents.

Users can search the entire digital document collection they manage by setting keywords for the conditions to be searched. Multiple documents containing the same keywords can also be browsed successively as one document. Links between browsed documents can be saved and looked at again as one new document the next time. This linked and newly summarized one arranges documents the individual has into a network form, and it will be a format that is easy to use. Here the system is created to handle ePub and PDF as the digital document formats.

3.1 PLS System Functions

The PLS system consists of the "Document Search", "Create Linked Document" and "View" functions (Figure 1).

Document Search Function

The Document Search Function is for searching whether a document contains keywords the user wants to find. Locations where the keywords are in the searched document are displayed, while word frequency in the document is also shown. Users can select documents by using the search results.

Create Linked Document Function

The Create Linked Document Function allows relevant pages of multiple documents to be read as one document. Pages with documents containing the same keywords can be linked. Only linked pages are grouped together, and can be saved as a new linked document. Those who have the same documents can also use the linked information by exchanging with each other.

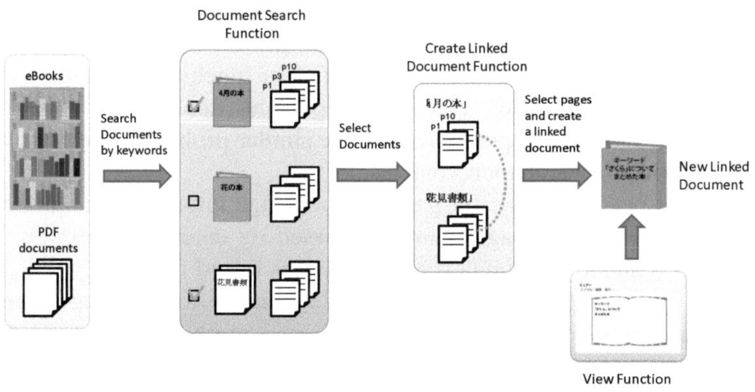

Fig. 1. PLS System Functions

View Function

The View Function is for browsing linked documents and viewing multiple documents in series. The "Keyword", "Document Name" and "Page Number" of linked pages can also be viewed in a list.

3.2 Flow of PLS System Use

The PLS system consists of "Search", "Search Results", "Create Linked Document" and "View" screens.

The Search screen displays documents located in the document collection and displays linked documents that have been created. Also, Users can enter a keyword to search documents containing them.

The Search Results screen lists documents containing keywords and allows the location containing the keywords and information on word frequency to be viewed. The Create Linked Document screen is launched when the document to be read from the search results list is selected (Figure 2).

The Create Linked Document screen is for selecting the pages contained in the new linked document from the search results list. The pages can be assigned while verifying them from the Preview screen. Selected pages are displayed in the linked page list area on the right side of the screen (Figure 3).

The View screen is for browsing documents and linked documents. These documents are displayed in the view area. The original documents can be browsed in a separate window when they are linked documents. Keywords used when a linked document is created are also shown.

4 Evaluation

Five (5) students and educators used the PLS system and we obtained their comments on the functions and user interface. Some of the evaluations were "it was useful for searching literature from many books", "You can easily search and select books you want to reference", "It can be used for work in grouping multiple documents together", "It would be useful if it could be linked to a digital library system." There were some comments of concern on improving the user interface such as "it was difficult to understand the operations method" and "it would be better to devise slightly a better method when putting information in the search results."

5 Conclusion

This paper proposes the PLS system for the effective use of many digital documents individuals possess, and evaluates it. Some improvements that can be made to the PLS system would be to support tablets and mobile devices, and improve user interface. Tests to evaluate the utility of the PLS system objectively are also being planned.

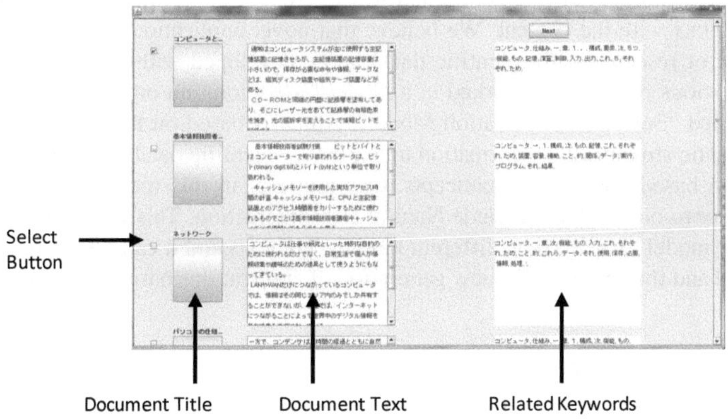

Fig. 2. The Search Result Screen

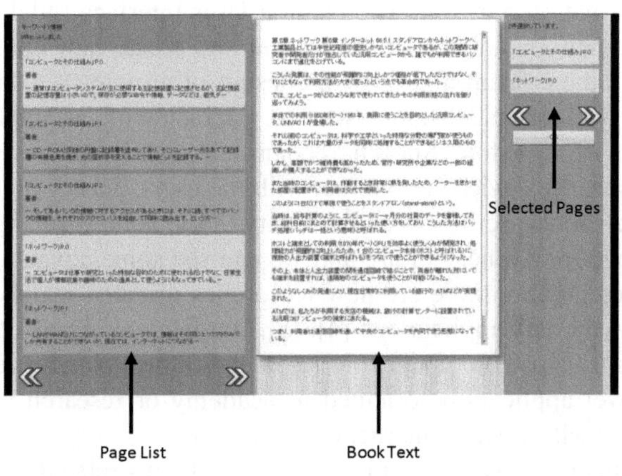

Fig. 3. The Create Linked Document Screen

Natural User Interface for Information Retrieval

J. Sergio Zepeda-Hernandez[1], Erick López -Ornelas[1], Rocío Abascal -Mena[1], Jovita Martínez[2], and Juan Carlos Estrada[2]

[1] Universidad Autónoma Metropolitana-Unidad Cuajimalpa., Av. Constituyentes 1054, Col. Lomas Altas, Del. Miguel Hidalgo, México, D.F.
[2] Centro de Investigación y de Estudios Avanzados del I.P.N., Av. Instituto Politécnico Nacional 2508, Zacatenco, Del. G.A. Madero, México, D.F.
{jzepeda,elopez,mabascal}@correo.cua.uam.mx,
{jmartine,jestrada}@cinvestav.mx

Abstract. The Natural User Interface (NUI) offers a great potential to create new paradigms of interaction and it also create new challenges about how we interact with the content. We believe that novel applications oriented to academy or research with scientific data can be developed with this paradigm. In a previous research we worked in a model for exploration on scientific databases called "Semantic Exploration Model", which is based on the use the small semantic structures of information to explore a scientific database thought navigation based on semantic concepts. Our proposal in this research is add a new layer to our model to include Natural User Interaction. This way, we can extend the model to be used on different kind the contexts and it can offer a new potential and the creation of a new generation of applications based on this paradigm.

1 Introduction

Nowadays there are several databases with important information available, but consequently there is also a need for new technics and more user-friendly interfaces oriented to information retrieval. The Natural User Interface (NUI) offers a great potential to create new paradigms of interaction and create new challenges about how we interact with the content and how the design of an interface should show the information [1]. NUI offers different way to interact with an application as: Touch Screen, Gesture recognition, Speech recognition and Brain-machine interface and each one with specific devices to interact with the users. Mistry in [2], with the Sixth-Sense prototype shows usefulness and viability of the natural hand gestures to interact with the information in a near future and we can see some advantage over traditional interaction styles [3]. So, there are new researches oriented mainly to develop video games or human therapy applications [4], [5]. But we look a lack of application based on NUI paradigm focused to data exploration and information retrieval. This way, we believe that novel applications oriented to academy or research with scientific data can be developed with gesture interaction paradigm.

To achieve this goal, we must solve several problems related to: gestural language for interaction, interface design, menus, presentation of contents and translation of

C. Stephanidis (Ed.): Posters, Part II, HCII 2013, CCIS 374, pp. 462–465, 2013.

gestural events on automatic queries. In this document we only present previously advance and how we are working in our objective, because still it is a work in progress with strong evidences to achieve good results.

2 Semantic Exploration Model

The interaction for retrieval information through NUI is not a trivial task, because all the applications are oriented mainly to traditional interaction (keyboard and mouse interaction). In a previous research we worked in a model for exploration on scientific databases called "Semantic Exploration Model (SEM)", which is based on the use the small semantic structures of information to explore a scientific database through navigation based on semantic concepts [6]. This model emerged of the necessity of come upon a new paradigm of interaction with scientific databases; so, we found a new way to interact with this kind of information. Our model is composed of three essential layers: Rich interaction, Control of behavior and Semantics of information.

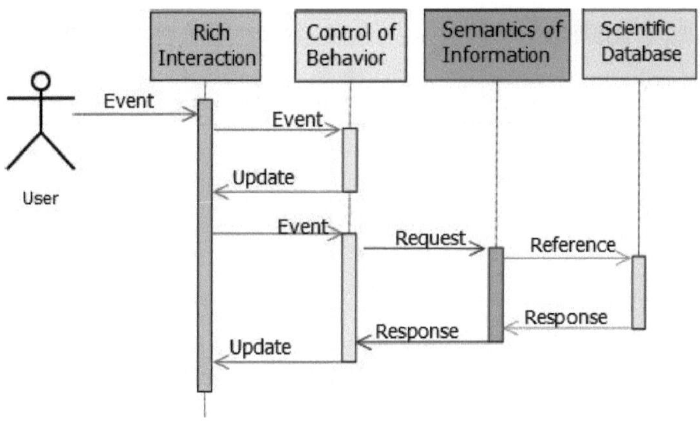

Fig. 1. The sequence diagram shows the communication and interaction between the three essential layers of Semantic Exploration Model (SEM)

The figure 1 shows the high-level abstraction of the model, each layer internally is composed of sub-layer with specific functionalities of interaction and communication. The layer named as semantic information is composed of small semantic structures belonging to the information of the scientific database.

The layer denominate as control of behavior update the interface with new content, it also offers control about all the events inside the interface, and it also translates the events on automatic queries through of the small semantic structures to retrieve information from the scientific database. Finally the layer labeled as rich interaction provides continuous updating of the interface on dynamic way using the semantic structures, it provides a rich interaction with the final user and it also offers transparent access to complex relationship of information in the database. This way, the final users can do exploration and retrieve information without to use the keyboard, because the interaction is through visual icons with a semantic meaning that layer semantics of information translates to traditional queries for web server. Here, we only offer a very general description of the Semantic Exploration Model part of this research, if it is necessary more information about the model we can to see [6], [7].

3 Integration of NUI with Semantic Exploration Model

Our model was design with the characteristic of flexibility for include future features and improvements to the model. In this research, our goal is add a generic new layer to our model and to include Natural User Interaction based on gestural recognition. So, this way we want to extend the model to be used on different kind the contexts and it can offer a new potential to develop a new generation of application based on this paradigm.

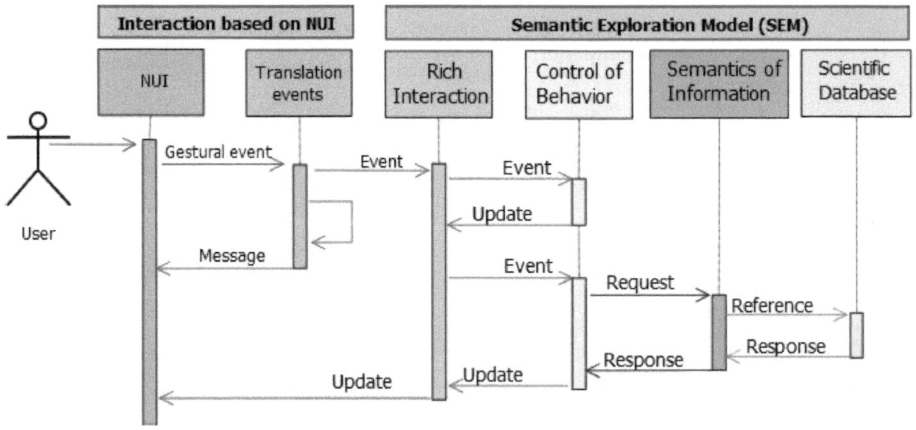

Fig. 2. The sequence diagram shows how the Semantic Exploration Model adds a generic layer to support the interaction based on a Natural User Interface

The figure 2 shows all the layers involved in this research, the sequence diagram is composed of two generic high-level abstraction layers (*Semantic Exploration Model and Interaction based on NUI*). The first is already built and the second is in the process of construction and initial testing. We can see in the figure 2, that we need a translation of gestural events, because the SEM was designed to mouse interaction based on traditional GUI and we need to adapt it to this new paradigm. So, the main idea is to have a translation engine of gestural events to traditional events, but during this research, we are considering to create a native layer of interpretation of gestural events to create automatic queries inside the model, we need to evaluate which of the two options is the most relevance, because we want to offer the better facilities to use the model in the largest number of contexts.

4 Conclusions

The goal of this research is to offer a Natural User Interface oriented to information retrieval, through a model previously developed by us. The main idea consists on adding the gestural events to our model, although it is not a trivial task, we are discovering some features not considered in the initial idea, because the integration of the SEM with NUI generates new questions and opens new possibilities. Therefore, we believe that this research can help to create a new generation of applications based on NUI in a near future.

References

1. Blake, J.: Natural User Interfaces. Manning Publications (2012)
2. Mistry, P., Maes, P.: SixthSense: A Wearable Gestural Interface. In: International Conference on Computer Graphics and Interactive Techniques (2009)
3. Rautherberg, M.: From Gesture to Action: Natural User Interfaces. Technical University of Eindhoven, Mens-Machine Interactive, Diesrede, pp. 15–25 (1999)
4. Song, Y., et al.: Continuous body and hand gesture recognition for natural human-computer interaction. ACM, Transactions on Interactive Intelligent Systems 2(1) (March 2012)
5. Regol, P.A., Moreira, P.M., Reis, L.P.: Natural User Interfaces in Serious Games for Rehabilitation. In: 6th Iberian Conference on Information Systems and Technologies, pp. 1–4 (2011)
6. Zepeda, J.S., Jiménez, H., Abascal, R., López, E., Martínez, J., Estrada, J.C.: Semantic Exploration Model for Scientific Databases. In: Advances in Computer Science and Engineering (accepted for publication, 2013)
7. Zepeda, J.S., Jiménez, H., Abascal, R., López, E., Martínez, J., Estrada, J.C.: Semantic Exploration based on Concepts for a Database with Microbial Information. Research in Computing Science (accepted for publication, 2013)
8. Stone, D., Jarret, C.: User Interface Design and Evaluation. Morgan Kaufmann Publisher, Elsevier (2005)

Part VII
Work, Collaboration and Creativity

Integrating Production Workers into User Interface Design for Diagnosis Devices in Automotive Production Environments: Field Experiences and Lessons Learned

Nikolaj Borisov, Annette Kluge, Wolfram Luther, and Benjamin Weyers

University of Duisburg-Essen, Duisburg
{nikolaj.borisov,annette.kluge}@uni-due.de,
{luther,weyers}@inf.uni-due.de

Abstract. In this paper, we present an exploratory case study regarding user interface design for test and diagnosis devices in automotive production environments. We report workers´ opinions concerning existing user interfaces and devices, as well as the use of innovative user interface and interaction concepts. Finally, we derive requirements for future use of modern interaction concepts and present a set of possible devices for future evaluation.

Keywords: Industrial production context, test and diagnosis, user interface design, user machine dialogue.

1 Introduction

Today's requirements for human-machine interaction should consider central aspects of human factors/ergonomics, usability, reliability, human-machine cooperation and a human-centered design. Innovative and future-oriented concepts to achieve an unambiguous interaction between humans and machines are furthermore needed in industrial production context in which they have been often neglected [1]. The purpose of the present study is to investigate the existing user interfaces and devices in an automotive production environment and to formulate requirements for future development. The challenges was the necessity of applying test benches for quality controls to improve existing user interfaces without radically changing existing workflows and induce negative side effects on the production process.

The study has been accomplished on production lines at two different automotive production locations. At these production lines, a car passes through several quality control stages where workers use mobile and stationary devices for checking certain electronic car features. The test duration depends mainly on the vehicle's configuration and the requirements of the countries they are exported to. Usually, the testing sequence begins with connecting a diagnosis device to the vehicle. Then, the worker starts the test sequence, which consists of automatic testing routines without interventions by the worker, as well as manual test procedures the worker has to carry out manually in and around the car. These manual test procedures contain visual examinations and/or interaction with the test device to confirm the well function of certain

C. Stephanidis (Ed.): Posters, Part II, HCII 2013, CCIS 374, pp. 469–473, 2013.

electronic car components by pressing a button on the device. All vehicles with at least one encountered error are sorted out and returned to overhaul, followed by a further quality check after resolving all errors. All cars leaving the production line have successfully passed all quality checks.

2 Methodology

We conducted a human factors centered exploratory case study based on semi-structured interviews with 36 production workers accompanied by field observations that were conducted in two production sites of a large German car manufacturer. The two sites used similar but not identical hardware concepts and thus also testing software. The working experience (tenure) of the workers varied from a few days up to 40 years. The interview was specially designed for being conducted in the field: at production lines during running production. Overall, each worker was asked 19 questions. Each question was rated on a 5-point scale from -2 (very negative) to +2 (very positive), and a zero as a neutral option. Topics addressed in the interviews were personal experiences with the existing equipment, especially their performance, software design and forms of assistance. In addition, workers were asked about information on non-functional elements, such as the use of multimedia stylistic elements. Finally, we proposed alternative user interface concepts to the workers, such as compact and handy sized terminals, headsets, head-mounted-displays, and gesture control. The workers were also asked about their requests and suggestions for new innovative diagnosis devices in the near future.

3 Results

The insights from the interviews with the workers at both production sites demonstrated the importance of user integration into the design process. According to our observations at two different locations with different diagnosis systems we encountered that the current diagnosis systems in use were primarily designed for diagnosis specifications and industry standards. The criterion of "user experience" was widely neglected. Analyzing the transfer of this assumption with regard to the definition of usability [2] we came to the conclusion that existing diagnosis systems were effective in terms of fulfilled specifications but not always efficient in terms of ease of use.

For example, diagnosis devices are very versatile with many features and many keyboard buttons providing a default layout. This can result in higher error rates by accidently pushing a wrong button, which may lead to the cancelation of the whole diagnosis process. Nevertheless, the interviewed workers have accustomed themselves to the current diagnosis system and use it properly and efficiently. We think that this is the reason for the low rating of proposed alternative devices presented to the workers, which show better condition concerning usability requirements. Other reasons for this negative outcome were difficulties of workers' ability to image the use of such devices and the work environment. For instance, wearing devices on the body foster hygienically problems and thus were rejected as a possible new class of devices. Furthermore, workers have no intention to use innovative interaction concepts unless there is a chance to increase ergonomic and usability aspects at the same time.

Below, we list important requirements and challenges for alternative diagnosis devices for production lines we gained from our exploratory case study:

- Compliance with the industry standards: heat resistance, stability, shock resistance, long battery life, mobility, short maintenance and service intervals, Safety and health aspect
- Compliance with company philosophy: Effectiveness and efficiency, high Availability and replaceable
- Flexibility: adaptable user interface on workers experience or cultural background
- Ergonomics and satisfaction, e.g. social acceptance, motivation, emotion, Communication features

3.1 Alternative and Innovative Diagnosis Devices

In this chapter we want to introduce various diagnosis devices and reactions to these alternatives, accompanied challenges arising from discussions with workers. Based on this study, the following results from interviews were obtained for devices with visual information representation with haptic controls, and alternative user interfaces such as gesture control, head mounted display and auditory input and output (i.e. headsets).

Handy sized terminals: These devices are usually equipped with touch screen and haptic controls. The great advantage of these devices is the common use of multimedia on graphical screens and audio capabilities. The haptic controls give also a better feedback feeling and safety versus touching screens. They can also be worn attached to an arm or pocket, hence it is in reachable range to read information and confirm incoming orders. Workers can interact with these devices only one-handed and use the other hand for interaction with the inspected vehicle. Graphical screens allow also customization and personalization for visual data representation due to user experience.

Negative aspects of such devices are a poor heat resistance, additional heat produced by operating a device, and current short battery life what is unsuitable for shifts up to 8 hours in production. To get further instructions during diagnosis process, a worker has to toggle his view between vehicle and diagnosis device, which implies high level of concentration.

Gesture-based interaction: For gesture-based interaction, devices such as sensor gloves should be used [3]. Thus, both hands can be used freely to interact with vehicle. If gloves are personalized for each worker also hygienic requirements are met. Furthermore, visual sensors can recognize workers' gestures without using any gloves or other wearing sensors for interaction [4].

But this kind of interaction has some challenges. The handling of such devices is not intuitive and workers would need to train available interaction commands [4]. Additional devices (i.e. acoustic, graphical interfaces, sensors) for input processing and incoming instructions are required.

Head-mounted displays: Devices such as Google Glasses [5] are at first glance one of the best alternatives which combines various technologies (i.e. display, camera, speaker and microphone) in one device. Workers do not need to toggle sight between vehicle and device. Visualized order and further information are always in focus without restrictions to the field of view and allows using a customizable graphical user interfaces.

Based on the workers statements, head-mounted displays are unsuitable for using on production lines. Head-mounted displays are predestinated to carry them on the body respective on the worker's head. Particularly, in summer and very hot temperatures of about 30 degrees Celsius (86 degrees Fahrenheit), this would be very unpleasant. The built-in computer devices would produce additional heat. Another issue is the hygienic of this device class. A further aspect is the heavy weight of many head-mounted displays, which may cause eyestrain and health problems [6].

Headset-based interaction: Interaction via headset also offers many possibilities for customization and personalization. To improve communication between workers and computer interface it is possible to create for each user own profile for voice input or language. Similarly, the output can be also adjusted to the user experience and language. Interaction with such devices is done by special acoustic signals and voice commands. Workers have both hands free to interact with a vehicle and the viewing direction must not be toggled anymore between diagnosis device and vehicle [7].

The main challenge of headsets would be to achieve a clear speech comprehension in noisy environment. Further, this kind of interaction depends on learning of correct pronouncing and encoded words to achieve a smooth interaction. Another unpleasant side effect of using such devices would be health and psychological aspects caused by permanent repetitive acoustic signals through excessive use.

On both production sides was confirmed that current used mobile devices are usable but are so far not ergonomically designed. All introduced alternative devices have also their challenges. Furthermore, the interviewed workers have confirmed that haptic controls were preferred over the touch-interfaces due to better physical feedback. Due to social acceptance and privacy violation, cameras are generally not possible. Therefore it is strongly recommended to carry out further studies to elaborate alternative diagnosis devices and further challenges for automotive production environments.

3.2 Software Challenges

In this case study we determined some usability issues in software design caused by overloaded screens with textual information and no use of multimedia elements, which may be important for less experienced workers. We also missed a feature to support workers on machine failures. On the production lines the diagnosis program is working very simple. Workers getting an order from the program what to do next (i.e. start engine, push button X, open/close doors, visual inspection of light sources, etc.), understand it and finally execute and/or confirm it. But once an error occurs, for example lost diagnosis communication to vehicle or important precondition due to accident prevention was not occurred. The worst case is when display still showing the same order, even if worker successfully finished or confirmed the order and nothing happens, because the diagnosis program lost connection to the vehicle. At this point, we need additional kind of software logic to compensate such situation by starting to report helpful user instructions after elapsed time for a task without noticed any user interaction. Among others, a very crucial insight was that workers constantly need an overview about what and why the software is doing what it does at a certain point in time and that support is needed to predict subsequent process states in accordance to workers' mental process model.

4 Conclusion

It was not easy to perform this study with interviews directly on the production line under time pressure. The quality of the survey can therefore be improved on outside of the production line. However, more important was to plan the worker integration in this study from the outset. Based on these experiences, we will develop a new approach of applying a human factors centered, worker-oriented approach of modeling user interfaces for human-machine interaction in automotive production environments. This modeling approach will be based on prior work in user interface modeling [8] and accompanied with the design of a new handy and versatile mobile interface, which will be developed comprehending production workers resulting in a structured and novel design for ease of use accordingly to the requirements revealed in the interviews and in ongoing case studies.

References

1. Backman, J., Helaakoski, H.: Mobile technology to support maintenance efficiency — Mobile maintenance in heavy industry. In: 2011 9th IEEE International Conference on Industrial Informatics (INDIN), pp. 328–333 (2011)
2. ISO 9241-11: Guidance on usability (1998)
3. Witt, H., Nicolai, T., Kenn, H.: Designing a wearable user interface for hands-free interaction in maintenance applications. In: Fourth Annual IEEE International Conference on Pervasive Computing and Communications Workshops, PerCom Workshops 2006, pp. 652–655 (2006)
4. Chu, T.-T., Su, C.-Y.: A Kinect-based handwritten digit recognition for TV remote controller. In: 2012 International Symposium on Intelligent Signal Processing and Communications Systems (ISPACS), pp. 414–419 (2012)
5. Google Glass, `http://glass.google.com`
6. Sage, C., Carpenter, D.O.: Public health implications of wireless technologies. Pathophysiology 16(2-3), 233–246 (2009)
7. Lee, K.B., Grice, R.A.: The Design and Development of User Interfaces for Voice Application in Mobile Devices. In: 2006 IEEE International Professional Communication Conference, pp. 308–320 (2006)
8. Weyers, B., Burkolter, D., Luther, W., Kluge, A.: Formal modeling and reconfiguration of user interfaces for reduction of errors in failure handling of complex systems. International Journal of Human-Computer Interaction 28, 646–665 (2012)

Improve of Business Intelligence Usage in Brazilian Chemical Industry in Global Crisis of 2008, 2009 and 2010

Tiago Vieira Carvalho and Renato Jose Sassi

Industrial Engineering Postgraduation Program, Nove de Julho University – UNINOVE.
São Paulo, SP, Brasil
tiagovc@gmail.com, sassi@uninove.br

Abstract. From 2008´s to 2010's a serious financial crisis forced many sectors to drastically review their production and sales plans. Sectors like the chemical industry were reorganized to deal with the challenging scenario found. This article's objective is to demonstrate how the world crisis from 2008 to 2010 was an opportunity to improve the business intelligence architecture usage, bringing benefits for a brazilian chemistry industry, helping the company on process standardization, data quality improvement and process automation.

Keywords: Chemistry Industry, Business Intelligence, Best Practices, Worldwide Crisis.

1 Introduction

On 2008 it began a global economic crisis born on the subprime real estate market in the United States. The crisis had consequences as deterioration of bank balance sheets and a strong reduction in interbank liquidity. As a crisis direct result there was a fall in industrial production and prices, which meant that capitalist firms had to postpone investment on new projects [11, 3].

The global economic crisis represented a turning point in the history of capitalism. Besides being the most severe economic crisis faced by capitalist economies since 1929, it was also a social crisis which, according to forecasts by the International Labour Organization, the number of unemployed increased from 20 million to 50 million by the end of 2009. The fall in income due to the crisis of the poor and the maintenance of international prices of food commodities at high levels, the number of undernourished people worldwide increased by 11% in 2009 and for the first time, surpassed one billion [10].

With the advancement in technology in recent years, companies started to operate with the support of Information Systems (IS) to achieve cost reductions and to create competitive advantage. One big trend in IS is the expansion of the system scope from a purely operational to support a broader scope, involving also support to decision taking process [2, 5].

C. Stephanidis (Ed.): Posters, Part II, HCII 2013, CCIS 374, pp. 474–478, 2013.

An IS example to support decision-taking is an architecture of Business Intelligence (BI). It provides assistance to identify situations in thousands of information. BI became something so popular in industries that it was cited as one of the highest priorities of the new millennium projects by more than half of the executives of information technology [6, 8].

Due to the recession, many companies did not have the financial capital for new investments. So, companies had to review their processes and information systems to remain competitive in a scenario of large cost savings.

In a Brazilian chemical industry this scenario of global crisis strengthened the dissemination of best practices in the use of Business Intelligence architecture. Were reinforced corporate governance rules, processes were improved and standardized, and the usage of the BI architecture by company's employees was increased.

As there was not enough money to invest on new projects, the global crisis created a great opportunity to increase the usage of BI architecture with the use of reporting tools like Business Objects (BO) and the Business Information Warehouse (BW).

2 Best Practices for Using a BI Architecture

The implementing and maintenance processes a BI architecture are similar. The vast majority of deployment best practices can also be considered as useful to ensure a good use of the architecture implemented. In the scenario of financial crisis, it was very important to apply best practices to encourage the use of the BI architecture of the company and thereby support decision-making.

Some of the best practices for deploying a BI architecture are: end-user involvement, to avoid proprietary architectures that are hard to integrate, to have the BI as a philosophy of work to be used by the company, to have the participation of experienced and practical consultants; the presence of an environment development, references to the tools of choice, training, participation in the design of an expert on multidimensional modeling, a team dedicated to DW [7, 12].

Communication is very important to define and encourage the use of a system. It is a complex process that involves issuing, receiving and understanding verbal and non-verbal messages. Interpersonal relationships are involved and often there may be incorrect understandings and other problems that make the message sent not properly understood [9].

BI should not be intended as something static, focusing on a few users, the scale factor is of utmost importance. The technologies used must allow growth in volume and queries [4].

The old models of relationship between employee and employer are currently being reviewed. More flexible strategies have been used to help reconcile the various types of professional work and professional interests. For these reasons, workers need to be constantly recycled to keep their knowledge up to date and develop other skills [1].

By studying the use of monthly indicators of BI architecture usage, it was possible to point out clearly who did not use the architecture and to work to understand the reason for nonuse. Among the reasons there were the following justifications: the lack of technical knowledge, distrust of information from and access no longer needed.

3 Methodology

We conducted a literature search with the keywords: Business Intelligence, Chemical Industry, Financial Crisis, Information Systems that found Master's dissertations, articles, books and web pages with relevant content. We accessed scientific databases like SCIELO, SCOPUS, EBSCO and WEB of Knowledge for retrieving searched topics' relevant articles.

Two tools were chosen to be analyzed, the tool BO and the tool BW (http://www.sap.com/brazil/solutions/sapbusiness objects/index.epx). Both tools are aimed at extracting reports from databases of the most varied subjects such as Sales, Purchasing, Production, Projects and others.

From the reports found on such tools, there are corporate (Core Reports) and not corporate (Non Core). Core Reports are standardized and used by a large number of people, areas and countries. Non Core Reports are users customized reports created because of special needs or exceptions that the core could not face.

Audit Databases were used to report how many times per month a user has accessed the tools BO and BW during all months of the years 2008 to 2010. If a user had used the system, there was no specific action taken with him. If he had not used, it was questioned why the non-use. The development of this paper is based on the study, revision and implementation of bio-inspired computing techniques for solving combinatorial optimization problems.

4 Results, Conclusion and Future Work

There was similar business analyzes with different results. To face this, all the data extraction criteria had to be analyzed, studying the reason for divergence. It was observed the importance to combat such groups of distrust to clarify myths and correct mistakes. Several meetings and trainings were done on such purpose and the benefits were amazing, the users really increased their trust on BI tools and data quality.

As a result of the work against these mistrust groups, there was an 8% increase of BW active users as showed in Fig. 1.

From 2009 to 2010, the number of active users on BW tool changed from 62 % to 70%. On BO tool, it went from 30% to 74%.

This study reinforced that monitoring the use of a BI architecture is as important as it is its implementation. BI architecture are very important for business processes automation, reducing the number of failures, minimizing rework and manual processing of information. Thus companies can gain in productivity and cost reduction. A BI architecture is used to support decision-taking and to speedup data collection and processing for the management of functional departments in several businesses.

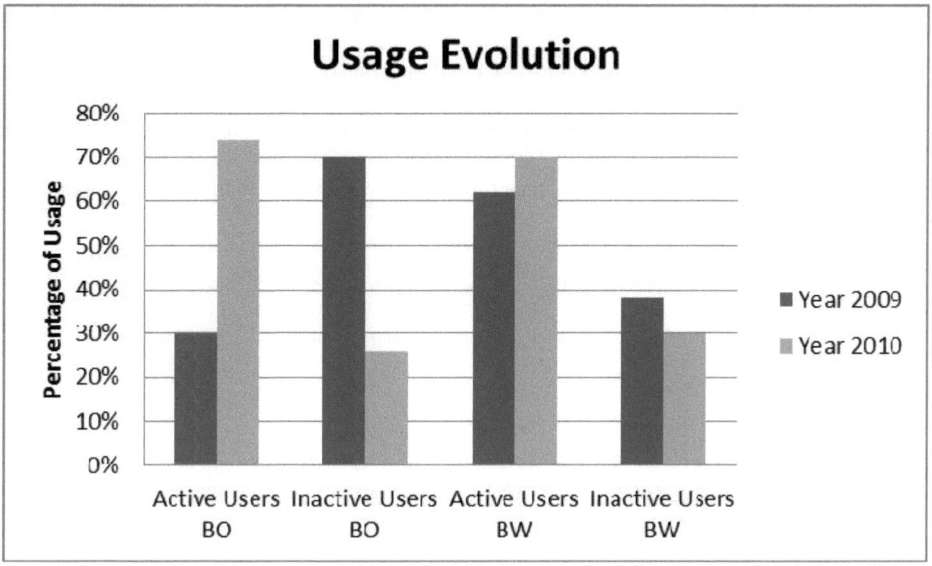

Fig. 1. BO and BW tools usage evolution between years 2009 and 2010

A continuation of this research is the study of other types of scenarios of economic or social circumstances where the use of BI tools can be beneficial as well as the application of similar studies in other sectors of the economy such as automobiles or services.

References

1. Cardoso, O.O.: Business Communication versus Organization communication: new theorycal challenges. Public Administration Journal 40(6) (November-December 2006)
2. Fleury, P.F., Wanke, P., Figueiredo, K.F.: Logistics business - the Brazilian perspective, vol. 9, pp. 284–321. Ed. Atlas, São Paulo (2000)
3. Lopes, R.S., Palmeira, E.M.: The global financial crisis: impact on Brazil. Economic Academic Journal (105) (2008)
4. Marques, A.S.: The Importance of Senior Management Training in the Implementation of Management Systems. Master dissertation, Univ. Federal Fluminense (2004)
5. Pighin, M., Marzona, A.: Data Value in Decision Process: Survey on Decision Support System in Small and Medium Enterprises. In: MIPRO, 2012 Proceedings of the 35th International Convention, pp. 1647–1654 (2012)
6. Rosa, R.N.: Scarcity of resources and imperial crisis. Portal Vermelho, http://www.vermelho.org.br/noticia.php?id_noticia=142599&id_secao=9 (accessed in March 04, 2012)
7. Sassi, R.J., Arrivabene, A.: An analysis of the application of best practices in the process of implementing a data warehouse project. In: XVII Production Engineering Symposium (2010)
8. Sen, A., Ramamurthy, K.R., Sinha, A.P.: A Model of Data Warehousing Process Maturity. IEEE Transactions on Software Engineering 38(2) (March/April 2012)

9. Stefanelli, M.: Communication with the patient: theory and teach, 2nd edn. Ed. Robe, São Paulo (1993)
10. Viana, N.: Financial crisis, state and regularization. Getulio Vargas Law Journal 5(2) (July/December 2009)
11. Wansett, R., Furtado, F.: Book Study about the Debt N° 2. Ed. Expressão, São Paulo (2008)
12. Weir, R.: Best Practices for Implementing a Data Warehouse. Journal of Data Warehousing 7(1) (Winter 2002)

Service-Learning Model of Cultural and Creative Talent Cultivation for the Bamboo Industry Cluster

Tsen-Yao Chang[1,*] and Kuo-Li Huang[2]

[1] Department of Creative Design, National Yunlin University of Science and Technology, Yunlin County, Taiwan
changty8908@gmail.com
[2] Visual Communication Design, Southern Taiwan University, Tainan, Taiwan
z3z@stust.edu.tw

Abstract. Action research was introduced in the design of learning services. Cultural and creative talent cultivation activities were completed to review the value of local cultural crafts, such as bamboo weaving, in a town. Young students participated in the creation of bamboo weaving crafts to investigate the threshold and difficulties of learning the art, and to build a feasible model of talent cultivation for traditional industries. Based on observation, learning, exhibition, and action reflection, this study established a feasible model in understanding the difficulties and opportunities of the cultivation of new cultural and creative talents. Moreover, the study built a sustainable concept framework for the cultivation of human resources of local industries.

Keywords: cultural crafts, cultural and creative talent cultivation, industry cluster, action research, clustering potential points, agglomeration economies.

1 Research Background

The bamboo industry was prosperous in the early days of Taiwan, and a bamboo industry-processing zone was even established in Zhushan Township, Nantou County. However, the development of high-tech industries, the mechanization of traditional handicraft industries, the popularization of plastic products, and the impact of globalization greatly reduced the use of bamboo products. Consequently, the bamboo industry in Taiwan shrunk with the establishment of a world economic market. Farmers abandoned bamboo groves or replaced the bamboo with high value cash crops..Bamboo industry manufacturers have relocated their production base in Mainland China and Southeast Asia because of cheap labor. The industry cluster has declined. The socio-demographic imbalance is evident in Zhushan Township because its young population has moved. Currently, the local government has adopted the sightseeing business for local industrial transformation. The strategy resulted in forced changes in the lifestyle of indigenous inhabitants, diminished culture and traditions, and the lessened the identity and self-confidence of the residents toward the town. Zhushan, which is the center of the development of bamboo handicrafts in Taiwan, felt the impact of these realities and the changes in consumption pattern.

C. Stephanidis (Ed.): Posters, Part II, HCII 2013, CCIS 374, pp. 479–483, 2013.

In addition, finding young successors to the master craftsmen became difficult. Therefore, the glorious industry of bamboo handicrafts was ignored, and thus, declined.

As the town of the bamboo industry is close to the university implementing the present study, visits and talks with local craftsmen were conducted. These visits identified core problems in the traditional bamboo industry to be aging workforce, difficult skills training, and inadequate familiarity or understanding of modern design among the craftsmen. Based on the needs and development potential of the local industry, a service-learning model for cultural and creative talent cultivation was established. This model emphasized local service and learning. Students from the Department of Design were guided in applying the design theories they learned to provide services for the town. Local residents were informed that the participation of the local artists in the learning activity would lead to the possible return of young people to the countryside. Craftsmen were provided with a new mode for teaching art. Creative effort, public concern for the bamboo craft culture, and student awareness for the bamboo craft and cluster industry were stimulated. Students were encouraged to consider how they could contribute to society based on what they learned in school.

2 Co-curricular Service-Learning into Action Research Process

This research incorporated service-learning into the cyclical nature of action research to develop creative learning for talent cultivation. In service-learning, the effect of the "learning" was obtained in the process of "service." Service-learning emphasizes experiential education. Students apply what they have learned, utilize the knowledge and skills, and complete the interactive service process to meet the requirements of social justice through participation in the services for the surrounding areas. Kolb's experiential learning cycle model comprises four stages, namely, experiential, reflecting, generalizing, and applying. Based on Kolb, design courses were established to encourage students to determine the causes of the decline of the local industry and to learn the local traditional bamboo weaving craft.

The case study on the bamboo industry in Zhushan enabled students to enter the field to learn and to understand the economic values and impact of modern design on the local industry. The present experimental curriculum was developed based on the four stages of the development of service-learning proposed by Fertmam, White, and White (1996). The implemented stages were preparation, service, reflection, and celebration. The corresponding activities were:

1. Mission Preparation: This stage included field exploration, surveys, and observation recording to establish the goals of the service-learning courses.
2. Service Import: The creative design service was introduced in the craft experience workshop to promote the teaching methods for cultural and creative talent cultivation based on the integration of design and crafts.
3. Reflection Fermentation: Participants (teachers, students, craftsmen of the community, local residents, and manufacturers) reflected on the positive interactions of the activities.

4. Result Sharing: The learning model was developed by exhibiting the school and community achievements, which expanded the interactions between the community and school.

In the present study, processes were established based on the spiral-type concept. Implementing situational teaching led to self-reflection. The concept was integrated with the activities of the four stages of action research. Teachers evaluated student learning at the end of the course, to improve future cultivation of cultural and creative talents of the community.

3 Curriculum Implementation Results

Practical experience included topic determination and four student exhibitions. Local newspapers and Internet media reported the overall results to provide the local government, industry manufacturers, and community the experience of the aesthetic nature of bamboo crafts and the valuable cultural resources of the community. The results of the responses of the participants are divided into four aspects corresponding to the contributions of this practical curriculum.

1. Service participation improved the practice of theories. The overall performance of the students enabled the teachers and craftsmen to discover the ideas and potential development capabilities of thc young generation with respect to traditional crafts.
2. Integration of design and crafts facilitated the transformation of the local industry. The double-instructor system was adopted in teaching. The teacher provided the students with a design guide, while the craftsman provided the technical training in craft production. The craftsman and the teacher worked together to inspire the students to stimulate their interest in the production of crafts, and to rethink possibilities of design and crafts integration. The creative ideas on the cultivation of the workforce of the traditional industry integrated with modern design increased.
3. Experiential learning promoted diversified learning. The exhibition of the achievements enabled the participants, local government, and residents to discover the power of design service. The students not only learned from the teachers and craftsmen, but also learned how to organize actively the exhibition, release information to the media, and to create more works to meet the local needs. This process indicated active learning, and was vital to the cultivation of comprehensive designers.
4. Self-experience and civic awareness cultivation. Student accomplishments included bamboo woven crafts and active participation in the preparation of publicity items, activity space, and media contacts. When the crowds and media reports appeared, the students had imperceptibly changed their original learning attitude and thought more on how to enable more people to see the power of the design in the new era through their design works. The process of the course and the follow-up extension enhanced civic awareness of students.

4 Conclusion

Service-learning was integrated in the local design learning services. A series of cultural and creative talent cultivation activities was completed to review and to recreate the values of local bamboo weaving crafts. Young students participated in the investigation of difficulties of learning the art and the problems of talent cultivation in traditional industries. To develop an adaptable model of the dynamic growth of cultural and creative talent cultivation, Fig. 1 summarized the innovative relationship for the sustainable development of local cultural industries. The relationship established practical and sustainable cooperation among the three elements (teachers, students, the local industrial participants) of cultural and creative talent cultivation. The teacher mediated between the students and the local community to create a learning platform for cultural and creative talent cultivation. Participation in the cultural and creative talent cultivation corresponded to the four-stage model of Kolb, and addressed the industry request for talent cultivation. Fig. 1 showed friendly environments could cultivate cultural and creative talents, and revive the industry and improve quality management. The model supported an interactive clustering environment to resolve the current difficulties of the industry cluster.

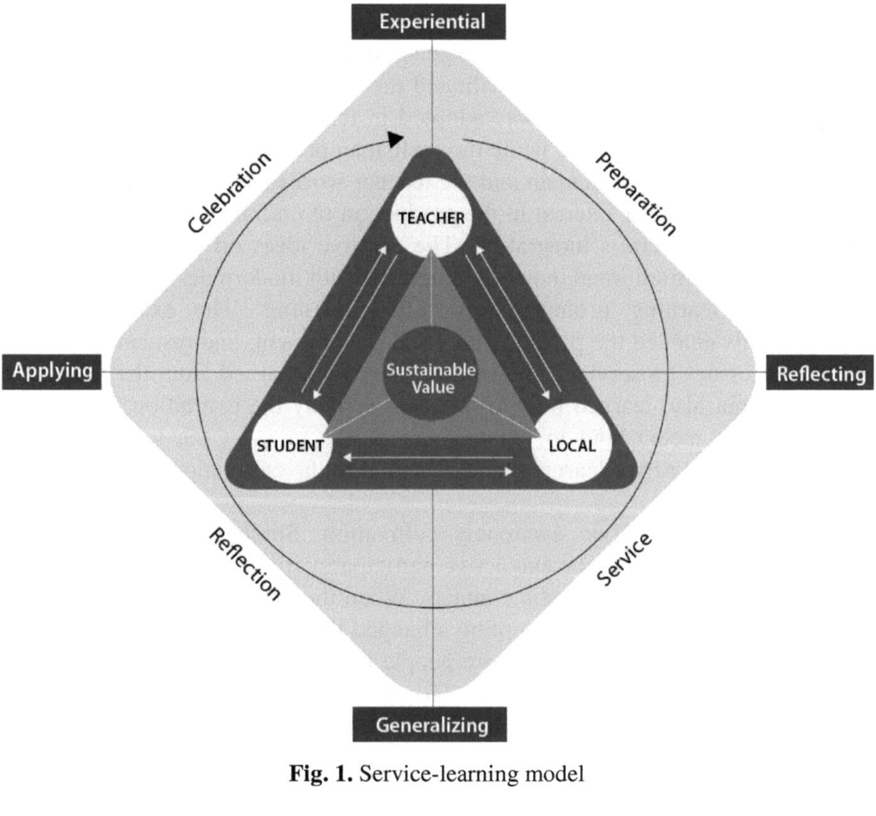

Fig. 1. Service-learning model

Acknowledgments. The authors gratefully acknowledge the financial support for this research provided by the National Science Council of Taiwan under Grants No. NSC-101-2410-H-224-04.

References

1. Fertman, C.I., White, G.P., White, L.J.: Service Learning in Middle School: Building a Culture of Service. National Middle School Association, Columbus (1996)
2. Kolb, D.A.: Experiential learning: experience as the source of learning and development. Prentice Hall, Englewood Cliffs (1984)

New Perspectives on Interactivity in Project Management Tools

Mirko de Almeida Madeira Clemente[1], Axel Berndt[1], Hannes Leitner[1], Mandy Keck[1], Ricardo Gaertner[2], and Rainer Groh[1]

[1] Technische Universität Dresden, Faculty of Computer Science, Institute of Software and Multimedia Technology, Chair of Media Design, 01062 Dresden, Germany
[2] queo GmbH, 01159 Dresden, Germany

Abstract. Software tools for project management are extremely complex desktop applications. Recently, we observe a shift from traditional project management where one project manager is responsible for creating the project plan and supervising its execution, towards a more agile multi-project management that involves project members early in the planning process. This shift demands the introduction of novel visualization and interaction techniques. This contribution summarizes our analyses of three typical scenarios and shows promising perspectives for the application of new interaction and visualization techniques. Our goal is to promote project management as an interesting and multifarious subject within HCI research.

1 Introduction

Project management in small and medium-sized companies is usually considered to be the responsibility of one person, the project manager. Project management software is designed for single users as conventional desktop applications. However, we observe a recent trend towards a more agile form of project management that integrates the whole team into early planning phases and crucial decision processes. Furthermore, a company usually runs more than one project. Its resources are thus concurrently demanded, which leads to conflicts that need to be resolved [1]. Hence, a computer-supported multi-project perspective on agile project management is required. Methods from the field of information visualization are rarely regarded within project management [2] and CSCW research but can be of great help to achieve this perspective.

In this paper, we describe results from the research project *Vizamp*, that aims to introduce novel interaction and visualization techniques to this scenario. The project is conducted in cooperation with a partner from industry, who develops project management tools and employs several project managers which were available to us for preliminary interviews. Little previous research is available on this subject. Thus, the main aim of this contribution is to characterize typical scenarios, analyze their demands and discuss existing applicable visualization and interaction techniques.

C. Stephanidis (Ed.): Posters, Part II, HCII 2013, CCIS 374, pp. 484–488, 2013.

2 Project Planning

The most traditional scenario in project planning is the creation of a schedule and the assignment of staff to the project team. This is typically done by a single user in a desktop environment. Some project managers tend to add very specific details to specify project phases and work packages. We regard this process as top-down approach. A central aspect of our research is the examination of agility in multi-project management. Since the project manager cannot know each detail of the project activities, we propose a middle-out approach by combining top-down and bottom-up processes. Thereby, potential conflicts caused by multi-project management (MPM) can be foreseen before they occur or efficiently handled if they do arise. In this case, the project manager is only concerned with the most important project information and asks the project members to clarify the details. Hence, the project planning is split into several levels of detail and the in-depth knowledge of all project members is incorporated. As the interviews with our industry partner revealed, this already takes place in practice through direct communication. Nevertheless, traditional applications for project management are hardly suitable for this highly agile and collaborative middle-out approach, as they do not adapt to different situations and devices with respect to interaction techniques and visualization methods. The detailed project planning can be regarded as a separate scenario, but to a certain degree it is part of all of the following scenarios.

Timelines are a well known visual metaphor used in the context of project scheduling to visualize time-oriented data. Several more sophisticated techniques have been developed based on Timelines [3,4,5,6]. Gantt charts in particular are occasionally criticized due to the use of a large amount of white space. However, this problem applies to all of the before mentioned methods. The middle-out approach seeks to mitigate this problem. The visual output does not necessarily need to depict every detail, only the details required in a particular context. Thus, our approach can be used to control the level of detail by semantic zoom techniques. Data can be stored in a hierarchical tree structure. Reducing the complexity of the graphical representation reduces the needed display space. The gained space can, for instance, be used to advance existing visualization methods towards multi-project visualizations.

3 Team Meeting

The team meeting is a highly collaborative scenario with interaction not only between project manager and team but also amongst the team members. The project manager is the session chair. The purpose of the team meeting is the refinement of the lower levels of the project plan's tree structure, i.e. work packages and tasks, and the assignment of staff to particular work packages. This also includes effort estimation for open and not yet finished parts of the project. In case of delays, the project plan has to be adapted or new planning content has to be created.

The team meeting is a typical roundtable situation and predestined for multi-touch tabletop interaction, since it allows meeting attendees to interact vis-à-vis.

Consequently, they foster communication as opposed to single-user systems, and a positive impact on task execution time is likely [7]. However, none of the traditional visualization techniques like Gantt charts are appropriate for this scenario since they require a one-sided orientation. The same applies to conventional applications for project management, which are in general controlled with pointing devices. AgilePlanner [8] supports face-to-face collaboration during planning meetings even though it is not designed for MPM. Tools coming from the CSCW research are mainly focused on interaction techniques and not on visualization. In the team meeting scenario, the project plan has to be intelligible and simultaneously editable from all directions. This suggests circular layouts, radial methods for information visualization [9], support for artifact orientation [10] and the manipulation of hierarchical data [11,12]. More promising insights for this scenario could be reached through the personalization of content depending on its location, the integration of a public and several personal areas [13], or the use of private interactive displays [14]. Even though several approaches already exist, some challenges still remain. A very particular problem in roundtable scenarios is textual information. As far as possible, text should be replaced by pictographic elements. Götzelmann [15] introduced several techniques to generate well-layouted annotations for interactive images. The main challenge in this scenario involves the combination of data-driven visualization methods and interaction techniques, which allow some sketchiness while planning. This may be a reason for the common creation of text documents during team meetings, and as a consequence, the additional effort to convert the documents into planning data. Figure 1 shows a conceptual sketch of the visualization and system functions.

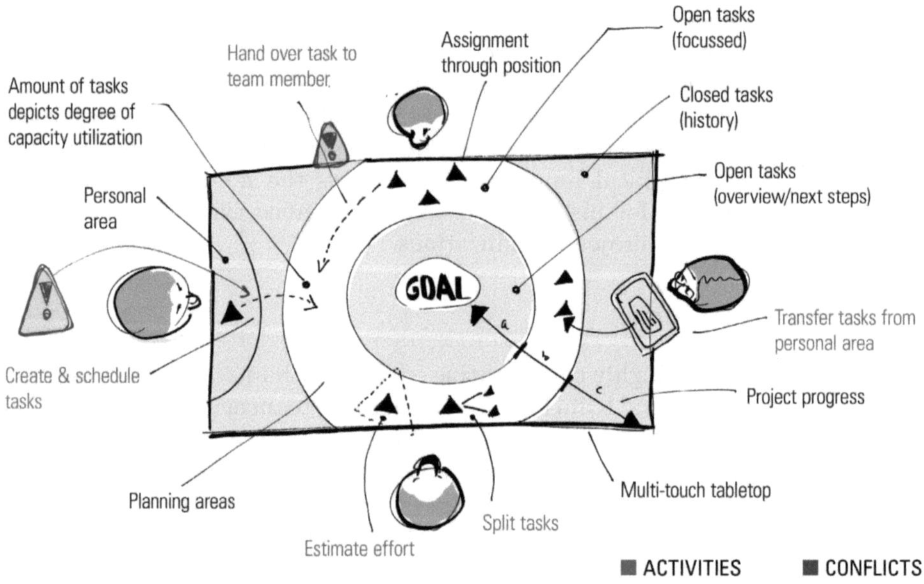

Fig. 1. Conceptual sketch of the team meeting scenario

4 Management Meeting

Another collaborative scenario is the management meeting. Its primary purpose is to resolve conflicts caused by managing multiple parallel projects. We focus on measureable and quantifiable conflicts, such as scheduling conflicts and the unbalanced distribution of workload. At our industry partner 5 to 8 of approximately 12 project managers participate in this meeting. The agenda of the meeting is a list of conflicts, which are processed consecutively. Every conflict may be related to different sub-groups of managers, so that the chair moderating the discussion has to change from time to time. We believe that communication is the most important aspect to resolve these conflicts efficiently. Thus, the system should be subtle supporting the conversation and a projection wall setting comes into consideration. To allow the changing chair to take control of the system, we have tested a gesture-based system which allows distant interaction without additional devices [16]. Recent work in this field has been applied to simple applications [17], but transferring these techniques to complex scenarios is challenging. Explicit and implicit interaction has to be combined in a way that allows reliable gesture recognition and natural behavior during conversation at the same time. A challenge with respect to the visualization is to reduce the complexity of the multidimensional data connecting projects, work packages, and resources. This can, for instance, be achieved by only taking the affected project managers into account.

5 Conclusion

In this paper we described three fundamental scenarios in the context of agile multi-project management. All scenarios feature high potential for collaborative work and are essential parts of the proposed middle-out approach. We stressed that conventional software for project management is not suitable for these scenarios. This does not only apply to the graphical representation but also to the corresponding interaction techniques. Part of our future work will be the further development and investigation of the described approaches. One of our main objectives is to bridge the gap between all scenarios and to bring together aspects from the fields of HCI, information visualization, and project management.

Acknowledgements. This research has been supported by the European Union and the Free State Saxony through the European Regional Development Fund (ERDF). We thank our colleagues and project partners from queo GmbH: Ricardo Gaertner, Daniel Wuttig, Dana Henkens, and Marcel Höhlig.

References

1. Payne, J.H.: Management of multiple simultaneous projects: a state-of-the-art review. International Journal of Project Management 13(3), 163–168 (1995)

2. Zhang, P., Zhu, D.: Information visualization in project management and scheduling. In: Proceedings of the 4th Conference of the International Society for Decision Support Systems (ISDSS 1997), pp. 1–9 (1997)
3. Gantt, H.L.: Work, wages, and profits. Engineering Magazine Co. (1913)
4. Chittaro, L., Combi, C.: Visualizing queries on databases of temporal histories: new metaphors and their evaluation. Data & Knowledge Engineering 44(2), 239–264 (2003)
5. Aigner, W., Miksch, S., Thurnher, B., Biffl, S.: PlanningLines: novel glyphs for representing temporal uncertainties and their evaluation. In: Proceedings of the Ninth International Conference on Information Visualisation, pp. 457–463 (July 2005)
6. Kosara, R., Miksch, S.: Metaphors of movement: a visualization and user interface for time-oriented, skeletal plans. Artificial Intelligence in Medicine 22(2), 111–131 (2001)
7. Kin, K., Agrawala, M., DeRose, T.: Determining the benefits of direct-touch, bimanual, and multifinger input on a multitouch workstation. In: Proceedings of Graphics Interface 2009, GI 2009, Toronto, Ont., Canada, pp. 119–124. Canadian Information Processing Society (2009)
8. Liu, L., Erdogmus, H., Maurer, F.: An environment for collaborative iteration planning. In: Proceedings of the Agile Conference, pp. 80–89 (2005)
9. Draper, G., Livnat, Y., Riesenfeld, R.: A survey of radial methods for information visualization. IEEE Transactions on Visualization and Computer Graphics 15(5), 759–776 (2009)
10. Barnkow, L., von Luck, K.: Semiautomatic and user-centered orientation of digital artifacts on multi-touch tabletops. In: Herrlich, M., Malaka, R., Masuch, M. (eds.) ICEC 2012. LNCS, vol. 7522, pp. 381–388. Springer, Heidelberg (2012)
11. Nguyen, Q.V., Huang, M.L.: EncCon: an approach to constructing interactive visualization of large hierarchical data. Information Visualization 4(1), 1–21 (2005)
12. Yang, J., Ward, M.O., Rundensteiner, E.A.: Interring: An interactive tool for visually navigating and manipulating hierarchical structures. In: IEEE Symposium on Information Visualization, INFOVIS 2002, pp. 77–84 (2002)
13. Scott, S.D., Carpendale, S.: Theory of Tabletop Territoriality. In: Müller-Tomfelde, C. (ed.) Tabletops—Horizontal Interactive Displays. Human-Computer Interaction Series, pp. 357–385. Springer, London (2010)
14. Rädle, R., Jetter, H.C., Reiterer, H.: TwisterSearch: supporting social search with tabletop and mobile displays. In: Reiterer, H., Deussen, O. (eds.) Mensch & Computer 2012 – Workshopband: Interaktiv Informiert – Allgegenwärtig und Allumfassend!?, München, pp. 509–512. Oldenbourg Verlag (2012)
15. Götzelmann, T.: Correlating Illustrations and Text through Interactive Annotation. VDM Verlag, Saarbrücken (2008)
16. Höhlig, M.: Kollaborative Konfliktbehandlung mittels Gestensteuerung im Kontext des agilen Multiprojektmanagements (2013)
17. Stellmach, S., Jüttner, M., Nywelt, C., Schneider, J., Dachselt, R.: Investigating freehand pan and zoom. In: Mensch & Computer 2012: Interaktiv Informiert–Allgegenwärtig und Allumfassend!? (2012)

Personal Risk Management

Hanna Gołaś

Poznań University of Technology, Department of Management Engineering,
ul. Strzelecka 11, 60-965 Poznań, Poland
hanna.golas@put.poznan.pl

Abstract. Outcomes of each organization functioning depend on personnel employed, and mostly on proper qualifications assigned to tasks, self-motivation and ability to communicate with co-employees. Thus, risk management system needs to take human factor into consideration as this is usually the weakest point of an organization.

Keywords: risk, beliefs, meta-program.

1 Introduction

The strategy of each company, regardless of its depth and scope, is prepared and implemented by the people (employees, contractors, managers). They are an important factor in determining strategy's success, having an impact on its shape and effects on both micro and macro levels. Therefore important determinants of reducing the risk of failure are the skills required and held by employees, as well as effective and proper communication. Hence, the process of personal risk management can be reduced to the elementary principles of cooperation and mutual relationships that are the result of both the organizational culture and the understanding of how the employee at the managerial and operational levels functions.

2 Personal Risk Elements

2.1 Tasks - Qualifications – Skills

The process of risk management in respect of the impact of staff on the strategy must therefore begin by defining tasks and deadlines for the scenarios, determining when they will have to be completed. At this point we do not specify what employees we have (assessing their strengths and weaknesses, features that make the difference), instead determining what we need. The lack of such approach means that either strategy is often changed or its objectives are not achieved. Identification of strategy is the priority instead of matching it to employees' competences.

The first step is to build a grid of skills needed to meet the goals and objectives defined in the strategy. This grid is a material input to the analysis of the human resources. At this point we define who is a resource, regardless of which position

C. Stephanidis (Ed.): Posters, Part II, HCII 2013, CCIS 374, pp. 489–493, 2013.

he/she currently holds. Confrontation of the current organizational structure and the target structure seems to be necessary and its analysis may lead to the conclusion that it will be necessary to offset positions in both divisions as well as in the levels of structure or even to employ new staff with the required skills.

Matching skills to the tasks performed is a priceless value in the long-term perspective of business management and strategy implementation. Top management cares about the culture of the organization and wants that employees were satisfied with their work, that there was no phenomenon of alienation and that employees were doing what was in line with their values, that they liked what they do and did do what they do best. The factors that contribute to job satisfaction include, among others professional respect for supervisors, good organization of work and jobs, safety, hygiene and ergonomics [1]. Every day, thousands of people worldwide struggle with mismatched workplaces, not wanting to risk losing their jobs or to trouble others (family, supervisor) they perform the tasks identified by the supervisor without complaint. This leads, consequently, to poor employee's psychophysical condition, which sooner or later will be reflected in productivity, absenteeism, stress and ultimately in worsened health. Building a corporate culture in which the employee has the courage to approach the manager and openly talk to him about it, is itself a great value. In this situation, it is possible that organization cannot offer a job that fits an employee and as a result that employee has to leave the company, but it may be valuable for each party involved. Advantage is brought to everyone: employee, because he will have the opportunity to find a job that will suit him and the employer because he will avoid mistakes made by a frustrated employee. Edward M. Hallowell [2] developed a Cycle of Excellence, which consists of five steps, and can help "alienated" employees. The cycle is constructed as follows:

1. Select: find the right job, task.
2. Create: derive the strength from those around you.
3. Have fun: exploit fantasy in your daily work.
4. Strive and develop: overcome the difficulties.
5. Impress: Make sure that you are appreciated.

Application of this cycle brings benefits to the employee but also to the employer. It is important that everyone performs his tasks well and is satisfied with it. Selection of job should be the result of three components: what someone likes to do, what he does best and what brings value to the company. If there is such job in a company employee currently works for, he is lucky. If not, changing position or even profession seems to be the best solution. Having the proper job, the next step is to create bonds at work. The approach has its supporters and detractors. However, studies prove [2] that employees having the best friend at work are seven times more likely to commit emotionally to the duties performed than others. Therefore, creating conditions for the development of emotional bonds in enterprises should be the priority for managers. If this approach is implemented as a personal risk management tool, we can be sure that employees are working at the appropriate positions, they are happy and can be entrusted with the increasingly ambitious tasks. They will be loyal employees which today is priceless.

2.2 Meta-Program

Implementation of the strategy depends on effective communication between employees and managers. Therefore an important element of reducing the likelihood of the risk of not achieving the objectives is listening to the words which employee uses to present his view of reality. When a manager asks a subordinate questions such as what is his suggested way of considering the problem? He hears the words, sentences, which show what subordinate's representation system is: visual, auditory or kinesthetic. Each of these systems can be reached, but only when using the correct phrases and expressions. Table 1 shows some useful examples.

Table 1. Types of clients of various representation systems

Representation system	Typical words	Example
visual	I see, look, have a glance, wide perspective…	After completing that task you will see your work in a different way
kinesthetic	Comfortable, warm	After achieving the goal you will feel great,
auditory	I will present an order, list it	You will have the following results: firstly …,

Beliefs and systems of representation are elements meta-program that every employee and manager has, what is more, each of them has its own individual meta-program. It is kind of a specific road map on which each moves. Ability to read employees' maps gives great potential to either manager or employee as they will be able to convince the others for their rations, will be able to argue better and motivate others to work, etc.

2.3 Illusion – Beliefs

Another aspect of effective communication in personal risk management is appropriate communication with each other. In every company there is an effective language (mother tongue, language adopted as the standard), which all use, hence, de facto employees and their supervisors should understand each other, and see reality in the same way. But in business practice it turns out that this is not sufficient because the manager cannot properly motivate workers to work more efficiently, "they are not on the same wavelength", do not see the same things in the same manner. The reason for this is that, regardless of their place in the organizational structure, the truth and the world for each of the parties are different. It turns out that this is a matter of belief. The conviction is the truth for the employee and the manager. Their truth. People talk only about their beliefs and use them to build their "world model" that they communicate through words. On every day basis, every employee uses various models of knowledge about the world. They are - more or less right - sets of beliefs [3]. Attempts to generalize behaviors are building additional models such as: "Boss is always right", "Women are not suitable for managerial positions." Realizing this fact, understanding it, causes people to tolerate other people's views, to be sympathetic to their mistakes, their emotions and approaches to reality. In the table 2 two sets of beliefs, according to which workers live and describe the world, are shown.

Table 2. Beliefs sets

Ilussion I	Ilussion II
World is evil and hostile	World is good and friendly
I want to defend against people	I trust people and myself
They offend me all the time	I am in various moods
Mistakes prove my weakness	Mistakes teach me
Stress limits me	Stress motivates me
I will not try again	I will try again

In both the first, and in the second example of thinking about the world, we are dealing with a set of beliefs and convictions only [3]. We call these beliefs illusions, lies, or truth. The issue is not naming, but answer to the question: which illusion, belief, the way of thinking is of my subordinate? Otherwise, the manager will talk with the employee living by the first or the second illusion. According to the illusion I we ask: what task you will fight with? And by the illusion II: on what you want to work to make customers satisfied?

Living either with the illusion I or II is a map. Each of our employees, as well as we, has the right to live according to one of them and no changes to these maps are required. Sometimes, however, the perception of the world causes problems to workers and influences their work results, which consequently leads to problems in relationships with colleagues and health. So it is worth checking whether what employees believe is right for them, healthy, useful and supportive. CM. Maultsby from Howard University (USA) suggested five questions that employees are to ask themselves (managers should also do this in reference to their beliefs)

Does this belief help me to protect myself, my life and health?
Does it allow me to reach closer and further goals?
Does it allow me to solve or avoid most of unwanted conflicts?
Does it help me to feel like I want?
Is my belief is supported by the facts? [4]

If the employee responded positively to three or more questions, then his approach is relatively healthy. However, if he answered "yes" to less than three questions, or to any of them, he should consider changing his beliefs which will contribute to improvement in their well-being, in the effects of work and private life.

3 Conclusions

The issues of personal risk management presented indicate that a worker who is the creator and executor of the strategy has individual characteristics and their recognition slowly leads to more effective achieving of the objectives. Issues concerning employee's satisfaction with his work, including which beliefs they live with and which system of representation is predominant in him, are essential elements of an effective personnel management in general, both in terms of strategy and daily work. Understanding these aspects of human functioning results in more effective work.

References

1. Drożyner, P., Mikołajczak, P., Szuszkiewicz, J., Jasiulewicz-Kaczmarek, M.: Management Standardization Versus Quality of Working Life. In: Robertson, M.M. (ed.) EHAWC 2011 and HCII 2011. LNCS, vol. 6779, pp. 30–39. Springer, Heidelberg (2011)
2. Hallowell, E.M.: Nauka o mózgu podpowiada nam, jak się doskonalić, Harvard Business Review Polska, Warszawa (2011)
3. Rożalski, M.: Mam przekonanie (October 13, 2009), że to prawda, `http://www.studencka.pl`
4. Rożalski, M.: Materiały z treningu Master in Art. of NLP – spotkanie pierwsze – Przekonania, Warszawa (2010)

Application of SMART Criteria in Planning Improvements to the Operating Conditions of Machinery

Adam Górny and Beata Mrugalska

Poznań University of Technology, Department of Management Engineering,
ul. Strzelecka 11, 60-965 Poznań, Poland
{adam.gorny,beata.mrugalska}@put.poznan.pl

Abstract. The use of work equipment generates substantial hazards for people involved in their operation and maintenance. The scope of improvements in the field should be selected with an eye to eliminating hazards and minimizing the impact of harmful, dangerous and onerous factors caused by the use of machinery. In order to develop solutions, implement them successfully and assess the results, it is advisable to apply the SMART criteria. Such criteria, which are widely known and commonly used in quality engineering, allow for the identification of crucial characteristics of specific technical and organizational solutions with a view to assuring safety.

Keywords: SMART criteria, improvement plan, technical and organizational devices, operation.

1 Introduction

Due to exposures to hazards of persons using technical machinery and equipment during their day-to-day operation and maintenance, there is a need to apply certain impact mitigation measures in keeping with the criteria set out in Directive 2009/104/EC [2].The prime responsibility for ensuring compliance with the relevant requirements rests with employers and persons in charge of securing worker safety in working environments [1]. The Directive itself stops short of specifying the technical and organizational measures required to ensure compliance with the minimum requirements. The scope and method of achieving improvements should be selected with the view to either eliminating risks or mitigating the impact of any deleterious, hazardous and onerous factors which come into play in the course of using work equipment. The measures should be designed to allow for effective deployment and to be acceptable by the concerned parties [5], [6], [8].In planning the effective deployment of appropriate solutions and, most importantly, in evaluating courses and outcomes of action, use may well be made of the SMART principles known from quality engineering. These help identify the desired significant scope of technical and organizational solutions designed to achieve safety objectives [3], [7].

C. Stephanidis (Ed.): Posters, Part II, HCII 2013, CCIS 374, pp. 494–498, 2013.

2 Description of the SMART Criteria

The purpose of evaluating improvement measures is to ensure that the desired objectives can be achieved. This is particularly true for evaluations designed to ascertain that technical equipment can be operated without exposing workers to hazards. Such evaluations are to provide clarity on whether the expected outcomes can in fact be attained.To this end, a methodology is needed for ensuring that the measures at hand will be assessed objectively. Evaluations of the proposed measures may rely on the SMART principle where each letter of the acronym stands for a specific concept [3], [7]:

- **S** as in specific (unambiguous identification) – the scope of measures corresponds to the scope of a company's operations, its mission, its position at a given time and the circumstances to be assessed,
- **M** as in measurable – wherever possible, outcomes should be assessed against specific numerical values or clear statuses to verify compliance,
- **A** as in agreed upon – evaluations based on objectives which workers accept and recognize as appropriate and likely to produce the expected results,
- **R** as in realistic – refers to objectives to be achieved – the objectives should be attainable and account for existing internal and external factors, including the available resources,
- **T** as in time-bound – having a clearly defined time horizon and tasks attainable within the anticipated time.

By adjusting the SMART principles to the specific health and safety requirements associated with the operation of technical equipment, it becomes possible to evaluate objectives (and the circumstances in which they are to be achieved) and consequently confirm the effectiveness of any planned measures.

3 Practical Application of SMART Criteria

3.1 Guidelines for Measures Aimed at Improving Machine Operation Safety

Before implementing improvement measures designed to achieve the desired level of safety, it is necessary to set objectives derived from conclusions from a prior assessment the existing system's compliance with minimum requirements [1], [8]. Such a plan should specify the scope of improvements and ways in which outcomes of improvement measures are be evaluated. Selected criteria for assessing the compliance of a plan with safety requirements and methods of implementation designed to achieve such compliance are given in Table 1. The assessment should also enable the assessor to ascertain whether:

- the proposed measures will contribute to mitigating the existing risks,
- any new risks may be triggered by deploying the proposed measures,
- any more effective and cost-efficient alternative arrangements are available,

Table 1. Selected criteria to be applied in assessing measures designed to improve the safety of conditions in which equipment is operated

- clearly formulate all necessary measures, - assign responsibility for the achievement of objectives to proper services, teams and persons, - specify the resources needed to achieve such objectives, - set a schedule for the achievement of the adopted objectives, - define indicators for the assessment of the degree to which the plan has been accomplished and the agreed objectives achieved, …

- the workers agree with the need to adopt the measures and regarding their effectiveness,
- the proposed measures will be put into practice.

Risks may be considered acceptable if their occurrence is communicated in keeping with applicable laws [3], [5].To select the scope to which technical and organizational measures designed to mitigate risks will be implemented, one needs to rely on well-tested guidelines which guarantee success. Before one can carry out the specific measures, it is essential to formulate clear detailed requirements ensuring interpretations beyond doubt and an assessment of implementation methods.

3.2 Application of SMART Criteria to Evaluate Equipment (Case Study)

By applying the SMART criteria, one can assess the potential for improving the conditions in which equipment is operated. The criteria help ascertain the achievement of the desirable status prescribed in risk assessment documentation concerning risks related to machinery operation. Once properly adjusted to suit the specific measures taken to improve operating safety, the SMART guidelines will facilitate the assessment of any proposed measures for effectiveness. In the case at hand, the assessment concerns a honing machine, as shown in Figure 1. A survey of the existing solutions suggested that multiple adjustments were needed to ensure the machine meets the minimum operating requirements set out in Directive 2009/104/EC [2]. Some of the selected measures undertaken in the case are given in Table 2.

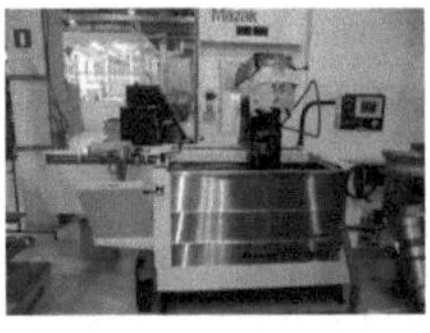

Fig. 1. Honing machine for which improvement measures have been identified

Table 2. Selected measures undertaken to ensure the machine satisfies minimum requirements as laid down in Directive 2009/104/EC

Organizational measure: - Train maintenance personnel charged with the day-to-day use of equipment and authorize the successfully trained workers to perform work. The training shall cover safe work guidelines concerning the use of the relevant equipment. Until the end of the current month, responsibility for achieving this measure shall rest with the Head of Training.
Technical measure: - Fit all equipment in use with guards preventing direct contact with moving parts. Such guards shall be designed not to hamper work or reduce efficiency. Until December 15 of this year, responsibility for achieving this measure shall be rest with the Head of Maintenance.

An assessment of the scope of measures (Table 2) designed to adjust equipment to minimum requirements is provided in Table 3.

Table 3. Assessment of solutions adopted to adjust the equipment for compliance with the minimum work safety requirements

Assessment criterion	Compliance assessment	Solution adopted
S specific	compliant	- technical equipment fitted with guards covering moving parts, - organizational solutions in place prevent the performance of work at equipment by persons unauthorized to work by employer
M measurable	compliant	- protective items fitted on all equipment in use, - maintenance workers authorized to perform work
A agreed upon	compliant	- workers trained in work safety and given access to protective items, - users of technical equipment aware of risks involved in wrong use
R realistic	compliant	- funds designated for deployment and guard fitting appropriated from overhaul budget, - the fitted guards improve safety without hampering work, - the fitted guards sufficiently protect workers from contact with moving parts, - only allowing duly authorized workers to work does not reduce the capacity to complete work and use equipment
T time-bound	compliant	- moving part guards to be fitted by 12/15/13, - workers to be authorized to perform work by the end of current month.

The assessment proved that the scope of improvements was compliant with the SMART principles. This, in turn, shows that once applied, the proposed solutions will bring the working environment into compliance with the minimum safety requirements.

4 Conclusions

Identification of the safety objectives needed to achieve the desired level of safety in the operation of technical equipment as well as the desired scope of preventive and corrective measures forms an integral part of technical equipment adjustments to mandatory legislative requirements [4], [6], [8].To guarantee the desired level of safety, it is essential to evaluate the adopted solutions. Evaluations should additionally extend to the planning and deployment of organizational and technical measures designed to rule out or minimize hazards and consequently improve working conditions. By using the SMART criteria to assess measures designed to improve conditions for the use of technical equipment, it is possible to gain certainty as to the effectiveness of the adopted measures. The end result is certainty as to whether the improvements in place are indeed appropriate.

References

1. Council Directive 89/391/EEC of 12 June 1989 on the introduction of measures to encourage improvements in the safety and health of workers at work, Official Journal L 183, 1–8 (June 29, 1989) (as amended)
2. Directive 2009/104/EC of the European Parliament and of the Council of 16 September 2009 concerning the minimum safety and health requirements for the use of work equipment by workers at work (second individual Directive within the meaning of Article 16(1) of Directive 89/391/EEC). Official Journal L 260, 5–19 (October 3, 2009)
3. Górny, A.: Application of SMART principles in planning occupational risk assessment objectives. In: Mondelo, P.R., Karwowski, W., Kaija, L.S., Swuste, P., Occipinti, E. (eds.) Proceedings of the VIII International Conference on Occupational Risk Prevention (ORP 2010: Creating Value Through Risk Prevention Management), Valencia (2010) (CD-ROM)
4. Jasiulewicz-Kaczmarek, M., Drozyner, P.: Preventive and Pro-active Ergonomics Influence on Maintenance Excellence Level. In: Robertson, M.M. (ed.) EHAWC 2011 and HCII 2011. LNCS, vol. 6779, pp. 49–58. Springer, Heidelberg (2011)
5. Reinhold, K., Tint, P.: Risk assessment in manufacturing: possibilities and results. In: Pacholski, L.M., Trzcieliński, S. (eds.) Ergonomics in Contemporary Enterprise, Proceedings of the 11th International Conference on Human Aspects of Advances Manufacturing: Agility and Hybrid Automation with 4th International Conference ERGON - AXIA, pp. 112–121. IEA Press, Madison (2007)
6. Mazur, A.: Shaping quality of work conditions. In: Health Protection and Ergonomics for Human Live Quality Formation, pp. 31–44. Poznan University of Technology, Poznań (2009)
7. Meyer, P.J.: Attitude Is Everything: If You Want to Succeed Above and Beyond. Meyer Resource Group, Waco (2003)
8. Misztal, A., Butlewski, M.: Live improvement at work. Publishing House of Poznań University of Technology, Poznań (2012)

The Effects of Online Multiuser Virtual Environments on Creative Motivation in Collaborative Design Studios

Seung Wan Hong[1], Yun Gil Lee[2], and Yehuda Kalay[3]

[1] Faculty of Architecture and Town Planning,
The Technion – Israel Institute of Technology, Israel
seungwan@berkeley.edu
[2] Department of Architecture, Hoseo University, Korea
yglee@hoseo.edu
[3] Faculty of Architecture and Town Planning,
The Technion – Israel Institute of Technology, Israel
kalay@ar.technion.ac.il

Abstract. Online Multiuser Virtual Environments (MUVEs) are online, immersive 3D environments based on anthropomorphic avatars and synchronous multiuser access. We investigated the effects of MUVEs on students' creative motivation in collaborative design studios. Based on qualitative analyses of two long-term and authentic collaborative architecture design studios in Second Life, a commercial MUVE platform, we found that the avatars' immersive experiences in the MUVEs, the presence of classmates' avatars, and co-presence with them allowed the students to evaluate the usefulness of the proposed buildings and organization of exhibition spaces. In addition, we found that the shared objects in the MUVEs encouraged the production of unexpected and new solutions. However, in the MUVEs, if any buildings were not in the immersive perception of the avatars, with respect to the body and views, students struggled to develop solutions.

Keywords: creativity, collaboration, design studio, Online Multiuser Virtual Environments (MUVEs).

1 Introduction

Architects have collaborated with other professionals to resolve architectural problems and develop pioneering solutions (Kalay, 2004). Furthermore, the mechanism of collaboration helps the production of creative solutions (Schön, 1983; Goldschmidt, 1995; John-Steiner, 2000). Since the importance of collaboration has been emphasized in the professional practice, design studio educators attempt to involve collaboration in their curriculum (Dunster, 1990). The use of Online Multiuser Virtual Environments (MUVEs) has been discussed in previous theories and studies as a method for supporting collaborative design studios (Maher & Simoff, 2000; Jeong & Trento, 2009). MUVEs are online, immersive 3D environments based on anthropomorphic avatars and synchronous multiuser access, such as Second Life.

C. Stephanidis (Ed.): Posters, Part II, HCII 2013, CCIS 374, pp. 499–503, 2013.

Previous studies have proposed the potential of MUVEs for collaborative design studios (Maher & Simoff, 2000) and the effects of MUVEs on collaborative behaviors and processes (Gu, Kim, & Maher, 2011; Koutsabasis, Vosinakis, Malisova, & Paparounas, 2012), but there is scarce research on the effects of MUVEs on creativity in collaborative design studios. Therefore, in this paper, we aim to investigate the ways in which MUVEs influence students' creative motivation in collaborative design studios.

2 Literature Review

Ijsselsteijn and Riva (2003) introduced three types of presence in a collaborative virtual environment (CVE): (1) physical presence, (2) social presence, and (3) co-presence. The authors argued that co-presence plays a critical role in CVE design by supporting users' social interactions, such as negotiations and community creation. The feeling of co-presence satisfies the concept of "Virtual Place" and possibly promotes social and psychological relationships amongst collaborators (Kalay, 2004, 2006). Harrison and Dourish (1996) also argued that the notion of place, which frames interactive behaviors, is valuable in supporting Computer Supportive Cooperative Work (CSCW).

To extend the aforementioned theories, first, we assume that users' immersive experiences in MUVEs possibly produce the feeling of being in the designated environment; thus, it may help designers in their search for new solutions. Second, we assume that the awareness of the presence of others, in the form of anthropomorphic avatars, and interactions with them may inspire new ideas. Finally, in MUVEs, users can synchronously share designated outputs with others, and this may facilitate communication, reflection-in-action, and joint decision-making amongst users for proposing creative solutions.

3 Methodology

Creativity is defined as a combination of novelty—new and inexperienced—and appropriateness—useful and suitable (Amabile, 1983, 1996; Sternberg, 1999; Kaufman, Plucker, & Baer, 2008). To investigate the effects of MUVEs on students' search for novel and appropriate solutions, we examined two cases of authentic, collaborative design studios in the Department of Architecture, University of California, Berkeley. Both studios targeted the design of a Virtual Smithsonian Museum using Second Life, a commercial MUVE platform, and other media (Fig. 1). The first design studio was held in the fall semester of 2008, and four students participated. The second design studio was held in the spring semester of 2010, and ten students participated. In both design studios, the students took charge of four theme museums and ultimately proposed one unified Virtual Smithsonian Museum.

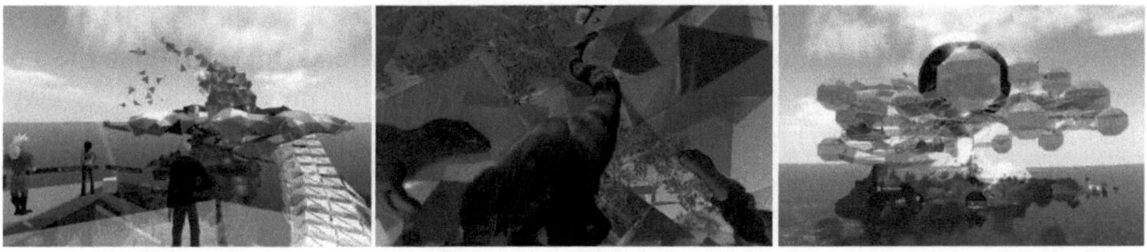

Fig. 1. Collaborative design studios in MUVEs: Virtual Smithsonian Museums

In the first studio, we collected the students' design products and observed their collaborative processes. After the studio, we provided a visual log of the students' outputs, dates, and media, and asked the students to select the dates when they thought they had produced novel and appropriate outputs. Based on the method, we systemically interviewed the students about the ways that the design media they had used on those dates had influenced their production of novel and useful outputs (Fig. 2). After the second studio, we administered an online survey to ask about what had influenced the MUVEs in the students' search for novel and useful design solutions, compared to sketches and physical models.

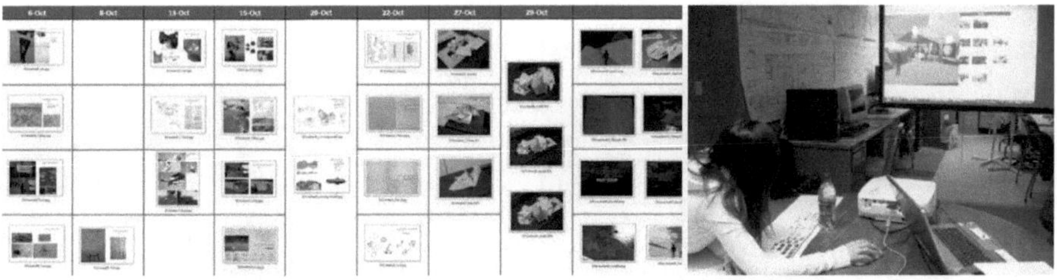

Fig. 2. The visual log and retrospective interview

4 Results

Based on the research method in the previous section, first, we found that the avatars' immersive experiences in the designated environment had motivated useful and appropriate designs. In the interviews, the students stated that the immersion in the first/third person view had enabled them to evaluate the organization of interior exhibition spaces and location of exhibits, thereby helping them search for useful solutions. The students also reported that the movements (e.g., sitting, standing, and walking) of the anthropomorphic avatars had allowed them to examine the usability of the museums (Fig. 3). However, if any designated space was not in the range of an avatar's immersive perception, it was difficult to perceive the collaborative design outputs and other classmates' distributed designs. Therefore, in the studios, the instructors allowed the students to use supplementary media, such as physical study models and a projector, to help them organize and integrate the different theme museums within the museum (Fig. 4). Second, in remote collaboration, the social presence of other avatars and co-presence with them had enabled the visualization of the classmates' participation and work progress. The students reported that the co-presence had helped them evaluate visitors' activities in the museums, such as way-finding and circulation (Fig. 5). Finally, in the MUVEs, the students were aware of their classmates' designed objects. The students stated that they had been motivated by the shared objects designed by their classmates in their search for new solutions (Fig. 6).

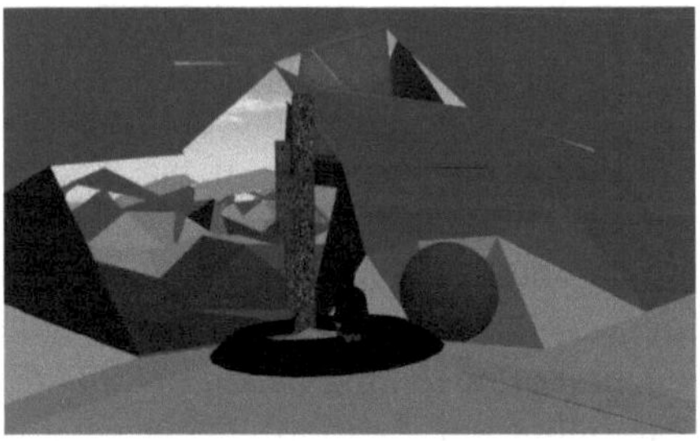

Fig. 3. Avatars' immersive experiences and activities in the designated environment

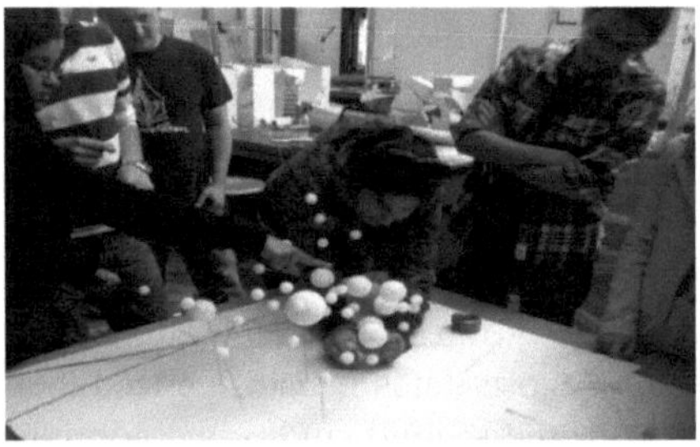

Fig. 4. Supplementary design tools

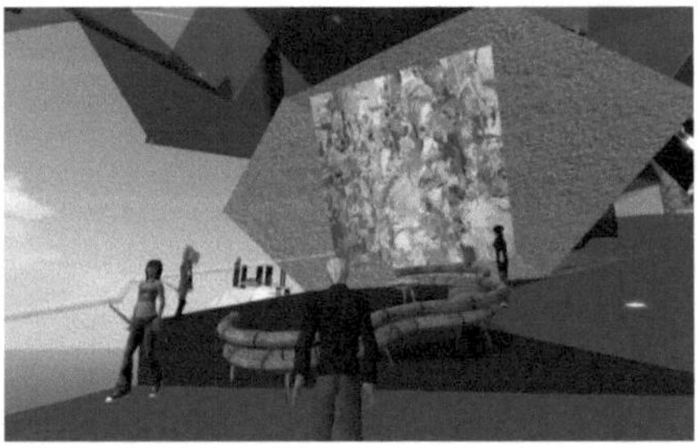

Fig. 5. Shared objects: experiencing others' design outputs

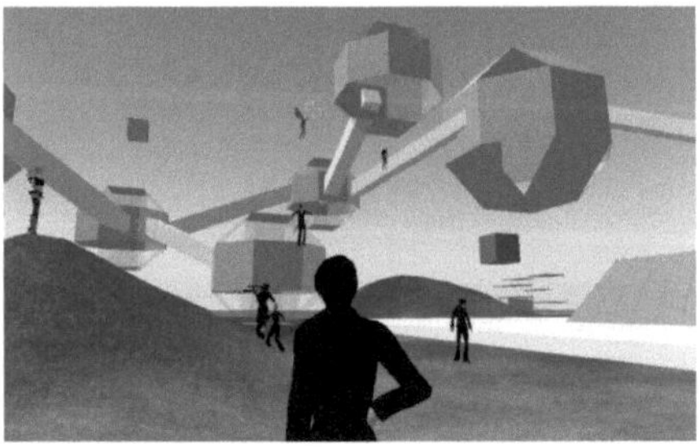

Fig. 6. Social presence of others and co-presence

5 Conclusion

In this paper, we investigated the effects of MUVEs on creative motivation, that is, the search for novel and appropriate solutions, in two authentic, collaborative design studios. We concluded that in the MUVEs, the anthropomorphic avatars' immersive experiences and their activities in the designated environment motivated the production of appropriate solutions. The co-presence of classmates also evaluated the museum visitors' activities and thus influenced the appropriateness of the design. In addition, the shared objects in the MUVEs motivated the students to produce unexpected and novel ideas. However, the avatars' immersive experiences in the MUVEs occasionally obstructed the integration of macro-scaled museums that were not in the avatars' body and view perceptions. We expect that this study is applicable for developing collaborative design studio pedagogy and creative collaboration tools.

Acknowledgement. This research is supported by the Technology Innovation Program(World Best Software Project, 10040794) funded by the Ministry of Knowledge Economy(MKE, Korea)

References

1. Amabile, T.M.: Creativity in Context. Westview Press, Unite State (1996)
2. Dourish, P., Harrison, S.: Re-Place-ing Space: The Roles of Place and Space in Collaborative Systems. In: Proceedings of the 1996 ACM Conference on Computer Supportive Cooperative Work 1996, pp. 67–76 (1996)
3. Dunster, D.: Collaboration in Education: The Diploma Project at the Bartlett School, 1988-89. Journal of Architectural Education 43(2), 14–21 (1990)
4. Goldschmidt, G.: The designer as a team of one. Design Studies 16, 189–209 (1995)
5. Gu, N., Kim, M.J., Maher, M.L.: Technological advancements in synchronous collaboration: The effect of 3D virtual worlds and tangible user interfaces on architectural design. Automation in Construction 20(3), 270–278 (2011)
6. Ijsselsteijn, W., Riva, G.: Being There: The Experience of Presence in Mediated Environment. In: Riva, G., Davide, F., Ijsselsteijn, W.A. (eds.) Being there: Concepts, Effects and Measurement of User Presence in Synthetic Environments, pp. 3–16. Los Press, Amsterdam (2003)
7. Jeong, Y.W., Trento, A.: A Web-based design environment to exercise collaboration in architecture studio. In: Carrara, G., Fioravanti, A., Kalay, Y.E. (eds.) Collaborative Working Environments for Architectural Design, pp. 177–192. Palombi Editori, Rome (2009)
8. John-Steiner, V.: Creative Collaboration. Oxford University Press (2000)
9. Kalay, Y.E.: Architecture's new media: Principles, theories, and methods of computer-aided design. The MIT Press, Cambridge (2004)
10. Kalay, Y.E.: The impact of information technology on design methods, products and practices. Design Studies 27(3), 357–380 (2006)
11. Kaufman, J.C., Plucker, J.A., Baer, J.: Essentials of Creativity Assessment. John Wiley & Sons, Inc., Hoboken (2008)
12. Koutsabasis, P., Vosinakis, S., Malisova, K., Paparounas, N.: On the value of Virtual Worlds for collaborative design. Design Studies 33(4), 357–390 (2011)
13. Maher, M.L., Simoff, S.: Collaboratively Designing within the Design. Proceeding of Co-Designing, 391–399 (2000)
14. Schön, D.A.: The Reflective Practitioner: How Professionals Think in Action. Basic Books (1983)
15. Sternberg, R.J.: Handbook of Creativity. Cambridge University Press (1999)

Studying Distributed Collaborations Using the Resource Allocation Negotiation Task (RANT)

Vincent F. Mancuso[1], Victor Finomore[2], Gregory Funke[2], and Benjamin Knott[2]

[1] Oak Ridge Institute for Science and Education,
vincent.mancuso.ctr@wpafb.af.mil
[2] Air Force Research Lab, Wright Patterson Air-Force Base, Ohio
{victor.finomore,gregory.funke,benjamin.knott}@wpafb.af.mil

Abstract. When conducting team research, the experimental task can have major effects on the interpretation and overall success of the study. While some researchers chose to use high-fidelity tasks to simulate an operating environment, an alternative perspective uses more simplified, metacognitive tasks. The purpose of this paper is to present a new metacognitive task, the Resource Allocation Negotiation Task (RANT), which aims to elicit complex and rich collaborations between distributed team members.

Keywords: Distributed teams, consensus tasks, collaboration.

1 Introduction

With an increased reliance on distributed teams in the workplace, understanding the cognitive and collaborative processes of such teams has become a critical need. In order to develop effective training mechanisms, intervention and collaborative support systems, it is essential that we first must achieve a holistic and complete understanding of the collaborative and cognitive work of these teams.

In much of this research, it is not uncommon to see experiments rely on synthetic task environments to simulate the complexities and context of the target domain. While these types of tasks help maintain ecological validity, they also introduce numerous confounds, making interpretation of the results more difficult. To account for this, researchers can utilize metacognitive tasks to hone in on the collaborative and cognitive demands of the task. In metacognitive tasks, the context and complexities are stripped away, and greater emphasis is placed on replicating critical elements of the task- and team- work within the environment. Metacognitive tasks such as group consensus tasks [1-3], who-done-it murder mystery [4], group recall [5], and collaborative assembly [6], have been successfully used to isolate various aspects of team cognitive behavior without the extra confounds of a complex target environment

In this paper, we will propose a new metacognitive task, the Resource Allocation Negotiation Task (RANT), designed to simulate team decision making in complex environments. In the following sections, we will present an overview of the theoretical development of RANT, an initial evaluation, and finally a discussion of future research directions.

C. Stephanidis (Ed.): Posters, Part II, HCII 2013, CCIS 374, pp. 504–508, 2013.

2 Resource Allocation Negotiation Task

2.1 Group Consensus Tasks

Group consensus tasks are a popular metacognitive task, which have been used in numerous team research studies. In group consensus tasks, teams are given a fuzzy problem and asked at coming to an agreement on the answer One of the more popular variations of this task type are group survival tasks such as "Lost in the Desert" [1], "NASA Lost on the Moon" [2], and "Lost at Sea" [3]. These tasks have been used widely in team research, with various foci such as designing collaborative systems [7] and training interventions [3,8], and studying the impact of group goals and time pressure [9], cognitive resource theory [10], interpersonal behaviors [11], cognitive motivation [12], and leadership [13], to name a few.

Group consensus tasks afford rich group discussions that require information sharing, negotiation, and team decision making. These critical elements make group consensus tasks a perfect platform for team cognition research.

2.2 Overview of Task

Building on previous work, we aimed to develop a new experimental task to enable basic team cognition research. In addition to developing a task that would afford the same rich collaborations, we wanted to develop a task that was more flexible for the purpose of experimental research.

In pursuit of this objective, we developed the Resource Allocation Negotiation Task (RANT). RANT is a metacognitive task that combines aspects of strategic decision making and group consensus. In RANT, teams assign resources across a set of targets based on a specific criteria. It is up to the group to come to an agreement on how many resources each target requires, as they have varying costs and/or demands. Like previous group consensus tasks, in RANT teams must negotiate their individual perceptions to come to an agreement of a final team answer.

While seemingly simple, the true utility of RANT comes in its flexibility. At its base, RANT is a simple consensus bidding task. However, upon this base, more complexities and manipulations can be introduced. When compared to previous group consensus tasks, RANT offers more extensibility, as well as greater data collection opportunities.

3 Initial Evaluation

3.1 Goals of Evaluation

In order to evaluate the utility of RANT, we designed and conducted an initial evaluation of various aspects of the task. Specifically, our goals were twofold, (1) to assess two different task-manipulations, and (2) to ensure that the content of the task has minimal effect on performance.

3.2 Experimental Design

To evaluate the utility of RANT in facilitating distributed team collaborations, we conducted an initial pilot study using a 2 x 2 within subjects design with independent variable manipulations for task type (finite vs. unlimited resources) and item sets (item set 1 and item set 2).

To manipulate the task types, we varied whether or not the participants had a set of finite resources they could allocate. In the finite resources condition, participants were given a fixed pool of money they could allocate, while in the unlimited resources condition there was no such constraint. The item set manipulation was a variation on two unique sets of 15 items. The two lists were balanced to have a similar total price ($610 and $670), and items with similar prices.

3.3 RANT Task

For the initial evaluation, participants receive two sets of 15 unique items, and tasked with coming to a group consensus on the price of each item (rounded to the nearest dollar). Keeping with the theme of previous group consensus tasks (i.e., lost in the desert, lost in the wilderness), each of the 15 items related to camping or survival. This decision was made as it was thought camping equipment (i.e., backpacks, tents, etc.) were accessible enough for regular participants, but foreign enough to elicit discussion and disagreement.

3.4 Participants

For this evaluation, 16 participants were recruited from available Air Force personnel and a subject pool. Each session included 4 participants, representing 1 team in the final data set (4 teams). During each experimental session, teams would complete two unique RANT tasks across the two within subjects conditions.

3.5 Measures

Performance was calculated using an average price ratio across all items for each of the conditions. The price ratio provides a normalized score calculated as a percentage based on the difference between the groups consensus price, and the actual price of the item.

In addition to performance, communications were captured and analyzed based on the total number across all participants

3.6 Procedures

Upon arrival, participants were assigned to a computer terminal. After an initial task briefing, one participant was asked to serve as the recorder and to track the team's final decision for each item. Prior to beginning the group discussion (via chat), each participant was given a paper packet that contained the directions of the task, and the list of the 15 items they would be discussing. In one condition, the directions included a total price they were permitted to spend across all items. Each team participated in two separate RANT sessions.

3.7 Results

Manipulation Check. To ensure that there was no effect of task content on performance, the two item sets were compared as a manipulation check. We found minimal difference across item list 1 (M = 50.90%, SD = 7.64%) and item list 2 (M = 54.85%, SD = 8.60%). Similarly, in a comparison of the total number of communications, we found minimal differences between item list 1 (M = 181.25, SD = 38.39) and item list 2 (M=184.25, SD = 60.84).

Effect of Task Type. Across the two variations of the task, for performance we found that teams, in general performed better in the unlimited resources condition (M=58.56%, SD = 2.44%) than in the finite resources condition (M=44.65%, SD = 0.48%). On the other hand, while they did not perform as well, team in the finite resources condition had more communications (M = 206, SD = 44.86) than teams in the unlimited resources condition (M = 159.5, SD = 28.62).

4 Discussion and Future Work

Based on these initial results, we can conclude that RANT offers a viable platform for future team research. While the teams did communicate more in the condition with the finite resources, due to the added complexity of the problem, for our own interests, we feel that the infinite resources variations will better support our research goals.

In our future research we plan to investigate the effects of spearphishing cyber-attacks on team cognitive biases. Spearphishing, a popular social-engineering attack, is when people are targeted by a message disguised as coming from a trustworthy source. Using RANT, during a team discussion of an item, we will inject seemingly trustworthy communications that suggest the items price is either higher or lower than its actual value. In this regard, in the infinite resources variation, each item can become its own unique trial. This will allow us to run a large number of trials and manipulations on the same participant base, as opposed to in the finite resources manipulation where each list would be a single trial.

Acknowledgements. The research conducted by author Vincent Mancuso was supported in part by an appointment to the Postgraduate Research Participation Program at U.S. Air Force Research Laboratory, 711 Human Performance Wing, Human Effectiveness Directorate, Warfighter Interface Division, Applied Neuroscience Branch administered by the Oak Ridge Institute for Science and Education through an interagency agreement between the U.S. Department of Energy and USAFRL.Energy and USAFRL.

References

1. Lafferty, J.C., Pond, A.W.: The Desert Survival Situation. In: Human Synergistics (1974)
2. Yetton, P., Bottger, P.: The relationships among group size, member ability, social decision schemes, and performance. Organizational Behavior and Human Performance 32(2), 145–159 (1983)
3. Nemiroff, P.M., Pasmore, W.A., Ford, D.L.: "The Effects of Two Normative Structural Interventions on Established and Ad Hoc Groups: Implications for Improcing Decision Making Effectiveness. Decision Sciences 7(4), 841–855 (1976)
4. Stasser, G., Stewart, D.D., Wittenbaum, G.M.: Expert roles and information exchange during discussion: The importance of knowing who knows what. Journal of Experimental Social Psychology 31(3), 244–265 (1995)
5. Wegner, D.M.: Transactive memory: A contemporary analysis of the group mind. In: Theories of Group Behavior, pp. 185–208. Springer, New York (1987)
6. Liang, D.W., Moreland, R., Argote, L.: Group versus individual training and group performance: The mediating role of transactive memory. Personality and Social Psychology Bulletin 21(4), 384–393 (1995)
7. Adams, S.J., Roch, S.G., Ayman, R.: Communication Medium and Member Familiarity The Effects on Decision Time, Accuracy, and Satisfaction. Small Group Research 36(3), 321–353 (2005)
8. Leshed, G., Hancock, J.T., Cosley, D., McLeod, P.L., Gay, G.: Feedback for guiding reflection on teamwork practices. In: Proceedings of the 2007 International ACM Conference on Supporting Group Work, pp. 217–220. ACM (2007)
9. Durham, C.C., et al.: Effects of group goals and time pressure on group efficacy, information-seeking strategy, and performance. Human Performance 13(2), 115–138 (2000)
10. Murphy, S.E., Blyth, D., Fiedler, F.E.: Cognitive resource theory and the utilization of the leader's and group members' technical competence. The Leadership Quarterly 3(3), 237–255 (1992)
11. Sundstrom, E., Busby, P.L., Bobrow, W.S.: Group process and performance: Interpersonal behaviors and decision quality in group problem solving by consensus. Group Dynamics: Theory, Research, and Practice 1(3), 241 (1997)
12. Scudder, J.N., Herschel, R.T., Crossland, M.D.: Test of a model linking cognitive motivation, assessment of alternatives, decision quality, and group process satisfaction. Small Group Research 25(1), 57–82 (1994)
13. Kickul, J., Neuman, G.: Emergent leadership behaviors: The function of personality and cognitive ability in determining teamwork performance and KSAs. Journal of Business and Psychology 15(1), 27–51 (2000)

TeamNETS: Scaled World Simulation for Distributed Cyber Teams

Vincent F. Mancuso[1] and Michael McNeese[2]

[1] Oak Ridge Institute for Science and Education
vincent.mancuso.ctr@wpafb.af.mil
[2] The Pennsylvania State University, College of Information Sciences and Technology
mmcneese@ist.psu.edu

Abstract. Cyber operations have become a significant interest to government, military and corporate entities. Unfortunately, the secure nature of cyber operations limits the access that researchers can obtain. Therefore, simulations that can mimic the operating environment are a critical need to push this research forward. The purpose of this paper is to present a human-in-the-loop, scaled world simulation, *teamNETS*, which is capable of simulating multiple types of cyber security tasks. *TeamNETS* simulates the cognitive and collaborative requirements cyber security work and serves as an effective platform to study varying aspects of individual and team cognition, as well as other issues in Human-Computer Interaction.

Keywords: cyber security, simulation, scaled world, team simulation.

1 Introduction

Over the last several years, cyber threats have begun to move to the forefront of the national security discussion. In 2012, a reported 42,887 cyber related incidents (117 incidents per day) resulted in data loss or theft, computer intrusions or privacy breaches[1]. In response to this, the federal government invested $13 Billion on developing effective cyber-operations over the last several years. Currently, much of the work and research has focused on the development of algorithms, and intelligent systems to detect and mitigate cyber threats.

While invaluable to our national goals, to obtain a fully secure cyber space, researchers must not only help improve the technology and algorithms that drive cyber security, but also must find ways to support the human operators. Unfortunately, due to the secure nature of the operating environment, it can be difficult, if not impossible, for human subjects researchers to gain access to the facilities and personnel necessary to develop a holistic and ecological understanding of the cognitive work.

---

[1] These statistics are taken from the August 21, 2012 of The George Washington University's "Face the Facts USA" program. Found at: http://www.facethefactsusa.org/facts/where-the-battle-lines-are-lines-of-code

C. Stephanidis (Ed.): Posters, Part II, HCII 2013, CCIS 374, pp. 509–513, 2013.

Without access, we must turn our attention to other, established methodologies, such as scaled world simulations, to help drive future human-computer interaction research in the context of cyber operations. Therefore, the purpose of this article, is to present a new team-based simulation, based off the NETS architecture [1], developed to simulate the individual and team cognitive requirements of cyber security work. In the following sections, we will present a new simulation, teamNETS and discuss its implementation and utilization in a human-computer interaction research program.

2 Simulating Cyber Operations

2.1 Ecological Grounding

Much of the previous work in scaled world simulations situates within traditional command and control environments such as battlefield operations and emergency response. While this research has provided us with invaluable knowledge on how individuals, teams, and technology operate in a multitude of contexts, the transfer from the physical to the cyber battlefield may be too drastic of paradigm shift. The cyber battlefield does not abide by the same laws by which the traditional battlefield operates. Traditionally, wars are fought against soldiers on a defined battlefield, during a set period. The cyber battlefield however, transcends army's and soldiers, and consists of civilians who possess the knowledge and resources to execute complex and costly multi-stage cyber-attacks across time and space. These inherent complexities of the cyber-environment create unique demands and stresses on the cognitive work and technologies operating within.

Leveraging these paradigmatic differences and ethnographic research by Tyworth et al. [2], attributes of the cyber environment were carefully extracted and implemented into teamNETS to provide a rich and immersive environment for human-computer interaction research.

2.2 The TeamNETS Simulation

History. TeamNETS builds upon the NeoCITIES Experimental Task Simulator (NETS) platform. The NETS platform is the newest iteration of the NeoCITIES simulation, which has been an effective test bed for team cognition research for close to 10 years [3-5]. Due to the scalability of NETS, and its ability to rapidly develop and deploy realistic cyber-security simulations, it offered a perfect platform for teamNETS.

TeamNETS Interface. Based on previous research of the design of simulation user interfaces [6] and an assessment of freely available cyber security tools, a simple user interface was designed. Careful consideration went into the design of the simulation user interface, as it is the player's only window into the state of the scaled world thus having a major impact on their performance. The final design (Figure 1) of the interface requires players monitor multiple resources, interpret complex data sets, and make multi-tiered decisions within the context of cyber-security.

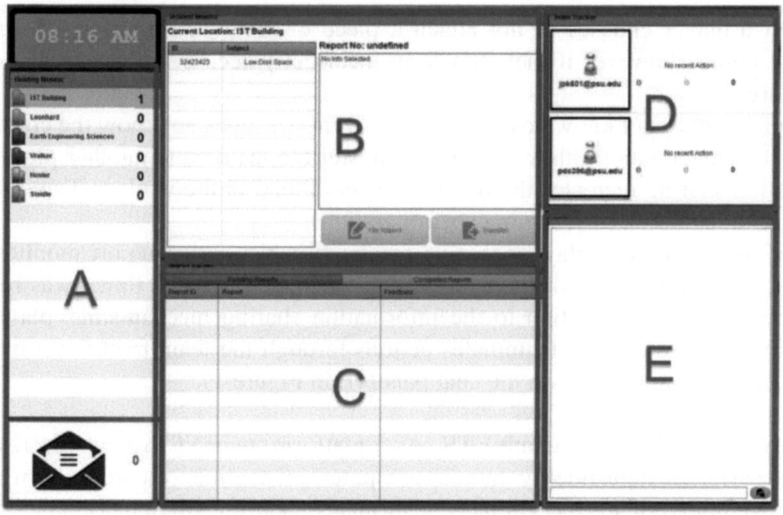

Fig. 1. teamNETS Interface

The main teamNETS interface consists of 5 components, the Location Tracker (A), Incident Report Monitor (B), Action Report Monitor (C), Team Monitor (D) and Chat (E). In addition to these components, there are pop-up windows to allow players to transfer information and file action reports. This interface allows players to monitor different locations on the simulated network, investigate or transfer emerging events, file action reports, and monitor individual and team progress in the simulation.

Playing teamNETS. In *teamNETS* simulations, teams include three participants. Each player is assigned a specific specialty, intrusion detection, malicious software detection, or policy management based off of the four primary functional domains found in Tyworth et al [2][2].

In *teamNETS*, players are responsible for monitoring locations for events, interpreting event descriptions, submitting action reports, and sharing information with their teammates. During a scenario, each player will receive reports of possible threats that are occurring on the network at varying time intervals. When a player recognizes an actual threat, in the location tracker (A in Figure 1), they must use the incident report monitor (B in Figure 1) to read the event description (in the form of a textual description and/or computer log file). Once they have identified the problem, they have two courses of action, try to mitigate the threat by filing an action report, or transfer the event to another player who may be better suited for that particular type of threat.

To mitigate a threat, players file action reports that consist of a categorization of the type of threat that it is and extra meta-data of specifics of the threat. Depending on how accurate the categorization, and meta-data is, their score will be either higher or

[2] Due to the constraints of the simulation, and focuses on reactive cyber operations, we removed threat landscape analysis from the final role structure.

lower. If a player chooses to not attach a piece of meta-data, they will receive no negative points, however if they attach an incorrect piece, it will negatively impact their score.

If a player does not know how to solve an event (i.e. does not know the correct meta-data or categorization), they can rather transfer the incident to another player. This information sharing recreates the report transfers found in the work of Tyworth et al. [2], and is a regular occurrence in cyber operations.

After filing a report, players receive feedback in the action report monitor (C in Figure 1) on the accuracy of their report and whether or not the threat was removed from the network. In addition to the information sharing mechanisims, players can maintain awreness of their teammates actions through the team tracker (D in Figure 1), as well as communicate via the chat panel (E in Figure 1).

Measuring Cognition in teamNETS. As a platform, *teamNETS* lends itself to conducting basic, to high-fidelity human-computer interaction research. At it's core, *teamNETS* is driven by the Human Performance Scoring Model [7], to assess the performance of individuals and teams within the cyber environment. The Human Performance Scoring Model is a multi-dimensional metric that accounts for accuracy and reaction time. This metric has been shown to be a useful measurement of various aspects of team cognition [3].

In addition to raw performance, *teamNETS* has built in data collection mechanisims to capture more abstract components of team cognition and collaboration. Metrics such as communication patterns and information sharing allow researchers to hone in on the behavioral aspects of the collaboration during each simulation. Finally, *teamNETS* has built in support for subjective measures of situation awarnesness (i.e. SAGAT [8]), workload (i.e. NASA TLX), and team mental models.

3 Conclusion and Future Work

In this paper, we have presented an overview of a new experimental platform for studying various aspects of team cognition in distributed cyber teams. Based off of a previously established simulation platform (NETS) we used ethnographic research of cyber security analysts to build a realistic task that can be used to study aspects of individual and team cognition, as well as other Human Computer-Interaction Issues, in a controlled laboratory setting.

Currently, *teamNETS* has been deployed in a study to assess how different types of team knowledge structures impact team performance and collaborations (Mancuso HFES), and assess the utility of shared virtual feedback in improving transactive memory systems for distributed teams [10]. Moving forward, we hope to expand the breadth of *teamNETS* to account for other functional domains within the cyber opperations space. In addition, we hope to continue to move forward with developing new, and introducing established metrics of cognitive and collaborative behavior within the simulation.

Acknowledgements. Work on this paper was partially supported by U.S. Army Research Office (ARO) MURI Grant "Computer Aided Human Centric Cyber Situation Awareness" W911-NF-09-1-0525. The Opinions expressed in this paper are those of the authors only and do not necessary represent the official position of the Army Research Office, the US Army, the Department of Defense or the Pennsylvania State University.

References

1. Mancuso, V.F., Minotra, D., Giacobe, N., McNeese, M., Tyworth, M.: idsNETS: An experimental platform to study situation awareness for intrusion detection analysts. In: 2012 IEEE International Multi-Disciplinary Conference on Cognitive Methods in Situation Awareness and Decision Support (CogSIMA), pp. 73–79. IEEE (2012)
2. Tyworth, M., Giacobe, N.A., Mancuso, V.: Cyber situation awareness as distributed socio-cognitive work. In: Proc. of SPIE, vol. 8408, pp. 84080F–1 (2012)
3. Hamilton, K., Mancuso, V., Minotra, D., Hoult, R., Mohammed, S., Parr, A., Dubey, G., McMillan, E., McNeese, M.: Using the NeoCITIES 3.1 simulation to study and measure team cognition. Proceedings of the Human Factors and Ergonomics Society Annual Meeting 54(4), 433–437 (2010)
4. Hellar, D.B., McNeese, M.: NeoCITIES: A simulated command and control task environment for experimental research. Proceedings of the Human Factors and Ergonomics Society Annual Meeting 54(13), 1027–1031 (2010)
5. McNeese, M.D., Bains, P., Brewer, I., Brown, C., Connors, E.S., Jefferson, T., Jones, R.E.T., Terrell, I.: The NeoCITIES simulation: Understanding the design and experimental methodology used to develop a team emergency management simulation. Proceedings of the Human Factors and Ergonomics Society Annual Meeting 49(3), 591–594 (2005)
6. Mancuso, V., Hamilton, K., McMillan, E., Tesler, R., Mohammed, S., McNeese, M.: "What's on "Their" Mind Evaluating Collaborative Systems Using Team Mental Models. Proceedings of the Human Factors and Ergonomics Society Annual Meeting 55(1), 1284–1288 (2011)
7. Wellens, A.R., Ergener, D.: The CITIES Game. Simulation & Gaming 19(3), 304 (1988)
8. Endsley, M.R.: Situation awareness global assessment technique (SAGAT). In: Proceedings of the IEEE 1988 National Aerospace and Electronics Conference, NAECON 1988, pp. 789–795. IEEE (1988)
9. Mancuso, V.F., McNeese, M.D.: Effects of Integrated and Differentiated Team Knowledge Structures on Distributed Team Cognition. Proceedings of the Human Factors and Ergonomics Society Annual Meeting 56(1), 388–392 (2012)
10. Mancuso, V.F.: An Interdisciplinary Evaluation of Transactive Memory in Distributed Cyber Teams. PhD diss., Pennsylvania State University (2012)

Application of Fuzzy Index to Qualitative and Quantitative Evaluation of the Quality Level of Working Conditions

Anna Mazur

Poznan University of Technology, Department of Management Engineering,
ul. Strzelecka 11, 60-965 Poznań, Poland
anna.mazur@put.poznan.pl

Abstract. Quality assessment can be performed with natural language (in descriptive form) or with numbers (in quantitative form). Such approach enables consideration of all the aspects and characteristics beyond quantification, difficult or impossible to assess with numbers, hence requiring linguistic representation. Application of fuzzy index to work conditions quality assessment provides objective identification of hazards and their influence on work conditions quality.

Keywords: quality of work conditions, quality characteristics, quality level.

1 Introduction

Man is a subject to every process of work and according to that human-centric paradigm he is the most important, the most active and decisive factor of production [1], [2], [5]. Thus considering man and his decisive role in manufacturing processes enterprises should strive for guaranteeing proper and safe work conditions that enable development of employees and performing their jobs in efficient and effective way [1], [3]. More complex analysis of the problem leads to the conclusion that safety and human-factor are just some of the factors influencing quality of work conditions [2]. Quality of work conditions is a complex term and it should reflect how many attributes connected with work influence satisfaction on health, professional life and supports increase of culture and morality of human environment in a company.

2 Quality of Work Conditions

Characteristics of quality of work conditions are not only limited to human-centric and hygienic aspects of work but also include some other areas of company's functioning [2]. They refer, for example, to reaction to changes, available resources, applied methods of assessment and improvement of work conditions, safety culture, managers' commitment and risk of managerial decisions taken, which are mostly caused by lack of knowledge about objectives, poorly determined goals, not noticing

C. Stephanidis (Ed.): Posters, Part II, HCII 2013, CCIS 374, pp. 514–518, 2013.

influences of the environment, incompetent or inadequate information or wrong advisers and experts [6]. Characteristics determining quality of work conditions are presented in the table 1.

Table 1. Selected characteristics of quality of work conditions

Reaction to changes:
A1 – how fast an organization can react to law changes
A2 – how fast an organization can react to work conditions changes
A3 – how fast an organization can react to a problem
Managers' commitment
E1 – clear strategy towards quality of work conditions improvement
E2 – planning actions improving quality of work conditions in manufacturing processes
E3 – setting goals (strategic, tactical and operational)
Risk of managerial decisions
F1 - managerial decisions have regard to improving the quality of working conditions
F2 - style of leadership decisions takes into account risk understood as a result of employees

The characteristics presented are partial results of research conducted in Polish manufacturing companies [5]. The level of meeting requirements defined by each characteristics will contribute to the total level of quality of work conditions. Quality assessment will hence include qualitative approach (descriptive, linguistics) and quantitative approach determinable in numeric form.

3 Qualitative and Quantitative Evaluation of the Quality Level of Working Conditions

3.1 The Fuzzy Index of Work Conditions Quality Level

The fuzzy index of work conditions quality level(FI_{WQCL})is based on linguistic variables and linguistic values, turned into triangular fuzzy numbers.

Fuzzy numbers derived from assessment procedure are aggregated into fuzzy weighted average with max-min paired eliminated method. The result, which is certainly the fuzzy number is then turned back into linguistic value, which makes its analysis clear and simple. Turning back procedure is based on the Euclidean distance method. Fuzzy weighted average, identifying fuzzy index of work conditions quality level (FI_{WQCL})is calculated with the following formula:

$$\mathrm{FI}_{\mathrm{WCQL}} = \frac{\sum_{j=1}^{n} W_i R_i}{\sum_{i=1}^{n} W_i} \qquad (1)$$

where:

R$_i$ - fuzzy rating i, **W$_i$** – fuzzy weighting i, **i** – index of a characteristics, **n** – number of the characteristics.

The membership function can be defined as follows [4]:

$$f_Y(y) = \text{sup.min } \{f_{Wi}(wi),\ f_{Ri}(ri)\},\ i = 1..n \text{ I } y = \frac{\sum_{j=1}^{n} W_i R_i}{\sum_{i=1}^{n} W_i} \tag{2}$$

where:
for each i=1,2..n f_{wi} i f_{Ri} are the membership functions of fuzzy number W_i i R_i respectively.

The membership function fy can be calculated with using an appropriate procedure [4] according to max-min paired eliminated method.

The calculated Fuzzy Index of Work Conditions Quality Level is a fuzzy number, which defines the level of work conditions quality. Hence the result of running the procedure is a fuzzy number, the next step should be translating it into an appropriate linguistic term.

To translate the index presented (FI_{WCQL}) Euclidean distance method is applied which consist of calculating the Euclidean distance from the given fuzzy number (which is the FI_{WCQL} calculated) to each of the fuzzy numbers representing the natural language expression set. Thanks to calculating the Euclidean distance it is possible to interpret the value obtained in the max-min paired eliminated method.

3.2 Application of the Fuzzy Index of Work Conditions Quality Level (A Case Study)

Evaluation of characteristics (examples of which were introduced in the table 1) is performed by a team of independent experts representing various fields. The level of meeting requirements defined with pre-determined criteria is qualitatively assessed with seven-level-scale including the following levels: **E** – excellent, **VG** – very good, **G** – good, **F** – fairly, **P** – poor, **VP** – very poor, **W** – worst. Determination of the index is based on transformation of linguistic parameters given by experts into fuzzy numbers according to the scheme: **E** in fuzzy number is (0.8, 1.0, 1.0), **VG** is (0.6, 0.8, 1.0), **G** is (0.5, 0.65, 0.8), **F** is (0.3, 0.5, 0.7), **P** is (0.2, 0.35, 0.5), **VP** is (0, 0.2, 0.4), **W** is (0, 0, 0.2).

Each of the predefined characteristics i also defined with an importance rate representing its influence on achieving a given level of quality of work conditions. The pre-mentioned importance rates were also assessed with the seven-level-scale and translated into fuzzy numbers (given in brackets): **TNI** - totally not important (0, 0, 0.2), **NI** - not important (0, 0.2, 0.4), **LI** - less important (0.2, 0.35, 0.5), FI - fairly important (0.3, 0.5, 0.7), **I** – important (0.5, 0.65, 0.8), **VI** - very important (0.6, 0.8, 1.0), **MI** - the most important (0.8, 1.0, 1.0). The example of assessment of predefined characteristics with linguistic variables is introduced in the table 2.

Table 2. Example of assessment of quality of work conditions derived by experts

ATRIBUTES Reaction to changes	LEVEL	WEIGHT
	G	I
	G	I
A1 – how fast an organization can react to law changes	F	VI
	G	VI
	G	VI
	P	LI
A2 – how fast an organization can react to work conditions changes	BN	NI
	F	I
	F	I
	G	LI
	F	VI
	F	NI
A3 – how fast an organization can react to a problem	G	I
	G	I
	F	VI

After linguistic analysis weighted level of quality of conditions of work FI_{WCQL} is calculated as a fuzzy number identifying quality level of work conditions.

For better interpretation of the research results the obtained number should be transformed into qualitative, linguistic assessment. Natural language scale for definition of work conditions quality level in an enterprise is defined as follows:

- **Level A$^+$** - The highest work conditions quality level, all the attributes are performed perfectly **– it is (1, 0.9, 0.8) in fuzzy numbers scale;**
- **Level A** - Very high work conditions quality level, though there are some characteristics that can be improved – **it is (0.9, 0.8, 0.7);**
- **Level A$^-$** - Very high quality of work conditions level, though there are some characteristics that need to be improved **– it is (0.8, 0.7, 0.6);**
- **Level B$^+$**- The company has numerous attributes of work conditions quality but their level is fairly low **– it is (0.7, 0.6, 0.5);**
- **Level B** - The average level, the company has some attributes of work conditions quality but most of them need to be improved **– it is (0.6, 0.5, 0.4);**
- **Level B$^-$**- The company has some attributes of work conditions quality but all of them need to be improved – **it is (0.5, 0.4, 0.3);**
- **Level C$^+$**- Low quality level, the company has some attributes of work conditions quality but their level is very low and numerous changes need to be implemented **- it is (0.4, 0.3, 0.2);**
- **Level C** - Very low quality level, there are no attributes of work conditions quality but there possibilities of their implementation **– it is (0.3, 0.2, 0.1);**
- **Level C$^-$**- The lowest level. There are no attributes of work conditions quality and the company is not willing to implement them **– it is (0.2, 0.1, 0);**

As a result of calculation procedure [6] the following results were obtained and illustrated with triangular fuzzy numbers as presented in the figure 1.

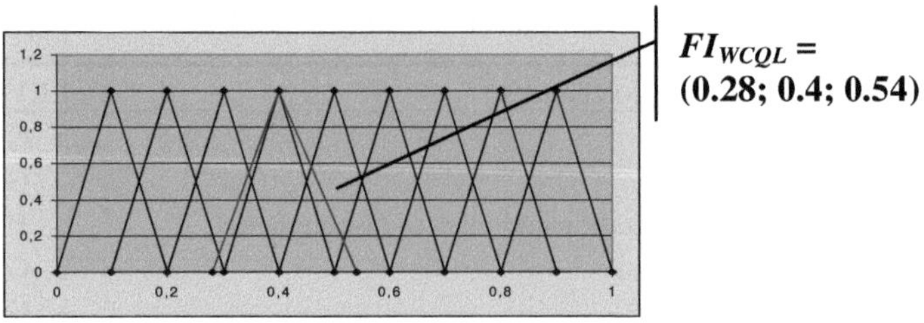

Fig. 1. Work conditions level assessment

Hence, the analysis led to the following conclusions: work conditions quality level in the company analysed can be defined as B- which means that the company has some attributes of work conditions quality but all of them need to be improved.

4 Conclusions

The attributes of quality are described with linguistic terms which makes fuzzy logic indispensable in quality measuring. Definition of the level of attributes of work conditions quality and consequently assessment of the quality level in the company allows to analyze the solutions applied in the work conditions quality area, as well as to make conclusions and improvement on the most requiring areas, analyze the influence of work conditions on the management quality, and analyze the influence of work conditions on the employees efficiency.

Companies can benefit from implementation of quality assessment performed as a calculation of the index presented as it provides them with detailed and holistic information in the same time. The components analysis indicates areas of necessary improvements, while the value of the index shows general level of quality. The index' structure enables repetitive analysis and results comparison, and experts team employed to assess the work system guarantees high standard of evaluation.

References

1. Gołaś, H.: O zarządzaniu ryzykiem personalnym inaczej, czyli porozumiewanie się ze szczęśliwym pracownikiem. Controlling 23 (2012)
2. Górny, A.: Ergonomics in the formation of work condition quality. Work: A Journal of Prevention, Assessment and Rehabilitation 41, 1708–1711 (2012)
3. Jasiulewicz-Kaczmarek, M.: Participatory Ergonomics as a Method of Quality Improvement in Maintenance. In: Karsh, B.-T. (ed.) EHAWC 2009. LNCS, vol. 5624, pp. 153–161. Springer, Heidelberg (2009)
4. Lin, C.-T.: Agility Index in Supply Chain. In: Proceedings of the 17th International Conference on Production Research Blacksburg, Virginia, USA, August 3-7 (2003)
5. Mazur, A.: Shaping quality of work conditions. In: Health Protection and Ergonomics for Human Live Quality Formation, pp. 31–44. Poznan University of Technology, Poznań (2009)
6. Więcek-Janka, E.: Decisions and games. Publishing House of Poznan University of Technology, Poznań (2011)

A Method of Team Communication Analysis Based on a Team Cognition Model and Task Analysis

Kohei Nonose, Taro Kanno, and Kazuo Furuta

Department of Systems Innovation, the University of Tokyo, Japan
nonose@cse.sys.t.u-tokyo.ac.jp

Abstract. Effective communication is believed to be essential for positive teamwork, and thus team communication has received much attention from human factor researchers for analyzing team cooperation. This study aims to propose a method of team communication analysis that can contribute to investigating changes of team cooperation in terms of team cognition possessed by a team member. In the beginning, a communication classification matrix that consists of the category of intentions derived from a team cognition model based on mutual belief and that of contents derived from a task analysis is developed. Subsequently, the matrix is applied to team communication data. Finally reasons behind changes of team cooperation are discussed according to the analyses. The results imply that the combination of both categories can contribute to understanding changes of team working in terms of team cognition.

Keywords: Communication analysis, teamwork, a cognition model in team, and task analysis.

1 Introduction

Effective communication is believed to be essential for positive teamwork, and thus team communication (verbal communications, gestures, etc.) has received much attention from human factor researchers for analyzing teamwork; a serious problem of traditional methods, including the number of utterances of each team member, the duration of communication, and social network analysis, is probably that the results from these methods can show superficial descriptions of team behaviors but cannot explain reasons behind the differences of team working in terms of cognition possessed by a team member, because the traditional categories are not based on any team cognition model possessed by a team member. To better understand and analyze team working in terms of team communication, it will be necessary to create communication categories derived from a team cognition model possessed by a team member. This study aims to propose a method of team communication analysis that can contribute to investigating changes of team behaviors and team cognition behind the changes of team cooperation. The next section explains a team experiment, which was conducted our previous study [1], that provides the team communication data to which that the proposed approach is applied to, because the explanation of a team task is necessary to explain our proposed method.

C. Stephanidis (Ed.): Posters, Part II, HCII 2013, CCIS 374, pp. 519–523, 2013.

2 Experiment

Task and Participants. An air traffic control simulator was used for a task. Participants were asked to route arriving and departing aircraft both safely and accurately. During the session, the aircraft randomly appeared on the display. Each two-person team comprised a "Selector," who had only a mouse, and a "Commander," who had only a keyboard. The standard operating procedures of the task were as follows: the Selector selected the aircraft to which they would give a command with the mouse. Then, the Commander would enter a command for the selected aircraft using the keyboard. Because the number of aircraft increased in the second and third sets, team members had to reallocate team resources in the sets; otherwise, they would fail to manage the aircraft. Twenty-two graduate/postgraduate students (11 teams) participated.

Instructions for Reflection, Procedures, and Team Performance Indices. Two-types of metacognitive instructions on cooperation were designed and applied. One was "Team-oriented instruction" whose instruction was "How is this task being operated by your team?" (6 teams), and the other one was "Self-oriented instruction" whose instruction was "How do you cooperate in this task?" The participants were asked to reflect on these instructions (5 teams). The participants practiced the operation until they could smoothly land and transfer an aircraft. The total trial duration was 15 min for all participants. The metacognitive instruction was presented every 7.5 minutes and the participants read it and wrote down their own cognitive status and beliefs twice in each set. When the instruction was presented, the display turned blank and the simulation was suspended. The participants sat face-to-face, and communicated freely with each other, except when they were responding to the instructions. Some teams could not participate in the third set because of their schedules. Two types of game score were used as team performance indices: safety violation time and number of aircraft successfully processed. Safety violation time was the duration in seconds of when the distance between two different aircraft was less than 1,000 feet vertically and 3 miles laterally. The number of aircraft successfully processed was calculated by subtracting the number of failed landings or improper exits from the airspace from the number of successful landings or successful transfers to other airspaces at the handoff points.

3 Development of Categories

In order to develop utterance categories that can represent the meanings of each utterance by a minimum number of categories, a communication classification matrix is created by combining the category of intentions derived from a team cognition model based on mutual belief [2] with the category of contents derived from a hierarchical task analysis. The category of intentions can examine the changes of intentions behind changes in team behaviors, while the category of contents can help identify subtasks where the changes in team behaviors occur.

The Category of Intentions. A team cognition model based on mutual belief describes team cognition as a set of three layers of mental processes and constructs, interaction between the different layers, and metacognition for cooperation. In a dyadic case (Agent A and B), the model is composed of the following three layers:

- The first layer (Ma/Mb) = an individual cognition that contains various mental processes and constructs except beliefs.
- The second layer (Ma'/Mb') = a belief in the partner's cognition.
- The third layer (Ma''/Mb'') = a belief in the partner's belief.

There are two types of interactions between different layers; intra- and inter-personal. Intra-personal interactions are manipulations of one's own mental components between different layers and are assumed to be involved in updating one's own cognition and in inferring a partner's cognitive status. Inter-personal interactions are communication and the direct or indirect observation of the behavior of others and can update the partner's layers. Metacognition for cooperation means monitoring and assessing the current status of each of one's own three layers in terms of, for example, sufficiency, conviction, and consistency. The metacognition for cooperation has been assumed as the beginning of team cognitive processes. Based on the metacognition, a team member could be motivated to increase sufficiency and conviction, or to maintain consistency among the status of each layer. In this study, these motivations are defined as communication intentions. The category of intentions is derived from the team cognition model (Table 1).

Table 1. The Category of Intentions

Intentions	Definition
Inform	To add new information to the partner's cognition/belief. To verify the partner's cognition.
Correct Cognition	To correct mistakes in the partner's cognition. To make the partner reflect about his/her cognition.
Correct Belief	To correct mistakes of the partner's belief. To make the partner reflect about his/her belief.
Check Cognition	To query others to check/complement his/her own cognition. To signal defects in his/her own cognition.
Check Belief	To query others to check/complement his/her belief on his/her partner's cognition (to elicit his/her partner's cognition).
Acknowledge	To agree with his/her partner. (Reply to "Inform.") To acknowledge "Inform". (Reply to "Inform.")
Interjection	To withhold his or her judgment. (Reply to "Inform.")

The Category of Contents. The category of contents is derived from hierarchical task analyses. The procedure of the task used in this study was as follows. In the beginning, participants need to understand the traffic situation such as positions and flight paths of aircraft. In addition, they need to check instructions given to aircraft.

Subsequently, participants need to give aircraft adequate instructions, including flight level control and flight direction, to route arriving and departing aircraft. The category is given in Table 2.

Table 2. The Category of Contents

Contents	Definition
Landing clearance	Decisions about clearance for landing aircraft and selecting appropriate runways.
Departing clearance	Decisions about clearance for departing aircraft.
Plan	Plans and instructions given to aircraft (flight direction and level).
Aircraft status	The status of instructions that aircraft have been given. Discrimination between arriving and departing aircraft.
Traffic situation	Positions of aircraft, the distances between aircraft, and appearance of new aircraft.

The Communication Classification Matrix. Based on both the category of intentions and the category of contents, a communication classification matrix is constructed (Table 3). The matrix is used to classify team communications for analyses of team cooperation.

Table 3. The Communication Classification Matrix

Intentions	Contents	Commander	Selector
Inform	Landing clearance		
	Departing clearance		
…	…		
Interjection	Traffic situation		

4 Results and Discussion

Table 4 shows the number of aircrafts successfully processed and safety violation time. The average number by the team-oriented instruction team improved in the second and third sets, while that of the self-oriented team remained the same. The average safety violation time of the team-oriented instruction team remained the same in the second and third sets, while that of the self-oriented instruction team increased in the second set. These results imply that team members in the team-oriented instruction changed their team behaviors to improve their team processes. We applied the proposed method to the communication data to investigate a part of reasons behind the changes. Although it is possible to compare the two conditions according the communication analyses by the method, this paper focuses on the transition of the measured "Check belief" ratios due to limitations of space (Table 5). The results imply that the "Check belief" ratio for "Plan" under the team-oriented instruction increased in the second and third sets. These results imply that some of the team members under team-oriented instruction became to give their partner initiative about making plans and actively check their partner's thoughts about plans to make a quick team decision in situation where team members have to deal with multiple tasks in parallel.

Table 4. Game Scores

	Team-oriented instruction			Self-oriented instruction		
	1st set	2nd set	3rd set	1st set	2nd set	3rd set
Number of Aircrafts Successfully Processed	3.67	7.50	8.33	5.80	6.00	5.00
Safety Violation Time	264.00	222.00	204.00	226.60	378.80	152.25

Table 5. "Check belief" Ratios

	Team-oriented instruction			Self-oriented instruction		
	1st set	2nd set	3rd set	1st set	2nd set	3rd set
Landing clearance	0.00	0.06	0.00	0.12	0.16	0.08
Departing clearance	0.62	0.73	2.02	1.26	1.04	1.23
Plan	1.75	3.16	2.69	1.06	0.78	0.60
Aircraft status	0.24	0.54	0.84	0.00	0.12	0.28
Traffic situation	0.08	0.20	0.32	0.08	0.00	0.08

5 Conclusion

In order to develop a method for investigating reasons behind changes of team cooperation in terms of team cognition, this study proposed a team communication matrix that consists of two utterance classification categories; one is the category of intentions derived from a team cognition model based on mutual belief, and the other is the that of contents derived from a task analysis. We applied the method to the communication data collected in our previous study. The analysis implied that the combination of both categories can enable systematic and detailed descriptions of characteristics of team cooperation in terms of team cognition possessed by a team member.

References

1. Nonose, K., Kanno, T., Furuta, K.: A Team Cognition Model Derived from Reflection on Cooperation. Cognition, Technology, and Work 14(1), 83–92 (2012)
2. Kanno, T., Furuta, K., Kitahara, Y.: A Model of Team Cognition based on Mutual Beliefs, Theoretical Issues in Ergonomics Science (2011) (in press, online available)

Methodology of Facility Automation Based on Audiovisual Analysis and Space-Time Structuring of Situation in Meeting Room

Alexander L. Ronzhin, Andrey L. Ronzhin, and Victor Yu. Budkov

SPIIRAS, 39, 14th line, St. Petersburg, Russia
{ronzhinal,ronzhin,budkov}@iias.spb.su

Abstract. Space-time context structurization is one of the key issues of the development of an automatic audiovisual monitoring system for meeting supporting and analysis of participants' behavior in a smart space. An analysis of accumulated data about participant's behavior including position in the meeting room, speech activity, and face direction allows monitoring system to generate participant profile, which is further used for predicting his/her behavior on successive meetings. It is also used for an adjustment of an audio and video recording and of multimedia devices controlling model in the smart room. In the experiment the main attention was paid to speaker localization in the chair zone with 32 predefined positions.

Keywords: Smart space, action recognition, speaker detection, audiovisual signal processing, space-time context structurization.

1 Introduction

Methods of multichannel audiovisual signal processing are widely used for analysis of participant's behavior in intelligent meeting rooms [1] and other prototypes of smart space [2]. The selection of key events and zones in meeting room helps to improve quality of meeting situation description as well as its formalization. The observation of the specific places in the meeting room (for instance, chairs, presentation zone, entrance area) during the work of a visual processing system allows a personification system to extract the main data, which are useful for creating and updating the participant profile., Additional characteristics to the participant profile (such as the frequency of the messages, their durations, the recorded speech itself) may be obtained by applying an audio localization system mainly to the main speaker in the presentation zone and to the speaking participants sitting in the chairs, and it is determined in advance by the visual processing system,. So, the proposed methodology of participant personification based on audiovisual analysis of meeting situation constituents limited in space and time accumulates data for the participant profile by means of his/her activity during the meeting and applies this knowledge for automatic control of multimedia and audiovisual recording facility as well as of personified participant service. The automation principles of the audiovisual facilities control taking into account equipment features and participant activities during the event in the smart meeting room are outlined in the next section.

C. Stephanidis (Ed.): Posters, Part II, HCII 2013, CCIS 374, pp. 524–528, 2013.

2 Automation of Audiovisual Monitoring in Smart Meeting Room

In a given research area of 8.85x7.15x4.80m located inside the institute building was reequipped for a smart meeting room [1]. The conference table for seating of participants of small meetings (round tables) up to 10 people is located on the left side of the hall. On the right side of the hall there are rows of seats, where up to 32 participants can seat. The main aim of an automatic audiovisual monitoring system in the smart space is generation of multimedia report during the meetings, which includes photographs A_F of participant's A_P faces as well as audiovisual records of speakers talk. We propose to use spatial-temporal structuring data about participants' behavior in an analyzed space during the process of audiovisual monitoring in the smart space. In particular, key time moments are detection of a new participant in the room, detection of occupied chair (moment, when non-registered participant sits in a chair), detection of the beginning and the end of speaker's talk (reporter or sitting participant).

First and foremost, for space structuring of the smart room certain zones are determined, which are different in functions (types of behavior) of participants located in it. Examples of such zones are presentation zone, entering/exiting zone, zone, where participants sit at conference table and zone, where participants sit in mounted chairs. For the control of soft-hardware audiovisual monitoring complex and for the receiving data for multimedia report $< A_F, A_R >$ a set of control commands C to audio F_a and video F_v recording devices have to be formed in time moments, which corresponds to the appearance of a new participant in the room, appearance of non-registered participant in a chair as well as beginning of reporter's talk or participant's question during the discussion. Data about the participant A_P, which were received during the meeting, are used for the formation of his/her profile A_H, which in follows used for predicting his/her behavior on successive meetings and for the adjustment of the audiovisual recording and multimedia devices controlling model in the smart room. The task of audiovisual situation monitoring in the meeting room could be defined as the following structure: $< F_a, F_v >, \mathrm{C}, A_P, < A_F, A_R >, A_H$.

A model for automation of audiovisual monitoring of participants in smart room provides multimedia report generation and collection of participant's personal data for adjustment of their profiles. Figure 1 presents a scheme of the model. Automation task consists in generation of the control commands C. To solve this task the detection of key time points during meeting on audiovisual data analyzing has to be developed. Sensor equipment of an intelligent room can be divided into two types - primary and auxiliary. Equipment of primary type is the sensor equipment that records events in the entire space of the room. Auxiliary equipment is used for a more detailed analysis of certain areas of interest, which were identified in the data recorded by primary equipment.

A panoramic ceiling camera F_{v_c} and a microphone array F_{a_r} are usually used in smart rooms as examples of main type sensor equipment. Auxiliary equipment includes an individual microphone F_{a_m} and a high resolution camera F_{v_h}, which services different zones of the room; an intelligent PTZ camera F_{v_p}, which is used for photography of participant face and recording their talks; integrated microphones in web-cameras, which are mounted on conference table etc. One of auxiliary equipment tasks is the analysis of certain room zones for receiving additional information for interpretation of particular objects in the room. Another auxiliary equipment task is the collection of audiovisual information about meeting participants.

Further we will consider a conceptual model that integrates both primary and auxiliary equipment and define the key events in the intelligent room. This model generates control commands for the equipment. On Figure 1 each of the considered equipment types is presented in a single sample, and this equipment is necessary for the designing of a minimal configuration of the automation model of audiovisual intelligent room monitoring. The proposed model allows the scalability of software and hardware resources at the increase of the room size, number of participants, number of observation zones, and number of requirements for activities logging, and this allows configuring the full range of equipment for a specific environment.

A microphone array F_{a_r} during monitoring process produces audio signal D_{a_r} multichannel recording, which used for determination data $D_{a\_r}^{loc}$ about sound source coordinates as well as start T_p^s and end T_p^f of presenters talk or participant question during discussion by sound source localization method [3] $M_{a\_r}^{loc}$ and speech activity spatial spectral analysis method [3] $M_{a\_r}^{vad}$ properly: $D_{a\_r}^{loc} = M_{a\_r}^{loc}(D_{a\_r})$; $C_a^{rec} = M_{a\_r}^{vad}(D_{a\_r})$, $C_a^{rec} = \{T_p^s, T_p^f\}$, where C_a^{rec} is a command to auxiliary audio recording equipment F_{a_m} about start T_p^s and end T_p^f of participant talk.

A ceiling panoramic camera F_{v_c} records video signal D_{v_c} with view of whole room. Video signal is used for receiving data about location of participants $D_{v\_c}^{cor}$ and data about occupied mounted chairs $D_{v\_c}^{chr}$ by detection and tracking method $M_{v\_c}^{cor}$ and detection of occupied mounted method $M_{v\_c}^{chr}$ accordingly [4].

An individual microphone F_{a_m} is an auxiliary equipment type and records audio signal D_{a_m} from one of the determined zones with one or several participants. At receiving control command C_a^{rec} microphone F_{a_m} records speech signal $D_{a\_m}^{sph}$ in a file during interval between time moment of speaker's talk start T_P^s and end by T_P^f recording method [3] $M_{a\_m}^{sph}$: $D_{a\_m}^{sph} = M_{a\_m}^{sph}(D_{a\_m}, C_a^{rec})$, i.e. data $D_{a\_m}^{sph}$ is speech segment of audio signal D_{a_m} in interval $[T_P^s, T_P^f]$.

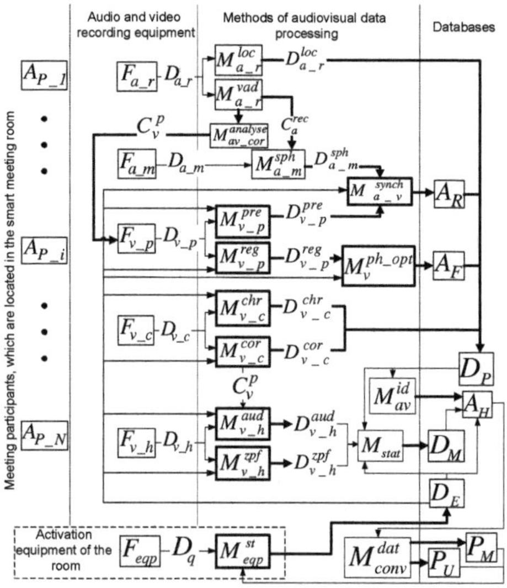

Fig. 1. Model of automatic audiovisual monitoring of smart meeting room

A high resolution camera F_{v_h} is used for processing of particular zones with several participants. Analysis of data, which were recorded by this camera, allows detecting object of interest and forming a control command to the camera F_{v_p} for pointing on this object. In particular, for servicing of participants, who sits in the chair zone, the camera F_{v_h} records video signal D_{v_h}, which is processed by a method $M_{v\_h}^{zpf}$ for determination of sitting participants' faces [4]. Data about detected participants (numbers of chairs, where participant face was found) are stored in a chairs data set, which includes information about occupied and free chairs. In addition, a high resolution camera F_{v_h}, which records video signal D_{v_h}, may be used for recording whole meeting process. When command C_v^{rec} appears the storing process of video signal $D_{v\_h}^{aud}$ in a file starts by recording function $M_{v\_h}^{aud}$. Video signal duration equal time interval between start T_m^s and end T_m^f of a meeting: $D_{v\_h}^{aud} = M_{v\_h}^{aud}(D_{v\_h}, C_v^{rec})$, $C_v^{rec} = \{T_m^s, T_m^f\}$, i.e. $D_{v\_h}^{aud}$ – is a segment of video signal D_{v_h} in an interval $[T_m^s, T_m^f]$.

An intelligent PTZ camera F_{v_p} is used for pointing and recording situation in particular zone or behavior of particular participant. In particular, in our research this camera is used for: photographing participants and recording their talks. The command C_v^p is used for pointing camera F_{v_p} on particular participant's face, after that process of recording video signal D_{v_p} starts, in which frames $D_{v\_p}^{reg}$ with participant's face are detected by face detection method and thus frames may be used as photographs A_F in multimedia report: $D_{v\_p}^{reg} = M_{v\_p}^{reg}(D_{v\_p}, C_v^p)$; $A_F = M_v^{ph\_opt}(D_{v\_p}^{reg})$, where estimation method $M_v^{ph\_opt}$ of camera F_{v_p} pointing on participant A_P face and selection best frames in photographs data base A_F.

In addition, intelligent PTZ camera F_{v_p}, which records video signal D_{v_p}, may be used for recording talks of meeting participants. At the command C_a^{rec}, which was formed earlier on the basis of the method $M_{a\_r}^{vad}$, another command C_v^p for pointing the camera to the speaker is formed by means of the method [5] $M_{av\_cor}^{analyse}$ for determining the nearest video object to coordinates of sound course. The recorded video signal $D_{v\_p}^{pre}$ is saved by function $M_{v\_p}^{pre}$ to a file with the duration equal to the time between the start T_p^s and the end T_p^f of a participant's cue: $C_v^p = M_{av\_cor}^{analyse}(C_a^{rec})$; $D_{v\_p}^{pre} = M_{v\_p}^{pre}(D_{v\_p}, C_v^p)$, $C_v^p = \{T_p^s, T_p^f\}$, i.e. $D_{v\_p}^{pre}$ – video signal D_{v_p} segment in interval $[T_p^s, T_p^f]$. Audio data $D_{a\_m}^{sph}$ – speech segment of audio signal D_{a_m} and $D_{v\_p}^{pre}$ – video signal D_{v_p} segmented in interval $[T_p^s, T_p^f]$, which were received during audiovisual signal processing may be used for forming of speaker's talk audiovisual records A_R by audio and video streams synchronization method [5]: $A_R = M_{a\_v}^{synch}(D_{a\_m}^{sph}, D_{v\_p}^{pre})$.

The data D_q about current state of activation equipment is presented on figure 1, are analyzed by method M_{eqp}^{st} and converted into data D_E with format, which satisfies one of the audiovisual data processing method, which requests current states of F_{eqp}.

Besides meeting multimedia report, which includes photographs and participant's cue, it consists of data about meeting participants A_P, which is accumulated in structure D_P during work of audiovisual monitoring methods. The structure D_P consists of data: $D_{v\_c}^{chr}$ – numbers of occupied chairs by participants; D_{stat} – their state; D_{role} – their role; $D_{a\_r}^{loc}$ – their speech activity; and $D_{v\_c}^{cor}$ – history of their movements. $D_P =< D_{v\_c}^{chr}, D_{stat}, D_{role}, D_{a\_r}^{loc}, D_{v\_c}^{cor} >$.

Stored data about participants D_P and equipment D_E is used by method M_{stat} for calculation characteristics of passed meeting M^j. This data includes meeting stages, total amount of presentation and other parameters, which may be received by statistical analysis of participant's behavior and used equipment: $D_{M^j} = M_{stat}(D_E, D_P)$.

In addition, data D_P, after processing by method M_{av}^{id} for analysis of audiovisual personal characteristics, are assigned an identification number of registered participant and then are converted into D_{P_id}. Then these data D_{P_id} with other data D_E and D_{M_j} are added to passed meetings database A_H : $D_{P\_id} = M_{av}^{id}(D_P)$, $A_H^j = (D_E, D_{P\_id}, D_{M^j})$.

At implementation of proposed model for automation of audiovisual monitoring of a smart room state of the art technologies of digital signal processing, pattern recognition were used [1, 2].

3 Conclusion

Methods of multichannel audiovisual signal processing are widely used for analysis of participant's behavior in intelligent meeting rooms and other prototypes of smart space. The selection of key events and zones in meeting room helps to improve quality of meeting situation description as well as its formalization. The main aim of an automatic audiovisual monitoring system in the smart space is generation of multimedia report during the meetings, which includes photographs of participant's faces as well as audiovisual records of speakers talk.

Acknowledgments. This research is supported by the stipend and the grant (#MK-1880.2012.8) of the President of Russia, the Ministry of Education and Science of Russia (contract No. 07.514.11.4139), the Russian Foundation for Basic Research (projects No.12-07-31128, No.13-08-00741).

References

1. Yusupov, R.M., Ronzhin, A.L., Prischepa, M.V., Ronzhin, A.L.: Models and Hardware-Software Solutions for Automatic Control of Intelligent Hall. Automation and Remote Control 72(7), 1389–1397 (2011)
2. Karpov, A.A., Lale, A., Ronzhin, A.L.: Multimodal assistive systems for a smart living environment. Proceedings of SPIIRAS 19, 48–64 (2011)
3. Ronzhin, A.L., Ronzhin, A.L., Budkov, V.Y.: Audiovisual Speaker Localization in Medium Smart Meeting Room. In: Proc. of the 8th International Conference on Information, Singapore (2011)
4. Ronzhin, A., Prischepa, M., Karpov, A.: A Video Monitoring Model with a Distributed Camera System for the Smart Space. In: Balandin, S., Dunaytsev, R., Koucheryavy, Y. (eds.) ruSMART 2010. LNCS, vol. 6294, pp. 102–110. Springer, Heidelberg (2010)
5. Ronzhin, A.: Audiovisual Recording System for e-learning Applications. In: Proceedings of the GRAPP 2012, Rome, Italy, pp. 515–518 (2012)

Part VIII
Text and Storytelling

How to Diagram a Dramatic Story

Sabah Al-Fedaghi

Computer Engineering Department, Kuwait University, Kuwait.
sabah@alfedaghi.com

Abstract. It has been proposed that UML diagrams are able to describe certain situations and can be used as instruments for reconstructing the dramatic progress of fictitious or real text. This paper claims that these diagrams are conceptually fragmented and proposes a new type of diagram for this purpose.

Keywords: conceptual modeling, UML diagrams, flow model.

1 Introduction

According to Tagliati and Caloro [1],

> *The problem of identifying new tools that the dramatist and/or director can use to analyze a text arises. Among these tools, it is important to select which is to be used in order to facilitate the sharing of the project among the different participants... The discipline of computer science can provide us with a valid solution to this problem, where comparable problems are, typically, solved by means of UML.*

Tagliati and Caloro [1] selected the episode Ecuador by Aristides Vargas, an Equadorian (see appendix A), in a work created by six Latin American dramatists to bring attention to the problem of thousands of abandoned children wandering the streets of big cities in the Third World. A short description of the text [2] is as follows. For the sake of brevity, only parts of the description are included.

> *A doctor, helped by his male nurse, trades in human organs, removed from innocent children. These organs are sold to him by their desperate parents...*
> *The male nurse, on the other hand ... is poor and miserable, though with a grain of conscience left... So ... [he] tells everything to the doctor's wife, who, unaware until that moment ...*

Tagliati and Caloro [1] analyzed the episode by first using semiotics tools to identify all the important elements. They then applied UML to the text to study "the possibilities of a dramatic interplay which can occur between set and technological displays, between natural and not natural language and between action on stage and systems" [1].

C. Stephanidis (Ed.): Posters, Part II, HCII 2013, CCIS 374, pp. 531–535, 2013.

2 The Flow Model (FM)

The flow model (FM) has been used in several applications [3-4]. A flow model is a uniform method for representing things that "flow," i.e., things that are created, processed, released, transferred, and received. "Things that flow" include information, materials (e.g., goods), and money. FM can be used to draw scenarios of events. A scenario is typically defined as a narrative or story that includes actors, activities, and objects. In FM, the basic structure of a scenario can be defined in terms of generic connected stages, with things flowing through this structure.

FM representation is a depiction of the structure of a scheme resembling a road map of components and conceptual flow. A component comprises spheres (e.g., those of a company, a robot, a human, an assembly line, a station) that enclose or intersect with other spheres (e.g., the sphere of a house contains rooms which in turn include walls, ceilings). Or, a sphere embeds flows (called flowsystems; e.g., walls encompass pipes of water flow and wires of electrical flow).

Things that flow in a flowsystem are referred to as flowthings. The life cycle of a flowthing is defined in terms of six mutually exclusive stages: creation, process, arrival, acceptance, release, and transfer.

Fig. 1 shows a flowsystem with its stages, where it is assumed that no released flowthing flows back to previous stages. The reflexive arrow in the figure indicates flow to the Transfer stage of another flowsystem. For simplicity's sake, the stages Arrive and Accept can be combined and termed Receive.

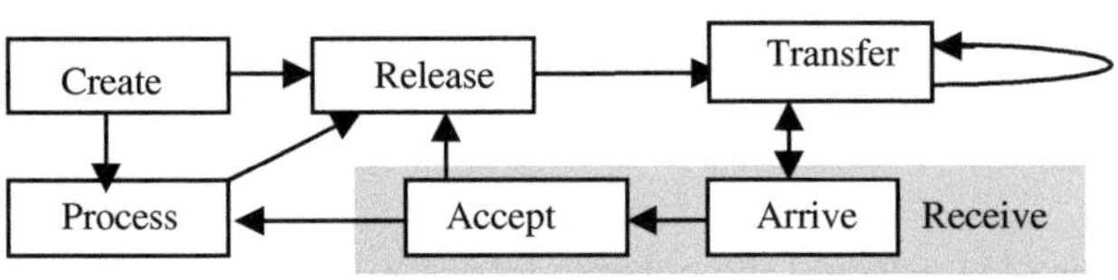

Fig. 1. Flowsystem

The stages of the life cycle of a flowthing are mutually exclusive (i.e., a flowthing can be in one and only one at a time). All other states or conditions of flowthings are not generic stages. For example, we can have stored created flowthings, stored processed flowthings, stored received flowthings, etc.; thus stored is not a generic stage. In contrast, there are no such stages as created received, or processed received stages. Flowthings can be released but not transferred (e.g., the channel is down), or arrived but not accepted (wrong destination).

In addition to flows, triggering is a transformation (denoted by a dashed arrow) from one flow to another, e.g., a flow of electricity triggers the flow of air.

Example: Formal models of narrative phenomena have been proposed in many applications, e.g., multimedia archives [5]. Schank (e.g., [6]) developed conceptual representations to be applied in story understanding systems, using a so-called conceptual dependency graph (CDG) to represent knowledge. The events of a narrative are represented abstractly through states that set the scene for the next event, and events impact states and cause new states to form. "*However … When encoding the events … narrative details may be lost and when reconstructing the event the original rendition of a scene is not always preserved*" [5].

Vassiliou [5] presents an example using a CDG of the film The English Patient in a scene that includes Hana (a nurse) losing her friend Jan in a jeep explosion. "The scene has 29 shots and is one minute and 40 seconds long" [5]. Fig. 2 shows the resultant CDG.

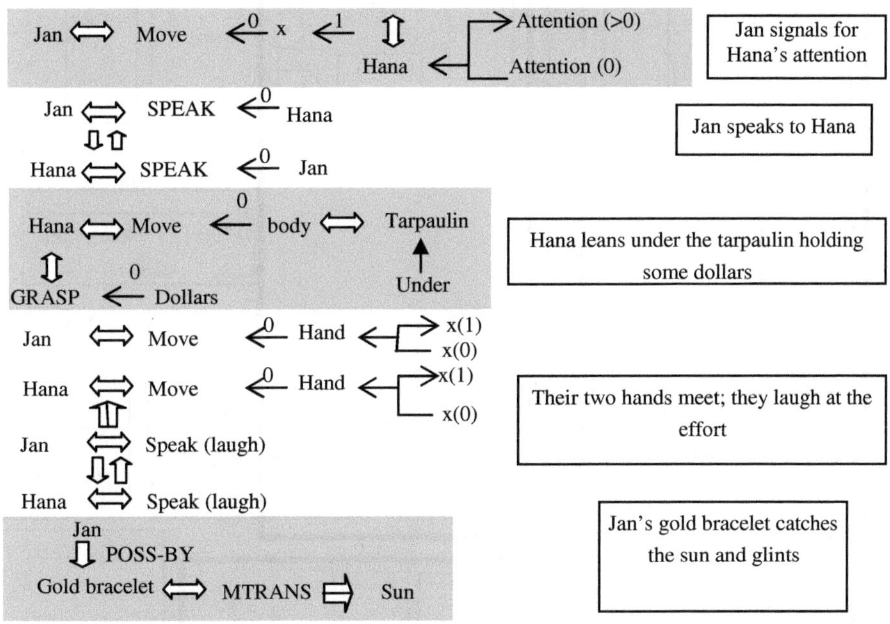

Fig. 2. A scene from *The English Patient* demonstrated in terms of Schank's conceptual dependency grammar (partial figure, redrawn from [5])

Fig. 3 shows the corresponding FM representation, with spheres of Jan (circle 1) and Hana (2). Hana is a subsphere of the JEEP sphere (3). Jan generates signals (4) that flow (5) to Hana, who processes the signals (6; e.g., recognizes them). Accordingly, her processing triggers (7) Hana to generate (8) a response (e.g., waving a hand) that flows (9) to Jan to be processed (e.g., 10, focusing her attention). This triggers Jan to speak (11) in speech that flows (12) to Hana to be processed (e.g., understood), triggering (14) a response (15) that flows (16) to Jan (17), who in turn creates a response (11). The rest of the diagram can be described in a similar manner.

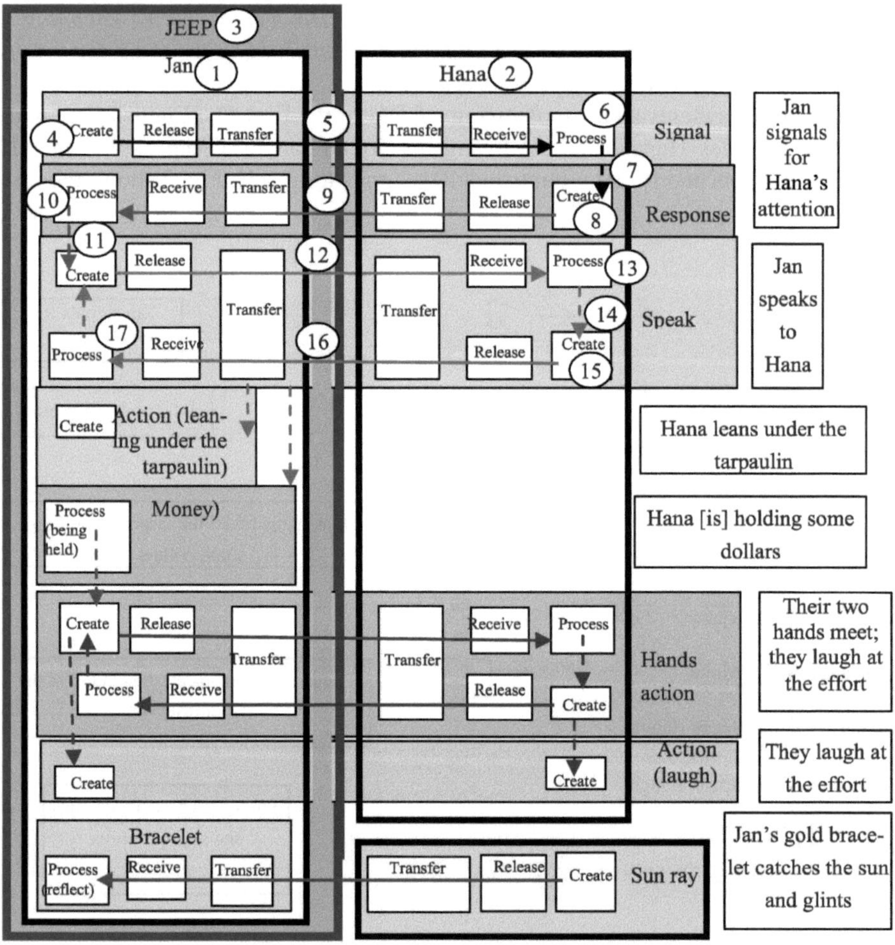

Fig. 3. A scene from The English Patient demonstrated in terms of FM

3 FM Representation of the Episode *Ecuador*

Fig. 4 shows the FM representation of the episode Ecuador, mentioned previously. It comprises seven spheres: child, doctor, buyer, parent, nurse , wife, and authority. We start the explanation at the child's sphere (circle 1 in the figure), which has one flow-system, in which the organ is the flowthing. The organ is processed, that is, removed, to flow to the doctor's sphere (circle 2). Receiving of an organ by the doctor triggers (3) a negotiation among the doctor, buyer, and parent. Note that the deal is also a flowthing that can be created, released, received, … The doctor creates a proposal (4) that flows to the buyer and/or the parent (5 and 6). When a buyer receives a proposal (7), he or she processes it (8), and may create a counter proposal (9), then sends it to the doctor (10). Similar communications occur between the doctor and the parent. The last acceptable deal is processed by the doctor, triggering (11) transfer of the organ to the buyer (12).

The nurse has a flowsystem of assistance (13) that is created and flows to the doctor (14). Note that assistance is a flowthing that can be created (generated) transferred, received, … Also, the nurse creates information (15) and releases it (16) to the wife. Upon receiving (17) this information, the wife informs (18) the authority. The authority receives (19) the information and processes it (20), and this triggers (21) sending (22) the doctor himself to jail (23).

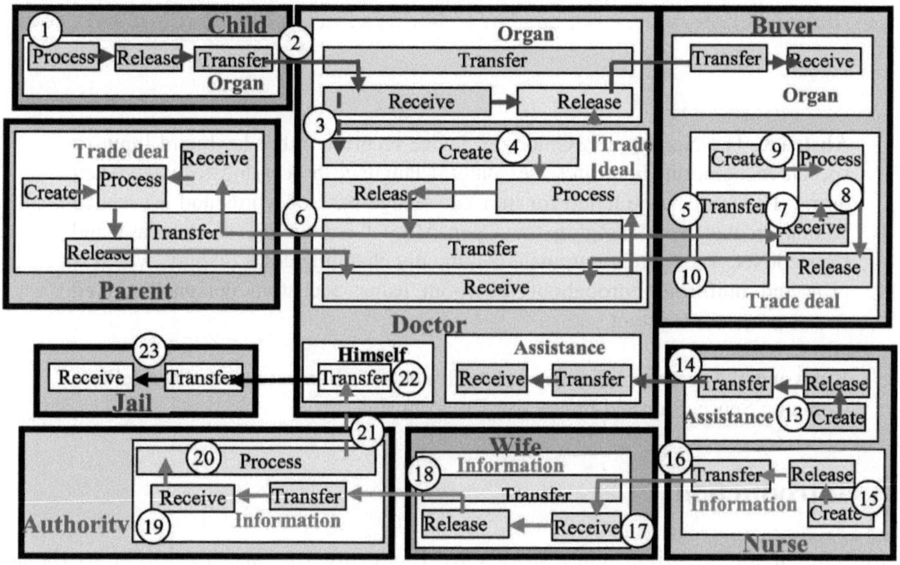

Fig. 4. FM representation of the episode *Ecuador*

References

1. Tagliati, L.V., Caloro, C.: UML and Object Oriented Drama. J. Object Tech. 7(1) (2008)
2. Barrionuevo, C., Espinoza, D., Jatahy, C., Nogales, I., Sanchis Sinisterra, J., Vargas, A., Viviescas, V.: La Cruzada de los Niños de la Calle. Sociedad General de Autores, Madrid (2001)
3. Al-Fedaghi, S.: Software Engineering Interpretation of Information Processing Regulations. In: IEEE Annual Computer Software and Applications, Turku, Finland (2008)
4. Al-Fedaghi, S.: Software System Development Based on Behavioral Aspects. Int. J. Inform. Processing Manage. 4(1), 86–96 (2013)
5. Vassiliou, A.: Representing Narrative in Multimedia Systems. PhD thesis, Department of Computing, University of Surrey (2004)
6. Schank, R.C.: Tell Me a Story: A New Look at Real and Artificial Memory. Scribner, New York (1990)

Narratarium: An Immersive Storytelling Environment

Kasia Hayden, Dan Novy, Catherine Havasi, Michael Bove, Santiago Alfaro, and Rob Speer

MIT Media Lab, Massachusetts Institute of Technology, Cambridge, MA, USA
{kmh,havasi,novysan,vmb,talfaro}@media.mit.edu, rspeer@mit.edu

Abstract. The Narratarium Colorizer device receives either keyboard input or speech recognition input and uses natural language processing to extract key terms. The terms are queried for in a knowledge base of words and associated colors, created by leveraging the Open Mind Common Sense database and ConceptNet. The system outputs a continually changing color display, which is projected uniformly throughout the room using a custom designed curved mirror projection system.

Keywords: Augmented Environments, Immersive Environments, Storytelling, Common Sense, Physical Interactive Environments.

1 Introduction

From camp leaders telling scary stories by flickering fire and flashlight to theater directors perfecting the blue hues of stage lighting on ocean wave props, storytellers across fields recognize the immersive effect of a good storytelling environment.

Whereas traditionally creating a tailored environment required some combination of preparation and skilled individuals, the Narratarium does so in real-time with no preparation or required skills. The effect of the Narratarium is to thematically augment the environment using color and images, and to create a hyper-immersive environment for storytelling. For instance, as a child tells stories about a jungle, the room is filled with greens and browns and foliage comes into view. A traveling parent can tell a story to a child and fill the room with images, color, and presence.

The Narratarium Colorizer is a device that takes in a source of words -- for example, keyboard input, speech recognition input, or song lyrics synchronized with music -- and connects to a knowledge base of words and associated colors. In real-time, it outputs a changing color display built from those words and the colors they are associated with, which are then displayed immersively in the room. The dynamically-generated canvas of colors, shapes and images is warped to fit the dimensions of the room and projected onto the walls of the room. The custom-designed projection system includes a frame to compactly house two projectors precisely calibrated at the correct distance from two curved mirrors and a small hard drive with a self-contained version of the required word association databases and image content.

C. Stephanidis (Ed.): Posters, Part II, HCII 2013, CCIS 374, pp. 536–540, 2013.

2 Software

The first version of the Narratarium prototype was originally built with Python and Javascript, and displayed in a web browser. Subsequently it was ported to C++ and OpenFrameworks. It uses the OpenGL libraries for the image manipulation requisite for proper 3D omni-directional projection. The backend calculation of color arrays most appropriately associated for a given word remains in Python. Here we outline the process involved in dynamically generating an aesthetically pleasing color scheme associated with the most recent words.

First the system receives a source of words, either in real-time or pre-recorded. It sends each word to a server running a REST API. The response that the frontend will receive from the server is a list of active colors. The server has access to a knowledge base that associates words with lists of colors that people identify with those words.

The server's job is to create an interesting set of colors associated with the words it has recently received. To do this, it treats the colors it receives from its knowledge base as "votes", and will hold an "election" to choose a color scheme of, for example, 8 colors. These votes are not necessarily equal; each vote is associated with a weight for how much it counts.

The more color data we have about a word, the more votes that word will get. If, for example, the word "tree" is associated with 1,000 different shades of green and brown, 1,000 new votes enter the system when the word "tree" appears; but if the word "quasar" has only been associated with a color twice, only two new votes enter the system. As these new votes enter, votes from previous words are not necessarily discarded. They are reduced in weight, and discarded when their weight crosses a minimum threshold. The goal of the election is to create an interesting color scheme, showing the range of colors represented by recent concepts. To accomplish this, the system holds the election using the Single Transferable Vote method of preference-based proportional representation.

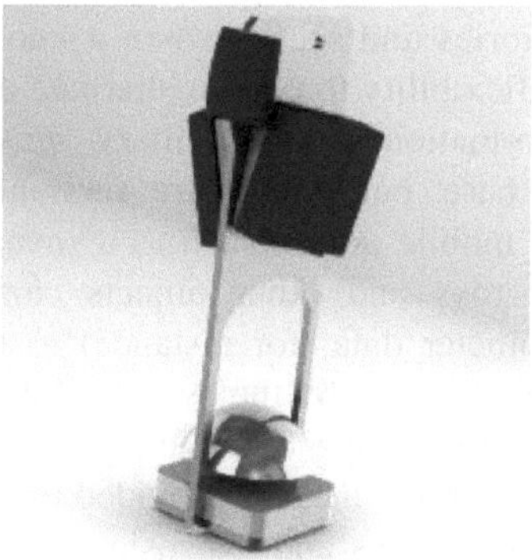

Fig. 1. Narratarium hardware setup, featuring two Optoma 500ML projectors, lasercut Acrylite GP frame, hemispherical mirror and Apple 2011 Mac Mini

The candidates in the election are chosen randomly from the voting colors. Each voting color produces a preference order of the candidate colors that are most perceptually similar to them (measured using the CIE L*a*b* color space). During the election, voting weights can be altered; for example, when some but not all of the colors have been elected, we can increase the voting weight of colors that complement them well according to color theory.

When the color scheme of 8 colors has been elected, the server returns two pieces of information to the frontend. The first is the list of RGB values of these colors. The second is a sample of RGB colors that relate specifically to the current word, showing which colors have newly been incorporated into the color scheme.

3 Hardware

Narratarium is a context-aware omnidirectional projector that combines sensing with intelligence and multimedia content to create an immersive environment.

The hardware component of Narratarium consists of a specialized omnidirectional projection system made of one or more projection engines and a hemispherical reflector. Our unit consists of two Optoma 500ML projectors, a transparent lasercut Acrylite GP frame designed in Solidworks and a hemispherical mirror. The base of the frame houses the computer, an Apple 2011 Mac Mini with an ATI GPU upgrade. The two projectors, one driven by the Mac Mini's native HDMI and the other driven by a Thunderbolt to HDMI adapter and hard drive are powered by a single power cord and On switch.

4 Future Work

Currently in development is the addition of an integrated sound database. Additionally, we are expanding on the natural language processing aspect of Narratarium so that it can determine story genre and setting for freeform oral stories, and can identify specific stories and scenes when a known story text is being read aloud. Narratarium has the flexibility to port to alternate designs and the capability to incorporate additional information from auxiliary sensors. The initial prototype contains a computer in its base, but in a future version Narratarium could also be constructed as a dock for a mobile device such as a smartphone or tablet. In another embodiment, instrumented toys and other objects can wirelessly report activity (button presses or accelerometer data, for instance) to the system and appropriate sounds and imagery can be produced by the system. Alternatively, an E-book reader can report to Narratarium which page of which book the reader is accessing and Narratarium can project appropriate imagery provided by the publisher.

In addition to hardware alterations and expansions, Narratarium's content sources are very adaptable. Narratarium's library of sounds and pictures can include both specific content (as might be provided by the publisher of a book or manufacturer of a physical product) as well as generic content for use with freeform story-genre recognition.

5 Previous Work

While various implementations of interactive storytelling environments have been developed to harness the power of immersive spaces, there is much variation surrounding cost for system setup, both financially and in terms of requisite technical expertise, portability, real-time capability, interaction complexity, ease of use and capability of expansion into new and wider content domains.

StoryRooms [1] is a collaboration between the HCI Lab at the University of Maryland, College Park and Sweden's Royal Institute of Technology's Centre for User Oriented IT Design to create room-sized interactive storytelling spaces for children. They emphasize children as authors rather than only participants and attempt to make accessible StoryRooms through the creation of StoryKits [2], a low-cost package of low-tech elements (such as cardboard boxes or Legos) and high-tech story elements (such as sensors, actuators and HandyBoard embedded computers). The StoryKits also contain "story starters," prompts for inspiring the story around which the props and entire experience are built.

Madame Bovary on the Holodeck [3] is a real-time immersive interactive storytelling system that uses CaveUT [4] software based on a commercial game engine (Unreal Tournament) and stereoscopic 3D animation featuring virtual actors projected in a 4-sided CAVE-like display. Users play a role as a character from the novel Madame Bovary, a famous 19th century novel by Gustave Flaubert. The user is outfitted with a head tracker to sync visuals and hand tracker to navigate through the virtual world. The system relies on an interactive storytelling engine to develop the narrative with interaction from the user, which has a limited range of allowable responses their story character would realistically give.

Each of the previous systems create immersive storytelling environments. Madame Bovary on the Holodeck is the most prohibitive to setup, in terms of financial cost, requisite technical expertise, dedicated space of a large room with blank walls for projection surfaces and equipment including projectors, head and arm trackers. StoryRooms is more accessible, incorporating low-tech equipment in addition to sensors and actuators. Using the high-tech equipment requires help from a technologically savvy person, although not a specialist. Narratarium, although not currently in a production state, is in the process of being explored for production by Hallmark, one of the Media Lab sponsors, which would place it as the most accessible of all, featuring a plug and play form factor and a friendly price point.

In terms of portability, both Madame Bovary on the Holodeck and StoryRooms require a dedicated staging area, although the latter can coexist in a playroom rather and can be erected and dismantled more quickly and easier than the former, which includes projectors installed into ceiling mounts. In contrast, Narratarium is instantaneous. As soon as a narrator begins telling their story the room around them is transformed. Unlike StoryRooms, there are no lasting physical props beside the Narratarium unit itself, which projects colors, lights and sounds, making the immersive environment temporary and immediately ready. Both StoryRooms and Madame Bovary on the Holodeck require significant preparation before use. StoryRooms differs from Narratarium in that the storytelling spaces are a longer-term project, collaboratively built by a group of children and adults. Madame Bovary on the Holodeck requires creation of virtual actors, analysis of a prescripted storyline and generation of responses and plot directions based on the user's possible responses to prompts. Narratarium is less complex than both systems, but has much higher ease of use and portability. Furthermore, it is able to quickly adapt and expand into new and wider content domains. In addition to adding new images, textures and sounds, it is also possible to add personalized word and content pairs.

References

1. Alborzi, H., Druin, A., Montemayor, J., Platner, M., Porteous, J., Sherman, L., ... Hendler, J.: Designing StoryRooms: Interactive storytelling spaces for children. In: Proceedings of the 3rd Conference on Designing Interactive Systems: Processes, Practices, Methods, and Techniques, pp. 95–104. ACM (August 2000)
2. Sherman, L., Druin, A., Montemayor, J., Farber, A., Platner, M., Simms, S., ... Lal, A.: StoryKit: tools for children to build room-sized interactive experiences. In: CHI 2001 Extended Abstracts on Human Factors in Computing Systems, pp. 197–198. ACM (March 2001)
3. Cavazza, M., Lugrin, J.L., Pizzi, D., Charles, F.: Madame bovary on the holodeck: immersive interactive storytelling. In: Proceedings of the 15th International Conference on Multimedia, pp. 651–660. ACM (September 2007)
4. Jacobson, J., Le Renard, M., Lugrin, J.L., Cavazza, M.: The CaveUT system: immersive entertainment based on a game engine. In: Proceedings of the 2005 ACM SIGCHI International Conference on Advances in Computer Entertainment Technology, pp. 184–187. ACM (June 2005)
5. Umaschi, M.: Soft toys with computer hearts: Building personal storytelling environments. In: CHI 1997 Extended Abstracts on Human Factors in Computing Systems: Looking to the Future, pp. 20–21. ACM (March 1997)
6. Umaschi, M.: Sage storytellers: Learning about identity, language and technology. In: Proceedings of the 1996 International Conference on Learning Sciences, pp. 526–531. International Society of the Learning Sciences (July 1996)
7. Bobick, A.F., Intille, S.S., Davis, J.W., Baird, F., Pinhanez, C.S., Campbell, L.W., ... Wilson, A.: The KidsRoom: A perceptually-based interactive and immersive story environment. Presence 8(4), 369–393 (1999)
8. Havasi, C., Speer, R., Alonso, J.: ConceptNet 3: a flexible, multilingual semantic network for common sense knowledge. In: Recent Advances in Natural Language Processing, pp. 27–29 (September 2007)

An Exploration of Figures and Text in Visual Narration: Visual Flow and Preference Factors

Chiwu Huang [1] and Miao-Hsien Chuang [2]

[1] Department of Industrial Design and Graduate Institute of Innovation & Design, National Taipei University of Technology, Taipei, Taiwan
chiwu@ntut.edu.tw

[2] Graduate Institute of Design, National Taipei University of Technology, Taipei, Taiwan
Department of Visual Communication Design, Ming Chi University of Technology, New Taipei City, Taiwan
joyceblog@gmail.com

Abstract. This study employed eye tracking and a questionnaire survey to investigate the relationship between plot-hinting advertisements and the image of characters in visual narration in order to identify the preferences of viewers. The results indicate the following. (1) Browsing time and two of the factors in our factor analysis (Recognition of Storyness and Imaginary Space) presented significant explanatory power in regression analysis. (2) Subjects without backgrounds in design spent more time viewing story-like advertisements than did subjects with a background in design. (3) The scanpaths showed alternating browsing patterns between the text and images in the story-like advertisement. The process of perceiving the face of the main character and the details of the image conformed to the tenets of constructivism. (4) Most subjects expressed praise for the plot-hinting and story-telling advertisement. The results of this study provide a valuable reference for the application of plot-hinting in advertisements and interactive interfaces.

Keywords: Visual narration, Eye tracking, Plot hinted text.

1 Introduction

Psychologists Heath & Heath (2008) claimed that for a piece of information to leave an impression, there are six qualities it may have: simple, unexpected, concrete, credible, emotional and story-like. Story-telling methods have been widely applied in many domains, such as television commercials, product marketing, and product design. This approach has also been employed in the design of print advertising. In the internet era, consumers are surrounded by a large number of images and many younger individuals are no longer used to reading text, unless the text is iconic or presented in a novel format. Text that is handwritten, doodled, documentary, plot-hinting, or character-introducing is more likely to be favored. Clearly, the relationship between images and text must be redefined.

C. Stephanidis (Ed.): Posters, Part II, HCII 2013, CCIS 374, pp. 541–545, 2013.

2 Objectives

Our objectives included the following: (1) examine the interactions between plot-hinting advertisements and the browsing behavior of viewers, (2) investigate the mutual relationship between browsing time and preference factors, (3) determine differences in the observation times between subjects with and without backgrounds in design, and (4) determine whether story-like advertisements and copies can stimulate interest and positive recognition.

Operational Definitions. Characters in visual narration: Images of characters with clearly presented facial expressions and body language in richly plot-hinting interfaces. Plot-hinting copy: Advertisement copy written or doodled or containing diaries or self-introductions rather than the advantages of products or other forms of promotion.

3 Literature Review

3.1 Eye Tracking

Visual Flow and the Center of Meaning. Visual scanpaths can reflect the process of attention shifting within observers. Treisman and Gelade (1980) compared the operation of visual attention to multiple packets that are continuously prepared by the visual system prior to the merging of information with its corresponding meaning manifesting in individual consciousness. When faced with a large amount of image and text information, individuals generally display more economical or preferential eye movements, according to their needs.

The Presentation of Text and Imagery and the Order of Detection. Finn (1988) claimed that images take priority over text. Of the time dedicated by viewers to observe print advertisements, the dominant illustration received focal attention, which was then followed by the headline and the copy. Experiments on explicit and implicit product presentation in advertisements have established that in terms of the latter type, viewers display more frequent saccades between images and text, spend more time on them, and exhibit more positive attitudes and greater interest (Radach, Vorstius, & Radach, 2001).

3.2 Interaction Requirements of Advertisements

Bendinger (1998) related that Ogilvy, often referred to as "The Father of Advertising", discarded the popular prototype of advertising in the 1960s and instead aspired to a unique story-like and individualized style described from the perspective of a particular individual. After the 1980s, storytelling became the mainstream form of visual presentation, in the hopes of inciting viewers through a comparison of experiences and active participation. With regard to the interaction between images and viewers, Kress and Leeuwen (2006) proposed two types of visual configuration: demand and offer. "Demand" enables viewers to create imaginary relationships from the gaze or physical movements of characters in the image, such as in the famous recruitment poster by Alfred Leete in 1914. In contrast, the image content associated with "offer" are merely regarded as data items or subjects of thought, such as in the 1953 Portrait of a Man by Jan van Eyck.

4 Methodology

The research methods employed in this study include eye tracking and a questionnaire survey. Using SPSS, we sought to determine whether differences existed among the subjects with different backgrounds in terms of browsing time and scanpaths. Furthermore, we examined whether a regression relationship exists between the two research methods.

4.1 Eye Tracking Method

Research Manipulation. Independent variable: advertisement copy; the sample for the experimental group was plot-hinting copy, whereas the sample for the control group was traditional copy. Dependent variable: total browsing time and scanpaths. Experimental control: identical images in the two samples and the two copies occupying similar amounts of area. Experiment samples: This study modified samples of an American Express credit card advertisement from the US magazine, Living. In Sample A (experimental group), the left half shows a touching scene of a mother and son in their daily life, while the right half presents self-introductory copy. The text in the copy indistinctly conveys the primary message of the advertisement—that the credit card is indispensable. In Sample B (control group), the image in the left half is the same as that in Sample A. In the right half is a traditional copy rewritten in Chinese by the author, introducing the various benefits that the main character has gained from accumulating points with her favorite credit card. Experimental equipment and participating subjects: This study employed Face Lab4 real-time face and fixation tracking device in conjunction with GazeTrail software analysis. The participants included 36 students in university and graduate school; 18 of the subjects had backgrounds related to design, while the remaining 18 subjects had backgrounds in other fields.

4.2 Questionnaire Survey

Objective and Subjects. Objectives: The objective of the questionnaire survey was to reveal the preferences of subjects in terms of visually narrative advertisements and enable comparisons with the results of the eye-tracking experiment. Subjects: In order for the factor analysis results to reach statistical reliability, we recruited 114 more participants in addition to the original 36 eye-tracking experiment subjects. Implementation process: We first explained to the subjects the differences between story-like advertisements (Sample A) and traditional advertisements. The subjects were then required to fill out the questionnaire based on their opinions of story-like advertisements. A seven-point Likert scale was employed in the questionnaire. Source of questionnaire items: The questionnaire items focused on two major factor characteristics of storyness in ads previously established by the author, the composition of the story-telling narrative and the emotional responses (Huang & Chuang, 2009).

5 Results and Discussion

5.1 Eye-Tracking Analysis

Browsing Time. To avoid the influence of memory, we adopted only browsing time data from the first sample viewed by the subjects. The browsing duration spent on the two samples was subjected to descriptive statistics. Viewing the mean values alone showed that subjects without a background in design spent more time than subjects with a background in design looking at the two samples. Furthermore, we discovered that the subjects spent more time browsing the story-like copy than browsing the traditional copy. Though the differences were not significant, the results corresponded to those of the pilot study.

Scanpaths. Sample A: The majority of the subjects first scanned the characters and background on the left before moving on to the text on the right and then returning to the characters and environment on the left. Sample B: The subjects displayed scanpaths similar to those of Sample A; however, they did not read the text as carefully as they did for Sample A. This may have been due to a lack of interest. Overall, the subjects presented zigzagging eye movements when viewing the two samples.

Alternating Browsing between Image and Text. Alternating browsing patterns between the image and text in Samples A and B were very obvious. The majority of the viewing moved from the left image to the right text before the subjects displayed back-and-forth sweeping between the two for comparisons. The looping patterns for Sample A were larger and more complex. This phenomenon corresponded to constructivist statements regarding the observation of images.

5.2 Factor Analysis and Regression Analysis

Factor Analysis. We first conducted item analysis and tests on internal consistency and reliability related to the 30 question items. After eliminating five items, we employed Varimax rotation for principal component analysis, the Bartlett test, and reliability analysis on the question items of each factor. Finally, we named the four factors Story Experience, Preferences and Expectations, Imaginary Space, and Link Between Product and Emotion. A single-sample t test was then performed to identify the mean preference of the subjects for the four factors. The mean score given by the subjects was significantly higher then 4 (no opinion), revealing that the story-like advertisement was praised by the subjects.

Regression Analysis. Regression analysis was performed on the sample browsing time and four factors to identify predictive variables in the time spent viewing the text on the right: Story Experience and Imaginary Space. For Story Experience, the standardized regression coefficient was negative, revealing that a stronger recognition of storyness led to shorter browsing time in the text on the right. This may mean that individuals who can understand the fun of the story need only a few glances rather than a long viewing time. In contrast, the standardized regression coefficient for imaginary space was positive, indicating that a stronger imaginary space was required a longer viewing period for text on the right. In other words, forming an imaginary space requires time.

6 Conclusions and Suggestions

This study investigated the relationships between story-like advertisements and their viewers in the context of postmodernism. We found that the browsing time displayed by the experimental group and two of the factors (Story Experience and Imaginary Space) presented significant explanatory power in the regression analysis: one positive and one negative. Subjects with different backgrounds exhibited slightly different browsing times when viewing different samples. The scanpaths presented alternating browsing patterns and the subjects generally praised the plot-hinting, story-like copy. The aim of this study was to derive more methods of story-telling, copy writing and layout in ads for a reference in the designs of print advertising and multimedia interfaces.

References

1. Bendinger, B.: The Copy Workshop Workbook. Wu-Nan Book, Taipei (1998); Zhang, P.J., Zhong, A.Z. (trans.): (Original work published 1993)
2. Finn, A.: Print Ad Recognition Readership Scores: An Information Processing Perspective. Journal of Marketing Research 25(2), 168–177 (1988)
3. Heath, C., Heath, D.: Made to Stick: Why some ideas take hold and others come unstuck. Arrow, London (2008)
4. Huang, C., Chuang, M.H.: The Analysis of Storyness in Visual Composition and Emotion Experience. In: Symposium Conducted at the Meeting of International Association of Societies of Design Research 2009, Seoul, Korea (2009)
5. Kress, G., Leeuwen, T.V.: Reading Images – The Grammar of Visual Design, 2nd edn. Routledge, New York (2006)
6. Radach, R., Vorstius, C., Radach, K., Heller, D.: Eye Movements in the processing of advertisements: effects of pragmatic complexity (2001), Abstract retrieved from: http://congress.utu.fi/ecem11/other_applied/radach.htm
7. Treisman, A., Gelade, G.: A feature-integration theory of attention. Cognitive Psycholgy 12(1), 97–136 (1980)

Computer-Based Character Creation in Storytelling: Prototyping and Testing of Random Character Creator

Ho Kyoung Im, YiKyung Kim, and Bong Gwan Jun

Graduate School of Culture Technology, KAIST, South Korea
imagine21c@hanmail.net, clarakkim@gmail.com,
bonggwan@kaist.ac.kr

Abstract. Since the concept of "Digital storytelling" was first introduced, concepts such as "digital platform for storytelling" as well as "storytelling for digital platform" have evolved. This study evaluates a computer-based story development tool, called Random Character Creator (RCC). Using this tool, the types of variables that can be considered while building a character in storytelling are set, and a database for each variable is established. Based on each variable and database, we developed a prototype of the RCC program, which allows the user to create a character sample with a combination of randomly/selectively chosen variables. Examples of results are evaluated.

Keywords: Digital storytelling, Screenwriting software, Digital storytelling software, Digital storytelling technology.

1 Overview

Most of the previously developed methods of providing creative support to story-authoring tools focused on simplifying the story-writing process. The authoring programs provide only a rudimentary support to the creation process itself. [1] This paper presents the development of a new computer-based story-writing tool, called the Random Character Creator (RCC), which helps the creator build characters for plays, screenplays, fiction, etc., in the field of storytelling.

2 Objectives of the Study

This study aims to develop a writing tool that supports character creation in the story-writing process. It breaks away from the traditional perspective that centered on maximizing the efficiency of the work processes and provides a new perspective of using a computer program for a useful and valuable work process. This new perspective will enable the creation of richer and more interesting characters for storytelling.
The objectives of this study are detailed as follows:

- Set the types of variables that can be considered to build a character in storytelling, and establish a database for each variable.

C. Stephanidis (Ed.): Posters, Part II, HCII 2013, CCIS 374, pp. 546–550, 2013.

- Based on each variable and database, construct a prototype of the RCC. program that allows the user to create a character sample with a combination of randomly/selectively chosen variables.
- Initiate the prototype and design a framework that can build up on the first character sample.

3 Method

3.1 Establishment and Classification of Variables for Character Creation

By referring to studies on factors influencing character creation by Adler [2], an American acting theorist, and Huh [3], we classified the variables to be used in the RCC. program as shown below Table 1.

Table 1. Classification of variables for character creation using a random module

Major variable	Dependent variable	Selective variable
(1) Occupation	(a) Social status	Age
	(b) Wealth	Gender
(2) Personality	(a) Animals that can be referred to for creating personality	Class location History
(3) Characteristic	(a) Disease	Periodical situation
(4) Motif [4][5][6]	(a) Action Verb	Place and background
	(b) Incident keyword	Habit, appearance

- Major variable: A variable that acts as the basic structure for character creation using the random module
- Dependent variable: A sub-variable that can be combined with other sub-variables according to the major variable
- Selective variable: A variable that can be used either as a major variable or a dependent variable depending on its genre or type; however, owing to the characteristics of this variable, the user can easily set this variable by observing the result of character creation

3.2 First Character Creation through Random Combination of Variables

When the user clicks the character creation button, random database values arbitrarily selected for the preset variables—occupation, personality, and motif—are combined to provide a result. Here, as many characters as the user has assigned are created. Among the first characters created, the user can choose the character where he or she wants to add variables or modify. Table 2 shows an example of the first character creation.

Table 2. Example of the first character creation

Random value	268 52 3 6 103	88 54 23 82 2	356 88 57 9 51	99 65 4 97 17	333 60 3 12 67
Occupation	Music producer	Animal trainer	Police	Carpenter	Paper-bag factory employee
Personality (Multiple selection)	Naive Arrogant Cowardly	Wicked Taciturn Think big	Good judgment Rough Messy	One-sided Old-fashioned Excellent	Narrow-minded Haughty Shy
Motif	Son	Family	Prostitution	Widow	disease
Random value	159 47 94 35 29	172 7 2 45 104	281 10 60 85 30	382 2 86 90 47	97 51 75 31 18
Occupation	Video shop staff	Ship maintenance Technician	High School Teacher	Computer programmer	Makeup Artist
Personality (Multiple selection)	Delicate Strong mind Frivolous	Straight Thoughtful Tough	Optimistic Petty Attentive	Easy-going Violent temper Poncey	Innocent Trustworthy Brazen
Motif	Miracle	Father	Dreams, Sea	Animals	Insanity

3.3 Second Character Creation through Selective Combination of Variables

After the creation of the first character discussed earlier, the user can move to the second character creation stage by qualitative selection or re-create the first character with more combination of variables. Once character selection is done for the second character creation, the user adds detail to the randomly built character through the below framework:

- Selective reproduction of chosen variables among the suggested variables
- Establishment of relationship between characters
- Connection with additional motifs for character and establishment of a plot
- Storytelling ideation using action verb variables and event keywords

3.4 Random Character Creator, RCC Prototype Result

In the prototype, three variables—occupation, personality, and motif—were selected. A total of 446 occupations [7], 136 personalities [8], and 160 motifs [4] were established in the database.

Using a computer program that generates a random value from a specified range, we generated a random value for each variable (range: 1 through the number of total variables). The character was then assigned attributes corresponding to the generated value, as shown in Table 3.

Table 3. Example of the prototype

	Total amount of variables	Randomly selected value	Substituting values with items (1st character creation)	Selective reproduction of selected variable (2nd character creation)
Occupation [7]	446	377	Computer programmer	Computer programmer (Random value 377) -> **Music producer (Random value 268)**
Personality [8]	136	52, 3, 6 (multiple selection)	Naive Arrogant Cowardly	Naive Arrogant Cowardly
Motif [4]	160	129	Cyborg	Cyborg (Random value 129) -> **Lost son (Random value 130)**

Through a qualitative variation in the combination of the final selection of variables, the user can obtain the character to be used in storytelling as well as the story line or the logline. This is illustrated in Examples 1 and 2 of Table 4.

Table 4. Example of results

[Example 1] 1st Character creation
Computer programmer, naive, arrogant, cowardly, cyborg ➔ *I know that the naive and cowardly computer programmer Lisa who seems arrogant is actually a cyborg.*
[Example 2] 2nd Character creation
Music producer, naive, arrogant, cowardly, lost son *Arrogant yet naïve and cowardly music producer Michael was visited by his son whom he has never seen before.*

4 Conclusion

Previous studies on story-writing tools acted on the writing mechanism of the scenario itself, so it was difficult to apply their findings efficiently to the qualitative aspects of the story and to actual creative work.

However, in this study, the prototype of the RCC program confirmed the possible number of selective combinations using previous random combinations. Thus, the benefits of the prototype for creating richer and more interesting characters for storytelling were also confirmed. This study has thereby prepared an index for future studies on the development of the story-writing tool with an interface that allows the user to choose between random combinations obtained computationally and selective combinations obtained manually.

References

1. Korea Creative Content Agency. Research trends and case studies, storytelling authoring tools. Culture technology reports (February 2012)
2. Adler, S., Kissel, H.: The art of acting. Applause Theatre & Cinema Books (2000)
3. Huh, Y.-H.: Acting and Actor training. Jipmoondang (2004)
4. Lee, S.J.: Das Anlegen von "Databases" zu Motiven der deutschen Literatur-Eine Studie zur Basis der "Storybank". Brecht and Contemporary Theater 20(Single Issues), 266–267 (2009)
5. Frenzel, E.: Motive der Weltliteratur, 5, überarbeitete und ergänzte Auflage. Kröner, Stuttgart (1999)
6. Daemmrich, H.S., Daemmrich, I.: Themen und Motive in der Literatur: ein Handbuch, Francke, vol. 8034 (1995)
7. Department of Labor, Job Classification Dictionary (1995)
8. Hampson, S.E., Goldberg, L.R., John, O.P.: Category-breadth and social-desirability values for 573 personality terms. European Journal of Personality 1(4), 241–258 (2006)

Genre Visualization Based on Words Used in Text

Hyoyoung Kim and Jin Wan Park

GSAIM, Chung-Ang University, Seoul, Rep. of Korea
the.kimyo@gmail.com, jinpark@cau.ac.kr

Abstract. Text visualization is one of sectors in data visualization. This study is on methods to visually represent text's contents, structure, and form aspects based on various analytic techniques about wide range of text data. In this study -as a text visualization study-, 1) a method to find out the characteristics of a book's genre using words in the text of the book was looked into, 2) elements of visualization of a book's genre based on verification through an experiment were drew, and 3) the ways to intuitionally and efficiently visualize this were explained. According to visualization suggested by this study, first, actual genre of a book can be understood based on words used in the book. Second, with which genre is closed to the book can be found out with one glance through images of visualization. Moreover, the characteristics of complicated genres included in a book can be understood. Furthermore, the level of closeness (similarity) of a genre -which is found to be a representative genre using the number of dots, curvature of a curve, and brightness in the image- can be assumed. Finally, the outcome of this study can be used for a variety of fields including book customizing service such as a book recommendation system that provides images of personal preference books or genres through application of books favored by individual customers.

Keywords: text visualization, data visualization, book genre visualization.

1 Introduction

Usually genres are defined by a librarian with a historical categorization method or by a publisher with market preferences. However, sometimes a book cannot be described as a single genre when it has multi-genres characteristics. This study suggests intuitive visualization technique that visualizes genre of a book based on the words used in it.

2 Method

We analyzed genre characteristics of each word in books and tried to substitute it with visual elements based on our algorithm which induces genre features. The process to represent genre uniqueness is designed as the following steps.

C. Stephanidis (Ed.): Posters, Part II, HCII 2013, CCIS 374, pp. 551–554, 2013.

a) Analyze as many books as possible to count the summed frequency of each word and to build an overall word-frequency dictionary (OWFD)-We processed four-thousand digital books-,

b) Select books that represent a specific genre and make a genre word-frequency dictionary (GWFD)-We chose 4 genres(Fantasy, Science Fiction, Philosophy, Classical Literature) based on our own discretion,

c) Compare the genre word-frequency dictionary (GWFD) with the overall word-frequency dictionary (OWFD) and find extraordinary words of more frequency in the genre word-frequency dictionary (GWFD), and with the selected extraordinary words make a genre-identity dictionary (GID).

To check the GIDs induced by the suggested process actually can reveal genre characteristics, we selected 7 books randomly from 4 genres and analyzed words used in those books. And we count 'Word Hit' which is the number of words correspond with the words in GIDs.

As we can see in Table 1, we found that the 'Word Hit' can judge genre of each book accurately. This method also successfully shows a mixed genre which cannot be defined as single conventional genre.

Table 1. Word-Hit

Book	Fantasy	Philosophy	S. F	Women's
Alice's Adventures in Wonderland	274**	188	108	229*
Solaris	127	374**	307*	243
Harry Potter (Book 3)	350**	128	120	208*
House Rules	86	145	115	270**
The Analysis of Mind	82	880**	355	467
Inquiry into the Nature	125	687**	288	600*
Little Women	190	267	153	525**

3 Visualization

For visualization, we chose each representative color for each genre randomly: Fantasy-orange/ Philosophy-purple/ S. F-blue/ Women's Fiction-yellow.

After that, we designed an algorithm to draw ellipses with color of each assigned genre when the words in any of 4 GIDs were found. The higher ranked words make the ellipses longer and brighter. And we used different curvature of Bazier curve to connect dots with same colors according to genre closeness. The words with a same color are connected to each other with Bezier curves to highlight the genre color. Also the genre with lower word-hit is hidden in a lower layer of whole image so that the genre color with highest word-hit can be stood out. And we applied more blur effect to the dots which have lower genre closeness to decrease visual sensitivity of them. In this way, the ellipses and curves which have the highest genre closeness can be stuck out. In the result, like Fig. 1, representative genre or complex genre elements which a book has can be identified at a look intuitionally.

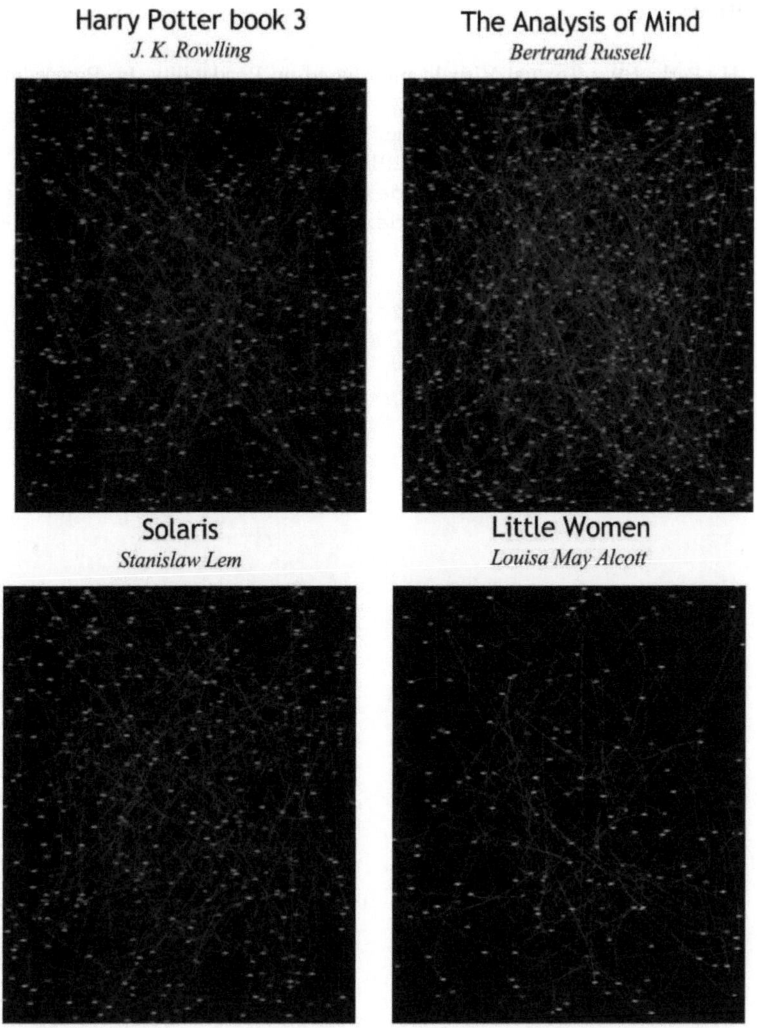

Fig. 1. Genre visualization images of Harry Potter(Book 3), The Analysis of Mind, Solaris, Little Women

4 Conclusions

The visualization technique suggested in the study visualizes books based on words used in books so that readers can grasp practical genre information or complex genre characteristics of books intuitionally. Furthermore, it can be used at book customizing (or book personalization) that helps a consumer look for books similar to their preferences.

References

1. Kim, H., Park, J.W.: Textual Visualization based on Readability. In: Proceeding of ACM SIGGRAPH Asia 2011 (2011)
2. Legan, T., Becker, L.: Visualizing the Text of Philip Pullman's Trilogy "His Dark Materials". In: Proceeding of NordiCHI 2010 (2010)
3. http://chrisharrison.net/index.php/Visualizations/BibleViz
4. http://itsbeenreal.co.uk/index.php?/wwwords/about-this-project

An Analysis of Composing Multiple Fictional Stories and Its Future Possibility

Mizuki Sakamoto and Tatsuo Nakajima

Department of Computer Science and Engineering
Waseda University
{mizuki,tatsuo}@dcl.cs.waseda.ac.jp

Abstract. There are currently many cases mixing existing multiple stories and their characters. A new special world is constructed by extending existing independent stories and a new mixed story in the special world provides audience vivid fresh experiences. However, if the mixed story loses the reality of the popular existing stories, it becomes unattractive to the audience. In this paper, we present a guideline when designing a good mixed story from multiple existing stories by analyzing a popular game title named *Super Smash Bros.*, which contains a mixed story derived from other popular games' stories. We believe that our guideline is useful when we design the services integrating various media presenting respective stories through the transmedia storytelling technique.

Keywords: Mixing multiple fictional stories, Reality, Transmedia storytelling, Game Design, Alternate Reality Game.

1 Introduction

There are currently many cases mixing existing multiple stories and its characters. Mixing multiple stories generates a new special world by extending the existing independent stories. Avengers[1] shown in 2012 as an American super hero film is one of typical examples of mixing multiple stories into one new story. The series of actions presented from multiple famous super heroes' stories increase the sense of thrills and excitements, and it provides a large amount of audience vivid fresh experiences. In addition, mixing stories can deliver audience the details of their ideological background messages. Transmedia storytelling [1] or Alternative Reality Game (ARG) [2, 7] is a promising approach to convey some ideological messages to people by using multiple channels and stories. In ARG, a fictional story is embedded into the real world game spread into multiple media to exploit a new story. It is possible to engage players' interests in the story because the original story is mixed with respective players' stories.

Once a player feels to favor a kind of game or other media, it affects his/her feeling and other activities in their real life in various situations. For example, if a player likes

[1] http://marvel.com/avengers_movie/

C. Stephanidis (Ed.): Posters, Part II, HCII 2013, CCIS 374, pp. 555–559, 2013.

a game, he/she may feel a sense of the closeness to a service including some contents related to the game. If he/she feels a sense of the game, it largely motivates him/her and becomes easier to affect his/her feeling or activities by using the service.

However, mixing existing stories is not an easy task, especially, if the original stories are well known. If the new mixed story loses the consistency with the original story, the reality of the original story is lost and its user decreases his/her interests on the new story. For example, a game named E.T. The Extra-Terrestrial[2] originated with E.T. which is a very popular American science fiction film, is one of famous failure examples. The goal of the game is finding parts of a communication device to send his help message to his colleague, and putting them together to let E.T. come back to his mother star. To find the parts, E.T. must fall into many pits. In [8], a player of the E.T.'s game says that "I've seen the movie, and I don't remember ET falling into one pit, much less 100!". This shows that there is no consistency between the original movie and the game produced later. It decreases the reality on the original story. Designing a service containing the reality is difficult, but a design guideline to mix several stories to maintain the original stories' reality is a powerful tool to increase the attractiveness of the service.

In this paper, we analyze a popular game named Super Smash Bros.[3], which includes a mixed story derived from other popular games' stories. Then, we present a guideline to which we should pay an attention when we mix multiple stories without losing their reality. Finally, we discuss about the future possibility of transmedia storytelling integrating with people's real experiential stories into existing stories.

2 Composing Multiple Stories

Super Smash Bros. series published by Nintendo is a battle-based action game, where four players can join the game at the same time. This series is a very popular game title in Japan, where three versions of the game as Super Smash Bros. series have put on sale and all of them have recorded million hit. Various famous Nintendo's characters such as Mario[4] from Super Mario Bros. and Pikachu from Pokémon[5] appear on the game, and a player can choose his/her favorite character and controls it to participate in the battle. Although each character has a different background story, it is natural that they battle with each other on the same stage in the world of Super Smash Bros., which let a lot of players enthusiastic in the world. It provides players not only the fun in the Super Smash Bros. world, but also the opportunity to notice other game titles mixed in Super Smash Bros. In fact, a lot of players of Super Smash Bros. become interested in other game titles which they have not been familiar with before.

[2] http://en.wikipedia.org/wiki/E.T._the_Extra-Terrestrial_%28video_game%29
[3] http://www.smashbros.com/en_us/index.html
[4] http://mario.nintendo.com/
[5] http://www.pokemon.com/

3 Analyzing the Reality of Composed Multiple Stories

We have observed several characteristics to mix multiple game stories in the game, Super Smash Bros. The important factors to realize a natural cross-story game are to maintain the reality on the original stories. We classified the reality into the following four patterns: Character's reality, World's reality, Goal's reality and Meta-concept's reality.

I. Character's reality: The features of a character in the original story

In Super Smash Bros., the existing features of each character are extremely clear and it is easy for players to notice them. Not only the character's visual and motion, but also the effect of the character's waza[6] should be reproduced. If each character's presence becomes weaker by coexisting with multiple characters, it loses the attractiveness of the existing game's fans.

II. World's reality: The background scene in the original story

The existing worlds where respective characters exist should be reproduced, too. There are some battle stages including gimmicks or items. For example, when a player who has played Pokémon plays Super Smash Bros., the stage related to Pokémon reminds him/her of some scenes in the Pokémon's story. It generates the nostalgic senses, which lead players to feel the experiential value. The scene of each stage plays a significant role as a metaphor to provide players the strong engagement.

III. Goal's reality: The goal of each character in the original story

In a game, each character has his/her own goal that needs to be also achieved by its player. When multiple stories in existing games are mixed, the goal of a character in the new mixed story should be consistent with his/her goal in the original game's story. The main theme of Super Smash Bros. is a battle among characters. Thus, all games mixed into the Super Smash Bros. story contain more or less battle factors. For example, Mario battles against his opponent within his adventure, and Pikachu helps his partner with the thunder power and fights against his opponent. Winning the battle is one of the important goals of these games. Thus, it is easy to maintain the consistency of the goal of a character in both Super Smash Bros. and the original story. The consistency of each character's goal both in a mixed story and the original story plays an important role to maintain the reality on the new game's mixed story.

IV. Meta-concept's reality: The plausible reason to gather the characters of he original stories in the new mixed story

There is an original story of Super Smash Bros. The story is that "Each character's figure in a toy box starts to move by magic." Usually, it is not natural for enthusiastic fans who like the existing games to look at many characters that have different backgrounds together in the same world of the mixed story's game. However, it is natural that many character's figures coexist in a toy box in our real world.

---

[6] A Japanese word that means "technique".

These realities work as a medium to reduce a sense of incongruity. If there are undesirable gaps between a player's impression in a fictional story's world and the impression in the real world, he/she might be upset about the gaps. On the other hand, a player tends to be persuaded by the story when he/she can feel the reality on the mixed story. Only mixing multiple stories inclines it to be chaos and vague the world of the mixed game, but as for Super Smash Bros., it presents the coherent reality in the various perspectives as described in this section.

4 Towards Transmedia Storytelling

A mixed story providing the well-defined reality leads audience to feel new additional values. We believe that our guideline would be a powerful tool to design services using existing stories based on transmedia storytelling, ARG, or character merchandising. Mixing multiple stories may raise subsidiary influences and offer a possibility to increase audiences' interests in other stories embedded into various media.

A fictional story can be combined with not only other fictional story but also audience's experiential daily stories, which contain more realistic factors. It is easy for us to memorize our own physical experiences in the real world. So, mixing fictional stories with the audience's story created from the real world activities helps to deliver the ideological messages in the fictional story. The message conveying the ideological value is important to motivate them intrinsically [3]. Integrating audience's story with the existing ideological story makes it possible to encourage them to increase their self-efficacy in the real world.

Mixing multiple stories as described in this paper will be essential in the near future when integrating a fictional story into the real world; it is unlikely that only using one story will attract most people because each user has a different personality [5]. In particular, each person has his/her own favorite stories according to his/her personality and past experiences. However, in this model, there is one serious problem in the real world that needs to be considered by everyone. Therefore, it will be important to mix multiple stories that each user likes. The discussions from Section 5 will be useful for achieving the composition of these stories.

5 Conclusion and Future Direction

This paper presents the guideline to which we should pay an attention when mixing multiple stories not for losing the reality of the original stories. Our approach offers a promising way to enhance their experiences by consistently integrating stories of multiple characters. In Japan, promoting consumer products with fictional animation stories is recently very common [6]. The collaboration of various attractive stories and its characters could make an extraordinary impact on our daily life. We believe that our guideline is useful when we design the services using transmedia storytelling because something in each story are embedded in different media can be integrated into one story through the transmedia storytelling.

References

1. Dena, C.: Transmedia Practice: Theorising the Practice of Expressing a Fictional World across Distinct Media and Environments. Dissertation Thesis, University Sydney (2009)
2. McGonigal, J.: Reality is Broken: Why Games Make Us Better and How They Can Change the World. Penguin Press (2011)
3. Sakamoto, M., Nakajima, T., Alexandrova, T.: Digital-Physical Hybrid Design: Harmonizing the Real World and the Virtual World. In: Proc. of the 7th International Conference and Workshop on the Design & Semantics of Form & Movement, DesForm 2012 (2012)
4. Sakamoto, M., Nakajima, T.: Augmenting Yu-Gi-Oh! Trading Card Game as Persuasive Transmedia Storytelling. In: Proc. of 15th International Conference on Human-Computer Interaction (2013)
5. Sakamoto, M., Alexandrova, T., Nakajima, T.: Analyzing the Effects of Virtualizing and Augmenting Trading Card Game based on the Player's Personality. In: Proc. of the Sixth International Conference on Advances in Computer-Human Interactions (2013)
6. Sakamoto, M., Nakajima, T., Akioka, S.: Promoting Consumer Products with Fictional Stories. In: Proc. of 15th International Conference on Human-Computer Interaction (2013)
7. Szulborski, D.: This is Not a Game: A Guide to Alternate Reality Gaming. Lulu.Com (2005)
8. Atari 2600 Reviews D-E by the Video Game Critic, http://videogamecritic.net/2600de.htm

Something Is Wrong with Us

Nicole Williams and Muharrem Yildirim

Media, Arts + Sciences / School of Arts, Media + Engineering
Arizona State University
{nmwilliams,myildirim}@asu.edu

Abstract. This paper describes the design and development of the interactive data visualization application *Something is Wrong with Us*. We discuss the experiential theory of Phenomenology as expressed through data aggregation and transmission. We analyze data visualization design as a process to express emotive data networks via sentiment analysis and what we term as "Density Effect." We conclude our analysis with a discussion on the value of emotive data visualization and discuss future developments of the application.

Keywords: Data visualization, wrongness, narrative, networks, experiential design, user interface design, sentiment analysis.

1 Introduction

"She's still not talking to me, what's wrong?"
- Anonymous blog post, 11/27/2011

"I feel like the wrong person will catch on to the fact that I'm living in my van and that could be dangerous."
- Anonymous blog post, 11/26/2011

"I feel like I'm actually on the wrong planet, and it's great when I'm in my garden but the minute I go out the gate I think: what the hell am I doing here?"
- Anonymous blog post, 11/26/2011

As we explore the existential concepts that mark the human experience, the question is not necessarily "what is the nature of our existence?" but rather, "who is asking the questions?" At the core of this inquiry resides the phenomenon known as *experience*, an innately personal process that colors our explorations of existential matters.

Throughout history, philosophers, social scientists, theorists, and artists have endeavored to define commonalities in the human experience, searching for communal and representational descriptions of subjective matters. This adherence to experiential categorizations is a distinguishing mark of the human condition. Our diverse experiences lead us to have certain presuppositions regarding how others will interpret our actions. These assumptions typically manifest themselves as binary roles: good vs. bad, right vs. wrong, etc. Examples of these comparative relationships are rampant

C. Stephanidis (Ed.): Posters, Part II, HCII 2013, CCIS 374, pp. 560–564, 2013.

within the World Wide Web. The internet is replete with users positing, asserting, decrying and pronouncing their beliefs under the scope of these binary relationships. *Something is Wrong with Us* is an application that explores this data, aggregating it based solely upon the concept of what internet users feel is "wrong." In approaching our analysis we chose to create an interactive data visualization to display a communal narrative of wrongness.

2 Visualizing Data

One method of gathering, analyzing, abstracting and displaying data is through Data Visualization. From the RSS news crawler of 10x10 [1] to the colorful nodes of websites as graphs [2] to the blue domes of the shape of a song [3], data visualizations communicate information through aesthetics and graphical compositions. They produce novel insights into current trends and global events, and they show how these data sets fluctuate over time.

But what of emotive data: the information pertaining to the subjectivity of the human experience? Emotions, beliefs, feelings and desires exist in some form or another all over the internet. How do we create graphical representations of these emotion-based datasets?

2.1 Sentiment Analysis

Sentiment analysis is one way to factor human experience into data abstraction. Not only does sentiment analysis give us a glimpse into the emotional status of the billions of end users on the web, it also prompts designers and programmers to craft novel methods for transmitting and displaying these emotive networks.

Past examples of sentiment analysis include the exploration of human emotions in Harris and Kamvar's *We Feel Fine* [4], the precarious nature of teenage love affairs in Golan Levin's *Dumpster* [5] and the search for love in the online dating scene in *I Want You To Want Me*, also by Harris and Kamvar [6]. These applications exemplify the process of expressing the subjective, ever-shifting nature of the human experience through computational analysis. *Something is Wrong with Us* follows in this tradition. It is a repository of experiential data, based solely upon the concept of wrongness. It is an interactive data visualization culling data from the blogosphere, data that is made of introspective thoughts, confessions declarations, and judgments. All of which are founded in the discussion and analysis of wrongness.

3 The Phenomenology of Wrongness

We define wrongness as a phenomenological experience. At its core reside the elements of randomness and deconstruction, each promoting the eradication of pre-conceived distinctions and borders. Wrongness occurs during the day-to-day operations of our lives, when suddenly an expected narrative (a habitual experience, an expected result, a belief system or a well-worn opinion) is disrupted, and subsequently altered. We encounter an object, person, or environment that unsettles us, attracting our full attention, and we consciously make note that the material (or data) associated with this experience is quite different from what we formerly supposed it should be. Wrongness sets the stage for that singular moment when we become fully engrossed in an experience because it does not compute with what we hold to be true.

These preconceived ideas or naturalized codes as Stuart Hall refers to them are "so widely distributed in a specific language community or culture, and learned at so early an age that they appear not to be constructed – the effect of an articulation between sign and referent – but to be 'naturally' given. [7]" These shifts from an a priori objectivity to an a posteriori wrongness range from the mildly amusing to the radically destructive. Whatever the efficacy of wrongness, one thing remains throughout; by introducing the unexpected into our lives, wrongness produces opportunities to re-evaluate our sense of self and to question those naturalized codes.

We define wrongness as phenomenological because wrongness is an experience; it is something that occurs in our consciousness. In his essay *Theoretical Foundations for Experiential Systems Design*, Mark Davis writes: "From phenomenology, we learn that experience is not a thing, but a process, and more particularly, a process that takes place in human minds/bodies. Therefore, experience itself is an inner psychic event which cannot be stored or transmitted, only the data we are reacting to and interacting with may be stored or transmitted. [8]" *Something is Wrong with Us* is a repository aggregating such data. It collects, analyses, and displays blog posts that reflect on the very materials that occasion the feeling of something being "wrong." These reflections entail introspective musings, provocative statements, humorous observations, and morality judgments. *Something is Wrong with Us* follows Davis' hypothesis that "we can only archive or transmit the materials (data) which occasion experiences in human minds, and every new interaction with these materials is itself a new experience. [9]"

4 Designing the Experience

Something is Wrong with Us is a data visualization of wrongness. From inception it was decided that the interface was to be minimalist, allowing the viewer to focus solely upon the data. As Davis states "choosing what data to record, when to record them, and from what point of view, and then choosing how to play back, sequence, visualize and interact with the data are all aesthetic choices [10]."

We chose to use the emotive database of the *We Feel Fine* API. It utilizes a sentiment analysis search engine, thus presenting us with a ready-made database of emotion from the blogosphere. We also chose to use smooth, natural animation as a navigational element in the form of vertical strings, or "tendrils," anchored to the base of the screen. These tendrils were animated (using Processing's *Perlin Noise* and Bezier curves) to move in a smooth continuous motion similar to a field of tall grass on a windy day. We chose to use this nonstandard navigation design to help create a visual clustering of wrongness. Each tendril represents a blog post, and when hovered over by mouse, its associated text renders onscreen.

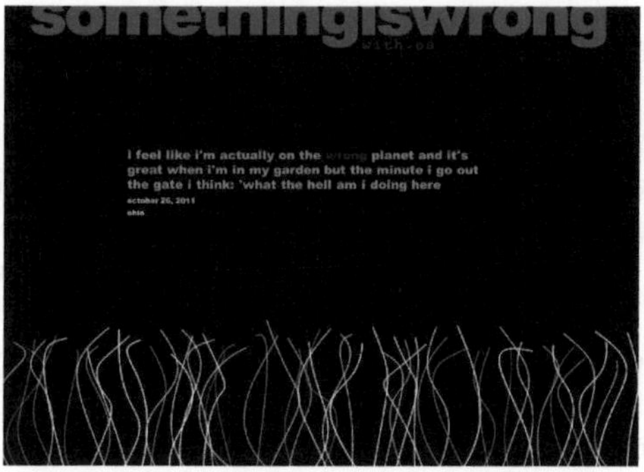

Fig. 1. Screenshot of the *Something is Wrong with Us* data visualization

4.1 Density Effect

What is unequivocally wrong to one person may be a minor infraction to another. We realized that the divergence in valuations of wrongness could lend themselves to interesting data visualizations. Thus we created what we term the *Density Effect.*

Traditionally, when visualizing relationships between data sets, designers connect nodes with linkages. The more lines the greater the amount of similarity. However, we chose to use a novel method to display the overall density of relationships. In *Something is Wrong with Us* tendrils glow with an intensity based upon their amount of similarity (a similarity that is determined by a word-by-word comparison of data.) As the user scrolls across the field of wrongness, the opacity of the tendrils fluctuate according to their similarities. The brighter the field the stronger the ties, the lighter the field the weaker the ties. This visual effect allows the user to quickly grasp the intensity of wrongness by the amount of glow in the tendrils.

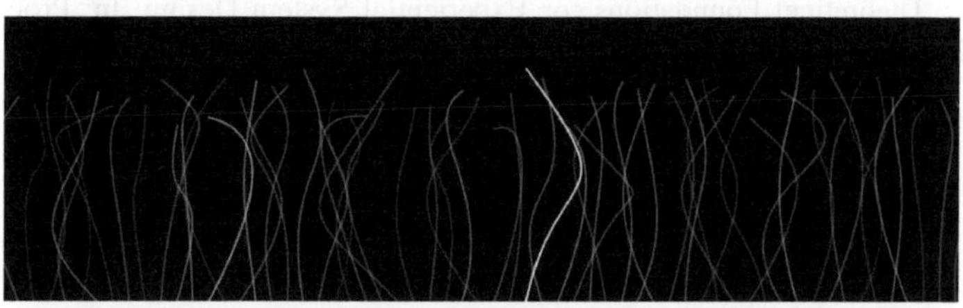

Fig. 2. A *low density* of relationships of wrongness

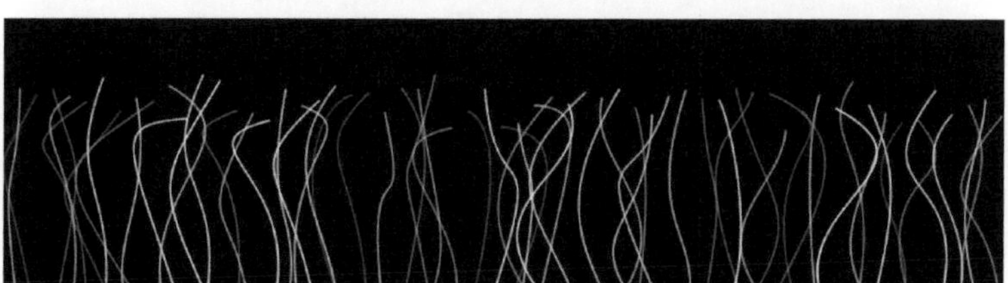

Fig. 3. A *high density* of relationships of wrongness

5 Future Work and Development

Future iterations of *Something is Wrong with Us* include expanding the data repository to include user input. Our goal is to create an interface that will allow users to post their thoughts and feelings of wrongness directly into the system. The database and interface will also be expanded to include imagery, video and audio. The tendril design will also be revised, aligning the height of the tendrils with the length of their corresponding blog posts. This will create a less constrained layout and also help to visually enhance the density effect.

Currently, the interface displays a maximum of 60 instances of wrongness. Future designs will include a browsable timeline, allowing users to sort through wrongness and view spikes and trends that may occur in tandem with global events. Cultural probes will also be designed to provoke dialogues about wrongness and to research how certain communities and cultures perceive wrongness.

References

1. Ten by Ten, `http://tenbyten.org`
2. Websites as Graphs, `http://www.aharef.info/static/htmlgraph/`
3. The Shape of Song, `http://www.turbulence.org/Works/song/index.html`
4. Harris, J., Kamvar, S.: We Feel Fine. In: Proc. WSDM 2011. ACM Press (2011)
5. Levin, G., Nigam, K., Feinberg, J.: The Dumpster (2005), `http://www.flong.com/projects/dumpster`
6. Harris, J., Kamvar, S.: I Want You to Want Me (2008), `http://iwantyoutowantme.org/`
7. Hall, S.: Encoding, Decoding. In: During, S. (ed.) The Cultural Studies Reader, pp. 507–532. Routledge Press, New York (1993)
8. Davis, M.: Theoretical Foundations for Experiential System Design. In: Proc. ETP 2003, pp. 45–52. ACM Press (2003)

Part IX
Agents, Avatars and Robots

An Investigation of Multimodal Metaphors in E-Book Assessment Interfaces

Dimitrios Rigas[1] and Amirah Algahtani[2]

[1] INSPIRE, University of West London, London W5 5RF, UK
Dimitrios.Rigas@uwl.ac.uk
[2] Faculty of Technology, De Montfort University, Leicester LE1 9BH, UK
Amirah@dmu.ac.uk

Abstract. This paper investigates the role of some multimodal metaphors in e-book assessment interfaces using avatar, images, visual text, and earcons in terms of efficiency, effectiveness and user satisfaction as well as learning performance. This experimental approach was evaluated using two different versions (one for a control group and another for the experimental group) of an e-book examination interface. The experiment was contacted by 30 users. The first version (VOEBT) that was based on text only to present the test questions and another version (VMEBT) that used avatars, images, text and earcons to present the same questions to users. The results of the experiment showed that the approach taken was effective to communicate additional supportive information for questions connected to the learning material and could indeed assist to enhance the usability of e-book assessment interfaces. It was observed that users taken less time to successfully complete tasks in a manner that facilitated ease of use and user enjoyment as well as making the interface more satisfactory. Furthermore, the use of images and avatars made the information communicated more memorable.

Keywords: avatar, e-learning, images, earcons, multimodal, virtual text e-book assessment.

1 Introduction

Nowadays, most of e-learning applications focus on the visual channel to communicate information in its interfaces. Multimodality is the natural method to human to communicate automatically using all diverse information and using dissimilar channels each day. Such as human can speak, write, listen and move at the same time [1 and 2]. However, other senses could be incorporated in a multimodal approach in order to communicate a larger volume of learning material either on their own or simultaneously. For example, combining graphics and diagrams with earcons has the potential to provide a richer user learning experience. This investigation therefore explores unique combinations of visual and auditory metaphors that are particularly applied in the communication of learning material. Research literature highlights the positive effects of images and avatar on the usability of interfaces in

C. Stephanidis (Ed.): Posters, Part II, HCII 2013, CCIS 374, pp. 567–571, 2013.

several domains including education." Some of these studies suggest that the use of multimodal metaphors such as speech sounds, non speech sound and avatar could improve the usability of computer interfaces in many different ways including e-learning application" [3, 4, 5 and 6]. However, more research is needed in order to the full capabilities and potential of multimodal metaphors in e-learning applications. The aim of this empirical study is to examine the impact of amalgamating and integrating different modalities using earcons, and avatars, images, visual text within an e-book assessment framework. This investigation was carried out by evaluating effectiveness, efficiency and user satisfaction of the multimodal designs introduced. Finally, a discussion of the obtained results and conclusion are provided.

1.1 Overall Aims and Methodology

The overall aim of this empirical study was to enhance the performance of e-book assessments as part of an e-learning system and to measure efficiency for learning tasks by measuring the time spent by users to perform the required task. This was achieved by measuring the effectiveness of the approach by counting the number of correctly completed learning tasks that in effect provide an indicator of the users' learning performance. User satisfaction and overall learning experience was also measured.

The methodology used for this research project comprised of a literature review and three experimental platforms. The data collection procedure was based on the experimental observations and questionnaires. The empirical measurements produced objective and subjective data. The objective data resulted from the observations and measurements such as effectiveness and efficiency. The subjective data were primarily user provided views and resulted from the questionnaires that were used to evaluate the user satisfaction and experience.

1.2 E-Learning

From an abstract point of view, e-learning could be defined as the learning material that can be offered, circulated, and accessed at anytime and anywhere by utilising electronic technology such as computers, networks and communications [7]. In (2007) e-learning uses new electronic media and gear and extends learning environment to personal computers and the internet. The growth has not yet ended and perhaps we will see cell phones and TV satellites as components of learning environment in the very close to future [9].

In addition scheduled delivery platforms such as video broadcasting, remote libraries, and virtual classrooms imitates real learning environments but with time and place limitations. This technology has been enhanced by the on-demand delivery platforms that facilitate anytime and anywhere learning in the forms of interactive training CD ROMs and web-based training. In comparison with the traditional learning, e-learning offers more flexible learning in terms of time and location that allows a better adaptation to individual needs [8].

There are several different views of definitions of e-learning one of these definitions in (2009) e-learning is a type of training or learning in which instructors and student interact at different times and different space gap and allowing learners to access training at their own pace and with methods that are convenient for them [2]. Another definition states that "e-Learning is defined by the programme itself as Learning facilitated and supported through the use of information and communications technologies (ICT)" [10].

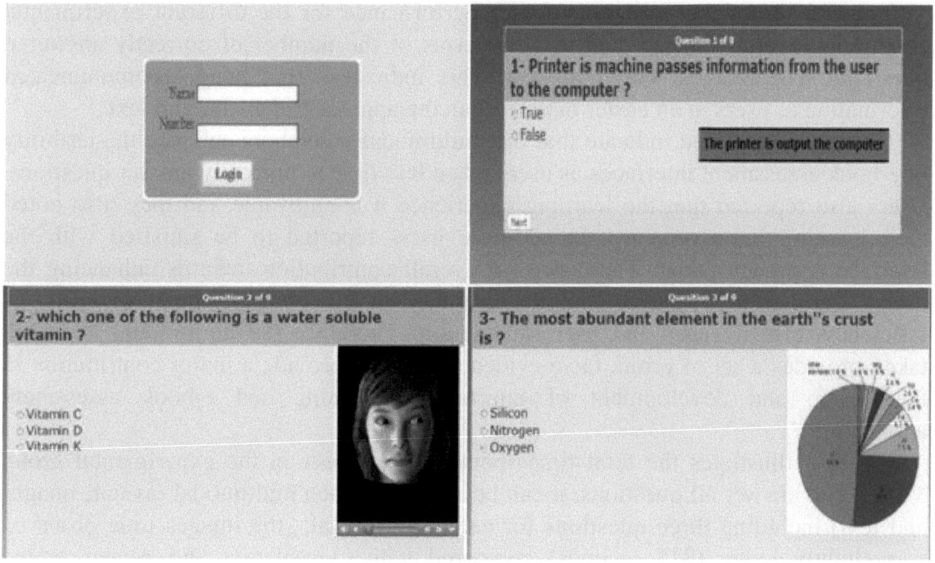

Fig. 1. Visual examples of the experimental platform of the e-book assessment

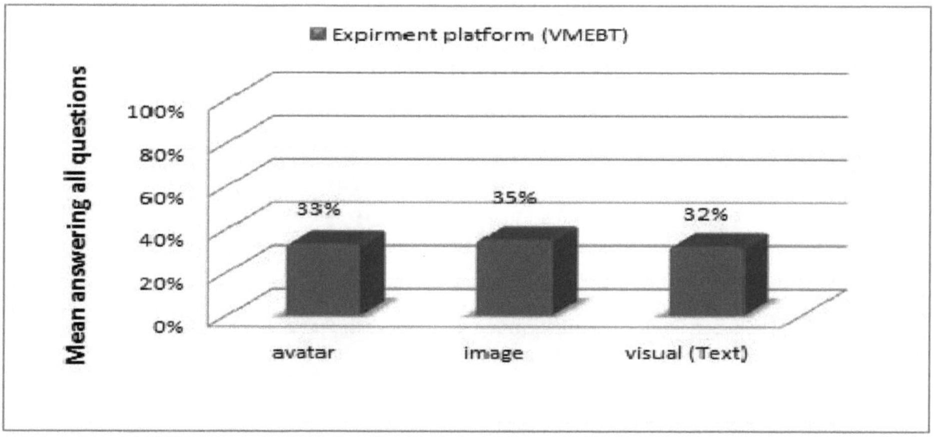

Fig. 2. Correct answers of all questions taken by users for each experimental condition

Two different versions of the experimental e-learning tool (see Figure 1) were tested by a group of 30 users for the first experimental work. The non-multimodal interface (VOEBT) is the text only version. It is the e-book assessment interface but with no multimodal communication metaphors. However, it provides the same functions in terms of examination and assessment, chapter order and level of questions. The second version used in the assessment interface introduces multimodal metaphors in terms of utilising avatar (sound and human-like expressions) with text, images and earcons as in a way that various parts of information are simultaneously presented to the users.

Figure 2 shows the variation of user performance for the different experimental conditions (avatar, images, and text) in terms of the number of correctly answered questions. The images scored highest. This indicates that images communicated information to users in an easier manner than the approach of avatar and text.

The results gathered indicate that the multimodal metaphors enhance the usability of e-book assessment interfaces as users taken less time to correctly answer questions. Users also reported that the learning experience was enjoyable and they also noted their learning improvement. In addition, users reported to be satisfied with the interface approach taken. There was an overall contribution towards enhancing the users' learning performance and the usability of e-book assessment in terms of efficiency, effectiveness and user satisfaction. Therefore the multimodal approach taken provides a set of prima facie evidence that can provide a major contribution in the design and development of interfaces e-learning and e-book assessment applications.

Figure 3 illustrates the total time spent via each user in the experimental group VMEBT to answer all questions, it can be shows for each multimodal (avatar, images and text) including three questions for each multimodal, the images time observed was slightly lower (815 seconds) compared with visual text and Avatar in the experimental group. The multimodal answering times were the avatar (966 seconds) and the difference between images and avatar were 151seconds.

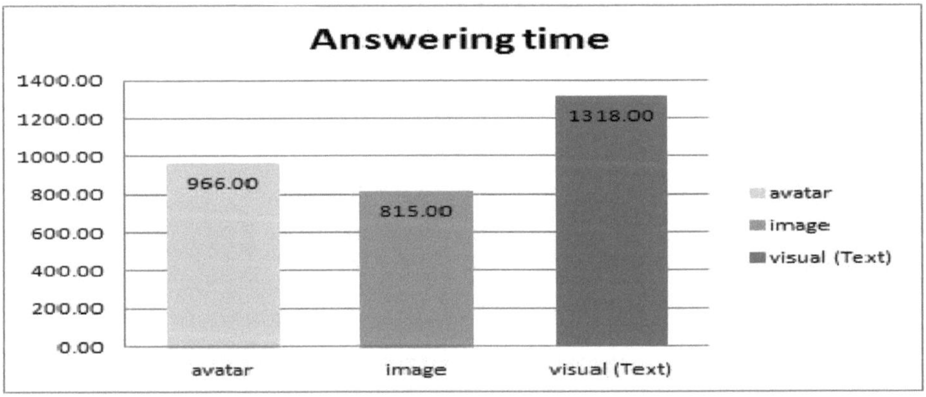

Fig. 3. Mean values of total time taken by users in multimodal to answer all questions

Finally, the textual approach was higher with 1318 seconds that were taken by users to answer and complete tasks among the conditions. In short, the images of the VMEBT were 815 seconds lower than textual and avatar approach in the VMEBT in terms of time taken by users to find the relevant information, answer the questions and complete their tasks.

2 Conclusion

This paper presented an overview of empirical experiments that aim to investigate the role of multimodal metaphors in interfaces for e-book assessment. This evaluation was focused on usability in terms of efficiency, effectiveness and user satisfaction. The obtained results showed that images and avatars are effective in communicating supportive information related to the presented learning material. Static images were also memorable by the users and provided an increased degree of user satisfaction.

References

1. Jokinen, K., Raike, A.: Multimodality– Technology, Visions and Demands for the Future. In: Proceedings of the 1st Nordic Symposium on Multimodal Interfaces (2003)
2. Baber, C., Mellor, B.: Using Critical Path Analysis to Model Multimodal Human-Computer Interaction. International Journal of Human-Computer Studies 54(4), 613–636 (2001)
3. Naidu, S.: Designing and Evaluating Instruction for e-Learning. Designing Instruction for Technology-Enhanced Learning (2002)
4. Clark, R., Mayer, R.: E-learning and the science of instruction: Proven guidelines for consumers and designers of multimedia learning. Pfeiffer & Co. (2007)
5. Rashid, S., Rigas, D.: A Proposed Approach for Investigating Note-Taking. In: Proceedings of the Sixth Informatics Workshop, Bradford, UK (2005)
6. Alseid, M., Rigas, D.: Utilising Multimodal Interaction Metaphors in e-learning Applications (2008)
7. Bleimann, U.: Atlantis University: a new pedagogical approach beyond e-learning. Campus-Wide Information Systems 21, 191–195 (2004)
8. Mikic, F., Anido, L.: Towards a Standard for Mobile E-Learning. In: International Conference on Systems and International Conference on Mobile Communications and Learning Technologies, International Conference on Networking ICN/ICONS/MCL 2006, pp. 217–222 (2006)
9. Ebner, K.: The impact of introducing e-learning. Grin verlag (2007); 3638701344, 9783638701341
10. Beetham, H.: Review: developing e-Learning Models for the JISC Practitioner
11. Communities, vol. 23 (retrieved January, 2004)

Estimation of User's State during a Dialog Turn with Sequential Multi-modal Features

Yuya Chiba[1], Masashi Ito[2], and Akinori Ito[1]

[1] Tohoku University,
Aoba 6-6-5, Aramaki, Aoba-ku, Sendai, Miyagi
yuya@spcom.ecei.tohoku.ac.jp
[2] Tohoku Institute of Technology,
Kasumicho 35-1, Yagiyama, Taihaku-ku, Sendai, Miyagi

Abstract. Spoken dialog system (SDS) is a typical speech application and sometimes regarded as one of ideal interfaces. However, most of conventional SDSs cannot help their user while waiting for input utterance since they treat a user's utterance as a trigger of processing. This architecture is largely different from the manner of human-human interaction and factor that makes the user feel inconvenience when they cannot respond to the system's prompt appropriately. To solve this problem, the system should be able to estimate the internal state of the user before observing the user's input utterance. In present paper, we proposed two-step discrimination method using multi-modal information to estimate the user's state frame by frame.

Keywords: spoken dialog system, user modeling, multi-modal information.

1 Introduction

Spoken dialog systems need to estimate the user's internal state in order to generate an appropriate response to the user. Many researches have been conducted so far [1-4], but they implicitly assume that the user always makes some response to the system's prompts. However, not all users can use the system proficiently. For instance, a user may abandon a session without uttering a word if he or she cannot understand the meaning of the system's prompt, or could take a long time to consider how to answer the prompt. We therefore considered that two internal states of a user who cannot make an utterance should be taken into account. The first one is the state where the user does not know what to input, and the second one is that where the user is considering how to answer the system's prompt. We call them state A and state B, respectively. We also assume state C, where the user has no problem answering the system. The purpose of this study is to discriminate these three states. Since the discrimination must be processed before the user's input, we denote them as the user's internal state "during a dialog turn." In our previous study [5], we made an attempt to distinguish these three states using an SVM and the features extracted from the whole video sequences. It worked well, but we cannot use the whole sequence as an input for the

C. Stephanidis (Ed.): Posters, Part II, HCII 2013, CCIS 374, pp. 572–576, 2013.

purpose to help the user who has difficulty to make an utterance. The present study proposes an automatic estimation method: we employed a two-step neural network to model the audio and visual information, and obtained the results of the estimation frame by frame.

2 Experimental Data

Experimental data were collected on the Wizard of Oz basis. The dialog experiments were conducted in a soundproof chamber. We implemented a question-and-answer task in which the system posed questions and the subjects answered them. The task was designed to make the user embarrassed as much as possible. The questions asked about common knowledge or a number memorized in advance. Additionally, an agent with a simple cartoon-like face was projected on the monitor to keep the subjects' attention. Figure 1 shows an experimental circumstance. We employed 16 subjects (14 males and 2 females). The subjects wore a lapel microphone. To record image of the subjects' frontal face, a CCD camera was installed above the monitor in front of the subjects. The operator remained outside of the chamber and controlled the agent remotely. The audio signal was recorded in PCM format at 16 kHz sampling, 16-bit quantization. The recorded video clips were stored as AVI files with 24-bit color depth, 30 frame/s. After the experiment, we separated the dialog into sessions; one session included one interchange of the system's prompt and the user's response. Here, we defined the length of the segment between the end of the system's prompt and the beginning of the user's input utterance as "latency". Sessions with more than 5.0 s latency were labeled by five evaluators. Table 1 shows the results of the evaluation. The label of each session was chosen by majority vote. The sessions shorter than 5.0 s were categorized as state C. One session was excluded because the acoustic feature could not be extracted due to overlapped utterances.

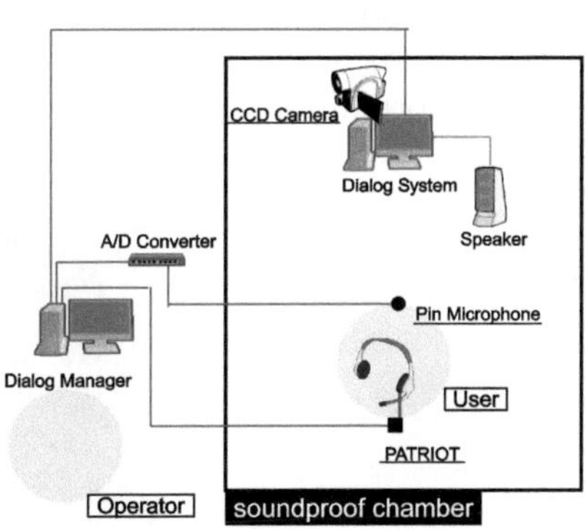

Fig. 1. Experimental circumstance

Table 1. Evaluation results

State A	State B	State C	Total
59	195	538	792

3 Discrimination Method

3.1 Hierarchical Discrimination

The system need incremental evaluation of the user's state to help just after detecting the user's embarrassment. Therefore, sequential features of the user are extracted and fed to the classifier frame by frame. The user's non-verbal behavior was recorded continuously during the dialog by the microphone and the CCD camera. Neural networks are used as the classifiers in the present paper. The front-end neural network outputs the scores of symbolic phenomena such as speech events or facial expressions. These outputs of the front-end network are used as the inputs of the back-end step. The back-end neural network outputs the definitive results, which are the scores of the states of the user.

3.2 Multi-modal Feature Selection

MFCC, fundamental frequency ($F0$) and zero cross ratio of the speech signal was employed as the low-level acoustic features. Here, MFCC contains their first and second derivatives and the total number of dimension was 39. $F0$ was calculated by cross-correlation method and first derivative was used for estimation. These audio features were extracted each 10.0 ms. The facial activity of the user is also important feature among the visual information. Therefore, feature points of the face were extracted by the method of Constraint Local Model (CLM) [6] and employed as the low-level visual feature. Figure 2 shows a model of feature points and Figure 3 is an example of the result of fitting. We used the relative coordinates of the feature points as the visual features. The number of feature points was 66 and the number of the dimensions of features was 132. The locations of feature points were normalized by the size of the facial region.

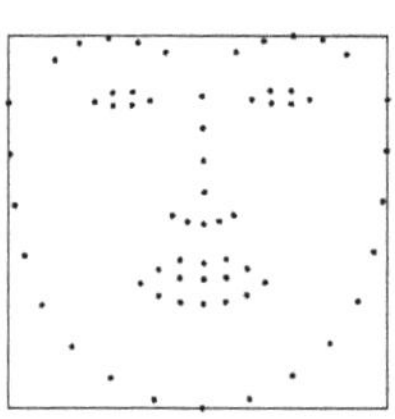

Fig. 2. Model of facial feature points

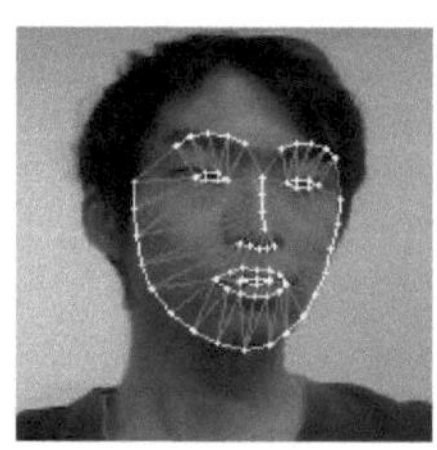

Fig. 3. Result of feature extraction

Table 2. Label of acoustic event

Acoustic events
System's prompt (AS)
Input utterance (AI)
Filler utterance (AF)
User's Aspiration or breath (AB)
Self speaking of the user (ASE)
Whisper of the user (AW)
Soundless segment (ASI)

Table 3. Label of visual events

Direction	Expression
Look on the system (DON)	Neutral (EN)
	Smile (ES)
Look out the system (DOF)	Odd face (EO)
	Wry face (EW)

Table 4. Discrimination results(%)

State A	State B	Harm.	Total
52.5	65.1	58.2	62.2

Some symbolic labels were defined as an intermediate feature of the hierarchical discrimination. Both the acoustic and the visual events were labeled manually according to the occasion of the event. These labels were used as the supervisory signal for training the front-end neural network. Tables 2 and 3 show the labels of the acoustic and the visual events. In addition to the single-frame score, the temporal dynamics of the scores are also important for estimation of user's state. Therefore, we incorporated the first derivative of the scores into the feature set. The total number of dimensions of the intermediate features including differential coefficients was 26.

4 Experiment

4.1 Experimental Conditions

All neural networks were three-layer networks having input, hidden and output layers including the bias unit. We employed a softmax activation function at the output layer in order to obtain the outputs as the probability of the above-mentioned class. The activation function of the hidden layer was a logistic sigmoid function and the number of hidden units were determined by preliminary experiments. All experiments were conducted based on 5-fold cross validation. Here, we examined two-class discrimination because state C and the rest (i.e. state A and B) were separated clearly by latency.

4.2 Discrimination Results

The definitive results should be decided considering the time variation of the outputs since the scores of the user's state change frame by frame. In this paper, we decided the definitive class $\hat{c}$ as follows:

$$\hat{c} = \arg\max_{c}(\max_{1 \leq t \leq T}(p_{tc})) \quad (1)$$

where, T is the length of the segment for which the state is estimated and currently set to equal to the duration of each session. Here, the total accuracy tends to increase as the determined class leans toward state B because the amount of data is not uniformly distributed (see Table 1), therefore harmonic mean (denoted as Harm.) were employed for measuring the performance. Table 4 shows the definitive result when the best harmonic mean was obtained; the total accuracy was 62.2%. Some of the results of the back-end classifier were closed to our intention. For example, the score of state B tends to be high in the filler or self speech segments, and the score of state A tends to rise when the user moves his/her head in a short period. However, the performance is not enough to apply our method to actual dialog systems. One problem of the present method is the lack of an important feature for the estimation. The results of previous human evaluations have shown that gaze action is efficient for recognizing the state of the dialog partner. Additionally, we need to consider how to model the temporal structure of the user's behavior.

5 Conclusion

We investigated a method to estimate the user's internal state frame by frame during a dialog turn. Sequential features including MFCC, $\Delta F0$, zero cross ratio of speech and facial feature points were extracted continuously, and were used for the estimation. From the results of two-step discrimination, we obtained about 62% accuracy of the definitive results. However, it is necessary to improve the performance of the classification in order to apply the method to actual systems. To enhance the accuracy of the results, we will make two improvements: employ a feature representing eye movement and examine the model for modeling sequential data.

References

1. Forbes-Riley, K., Litman, D.: Benefits and challenges of real-time uncertainty detection and adaptation in a spoken dialogue computer tutor. Speech Communication 53(9), 1115–1136 (2011)
2. Schuller, B., Müller, R., Eyben, F., Gast, J., Hörnler, B., Wöllmer, M., Rigoll, G., Höthker, A., Konos, H.: Being bored? Recognising natural interest by extensive audiovisual integration for real-life application. Image and Vision Computing 27, 1760–1774 (2009)
3. Morrison, D., Wang, R., Silva, L.C.D.: Ensemble methods for spoken emotion recognition in call-centres. Speech Communication 49, 98–112 (2007)
4. Devillers, L., Vidrascu, L.: Real-life emotions detection with lexical and paralinguistic cues on human-human call center dialogs. In: Proc. INTERSPEECH, pp. 801–804 (2006)
5. Chiba, Y., Ito, M., Ito, A.: Estimation of User's Internal State before the User's First Utterance Using Acoustic Features and Face Orientation. In: Proc. HSI (2012)
6. Saragih, J., Lucey, S., Cohn, J.F.: Deformable model fitting by regularized landmark mean-shift. Int. J. Computer Vision 91, 200–215 (2011)

Your Own Facial Parameter Generation for a 3D Avatar Interface Using an MRI Medical Image

Hiroshi Dohi, Hitoshi Iba, and Mitsuru Ishizuka

Dept. Information and Communication Engineering,
School of Information Science and Technology, University of Tokyo, Japan
dohi@mi.ci.i.u-tokyo.ac.jp

Abstract. This paper describes empirical study to make your own facial model for a 3D avatar interface using an MRI medical image. Our idea is that we make use of the MRI medical image as the reference face, then decide more than 50 morphing parameter values automatically to design your original avatar face that resembles a real person. MRI data is also useful for 3D human face/body modeling, although it has been used for medical diagnosis only as a general rule.

1 Introduction

In a 3D avatar interface, a user controls his/her own avatar, and communicates with other avatars (users) in common 3D virtual world. This is same as our communication style in our daily life. We can use arbitrary types of characters as the avatar. e.g., a realistic human, an animation hero/heroine, an animal, a robot, a monster, and so on.

In our real life, "identity" has an important meaning. The human has superior discrimination capability for human faces. The realistic face, of course, is not necessarily critical for avatar communication. However, especially in business field, it is very important that others remember your name and your face.

It is often difficult to make your own avatar face that resembles a real person.

3D shape modeling. It generally requires both artistic sense and computer graphics skills for creating the fascinating avatar.

facial control mechanisms. In addition to the accurate shape modeling, we need to apply some facial control mechanisms such as various facial expressions, lip synchronization, and blinking eyes.

3D avatars working over network connection. There are some constraints in order to decrease network load and network delays.

As the 3D avatar interface platform, we adopt the OpenSimulator (OpenSim) server[2]. OpenSim is an open source multi-user 3D application server[5]. It can be used to simulate virtual 3D environments similar to the SecondLife[6].

In order to generate a realistic 3D avatar face, it is a simple way to move each vertex and fit the facial model to the shape of the actual face. For example, Morishima[4] developed a superior 3D avatar with the realistic face. A generic face model is manually adjusted to captured images.

C. Stephanidis (Ed.): Posters, Part II, HCII 2013, CCIS 374, pp. 577–581, 2013.

On the other hand, OpenSim defines not only the facial control but also the shape of the face using the combination of more than 50 morphing parameters. It isn't allowed to move any vertices of the facial model directly. Therefore, we need to encode vertex position information to morphing parameters.

In our previous paper[3], we have proposed the automatic 3D facial fitting technique for 3D avatar on OpenSim using a well-sculpted voxel image. In this paper, we have applied the technique above to true MRI medical images.

2 3D Avatar Face Modeling on OpenSim

The OpenSim server delivers information for the 3D virtual environment to all clients over network connection. In order to reduce transmission data, the server sends morphing parameters instead of vertices position data. Each client (viewer) has the common 3-D wire frame base model of the avatar face in local storage, and then calculates the shape with facial control using received parameters.

- There are more than 50 morphing parameters for facial shape deformation. The parameter range is usually "0 to 100" (or "-50 to +50") and it is restricted to be integer values.
- One parameter moves a group of vertices. Each vertex moves independently to different directions with different speeds in 3-D space.
- One vertex may belong to many morphing groups. That is, more than 40 parameters may have relation to the position of one vertex.

The new position $\boldsymbol{V_n}$ of the vertex n is determined by following equations.

$$\boldsymbol{V_n} = f(\boldsymbol{v_n}, p_1, \ldots, p_m) \quad (1)$$

$$= \boldsymbol{v_n} + \sum_{i=1}^{m} w_i(p_i) \cdot \boldsymbol{d_{i,n}} \quad (2)$$

$\boldsymbol{v_n}$ is the base position of the vertex n. p_m is a parameter value of morphing m, and it is restricted to be integer values. $\boldsymbol{d_{m,n}}$ is a morphing unit vector for vertex n on morphing m. $w_m(p_m)$ returns the weight (coefficient) of each vector.

Our problem is to get a set of parameter values $(p_0, p_1, \ldots p_m)$ that achieve the lowest errors below.

$$Errors = \sum_{j=1}^{n} |V_{j}.\mathrm{Y} - D(V_{j}.\mathrm{X}, V_{j}.\mathrm{Z})|$$

$D(x, z)$ is depth information of the reference face (MRI data).

In order to decide the set of parameters, we adopted a simple hill-climbing algorithm.

1. Choose one of morphing parameters p in random order.
2. Change the parameter value from 0 to 100, and calculate each error value.
3. If error value is lower, update the parameter value.
4. Iterate above steps until all parameters are not changed.

3 MRI Medical Image

We make use of MRI medical image in order to get accurate shape data of actual human face as the reference target.

MRI (Magnetic Resonance Imaging) is a medical imaging technique to visualize an internal human body. It doesn't use ionizing radiation unlike X-rays technique, and it is non-invasive measure method. Hence it becomes rapidly popular for health care as well as medical diagnosis,

MRI can get high-resolution voxel images. It doesn't have the occlusion problem, nor blind spots. We can get the accurate head/facial shape, regardless of the hairstyles and the hair color.

Traditional scanning devices, e.g., stereo cameras and a range finder, are suitable for getting depth information from one viewpoint. But side surfaces of the target object are not clear. It isn't easy to merge depth information from multi viewpoints. Also, these devices are easily influenced by lighting condition and diffused reflection of the target surface.

We think that MRI data is stable and is also useful for 3D avatar modeling. It is true that the MRI system is a special device dedicated for medical use and is very expensive. However we can reuse MRI data captured for medical / health care. So far, MRI data is used for medical diagnosis only as a general rule, and has been usually discarded without being reused for any other purposes.

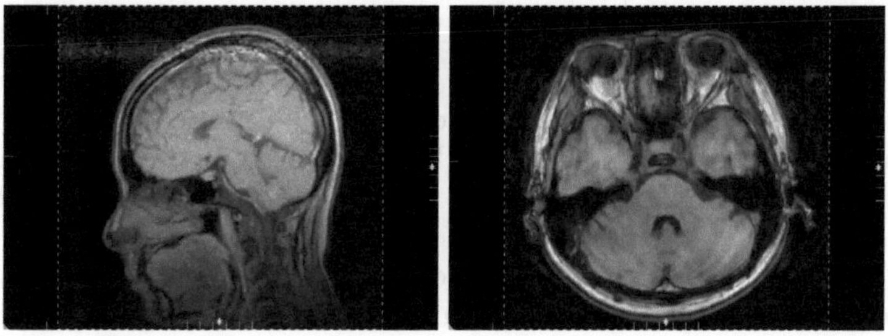

Fig. 1. MRI scanned image (left: sagittal plane, right: axial plane.)

Figure 1 shows an example of our MRI scanned image. The left is in sagittal plane, and the right is in axial plane.

The resolution is 256 x 256 [pixels] and its pitch is 0.75 x 0.75 [mm]. We captured 120 slices (images) in axial plane with 2.0 mm spacing from the top of the head to the neck (240 mm). Due to the limitation of our MRI system, it isn't an isotropic voxel data.

Our MRI system uses modest magnetic field (0.2 tesla), then it takes about 20 min in this scanning. However, its operation is automatic. Scanning-time depends on its resolution and the number of slices. It can capture high-resolution images in a short time by using strong magnetic field. A 3-T (3.0 tesla) MRI system is widely available for medical use.

4 Evaluation

Weak noise is observed on both sides of the head in Fig.1, but it is clear in front of the face. Hair may affect the image. Therefore we can cut out the head region using the bounding box and simple threshold level.

Figure 2 shows an example of fitting results. White area is good fitting. Red area (e.g., upper right) has plus errors (convex), and blue area (e.g., top and left) has minus errors (concave). In black area (jaw), MRI data is missing since these MRI images are captured for brain diagnosis. Gray area is not evaluated.

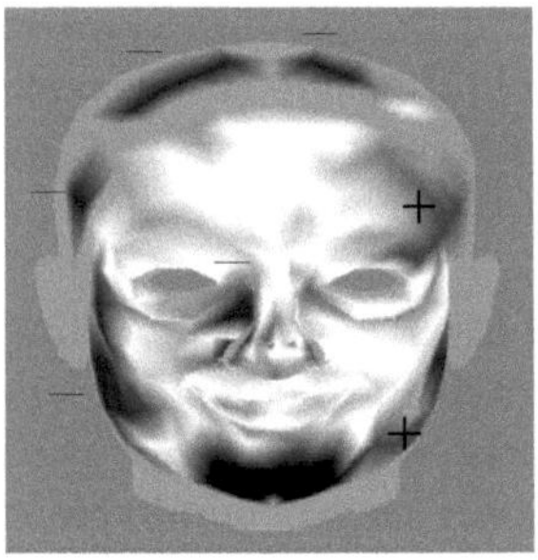

Fig. 2. fitting result

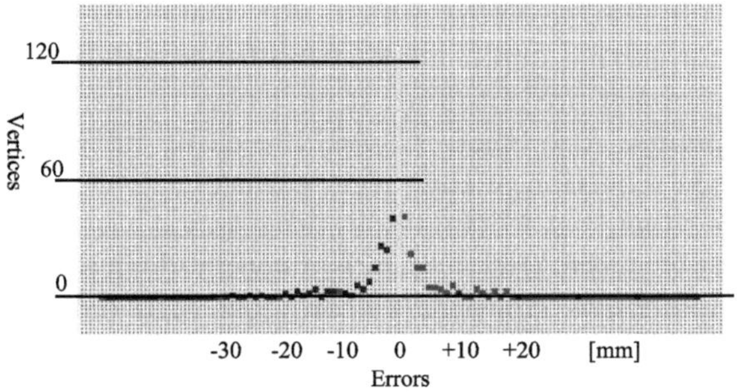

Fig. 3. histogram

In our preliminary experiments[3], we used well-sculpted voxel data[1]. The resolution is 2 x 2 x 2 [mm]. And we have achieved that more than 50 % of vertices are just on the reference target voxels, and more than 85 % of vertices are fitted within $\pm$ 2 mm of errors.

In this experiments, we have applied to actual MRI data. It includes noise and a part of data is missing. The fitting result is modest yet (Fig.3), and there may be still a room for improvement. There are many local minimums (candidates for fitting).

MRI facial data may slightly rotate about the center axis of the face. Although it is well known that real human face isn't symmetry, most of morphing parameters affect equally both sides of the face on OpenSim.

Figure 4 shows the MRI image as the reference face (left) and the generated 3D avatar (right).

The top of the head looks too flat. It is because parameter ranges are restricted. The initial scale of the facial model may also affect fitting results. However it isn't a serious problem since the avatar usually wears another hairstyle object on the head.

The morphing parameter can control the shape of ears, however the position of ears are fixed.

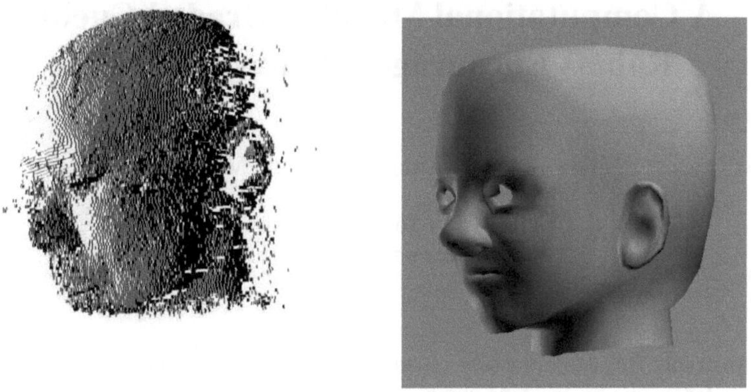

Fig. 4. MRI image (left) and generated 3D avatar face (right)

5 Conclusion

In this paper, we have described empirical study of our own facial parameter generation for 3D avatar face using an MRI medical image. MRI is an interesting technique to visualize the internal human body. We can get accurate voxel images that differ from pervasive camera image. MRI data is very useful for the computer graphics field, includes 3D avatar modeling. However, it has been used for medical diagnosis only, and usually discarded. We hope we can get our own raw MRI data easily.

References

1. Nagaoka, T., Watanabe, S., Sakurai, K., Kunieda, E., Watanabe, S., Taki, M., Yamanaka, Y.: Development of Realistic High-Resolution Whole-Body Voxel Models of Japanese Adult Male and Female of Average Height and Weight, and Application of Models to Radio-Frequency Electromagnetic-Field Dosimetry. Physics in Medicine and Biology 49, 1–15 (2004)
2. Dohi, H., Ishizuka, M.: An Interactive Presentation System in a 3D Virtual World using an OpenSimulator Server. In: Proc. Image Electronics and Visual Computing Workshop 2010 (IEVC 2010), vol. 3A-1 (2010)
3. Dohi, H., Ishizuka, M.: Automatic 3-D Facial Fitting Technique for a Second Life Avatar. In: Shumaker, R. (ed.) Virtual and Mixed Reality, Part II, HCII 2011. LNCS, vol. 6774, pp. 227–236. Springer, Heidelberg (2011)
4. Morishima, S.: Face Analysis and Synthesis – For Duplication Expression and Impression. IEEE Signal Processing Magazine, 26–34 (May 2001)
5. OpenSimulator (OpenSim) official site, `http://opensimulator.org/`
6. SecondLife official site, `http://secondlife.com/`

A Computational Model of Graded Cueing: Robots Encouraging Behavior Change

Jillian Greczek, Amin Atrash, and Maja Matarić

University of Southern California, USA
{greczek,atrash,mataric}@usc.edu

Abstract. This work presents a model of the occupational therapy technique of *graded cueing* for teaching and practicing desirable health and social behaviors adapted for use in socially assistive human-machine interaction. Graded cueing is represented as a probabilistic model of first prompt choice based on the perceived user ability level. The model is used to increase imitation proficiency of children with autism spectrum disorders through a "Copy Cat" imitation game.

1 Introduction

Socially assistive robots have the potential to augment therapy and rehabilitation by providing personalized care at any time and for as long as is needed. Studies are beginning to show how robots can invoke behavior change in humans over long-term interactions (e.g., [9]). In this work, we model the occupational therapy technique of *graded cueing* to provide a general framework for teaching and practicing desirable health and social behaviors over many human-machine interactions. The potential benefit of our approach to long-term interaction is the ability to adapt to and affect the user's behavior over time.

Graded cueing is a process of behavior shaping that uses increasingly specific cues, or prompts, to help improve people's skills at everyday tasks during recuperative therapy [2]. It is used in treatments for individuals who have lost skills, such as through a brain injury, or need to learn new skills, such as social skills of individuals with autism spectrum disorders (ASD). In graded cueing, the therapist asks the patient to perform a task, then prompts the patient with increasing specificity based on how much the patient struggles with the task. The goal is to increase both patient task performance and autonomy in performing the task, through minimal therapist intervention.

Our graded cueing framework is instantiated in a "Copy Cat" imitation game played between a NAO robot and a child with ASD. Our work is motivated by the evidence that children with ASD are often behind in their development of imitative behavior [11], and that practicing through repeated interactions with a therapist can improve imitation abilities [13]. Our model approximates those effect with a socially assistive robot in order to use technology to broaden access to ASD therapy.

C. Stephanidis (Ed.): Posters, Part II, HCII 2013, CCIS 374, pp. 582–586, 2013.

2 Related Work

Our approach uses a probabilistic graphical model of graded cueing capable of adapting a socially assistive robot's behavior along with the changes of the user's performance over time. Probabilistic graphical models have been shown to be effective tools for representation in human-centric domains such as assistive technologies [7], including nurse robots [15] and autonomous wheelchairs [14]. Research has also addressed learning of parameters over these models through human interaction [15, 1, 10], allowing for their use in human-robot interaction (HRI) domains.

Robots are good candidates for ASD therapy because of their apparent appeal to some children with ASD, and their ability to provide predictable, concrete feedback. Larson found that children with ASD prefer concrete feedback such as lights, colors, and sounds, which can be measured and quantified [12]. Ingersoll reported that multimodal feedback is more effective than any single feedback alone [8]. Thus, the NAO robot in our study uses lights, colors, and sounds as feedback modalities to indicate to the children how well they are imitating. The NAO has previously been used in a study where a child with ASD imitates a robot, but the focus was modeling human motion rather than affecting child imitation behavior [6]. Although our initial study utilizes the NAO for interaction with the children, the framework is not dependent on a specific platform or user population.

Various robots have previously been used to shape child behavior [16, 3, 5]. Robins et al. [16] found that four children with ASD imitated a doll-like robotic toy, often without any initial prompting; they attributed this to the robot's "simpler" physical appearance. Duquette et al. [3] found that a humanoid robot elicited more shared attention between two children with ASD than a human mediator. Ferrari et al. [5] presented the IROMEC robot as a social mediator in interactive play between a child with ASD and a parent, teacher or therapist. Our work extends previous work by Feil-Seifer and Matarić, which introduced the use of graded cueing applied to socially assistive robots interacting with children with ASD [4]. There, graded cueing was implemented as a finite state machine in the context of a Simon Says imitation game of arm postures.

3 Methods

Tasks amenable to graded cueing are characterized by their ability to be broken down into discrete steps. The simplest tasks consist of a single step, while more complex tasks may require a long series of steps. For each step of the task, there is a series of increasingly specific prompts that provide the therapy patient assistance with that particular step. The prompts are meant to be tailored to the patient's specific abilities in the given task, so that the process is neither frustrating nor patronizing. In computational terms, the therapist seeks to minimize the number and specificity of prompts while maximizing patient progress.

The Model. This work aims to contribute a general framework for graded cueing, based on a probabilistic model of prompt choice. The model consists of N states, one for each level of the user's task ability. Higher levels of ability are associated with increased prompt specificity. For example, specificity level 4 would be the best action for ability level 4. An N+1 state (P0) represents the success state. The goal of our model is to select the *first* prompt to give to the user depending on the user's ability level. From that initial prompt, any subsequent prompt required is the next most specific prompt. An example of this model for four levels of prompt specificity in shown in Figure 2. During execution, the robot uses the child's responses to maintain a distribution over the ability level, and then to select appropriate actions based on a policy calculated over the model. To compensate for few available data points that are typical of HRI contexts, the probabilistic model must be able to adapt quickly to the changing user state. To achieve this rapid adaptation, we use a Bayesian approach, wherein the model maintains a distribution over the states, updates based on the responses, and selects actions by sampling from the distribution.

The Application. The above-described probabilistic representation of graded cueing is implemented in a "Copy Cat" imitation game played between a NAO robot and a child with ASD. In the game, the robot poses its arms and asks the child to copy its pose. If the child successfully copies the robot's pose, the robot gives positive verbal feedback, nods, and flashes its eyes green. If the child does not successfully copy the robot's pose, the robot gives a starting prompt as determined by the model. During the first interaction, the starting prompt specificity is P1, but for each subsequent round of interactions over the entire study, the starting prompt is determined by the model. From there, if the child requires further prompting, the robot moves up within four levels of prompt specificity in this particular implementation, corresponding to the following five states:

P0. no prompts are given (success)
P1. words ("Are you sure?")
P2. words + gesture ("Look again at your left arm." + arm movement)
P3. specific words + gesture ("Bend your right arm." + arm movement)
P4. specific words + specific gesture ("You look like this." + imitation of child)

Fig. 1. The five states that dictate the actions of the robot based on the perceived imitation ability of the child. The verbal prompts were designed by an ASD therapist.

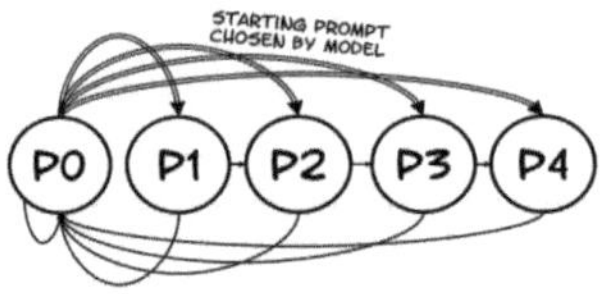

Fig. 2. The graded cueing implementation of the model. The double lines represent the starting prompt chosen by the model.

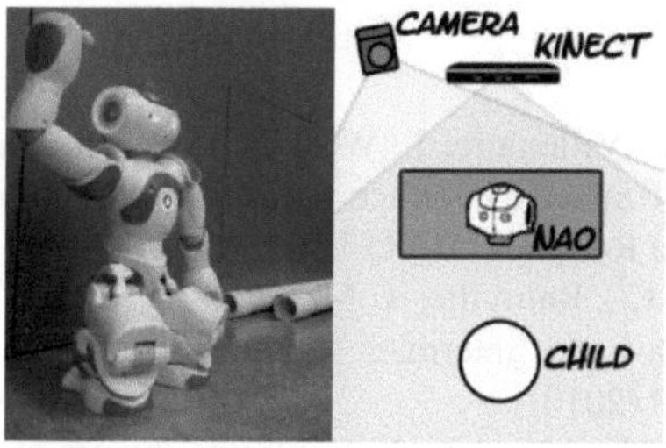

Fig. 3. The NAO during the imitation game (left) and the experimental setup (right)

The Pilot Study. A pilot study is being conducted to validate the described model with children with ASD at a local elementary school. The expected sample size is 12 participants, drawn from an ASD-only class of students between the ages of 7 and 10. The participants are split into two groups: one receives graded cueing feedback from the robot, the other (control group) receives constant feedback, P4, from the robot in each round. The constant-P4 condition represents a lack of cueing, which is expected to result in a lack of generalization of the imitation skills learned by the child despite descriptive feedback. The study is being conducted over 2.5 weeks, with each child receiving two fifteen-minute interactive play sessions with the robot per week.

The experimental setup, shown in Figure 3, above, consists of the NAO robot placed on a table in front of the seated child so that it is approximately at the child's eye-level. Behind the robot, a Microsoft Kinect is used for sensing the child's pose. A teacher or aide may also be in the room for comfort or safety. The teacher or aide does not interact with the child during the experiment, but may assist the child during setup or after the experiment. The relevant outcome measure of the study is the increase in the child's imitation ability. This measure will be evaluated both within and between sessions. No statistical significance is necessarily expected given the small size of the pilot study, but trends in the outcome measure are expected. Specifically, we expect an increase in the average correctness of the child's pose, measured as a decrease of the child's deviation from the robot's pose, a decrease in the level of prompt specificity the child needs for successful imitation of the robot, and a decrease in the number of prompts the child needs for successful imitation of the robot.

4 Future Work

At the time of this submission, the pilot study of the effectiveness of the presented model is near completion. Improvements of the model will be based on the insights gained from the study results.

Acknowledgements. We thank Dr. Sharon Cermak of USC HSC for lending her expertise to our implementation of graded cueing.

References

1. Atrash, A., Kaplow, R., Villemure, J., West, R., Yamani, H., Pineau, J.: Development and Validation of a Robust Speech Interface for Improved Human-Robot Interaction. International Journal of Social Robotics (IJSR) 1(4), 345–356 (2009)
2. Bottari, C.L., Dassa, C., Rainville, C.M., Dutil, É.: The IADL Profile: Development, content validity, intra- and interrater agreement. Canadian Journal of Occupational Therapy 77(2), 90–100 (2010)
3. Duquette, A., Michaud, F., Mercier, H.: Exploring the use of a mobile robot as an imitation agent with children with low-functioning autism. Autonomous Robots 24(2), 147–157 (2007)
4. Feil-Seifer, D.J., Matarić, M.J.: A Simon-Says Robot Providing Autonomous Imitation Feedback Using Graded Cueing. In: Poster paper in International Meeting for Autism lResearch (IMFAR), Toronto, On, Canada (May 2012)
5. Ferrari, E., Robins, B., Dautenhahn, K.: Therapeutic and educational objectives in robot assisted play for children with autism. In: IEEE International Symposium on Robot and Human Interactive Communication (RO-MAN 2009), pp. 108–114. Toyoyama International Conference Center, Japan (September-October 2009)
6. Fujimoto, I., Matsumoto, T., Silva, P.R.S., Kobayashi, M., Higashi, M.: Mimicking and Evaluating Human Motion to Improve the Imitation Skill of Children with Autism Through a Robot. International Journal of Social Robotic (IJSR) 3(4), 349–357 (2011)
7. Hoey, J., Poupart, P., Boutilier, C., Mihailidis, A.: POMDP models for assistive technology. In: ACM/IEEE International Conference onHuman-Robot Interaction (HRI), Washington DC, pp. 65–72 (March 2007)
8. Ingersoll, B., Schreibman, L., Tran, Q.H.: Effect of sensory feedback on immediate object imitation in children with autism. Journal of Autism and Developmental Disorders 33(6), 673–683 (2003)
9. Kidd, C.D., Breazeal, C.: Robots at home: Understanding long-term human-robot interaction. In: Int. Conf. on Int. Rob. Sys. (IROS), Nice, France (2008)
10. Koenig, N., Takayama, L., Matarić, M.: Learning from Demonstration: Communication and Policy Generation. In: 12th International Symposium on Experimental Robotics (ISER 2010), Delhi, India, pp. 1–15 (December 2010)
11. Larson, J.C.G., Mostofsky, S.H.: Motor Deficits in Autism. Autism: A Neurological Disorder, 231–247 (2006)
12. Larson, M.J., South, M., Krauskopf, E., Clawson, A., Crowley, M.J.: Feedback and reward processing in high-functioning autism. Psychiatry Research 187(1-2), 198–203 (2011)
13. Nadel, J.: Imitation and imitation recognition: Functional use in preverbal infants and nonverbal children with autism. In: Meltzoff&, A.N., Prinz, W. (eds.) The Imitative Mind: Development Evolution, and Brain Bases, pp. 42–62. Cambridge University Press (2002)
14. Pineau, J., Atrash, A.: Smartwheeler: A robotic wheelchair test-bed for investigating new models of human-robot interaction. In: Assoc. Adv. Artif. Intell. Spring Symp. (AAAI), Vancouver, British Columbia, Canada (July 2007)
15. Pineau, J., Montemerlo, M., Pollack, M., Roy, N., Thrun, S.: Towards robotic assistants in nursing homes: Challenges and results. Robotics and Autonomous Systems 42(3-4), 271–281 (2003)
16. Robins, B., Dautenhahn, K., Boekhorst, R.T., Billard, A.: Robotic assistants in therapy and education of children with autism: can a small humanoid robot help encourage social interaction skills? Universal Access in the Information Society 4(2), 105–120 (2005)

Developing a Human Figured Agent Interacting to Architectural Context for the Advanced Simulation of Human Behavior in the Built Environment

Yun Gil Lee[1] and Changhoon Park[2]

[1] Department of Architecture, Hoseo University, Korea
[2] Department of Game Engineering, Hoseo University, Korea
{Yglee,chpark}@hoseo.edu

Abstract. In architectural design, architects conventionally rely on their previous knowledge and experience, and building codes to evaluate their design alternatives. These factors for the evaluation of designs normally focus on the physical information of building such as size, shape, color and so on. Recently, there have been several attempts to evaluate the performance of the buildings such as light, energy, heat, structural stability and so on. However, building and space contains more complicated information than what we have seen and what these attempts have focused on. Especially, human behavior is one of the most important factors to evaluate the performance of built environment. In this manner, we intend to suggest the advanced simulation model for human behavior in the built environment. It is a kind of human figured agent which interacts with physical, semantic and social information of the built environment.

Keywords: Virtual Reality, Artificial Intelligence, Building Information Modeling, Simulation, User Behavior Evaluation.

1 Introduction

Computational support has become one of the important research issues in the field of information visualization. Moreover, in the field of architecture, the computational representation of the designed alternatives for the construction of building has become a general task in the practical design process. This might be quite useful to figure out the three dimensional shape of the designed result in the future and conveniently persuade the clients. However, it is not enough to evaluate the ultimate values of building and spaces because these visualization conventionally handle the physical information of the buildings. building and space contains more complicated information than what we have seen and what these attempts have focused on. Especially, human behavior is one of the most important factors to evaluate the performance of the built environment because it is the fundamental standard of judging the quality of building and spaces. Doursh(2003) introduced three types of information to visualize in the building simulation such as: physical, semantic and social. It is not easy to see the previous attempts of simulation to handle the physical as well as semantic and social.

C. Stephanidis (Ed.): Posters, Part II, HCII 2013, CCIS 374, pp. 587–590, 2013.

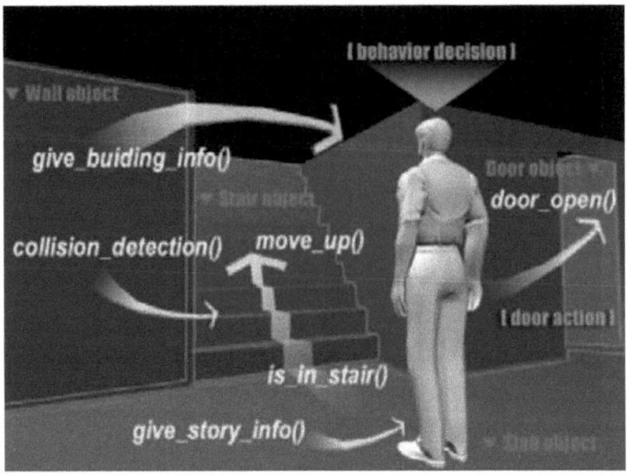

Fig. 1. The Concept of the Proposed Intelligent Virtual Place

In this manner, we intend to suggest the advanced simulation model for human behavior in the built environment. It is a kind of human figured agent which interacts with physical, semantic and social information of the built environment. In order to realize the autonomous agent which behaves in the built environment freely, we developed the data model that can describe the architectural context regarding to physical, semantic and social context. And we also propose the technological framework of so-call intelligent virtual environment based on autonomous human-figured agent.

2 Data Modeling for Physical, Semantic, and Social Information Visualization

Traditionally, in the field of CAAD(Computer Aided Architectural Design), the modeling and visualization of physical data related to building and its elements has been studied for a long time. Architects have been enjoy to use the physical information in the design process for form generation, presentation, evaluation and so on. Recently, the advent of BIM(Building Information Modeling) might be a sensational influence to change the conventional practice of architectural design and construction. BIM is the process of generating and managing building data during its life cycle.(Lee, G., Sacks, R., and Eastman, C. M., 2006) BIM might be one of the most and latest well-defined solution of the physical data regarding the building and its components. And also, in BIM, there are crucial possibilities to contain not only physical data but also semantic data which can be selected CAD behaviors, relationships, constraints, reference and so on.(Yang and Zhang 2006) However, BIM still cannot hold the data of user's behavioral response to the built environment. It is one of the most important information to evaluate the quality of the buildings. There is no room to contain these information in the existing data model of BIM. So, with BIM which might be the most advanced solution of building data modeling, architect cannot visualize and evaluate the inhabitant's behavior in the designed alternatives.

In the practical field of architecture, the user's behavior is conventionally considered by relevant design criteria as building codes. However, it is not enough to predict and evaluated the building performance of user's behavior as the minimum of standard. And also, once building codes are codified, it become quite hard to change. To overcome the limitation of building codes, there have been actual experience-based attempts using the real user and space for the evaluation of user's behavior. More recently, advances of Virtual Reality(VR) have begun to enable more rapid and easy simulation of the design alternatives. However, it takes too much time and efforts and the result of simulation is not easy to apply the design process because the design process is separated to the simulation process.

In order to realize the simulation environment interacting with the design process, we need the design tool based on the advanced data model which contain not only physical and semantic but also social information. In this study, we defined social information as the action possibilities of building and its components. Gibson called it 'Affordance'.(Gibson, 1977) Moreover, 'Affordance' can be extended to the perceived action possibilities which was concerned with the complicated context related to society, history, culture and so on. To make data model of 'Affordance', we need to adapt the rule-based data modeling as well as ontology because their complicated relationship of data cannot be easy to build up.

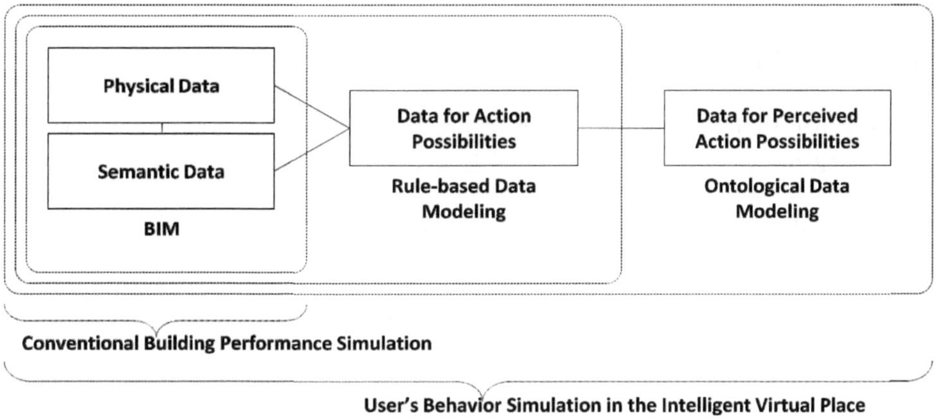

Fig. 2. The Concept of The Proposed Data Model

3 Concept and Technologies of Intelligent Virtual Place

Virtual place based on previously stated data model is enable to realize the so-called intelligent virtual environment which is the more advanced technologies than the existing VR using rule, FMS(Finite State Machines), Fuzzy Logic, Neural Networks and so on. In the intelligent virtual place, the human figured agent automatically interact with the objects and context which mimic physical world.[5] To utilize it in the design process, the designed alternatives based on BIM should be converted to the data for the intelligent virtual environment. It means that all of objects contain

'Form' to visualize, 'Meaning' to recognize and retrieval, and 'Rule' to behave and interact. And also, these objects should be ontologically structured to illustrate the complicated context.

Also, in order to realize the proposed intelligent virtual environment, the role of human figured agent is significant. We can call it 'Intelligent Virtual User(IVU)'. IVU should autonomously behave and interact with objects in the intelligent virtual environment. For this intelligent behavior of IVU, we need to consider to apply several technologies showing table1 to the intelligent virtual environment.

Table 1. The significant technologies of the proposed intelligent virtual environement

Technology	Direction	Component
Navigation	Optimal Path Planning	Global & Local Mission User profile-based Navigation Spatial Semantics
Steering Behavior	Social Interaction	Social Semantics Situation-based Behavior
Manipulation	Semantic Interaction	Evolving Manipulation Distributed Intelligence Affordance

4 Conclusion and Discussion

In this paper, we intend to illustrate the entire vision of intelligent virtual environment interacting the architectural design tool to evaluate inhabitant's behavior in the designed alternatives for building. The proposed ontological data modeling and autonomous behavioral agent based on the suggested technologies could be helpful to realize the intelligent virtual environment. Although this study is only the early stage of entire research, there is no doubt that the result of this study can provide the fundamental framework to develop the intelligent virtual environment.

References

1. Dourish, P.: Where the Footprints Lead: Tracking Down Other Roles for Social Navigation, pp. 273–291. Springer, London (2003)
2. Lee, G., Sacks, R., Eastman, C.M.: Specifying parametric building object behavior (BOB) for a building information modeling system. Automation in Construction 15(6), 758–776 (2006)
3. Yang, Q.Z., Zhang, Y.: Semantic interoperability in building design: Methods and tools. Computer-Aided Design 38, 1099–1112 (2006)
4. James, J.G.: The Theory of Affordances. In: Shaw, R., Bransford, J. (eds.) Perceiving, Acting, and Knowing (1977)
5. Aylett, R., Cavazza, M.: Intelligent Virtual Environments - A State-of-the-art Report. In: Eurographics Conference, Manchester, UK (2001)

Automating the Mentor in a Serious Game: A Discourse Analysis Using Finite State Machines

Brent Morgan[1], Fazel Kehtkar[1], Athur Graesser[1], and David Shaffer[2]

[1] University of Memphis, Psychology, Institute for Intelligent Systems, 365 Innovation Drive, Memphis, TN 38152, USA
[2] University of Wisconsin-Madison, 1025 West Johnson Street, Room 1065, Madison, WI 53706, USA
{brent.morgan,graesser}@memphis.edu,
{fazelk,david.williamson.shaffer}@gmail.com

1 Introduction

Serious games are increasingly becoming a popular, effective supplement to standard classroom instruction [1]. Similar to recreational games, multi-party chat is a standard method of communication in serious games. As players collaborate in a serious game, mentoring is often needed to facilitate progress and learning [2, 3, 4]. This role is almost exclusively provided by a human at the present time. However, the cost incurred with training a human mentor represents a critical barrier for widespread use of a collaborative epistemic game. Although great strides have been made in automating one-on-one tutorial dialogues [5, 6], multi-party chat presents a significant challenge for natural language processing. The goal of this research, then, is to provide a preliminary understanding of player-mentor conversations in the context of an epistemic game, Land Science [7].

1.1 Land Science

Land Science is an extension of the epistemic game Urban Science, created by education researchers at the University of Wisconsin-Madison [7], designed to simulate an urban planning practicum experience. Young people role-play as professional urban planners in an ecologically-rich neighborhood to develop new ways of observing and acting in the world they inhabit. Players are assigned to one of three planning teams, each of which represents a stakeholder group (e.g., People for Greenspace). Players conduct a virtual site visit to learn about the issues their Non-Player Character (NPC) stakeholders care about. The players ultimately submit and defend a new plan for the city that aims to meet the needs of the community. During the game, players communicate with other members of their planning team, as well as with an adult mentor role-playing as a professional planning consultant.

These conversations between the mentor and players were analyzed with respect to meaning, syntax, and discourse function by classifying contributions into individual speech acts. The categorized speech acts were then analyzed to identify speech act sequences in the conversations, represented as Finite State Machines (FSM).

C. Stephanidis (Ed.): Posters, Part II, HCII 2013, CCIS 374, pp. 591–595, 2013.

1.2 Speech Act Classification and Finite State Machines

We selected a system for classifying speech acts [8]. Analyses of a variety of corpora, including chat and multiparty games, have converged on a set of speech act categories that are both theoretically justified and that also can be reliably coded by trained judges [9]. Our classification scheme has 8 broad categories:

- **Statements** are verbal reports on scientific facts, the status of the game activities, or other information about the Land Science domain (e.g., "Each of the stakeholders needs to give you feedback on your preference survey").
- **Requests** include asking other participants in the conversation to provide information or to take some action (e.g., "Please check your inbox").
- **Questions** are queries for information from the addressee (e.g., "Tina, have you finished your intake interview?").
- **Reactions** are short verbal responses to requests or questions (e.g., "Yes, Frank").
- **Expressive Evaluations** consist of feedback regarding the players' performance or feedback from the players on the program or activity (e.g., "That's a great idea").
- **MetaStatements** are statements about the communication process or the metacognition of participants (e.g., "Oops. Sorry for the double chat", "I'm lost.").
- **Greetings** are expressions regarding any party's entrance to or exit from the conversation (e.g., "Hi Janet and William!", "So long, folks").
- **Other** represents speech acts which did not fit into the above categories (e.g. nonsensical contributions).

Our assumption is that there are patterns in multi-party conversation that can be captured in sequences of speech acts, and that FSMs provide a first step to discover these patterns. For example, FSMs can identify particular nodes (i.e., speech acts) which are frequently connected to other nodes in the chat room. Sequences of speech act categories can be quite enlightening even when the content of the speech acts is not analyzed. Our goal is to identify the conversational patterns in multi-party conversations in a serious game (such as Land Science) with the ultimate objective of automating the mentor's role.

2 Methods

2.1 Participants

Players participated in the epistemic game, Land Science, which enabled them to complete an urban planning internship for a fictitious urban planning firm. During the game, participants worked in different teams and interacted with mentors who were trained in the urban planning profession, the game's activities, and preferred mentoring strategies. The primary task of the players was to redesign the Northside neighborhood in Madison, WI.

2.2 Procedure

Players participated in the epistemic game, Land Science, which enabled them to complete an urban planning internship for a fictitious urban planning firm. During the game, participants worked in different teams and interacted with mentors who were trained in the urban planning profession, the game's activities, and preferred mentoring strategies. The primary task of the players was to redesign the Northside neighborhood in Madison, WI.

Players completed three phases of Land Science: Introduction, Stakeholder, and Final Plan. The three phases were subdivided into 19 stages, with each stage requiring different tasks, skills, and goals. Across all three phases, players conversed with their planning team and a human mentor via a chat window.

2.3 Automated Speech Act Classification and STN Creation

Player and Mentor contributions were automatically categorized into speech acts using the Naive Bayes classification algorithm on word features. The classification compares favorably to trained human coders with a kappa of 0.677, compared to a kappa of 0.797 between two humans [10].

STNs were created by calculating the conditional probability of each transition between speech acts as well as the overall frequency of each speech act in the corpus. For example, a mentor statement might be followed by a player reaction 28% of the time, and a player reaction might constitute 0.8% of the entire corpus. For each transition, a minimum conditional probability threshold of 15% was used for inclusion in the network, as well as an overall frequency of 0.3%. Additionally, although there are only two roles in the game (player and mentor), one crucial piece of information that the STNs can provide is the identity of the speaker. Specifically, in the case of adjacent player contributions, it is critical to distinguish whether the response is a follow-up from the same player ("P → P") or whether it is a reply by some Other Player ("P → OP"). This distinction helps in identifying player collaborations.

3 Results and Discussion

An overall FSM for Land Science is shown in Figure 1. One important pattern to note is a "Question → Response → Feedback" sequence (Mentor Question, followed by a Player Statement or Reaction, followed by a Mentor Statement). This didactic pattern is common and aligned with previous research [11]. Overall, two distinct epistemic networks emerged: scaffolding and collaboration. Scaffolding occurs when mentor responses to player contributions help guide players to the next step. This is necessary to facilitate goal completion throughout the game. Conversely, collaboration represents meaningful interactions between players. These player-player interactions are essential for collaborative problem-solving as members of a team.

M = Mentor; P→P = follow-up by same player; P→OP = reply by some Other Player

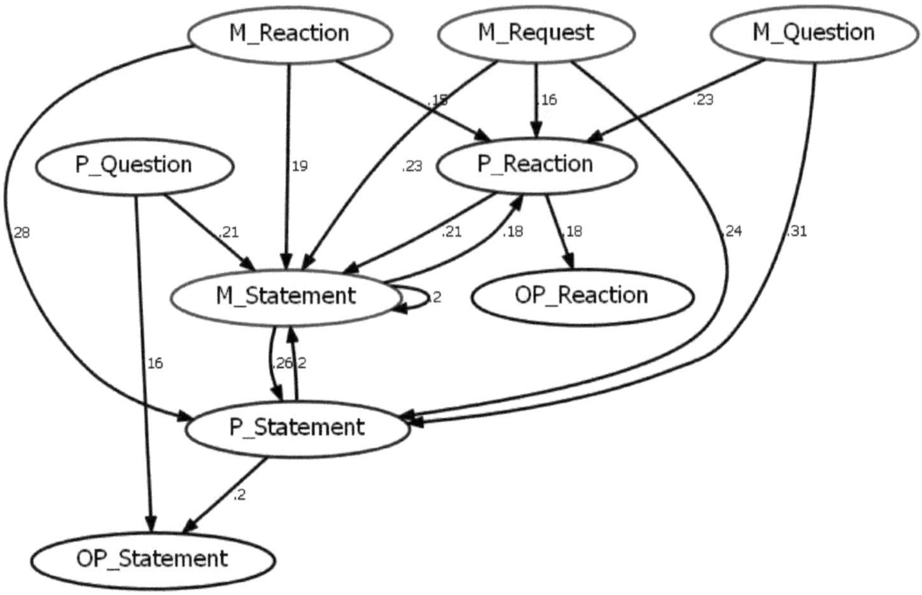

Fig. 1. Finite State Machine for Land Science

These data are applicable to a number of current and future investigations. First, we are currently analyzing additional chat room interactions between players and mentors in order to replicate these findings and allow for additional data mining. This includes predicting points in the conversation where a mentor should provide a contribution, as well as the appropriate speech act at a given point. Recurrence connectionist models can be used to predict the generation of speech act category N+1 on the basis of category sequences 1 through N. Additionally, the chat room conversations can be analyzed by human coders to link each contribution to its intended recipient. If sequential mismatches or breakdowns end up being more frequent than expected, additional context is needed to improve our understanding of chat room dynamics.

In analyzing these transitions between speech acts, the goal is to ease the burden of training human mentors and the accompanying logistical constraints. Even a semi-proficient automated mentor would represent significant progress, as fewer human mentors would be needed for each instance of gameplay. Hence, the current findings, combined with other analyses will help guide the implementation of an AutoSuggestor. The AutoSuggestor program will aid human mentors by providing recommendations for mentor contributions at various points in the conversation. In addition to making the human mentor's role easier, the human mentors can rate the quality of AutoSuggestor's recommendations. These ratings can then be analyzed to improve the quality of AutoSuggestor's contributions, and progress towards fully automating the role of the mentor in an epistemic game.

Acknowledgments. This work was funded in part by the Macarthur Foundation, National Science Foundation (REC-0347000, DUE-091934, DRL-0918409, DRL-0946372, BCS 0904909, DRK-12-0918409), the Gates Foundation, and U.S. Department of Homeland Security (Z934002/UTAA08-063). Any opinions, findings, and conclusions or recommendations expressed in this material are those of the authors and do not necessarily reflect the views of these funding agencies, cooperating institutions, or other individuals.

References

1. Ritterfeld, U., Cody, M., Vorderer, P. (eds.): Serious games: Mechanisms and effects. Routledge, New York (2009)
2. Bagley, E.S., Shaffer, D.W.: When people get in the way: Promoting civic thinking through epistemic gameplay. International Journal of Gaming and Computer-Mediated Simulations 1(1), 36–52 (2009)
3. Kirschner, P.A., Sweller, J., Clark, R.E.: Why minimal guidance during instruction does not work: An analysis of the failure of constructivist, discovery, problem-based, experiential, and inquiry-based teaching. Educational Psychologist 41(2), 75–86 (2006)
4. Nash, P., Shaffer, D.W.: Mentor modeling: The internalization of modeled professional thinking in an epistemic game. Journal of Computer Assisted Learning 27(2), 173–189 (2011)
5. Graesser, A.C., D'Mello, S.K., Cade, W.: Instruction based on tutoring. In: Mayer, R.E., Alexander, P.A. (eds.) Handbook of research on learning and instruction, pp. 408–426. Routledge, New York (2011)
6. Graesser, A.C., D'Mello, S.K., Hu, X., Cai, Z., Olney, A., Morgan, B.: AutoTutor. In: McCarthy, P.M., Boonthum, C. (eds.) Applied Natural Language Processing and Content Analysis: Identification, Investigation and Resolution, pp. 169–187. IGI Global, Hershey (2012)
7. Bagley, E.: Epistemography of an urban and regional planning practicum: Appropriation in the face of eesistance. In: WCER Working Paper 2010-8. University of Wisconsin Center for Education Research, Madison (2010)
8. Moldovan, C., Rus, V., Graesser, A.C.: Automated Speech Act Classification For Online Chat. In: The 22nd Midwest Artificial Intelligence and Cognitive Science Conference (2011)
9. D'Andrade, R.G., Wish, M.: Speech act theory in quantitative research on interpersonal behavior. Discourse Processes 8(2), 229–259 (1985)
10. Rus, V., Moldovan, C., Witherspoon, A., Graesser, A.C.: Automatic Identification of Speakers' Intentions in A multi-Party Dialogue System. 21st Annual Meeting of the Society for Text and Discourse (2011)
11. Sinclair, J., Coulthart, M.: Towards an analysis of discourse: The English used by teachers and pupils. Oxford University Press, London (1975)

Reasoning, Planning, and Goal Seeking for Small Combat Unit Modeling and Simulation

Daniel Rice[1], Medhat Korna[1], Peter Amstutz[1], and Dale Malabarba[2]

[1] Technology Solutions Experts, Inc., Natick, MA
[2] U.S. Army Natick Soldier Research, Development, and Engineering Center, Natick, MA
{daniel.rice,peter.amstutz,medhat.korna}@tseboston.com,
dale.malabarba.civ@mail.mil

Abstract. The current state of Modeling and Simulation (M&S) scenario creation is difficult, requiring too much time and effort on the part of Subject Matter Experts (SMEs) and analysts to produce scenarios that are sufficiently realistic for valid analysis, as well as a need for more realistic M&S agent behavior and decision making in simulation. Additionally, there also is a critical need for decision support tools to support Soldier and Small Unit (SU) decision making in the field. TSE is currently developing algorithms for the automation of combat operation simulation behaviors on the individual Soldier and SU level that may also be leveraged for Soldier and SU decision support tools to meet these critical Computer-Human Interaction (CHI) domain problems. TSE is researching and developing the Reasoning, Planning, and Goal-Seeking (RPGS) architecture, which is targeted at the next generation of constructive simulations requiring autonomous and intelligent agents that are capable of problem solving; considering multiple courses of action; coordinating with friendly forces; following chain of command; and using Tactics, Techniques, and Procedures (TTPs) to guide operations. Intelligent agents guided by RPGS methodologies and algorithms will be able to execute complex tasks given mission goals, initial/boundary conditions, constraints, and access to a battlespace knowledge base. TSE is creating a formal model of the Soldier and SU battlespace on which reasoning can be conducted. TSE will integrate two technical standards into the battlespace knowledge model; the Joint Consultation, Command, and Control Information Exchange Data Model (JC3IEDM) and the Coalition Battle Management Language (C-BML). This paper discusses the application of these standards and the design and development of a battlespace knowledge base and new RPGStechnologies.

Keywords: reasoning, planning, goal selection, autonomous behavior, constructive simulation.

1 Background

Technology Solutions Experts, Inc. (TSE) develops the Infantry Warrior Simulation (IWARS) system for the U.S. Army Natick Soldier Research, Development, and Engineering Center (NSRDEC). TSE is researching and developing algorithms for

C. Stephanidis (Ed.): Posters, Part II, HCII 2013, CCIS 374, pp. 596–600, 2013.

Soldier and Small Unit (SU) combat operation behaviors for use in constructive simulations such as IWARS. The primary goal of this research is to develop methodologies and algorithms for improving the scenario-generation process in simulations by reducing the dependence on textual or graphical scripting languages. Currently, analysts must plan behaviors in great detail in order to construct large, realistic, and valid simulation scenarios with scripted behaviors. Scripting inherently requires the analyst to anticipate every situation that could occur during the scenario and ensure there is a decision process to produce a response. An early result of this research was the creation of a conceptual design for the Reasoning, Planning, and Goal-Seeking (RPGS) framework, a cognitive approach for SU constructive simulation [1].

Currently, TSE is creating new approaches to model agent behavior capable of responding to unanticipated battlefield conditions [2]. TSE's approach is to improve the autonomous decision-making capability of the Soldier agent, which will reduce the analyst's burden of inputting and scripting realistic Soldier and SU behaviors. To this end, intelligent agents are enabled to process assigned goals and to apply cognitive and problem-solving methodologies to assess the situation and to determine, autonomously, the optimal means to accomplish its goals. TSE also is extending this research into the next generation of constructive simulations for intelligent agents that are capable of problem solving; considering multiple courses of action; coordinating with friendly forces; following chain of command; and using Tactics, Techniques, and Procedures (TTPs) to guide operations. The goal is to develop intelligent agents guided by RPGS methodologies and algorithms that can execute complex tasks given only mission goals, initial/boundary conditions, and constraints. These new technologies and capabilities will provide significant contribution and innovation in human behavior representation for military and commercial constructive simulations by reducing scenario construction time and providing more realistic Soldier agent behavior and scenario outcomes.

The RPGS framework has been influenced by the widely used Belief-Desire-Intention (BDI) model [3]. TSE refines the BDI model in RPGS with explicit rule-based reasoning to establish belief, goal-selection rules that reflect desire, and dynamic planning to establish intention.

2 Reasoning, Planning, and Goal Seeking

TSE designed the RPGS framework to allow intelligent agents to complete problem solving, consider multiple courses of action, coordinate with friendly forces, follow chain of command, and use TTPs to guide operations. RPGS methodologies and algorithms allow agents to execute complex tasks given only mission goals, initial/boundary conditions, and constraints, and allow them to access to an underlying battlespace knowledge base.

"Reasoning" is the act of adding new facts to the agent's knowledge base and using these facts to select the agent's goal. This includes perception of the environment, spatial reasoning, and the application of knowledge rules to determine new facts. The battlespace knowledge model is a key component of the RPGS system, providing the foundation for knowledge-based understanding and reasoning. The U.S. Army has invested heavily in the development of battlespace knowledge systems, and TSE is leveraging existing system models including Command and Control (C2) models such as the Joint Consultation, Command, and Control Information Exchange Data Model (JC3IEDM), knowledge portals such as the Army Knowledge Online (AKO), battlespace languages such as the Coalition Battle Management Language (C-BML), and training documents such as the U.S. Army Training and Doctrine Command (TRADOC) Pamphlet 350-70-6 [4].

"Planning" is the process of finding a sequence of actions that will achieve a goal. By understanding and anticipating the outcomes of specific actions and acting with intent, the agent can engage in problem solving, which is difficult with scripted behaviors.

"Goal Seeking" links the reasoning and planning processes to actual behavior, translating planning operators into actions in the underlying simulation. TSE identified the operator precedence selection mechanism that exists in the Soar cognitive architecture [5] as a promising basis on which to design a preference system for action selection. TSE will combine this system with existing technical standards for battlespace knowledge systems such as JC3IEDM [6] and C-BML [7]. Leveraging these systems provides the analyst with a way to express preferences and priorities for agents in determining how to execute mission orders.

3 Battlespace Knowledge

3.1 Battlespace Knowledge Models

JC3IEDM and C-BML are the two technical standards TSE identified for direct integration into the battlespace knowledge base. JC3IEDM is a North Atlantic Treaty Organization (NATO) standard database schema used to enable interoperability of C2 systems, and it is capable of describing many knowledge items of military interest, such as troop locations, materiel, hazard zones, and key events. The JC3IEDM contains three data models: a conceptual data model, a logical data model, and a physical data model. The conceptual model represents the view of information in generalized terms, such as "actions," "organizations," "materiel," "features," and "locations." The logical model breaks these generalized concepts into specific information that follows human reasoning patterns. The physical model is the physical schema that defines the structure of a relational database. JC3IEDM provides an extensible base for representing information about battlefield entities. C-BML, which has already been integrated with JC3IEDM, is a formal language for specifying orders and reports by specifying the "who, what, when, where, and why" of a mission order. C-BML provides an abstracted representation of the information in JC3IEDM that is closer to how humans create plans, using goals and objectives to define final and intermediate results and the mission contingencies that need to be followed. As a formal language, C-BML is well suited for use with the RPGS battlespace knowledge model because it eliminates the ambiguity of free text associated with human-written orders and plans.

TSE will leverage C-BML to describe mission goals and constraints that the analyst gives to agents allowing the RPGS behavior engine to generate autonomous agent behavior.

3.2 Battlespace Knowledge Rules

Battlespace knowledge rules are being developed in the context of JC3IEDM and C-BML. TSE currently is mapping the IWARS underlying information model to both JC3IEDM and C-BML and is discovering the existence of knowledge gaps. TSE is leveraging enabling standards and technologies such as the World Wide Web Consortium (W3C) recommended Semantic Technology standard languages of Resource Definition Framework (RDF), RDF Schema (RDFS), and the Web Ontology Language. These standards and languages are being used to codify behavior rules and a common vocabulary. TSE created a custom triple store, user interface, and integration with IWARS that enables a battlespace knowledge base and the RPGS behavior engine.

4 Conclusions and Future Work

TSE currently is developing the RPGS framework, shown conceptually in Figure 1. The RPGS framework will enable agent behaviors based on inference of the logical consequences of asserted facts or axioms, and the implementation of a set of inference rules specified using a declarative logic programming language. The RPGS Reasoning Engine will perform reasoning using first-order predicate logic and inference through both forward and backward chaining.

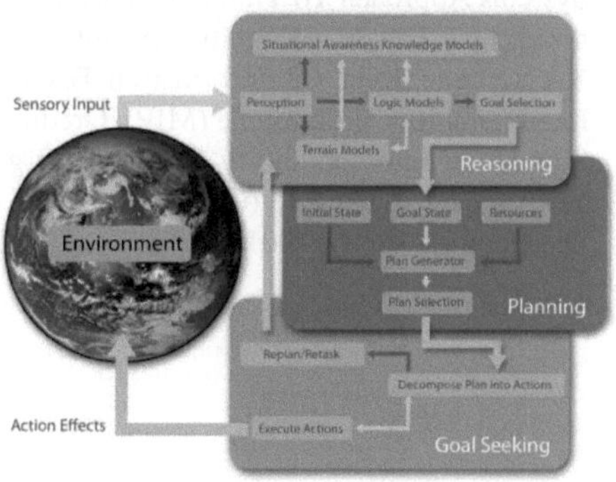

Fig. 1. The Reasoning, Planning, and Goal Seeking Framework

Figure 2 shows how TSE will use its research results to generate the RPGS behaviors. TSE is using JC3IEDM as the common vocabulary to define the tasks, and TSE is using C-BML as the language to express those tasks to the agents. The terrain representation includes semantic information for terrain reasoning and the terrain reasoning algorithms use that information to provide realistic military use of the terrain. Along with military doctrine, the C-BML plans and terrain reasoning will provide the

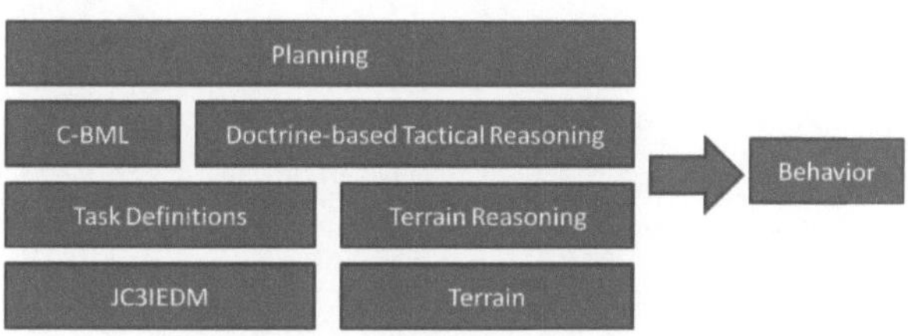

Fig. 2. RPGS Framework to Behavior

overall tactical reasoning that the planning system will use for initial scenario generation as well as monitoring and potential re-planning during mission execution.

The RPGS framework is a promising approach to developing autonomous agent behavior for constructive military simulation. The ability to build reusable, portable, dynamic behaviors demonstrates there is significant potential in improving the flexibility (and thus the realism) of agent behavior. The composition of operations enables users to generate increasingly sophisticated and reusable collections of behaviors.

Acknowledgements. This work is funded in part by the U.S. Army Natick Soldier Research, Development, and Engineering Center (NSRDEC) and the Small Business Innovation Research (SBIR) program under contract W911QY-12-C-0056.

References

1. Amstutz, P., Andra, M., Rice, D.: Reasoning, Planning, and Goal Seeking: A Cognitive Approach for Small Combat Unit Constructive Simulation. In: 2012 Spring Simulation Multiconference. The Society for Modeling & Simulation International, Orlando (2012)
2. NATO Research and Technology Organisation: Human Behavior Representation in Constructive Simulation Technical Report RTO-TR-HFM-128 (2009)
3. Rao, A.S., Georgeff, M.P.: BDI Agents: From Theory to Practice. In: Proceedings of the First International Conference on Multi-Agent Systems (ICMAS 1995), San Francisco (1995)
4. Systems Approach To Training Analysis, TRADOC Pamphlet 350-70-6 (2004)
5. Laird, J.E.: The Soar Cognitive Architecture. The MIT Press, Cambridge (2012)
6. NATO: The Joint C3 Information Exchange Data Model (JC3IEDM Main) Multilateral Interoperability Programme (MIP), Greding, Germany (2011)
7. Simulation Interoperability Standards Organization (SISO): Standard for: Coalition Battle Management Language (C-BML) Phase I Coalition Battle Management Language Product Development Group (2012)

Dialog Systems and Their Inputs

Darren Scerri and Alexiei Dingli

Department of Intelligent Computer Systems, Computer Building,
University of Malta, Msida, Malta
{dsce0006,alexiei.dingli}@um.edu.mt

Abstract. One of the main limitations in existent domain-independent conversational agents is that the general and linguistic knowledge of these agents is limited to what the agents' developers explicitly defined. Therefore, a system which analyses user input at a deeper level of abstraction which backs its knowledge with common sense information will essentially result in a system that is capable of providing more adequate responses which in turn result in a better overall user experience. From this premise, a framework was proposed, and a working prototype was implemented upon this framework. The prototype makes use of various natural language processing tools, online and offline knowledge bases, and other information sources, to enable it to comprehend and construct relevant responses.

Keywords: Dialog Systems, External Knowledge Acquisition, RDF, Knowledge Bases, Chatterbots.

1 Introduction and Background

Conversational agents are deployed in various forms and designed to cater for different domains and goals, ranging from automated hotel-booking agents, to personal assistants, companions, and agents designed simply for entertainment purposes. Moreover, one can categorize conversational agents into two main types based on how these process the input and generate their output. These two types can be realized as being chatterbots and dialog systems [1].

The main difference between these two types of conversational agents lies in what these systems are designed to model. Chatterbots model, or rather simulate a conversation in its basic sense, and intend to fool the user that he is communicating with an intelligent entity that does in fact understand what is being said. On the other hand, dialog systems attempt to model the actual dialog process which also incorporates the task of analyzing and understanding the input, which in turn aids in the generation of an adequate dynamic response.

2 Aims and Objectives

The aim of this project is to provide a proof-of-concept generic-conversation framework for conversational agents, and a working prototype that can be categorized as being a hybrid between a chatterbot and a dialog system.

C. Stephanidis (Ed.): Posters, Part II, HCII 2013, CCIS 374, pp. 601–605, 2013.

"Building a system that could understand open-ended natural language utterances would require common sense reasoning, the huge open-ended mass of sensory-motor competencies, knowledge and reasoning skills which human beings make use of in their everyday dealings with the world" [2].

With regards to this hypothesis, the system makes use of modern natural language processing technologies and tools to analyze user dialog input while simultaneously using information that is obtainable from external sources to attempt to further understand the input and ultimately generate appropriate responses to the user. Another goal is to merge these various sources to create a single, local, knowledge base which enables the system to keep track of the world of the user, i.e. the relationship and interaction of the user with various entities. These sources include content and information on different entities and concepts, including common sense knowledge and knowledge about specific people and world entities.

The aims and objectives of this project can be summarized as follows:

1. To build an expandable proof-of-concept system that provides a syntactic, semantic and pragmatic understanding of input.
2. To simulate intelligence by providing adequate output and logical conclusions derived from dialogue input and local and external knowledge bases.

Moreover, the proposed system will be as customizable, flexible, and modular as possible, so that it would require minimum effort to upgrade and adapt the system to handle input of varying complexity and topics.

3 Design

The developed prototype consists mainly of three phases: Natural Language Understanding (NLU) phase, intermediary processing phase, and finally the output generation phase.

The NLU module is primarily makes use of ChatScript [3], an award-winning chatterbot engine. ChatScript employs various linguistic technologies to enable support for more flexible linguistic input in terms of syntax and semantics, and more expressive and semantics-oriented pattern matching rules, where matching patterns of meaning (semantics and pragmatics) is considered more important than matching patterns of words (syntax). These technologies and processes include the use of WordNet as a semantic network, Part-of-Speech tagging, pronoun resolution, conceptual relations, and preprocessing abilities.

ChatScript is used by the system mainly as a "normalization phase". This phase is essentially a mapping process that maps natural language input into a more formal representation using XML. This is essential in order to allow the creation of rules that allow matching of a number of input utterances that are effectively semantically equivalent. This phase is analogous to how Façade maps text to discourse acts.

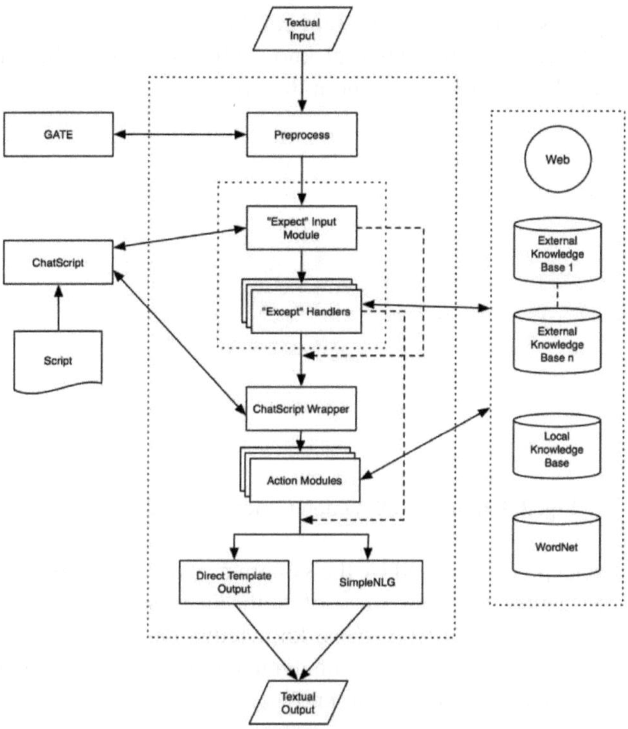

Fig. 1. System Block Diagram

Input is preprocessed using two approaches. Using GATE and ANNIE [4][5], the system attempts to resolve pronouns into their respective named entities. Moreover, ChatScript includes a preprocessing phase in itself, performing actions such as spell checking and term substitution.

The normalization phase allows the system to perform further intermediary processing on the input, such as querying local and external knowledge bases to allow to better understand and respond to the input. This is achieved by a number of processing modules that can be developed to handle specific types of input. The system's dialog manager employs a similar technique used in CONVERSE [6] with regards to these processing modules. The system incorporates a polling technique for which the input is passed through all implemented processing modules, or "Action Modules", for which each module advertises a score indicating how much it is confident to process the input.

Each action module is able to perform various tasks, include querying and managing local and external knowledge bases through global wrappers, triggering other action modules, querying ChatScript for further normalization, adding and retrieving topics from the dialog manager, generating output and alerting the dialog manager that the subsequent user utterance is expected to contain certain type of information (such as names, feelings, numbers, etc.).

The knowledge bases used in the system can be grouped into two types: the local RDF knowledge base, and other external knowledge bases (can be either offline or online), which are all accessible throughout the system.

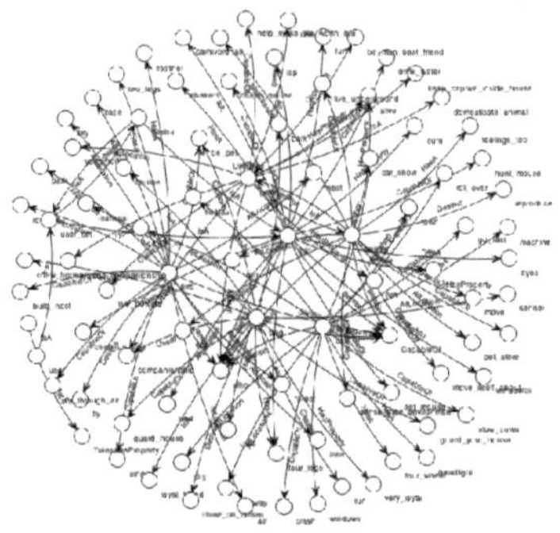

Fig. 2. Example RDF Graph Generated by the System

YAGO and ConceptNet are used by the system as external knowledge bases allowing the system to gather and make use of both entity specific and common sense knowledge. The retrieved data from these knowledge bases can be merged with the local RDF knowledge base to create an amalgamated network of knowledge, combining the "world of the user" with external knowledge.

4 Implementation and Evaluation

A prototype system was developed upon the described framework. This prototype included the development of a number of action modules, in conjunction with their respective ChatScript script which attempt to handle a specific set of user utterances, ranging from possession and sentiment statements, to questions regarding general and specific world entities.

The evaluation was carried out two-fold: hands-on conversation with the system (prototype), and a questionnaire filled by a number of users who engaged in a dialogue with the system, following a pre-defined context and a set of example tasks, tested this prototype and answered questions on a five-point Likert scale which were aimed to be conclusive in whether the system actually achieved its aims and objectives. All results were biased towards the higher end (mean values for answers: 1 - 2.05%, 2 - 6.77%, 3 - 25.84%, 4 - 49.73%, 5 - 15.54%), which imply that the overall result is positive.

The following example shows the system's ability to keep track of user-defined information and depicts a level of understandability:

- User: I have a red car.
- System: OK, noted!
- User: What is the color of my car?
- System: Red.
- User: I also have a cat named Simba.
- System: Glad to know that you have a cat named Simba.

- User: Do you know who is Simba?
- System: Simba is your cat.
- User: Do you know who is Barack Obama?
- System: Barack Hussein Obama II is the 44th and current President of the United States. Also, I have heard a lot of positive things about Barack Obama. What's your view?
- User: I think he is a great president .
- System: Why do you think that Barack Obama is great?
- User: Because he is an exemplary politician.
- System: Ok then, so you think that Barack Obama is great, because he is an exemplary politician.
- User: Are cats capable of chasing mice?
- System: Yes
- User: Can cats fly?
- System: No, I don't think so
- User: Is a cat an animal?
- System: Yes
- User: Is it a machine?
- System: No
- User: Do you know anything about Bill Gates?
- System: Bill Gates is born on date 1955-10-28.
- User: Anything else?
- System: Bill Gates is married to Melinda Gates.
- User: Tell me about cats
- System: Cats are capable of eating meats, killing birds, drinking milks, eating mice, sleeping, climbing up trees and chasing mice.

It can be concluded that the system is regarded as having potential to expand and improve to further achieve higher quality results and ultimately fulfill the aims and objectives in a greater sense. Naturally, there are still possible areas for improvement since the evaluation was done on a prototype with strict boundaries.

The system's ability to make use of external sources to support and enhance its knowledge of the real world can be considered as being a step forward towards the implementation of more natural and human-like conversational systems. The system is able to exploit the vast amounts of data found in structured knowledge databases that are consulted to both understand, and answer in a natural and informed manner.

References

1. Klüwer, T.: From Chatbots to Dialog Systems. International Journal, 1–22 (2011)
2. Mateas, M., Stern, A.: Natural Language Understanding in Façade: Surface-text Processing (2004)
3. Wilcox, B.: Suzette, the Most Human Computer (2011)
4. Bontcheva, K., Cunningham, H., Maynard, D., Tablan, V., Saggion, H.: Developing Reusable and Robust Language Processing Components for Information Systems Using Gate. In: 3rd International Workshop on Natural Language and Information Systems, pp. 223–227 (2002)
5. Cunningham, H., Humphreys, K., Gaizauska, R.: GATE - a Tipster-Based General Architecture for Text Engineering. In: Proceedings of the TIPSTER Text Program (Phase III) 6 Month Workshop (1997)
6. Levy, D., Batacharia, B., Catizone, R., Krotov, A., Wilks, Y.: CONVERSE: a Conversational Companion. In: Proceedings of the 1st International Workshop on Human-Computer Conversation (1997)

A Dress Coordination Robot System Which Can Improve User's Ability by a Dialogue Robot

Aoi Shimizu, Yu Suzuki, and Hirotada Ueda

Division of Frontier Informatics, Kyoto Sangyo University, Motoyama, Kamigamo, Kita-Ku, Kyoto-City 603-8555, Japan
{i1258069,ueda}@cc.kyoto-su.ac.jp

Abstract. People who are not good at coordination of apparel tend to wear similar clothes many times. Unless they notice this fact, they won't be able to change. Therefore, We developed a dress recommendation system that can cope with this problem by a conversational robot. A big screen displays life-size clothes and the robot explains the recommendation Dress is divided into three parts, an inner, an outer, and bottoms and recommended as a combination of those three. When it is not user's favorite combination, user can ask a robot the reason for recommendation. We propose two dialogue strategies, blind spots pointing and chance discovery mechanism, to improve the user's coordination power. The system adapts to the user through the interaction. Furthermore, since the robot explains the user reasons of the recommendation and blind spot pointing, user can easily carry out the chance discovery. Thus, user's dress coordination power is improved.

Keywords: dress coordination, robot system, dialogue robot, dialogue strategy, chance discovery.

1 Introduction

Recently, some research of dress coordination systems has been proposed. They are mainly fitting simulation systems. For example, in the case of a system named Talkin' Closet, a computer in the closet selects a proper coordination depending on the mood of the day that the user tells and the clothes appeals "I want to be wear."[2]. A system named MagicCloset [3] recommends a dress suitable for the purpose considering the attributes of the clothes. We paid attention to the fact that people who are not good at coordination of apparel tend to wear similar clothes many times. Unless they notice this fact, they won't be able to change. Therefore, we developed a dress recommendation system which can cope with this problem by a conversational robot.

2 Outline of the System

Our system is installed in our experiment house. As shown in Figure 1, the big screen in the living room displays the recommended clothes, and the robot in front of the screen explains them to user with gesture. Dress is divided into three parts, an inner,

C. Stephanidis (Ed.): Posters, Part II, HCII 2013, CCIS 374, pp. 606–610, 2013.

an outer, and bottoms and recommended as a combination of those three. When the user shows the robot a cloth that the user wants to wear, the robot recommends to the user the remaining parts that are much to it. User decides a best coordination on the day while talking with the robot and watching the recommendations.

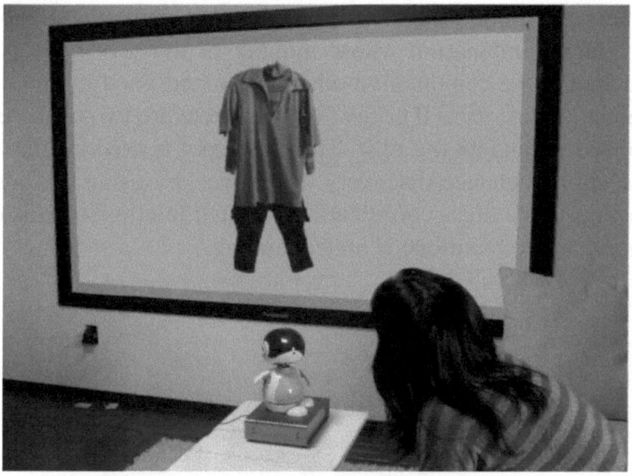

Fig. 1. System appearance

The recommendation of the clothes is decided referring to the attributes values of clothes. Evaluation attributes are color, collar shape, sleeve length, and texture. Each attribute value is out of three kinds; good, fair, bad, and stored in the decision matrix. These values are assigned subjectively at this developing stage. The user may answer to wear or ask the robot the reason of the recommendation. For example, the robot says "This dress was judged to match color combinations. Do you think the color combination is no good?" If user is not satisfied, the evaluation value of the decision matrix is changed 'bad'. Thus the decision of the robot is adapted to the user and the user is more likely to trust the system.

3 Interaction Design

3.1 Chance Discovery Dialog Strategy

It is said that three steps (noticing, understanding, conviction) is important for the chance discovery or innovation[5], [6], [7]. These three steps are defined as follows. In the notice step, the user's point of view changes, this is to facilitate the decision-making. In the understanding step obtaining accurate information is important. In the understanding step the user accepts the changed viewpoint. In this study, we used as the basis for a dialogue strategy this chance discovery mechanism. As the noticing, the robot presents a combination of clothes that the user did not wear. As the understanding, the robot provides information for the right decision. As the conviction, User wears a combination of clothes recommended by the robot.

3.2 Pointing User's Blinds Points

The combination which was not worn is called a blind spot although a user had not worn in the past in this research. For example, Fig. 2 shows the history of the dress which the author wore for 48 days from June 15, 2012. A horizontal axis expresses the color of inners and bottoms and a height axis expresses the number of times of wear. There is much combination whose number of times of wear is zero. Among these, the blind spot is the combination which is judged good by the decision matrix and a recommendation history is 0 or few. When there are two or more blind spots, 1 set is recommended at random out of it. The blind spot is used for the "noticing" step of the above-mentioned chance discovery. Moreover, by using this histogram, since the deviation over a user's dress coordination is found intelligibly, this can be used as information for the above-mentioned "understanding."

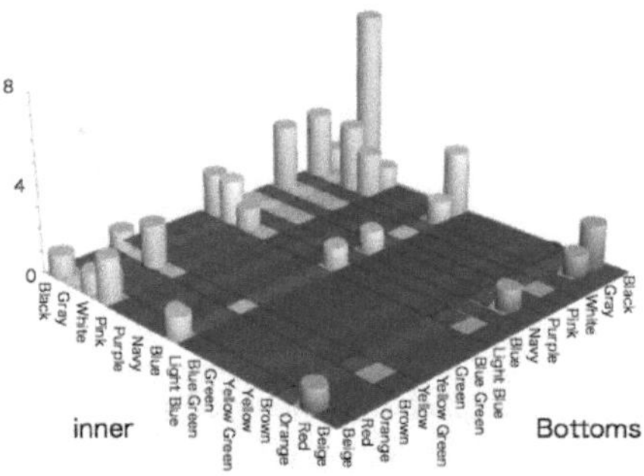

Fig. 2. Histogram of user's worn history(Frequency combination of inner and bottoms)

4 Subject Experiment

4.1 Method of Experiment

We had performed an experiment with two hypotheses. Hypothesis 1: This system's recommendation is useful. Hypothesis 2: By continuing to use the recommendation system user is getting to extend the power of coordination. Experimental period is divided into three period A, B, and A'. In period A and A', subject is asked to decide on its own dress daily by oneself. In period B, subjects are asked to decide it using the system. We checked the wearing history and evaluation questionnaire after these three periods. In order to verify the hypothesis 1, subjects record whether combination it wanted to wear did appear, and what subjects thought at any stage of the recommendation for coordinate system every day. In order to verify 2, we compare the history of clothes worn in each period. Subjects are 2 people, and subject 2 is the author.

4.2 Results of Experiment

In order to validate the hypothesis 1, we searched a wearing log and every day questionnaire in period B. From survey of period B, we got the comment about reason subject decide, such as "I thought it was favorite." and "I thought its tint is good."Since there were many favorite comments, we judged that subjects. However, there are also some non-positive comments such as "It was better than what was recommended in the other." and "I thought no problem." Figure 3 shows average number of clothes recommendation until subject decides to wear. Both subjects decided at the presentation of the four or five times. These numbers are reasonable as a recommendation system.

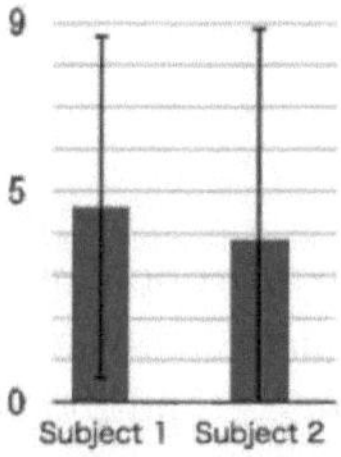

Fig. 3. Number of recommendations until subjects decision

Table 1. How many kinds of coordination subjects wore in each period

	Subject 1	Subject 2
Only Period A	8	14
Only Period B	8	12
Only Period A'	2	12
Both A and B	1	2
Both B and A'	1	3
Both A and A'	3	1
All Periods	1	0

Regarding the hypothesis 2, the clothes that subjects had worn in each period are compared. The questionnaires after the end of the entire period are also surveyed. Table 1 is a comparison of the combination that subjects wore in each period. It shows that which subjects wore how many combinations in which period. There are rather large number of items in period A both subjects, is because the experimental period has been 31 days instead others are 19 and 20. For example, subject 1 wore three sets of combination in both periods A and A'. Since there are slightly more combinations common in period A and A' about subject one, It is not clear whether subject 1 improved its coordination by the system from this data. But, since there are also eight sets that exist only in the period B, we say that subject 1 increased the coordination range when using this system. About subject 2, there are respectively twelve sets in only B period and in only A' period, we judge that subject 2 had realized new possibilities by this system and improved its dress coordination power through the usage of the proposed system.

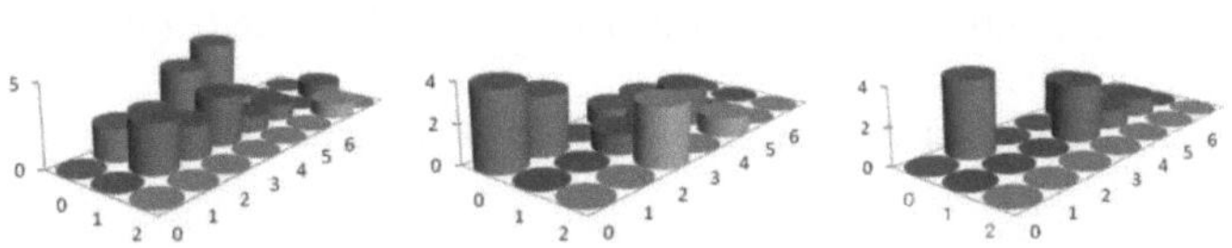

(a) duaration A (b) duaration B (c) duaration A'

Fig. 4. Change of the number of times of clothes worn (Subject 1)

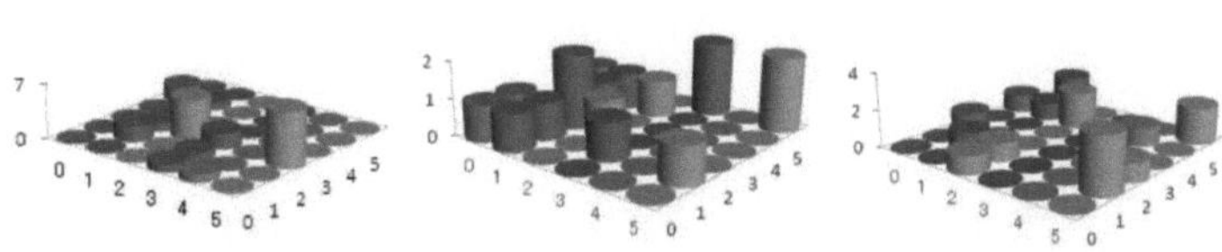

(a) duaration A (b) duaration B (c) duaration A'

Fig. 5. Change of the number of times of clothes worn (Subject 2)

Fig. 4 and Fig. 5 show the number of times of wear of the dress combination in the three periods. The horizontal axes are the identification numbers of the outers (left) and the bottoms (right), and height axis is wearing frequency. It turns out that the places of a mountain, places of the frequently worn combination, was sifted. Especially for subject 2, similar peaks are observed in the period B and A'. It shows that the period B has affected the period A'. It can be said that the proposed dialog strategy is practical and the latitude of the coordinating clothes of users had been expanded.

5 Conclusion

In this paper, we proposed a recommendation system with robot interaction to improve the ability of user's coordination power. We designed the system based on the unique dialog strategy that consists of the blind spot pointing and the chance discovery. The robot also explains the user reasons of the recommendation and the blind spot pointing, user can easily carry out the chance discovery. As a subjective experiment result, it was found that user's dress coordinating power is improved.

References

1. Masuko, S., Myagmarsuren, S., Sakamaki, R.: KiTeMiROOM:Fashion Coordinate System for Online Shopping. In: Interaction 2012, JAPAN EXB-07, pp. 807–812 (2012)
2. Fukuda, M., Yonezawa, Y., Nakatani, Y.: Talkin' Closet: Clothes Recommend Themselves from Their Sales Points. In: Human Interface Symposium 2010, Japan Interactive Presentation 2507, pp. 617–620 (2010)
3. Si, L., Jiashi, F., Zheng, S., Tianzhu, Z., Hanqing, L., Changsheng, X., Shuicheng, Y.: Hi, Magic Closet, Tell Me What to Wear! In: Proceedings of the 20th ACM International Conference on Multimedia, pp. 619–628 (2012)
4. Shimizu, A., Ueda, H.: A System which Determines the Combination of a Dress by a Conversational Robot. In: Human Agent Interaction 2011, Japan III-2A-5 (2011)
5. Shoji, H., Hori, K.: Creative communication for chance discovery in shopping. New Generation Computing 21(1), 73–86 (2003)
6. Ohsawa, Y., McBurney, P.: Chance Discovery. Advanced Information Processing. Springer, Berlin (2011)
7. Konno, N.: Social Innovation Design, Nihon Keizai Shinbun Shuppansha (2007)

Specification of Daily-Life Objects Places for "Tidy-Up" Robotic Service

Weerachai Skulkittiyut[1], Haeyeon Lee[2], Trung Ngo Lam[1], and Makoto Mizukawa[1]

[1] Graduate School of Engineering, Shibaura Institute of Technology
[2] Partner Robot Division, Toyota Motor Corporation
{m710502,m709507,mizukawa}@shibaura-it.ac.jp,
haeyeon_lee@mail.toyota.co.jp

Abstract. In this paper, we focus on the "Tidy-up" robotic service which needs extremely complex and enormous kinds of knowledge about objects, environments, places, and user's status. Especially, we have tried to find the way for specifying of appropriate places of daily-life objects for the "Tidy-up" robotic service. As the first phase, we categorized daily-life objects into three categories: Trashable, Reusable, and Washable. In the specification of an appropriate place, there are two methods: object category based and individual object trajectory based. For the first method, object state machine has been provided for each object category. In the second method, the object trajectories in term of places have been collected. Based on these historical trajectories, we could recognize the trajectory pattern and use it to provide and appropriate place for individual object.

1 Introduction

In this research, we are working on the "Tidy-up" robotic service. Especially, we have tried to find the way for specification of appropriate places of daily-life objects for the "Tidy-up" robotic service. Comparing with "Bring something" service [1] which can be delivered straightforward process, "going to the object's place" → "fetch the objects" → "return to the user's place". However, in "Tidy-up" service, robot needs to decide the way depending on the object's properties, One example is shown in Fig. 1 in which the robot is asked to tidy-up the table. The service requires the robot to perform different tasks with different objects on the table. For example, the books should be brought to bookshelf for storing, and the noodle cup and disposable chopstick should be brought to the trash bin. We have defined three categories of objects that are necessary for the "Tidy-up" service, namely Trashable, Reusable, and Washable. These categories will help to identify the tasks that robot need to do with each object during a "Tidy-up" service scenario. Reusable objects can be returned to their storage area after each use. Washable objects are needed to be washed before returning to storage area. Trashable objects can be trash of directly. The main issue in this research is how automatically specify the appropriate place for each object. In this paper, we propose to use daily-life object properties including categories, usage status and trajectory in term of real-time and historical information to decide and specify an appropriate place for object.

C. Stephanidis (Ed.): Posters, Part II, HCII 2013, CCIS 374, pp. 611–615, 2013.

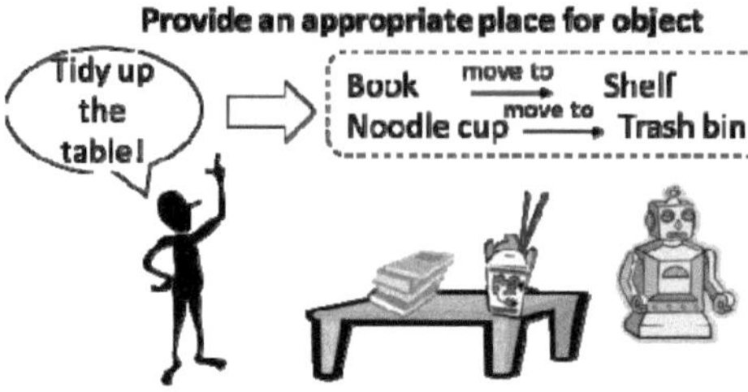

Fig. 1. Example of "Tidy-up" Robotic Service

2 Daily-Life Object Information Management

To provide an appropriate place for "Tidy-up" service, object categories, object usage status and trajectory information is needed. In [2, 3], we proposed a daily-life object information management system to collect, preprocessing and manage the necessary systematically. It has five parts: hardware, software, applications, server and database.

- *Hardware*: RFID reader, RFID tag, ultrasonic transmitter and ultrasonic Receiver attached to receive object ID, object position and usage status information and send it to software layer.
- *Software:* Object information management system has four main modules: object events detection, positioning, and usage status detection and object identification. These modules provide preprocessing raw data that receive from the hardware module then send processed data to the applications layer.
- *Applications:* Appropriate place specification module with object usage status and object position information, this application provided an appropriate place for storing an object or the place to do the next required task. For example, the system will suggest the storing place for the book when we finished read it or suggest the kitchen for used dishes when we finished having lunch.
- *Server & Database:* Server is the center for collecting and processing the data. The database has been used to collect and built the trajectory log.

3 Appropriate Place Specification

Appropriate place specification is a service which automatically provides an appropriate place for individual object based on object current status, place and object type. For the first method, object state machine has been provided for each category of object. In the second method, the object trajectories in term of places have been collected in term of historical data. Based on these historical trajectories, we could recognize the trajectory pattern and use it to provide and appropriate place for individual object.

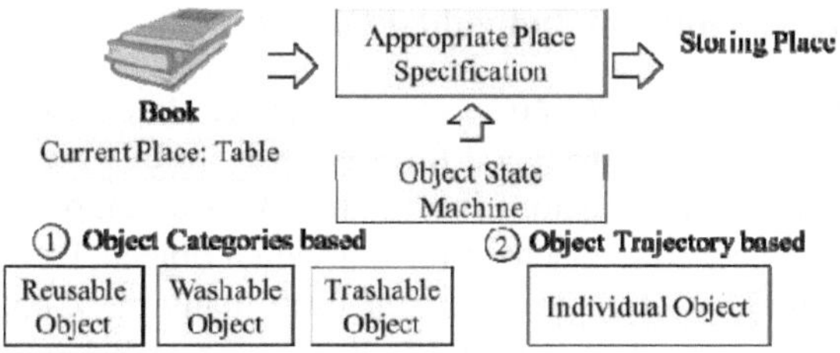

Fig. 2. Appropriate Place Specification Overview

3.1 Object State Machine for Each Category

In this paper, object state machine in terms of place is realized. The following will explain object state machine in detail for each object type.

- **Reusable Object:** A reusable object is an object, equipment or tools in daily life that we can use more than one times e.g. remote control, cell phone. The states of reusable object is most straightforward and have only two state *"Current Place"* After finished the object, or user request appropriate place, the object state change to *"Storing Place"*. Moreover, after the object moved to the *"Storing Place"*, it could be moved to other *"Storing Place"*. Fig. 3a) shows a general state machine of reusable object.
- **Washable Object:** A washable object is an object which could be/ need to be washed e.g. Cup, dish, and towel. The state of washable object consists of "*Current Place*", "*Washing Place*" where represents the place for washing the object, and *"Storing Place"* where represents the place for storing an object. Fig. 3b) shows a general state machine of washable object. The object might be moved to "*Washing Place*" and then moved to "*Storing Place*" or skipped "*Washing Place*" and go to "*Storing Place*" directly.
- **Trashable Object** A trashable object is an object that could be trash. The state of trashable object consists of "*Current Place*", "*Storing Place*" where represents the place for storing the object, and "*Trashing Place*" where represents a place for trashing an object. Fig. 3c) shows a general state machine of trashable object.

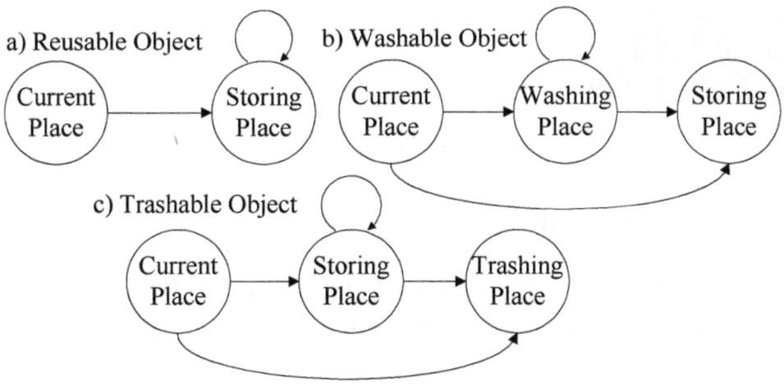

Fig. 3. State Machine of Washable Object

3.2 Object State Machine for Individual Object

In the previous method, we have proposed the object state machine depending on object category. However, it is designed for a general. In this method, the individual properties of the object e.g. trajectory information will be emphasized and used for providing a specific object state machine for individual object. To reduce the effort of collecting the trajectory in a real environment from many participants, the questionnaire approach has been used to ask and collect the real behavior when the users tidy-up the object in the real environment. PrefixSpan [3] algorithm has been used to extract and mining sequential pattern from the answer of the participant. At last, the object state machine for an individual can be build. Fig. 4 shows overview of object state machine building.

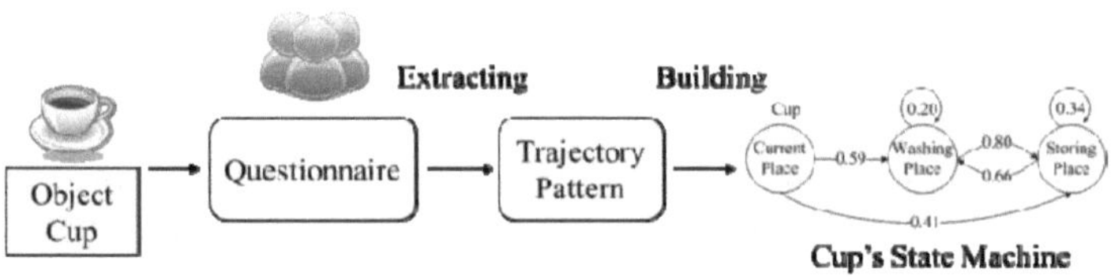

Fig. 4. Building of Object State Machine Overview

1. "Tidy-up" Questionnaire

A questionnaire about "*how users tidy-up the object in a real situation*" has been conducted. As shown in Fig. 5, the questionnaire show the object which put on the table and ask the participant to provide a sequential of place for tidy-up. Participants are freely to choose the sequential of place at from one to three places. The results from questionnaires are the object trajectory and related places. For example in Fig.5, trajectory of the cup from this participant is start from table to dishwasher, sink and finally at shelf; Cup trajectory = table → dishwasher → sink → shelf.

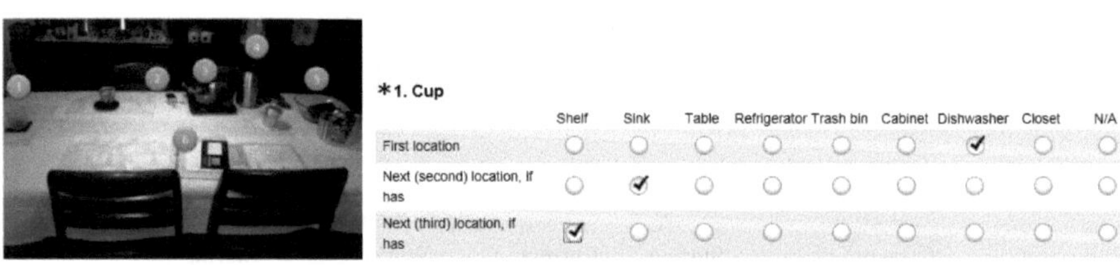

Fig. 5. Example of "Tidy-up" Questionnaire of Cup

2. Extracting Trajectory Pattern

In the second step, the object trajectory of each user will be collect and combined. Using PrefixSpan algorithm [3] we could get the sequential of object trajectory and number of support.

3. Building Individual Object State Machine

In this step, the object state machine would be constructing based on extracting sequential pattern. The places would be merging together based on the place type. Shelf, Table, Refrigerator, Cabinet and Closet are "*Storing Place*", Sink and Dishwasher are "*Washing Place*", and Trash bin is *"Trashing Place"*. For example, sequential pattern Table → Sink, Table → Dishwasher is Table → Washable Place, so we could merge and combine it together. Applying this approach to the entire sequential pattern, we will able to build the object state machine including the transition probability as shown in Fig. 6.

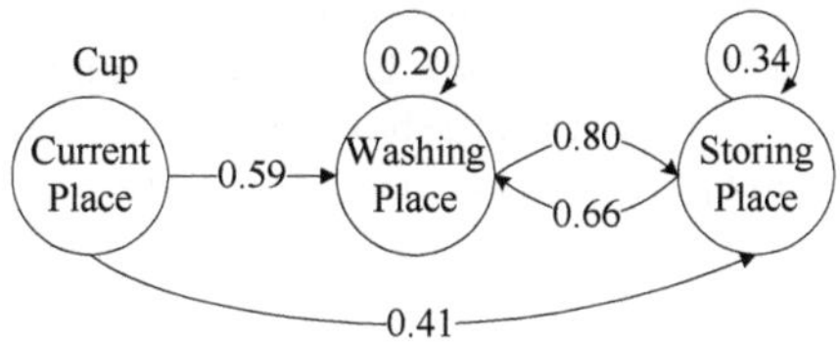

Fig. 6. Object State Machine of Object Cup

4 Conclusion and Future Work

In this paper, we proposed an appropriate place specification method for "Tidy-up" service. We have categorized daily-life objects into three categories namely Trashable, Reusable, and Washable. In the specification of an appropriate place, there are two methods: For the first method, object state machine has been provided for each category of object. In the second method, the object trajectories in term of places have been collected from the questionnaire. Based on these trajectories, we found that the object state machine of individual object was more precise than categories based. It provides a finite state machine including a probability of transition each path. On the others hand, the object state machine for each category describes object state machine in general. The object state machine allows the service robot to know an appropriate place of each object. Our future work will focus on the implementation of "Tidy-up" service in a real experiment with the actual robot system.

References

1. Lam, T.N., Lee, H., Mizukawa, M.: Automatic Building Robot Technology Ontology Based on Basic-Level Knowledge Network. Journal of Roboticsand Mechatronics 23(4), 515–522 (2010)
2. Pei, J., et al.: PrefixSpan: Mining Sequential Patterns Efficiently by Prefix-Projected Pattern Growth. In: Proc. of International Conference of Data Engineering, pp. 215–224 (2001)
3. Skulkittiyut, W., Mizukawa, M.: Daily Life Object Management System in Intelligent Space. In: Third International Conference on Advances in Computer Engineering ACE 2012, pp. 29–34 (June 2012)
4. Mayama, K., Skulkittiyut, W., Ando, Y., Yoshimi, T., Mizukawa, M.: Proposal of object management system for applying to existing object storage furniture. In: 2011 IEEE/SICE International Symposium on System Integration (SII), December 20-22, pp. 279–282 (2011)

Safe Physical Human-Robot Interaction through Sensorless External Force Estimation for Industrial Robots

Axel Vick and Jörg Krüger

Technische Universität Berlin, Department of Industrial Automation Technology,
Pascalstr. 8-9, 10587 Berlin, Germany
vick@iwf.tu-berlin.de
http://www.iwf.tu-berlin.de

Abstract. The presented research work introduces the safe limitation of contact forces between an industrial robot and its human operator during physical collaboration. While estimating these contact forces with a physics algorithm in the robot control software, they can be easily limited before getting harmful. The developed algorithms allow the user to stop and move the robot arm with moderate effort and therefore he feels safe during interaction. Through bypassing and redesigning the position feed-back controllers of the robot, the drive output torques can be held under the critical threshold calculated via Newton-Euler dynamics.

Keywords: human-robot interaction, robot safety, control algorithms.

1 Introduction

Industrial robots can appear in different kinematic and dynamic configurations, however, a six- or seven-degree-of-freedom articulated robot arm type is used for most industrial tasks. Recent research studies concern the collaboration of humans and robots within the industrial field and the related safety issues [1-3]. The collaboration include teach-in programming or workplace-sharing where the human operator touches and pushes the robot. However, the robots are optimized for path accuracy by powerful drives, high gear ratios and stiff controller parameters. Their use for physical human-robot interaction tasks may implicate certain risks for the operators health. As the electro-mechanical construction of an industrial robot is fixed, additional hardware like in [4] or an adaption of the control software is able to decrease the specific risks. The following sections describe the conducted work for conception and implementation of such a control software extension. The results of experiments with an industrial robot system introduces possible applications in human-centered assembly and processing automation [5-7].

C. Stephanidis (Ed.): Posters, Part II, HCII 2013, CCIS 374, pp. 616–620, 2013.

2 Methodology

2.1 Risk Analysis

As recommended by ISO 10218 norm, a detailed risk analysis has been carried out for a standard articulated robot arm to be used for physical human-robot interaction. The most common risks were identified and a strategy for their decrease had been formulated. As a result, the hazards from squeezing, clamping or pushing the human body can be reduced by limiting the exposing force from the robot to a maximum of 150 N and the overall power output to 80 W besides an endeffector speed limit of 0.25 m/s. In case of a collision between human and robot, the robot shall stop moving or give way if neccessary.

2.2 Robot Dynamics Modeling

The fundamental equation for the dynamics of a robot interacting with the environment can be denoted with

$$H(q)\ddot{q} + B\dot{q} + h(q,\dot{q}) + g(q) + \tau_C(\dot{q}) = \tau_q + J(q)^T F_{ext}, \tag{1}$$

where H is a symetric inertia matrix of the composited rigid robot body with dimension corresponding to the robots number of joints $(n \times n)$, B is a diagonal joint damping matrix, h is a nonlinear vector funtion of centrifugal and Coriolis effects, g is a vector of gravitational torques, τ_C is a vector function of Coulomb friction; where for all terms, q is the vector of robot joint positions. The vector τ_q describes the joint driving torques and $J(q)^T F_{ext}$ is the vector of resulting torques from external forces at which $J(q)$ is the Jacobian function $(n \times 6)$ for the robot arm. With

$$\tau_q = \hat{H}(q)\ddot{q}_0 + \hat{B}\dot{q} + \hat{h}(q,\dot{q}) + \hat{g}(q) + \hat{\tau}_C(\dot{q}) + \tau_{pid} \tag{2}$$

the joint driving torques τ_q consist of a feed-forward control torque compensating estimated $(\hat{\cdot})$ robot dynamics and a feed-back control torque τ_{pid}. The estimation model parameters are based on CAD data and dynamic experiments on joint level. The term $\ddot{q}_0$ is the vector of nominal joint accelerations from a path interpolator. With (2) in (1), compensating model uncertainty and the so far unknown external forces F_{ext}

$$\tau_{pid} = -J^T F_{ext} + \varepsilon. \tag{3}$$

Now, even assuming ε to be very small and bounded, the inversion of J^T is difficult for robots with more than six joints and actually ominous for singular configurations.

2.3 External Force Estimation and Limitation

The main goal of the sensor-less force estimation and limitation is to prevent high controller output to be applied to the drives. In sensor-based safety control

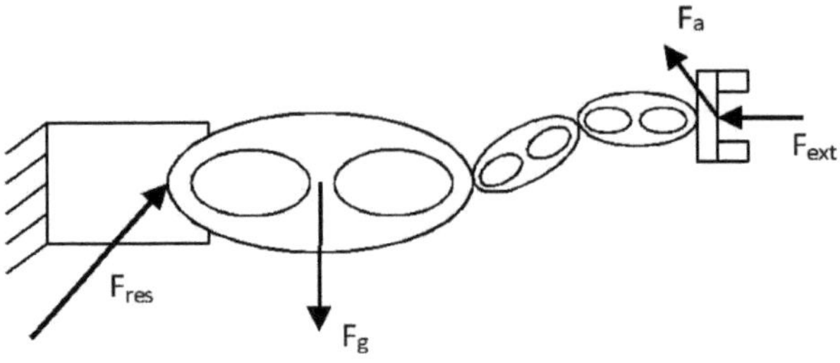

Fig. 1. Robot Reaction Force Scheme

the high forces may taking effect on the environment or the human before they are measured. Very high bandwidth is required to duly detect fast rising forces e.g. in stiff contact situations. The force estimation may be simplified by using an efficient Newton-Euler inverse dynamics scheme. In the considered actual robot arm position, a virtual system dynamic is assumed with zero velocity, zero gravity and virtual joint accelerations $\ddot{q}_v$ from drive torques τ_{pid} via an inverse inertia matrix $\hat{H}^{-1}$ with

$$\ddot{q}_v = \hat{H}^{-1}\tau_{pid}. \tag{4}$$

From $\ddot{q}_v$, the corresponding robot base reaction force F_{res} (Fig. 1) is caculated via the simplified Newton-Euler model

$$F_{res} = \sum_{k=n}^{1} m_k \cdot \sum_{i=1}^{k} e_{i-1}\ddot{q}_{v,i-1} \times l_{i-1} + e_i\ddot{q}_{v,i} \times c_i \tag{5}$$

with l_i and c_i as the joint length and center of gravity. The gravity force F_g is compensated by the feed-forward control. The force F_a from nominal acceleration must not be compensated since all motion should be stopable by external forces. The force $-F_{res}$ then represents the external force F_{ext} at the end-effector or even any other contact point on the robot structure as the actio-reactio relation to the controller output τ_{pid}. The needed constraints for controller output are defined through a scaling proportional to the force excess ratio

$$\tau_{max} = \tau_{pid}\frac{|F_{max}|}{|F_{ext}|} \tag{6}$$

with $|F_{max} = 150N|$. The output torques τ_{max} can then be transformed to motor currents and applied to the robot joint drives. That will result in a limited external force effect.

2.4 Robot Control Algorithms Implementation

The implemented robot control architecture follows the scheme in Fig. 2. The position lag monitoring algorithm (PLM) effects the interpolation (IPO), if a position error maximum is exceeded through external forces, by slowing or stopping

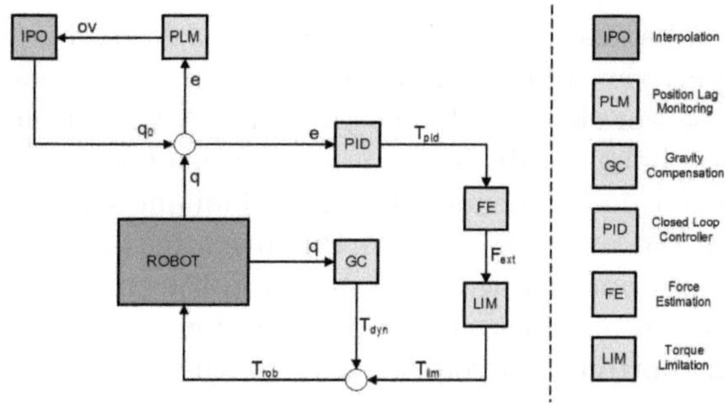

Fig. 2. External Force Estimation and Torque Limitation Scheme

the nominal motion. The dynamic feed-forward control with gravity compensation (GC) compensates non-linearities like gravitational, centrifugal and Coriolis effects. The position control (PID) for the robot joint drives is redesigned with a PID feed-back controller, whose parameters are adjusted to the estimated robot dynamics model. The controller output is used to estimate external forces (FE) and, if necessary, to limit the joint drive torques (LIM) to ensure a safe human-robot interaction.

3 Experiments and Results

The following experiments have taken place with the 7-DOF PISA dual-arm Workerbot [5-6] and a human. In order to evaluate the sensor-less force estimation approach, a force sensor was mounted at the wrist joint. In the first scenario, the robot feed-back control is supposed to hold a position. Meanwhile the human touches the robot two times at any point of the structure with a force of more than 150 N. As expected, the robot can hold the position until the force limit

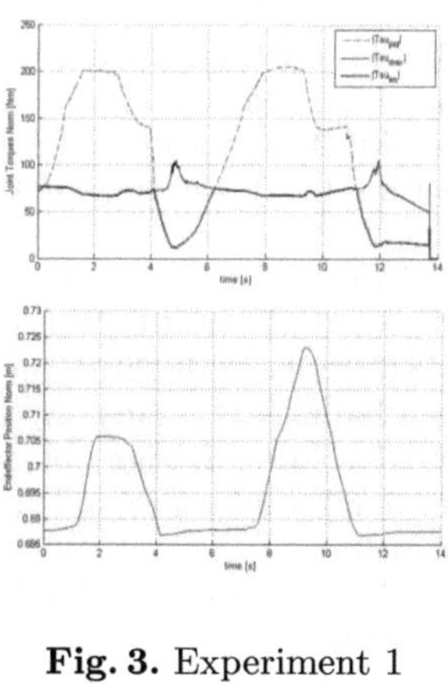

Fig. 3. Experiment 1

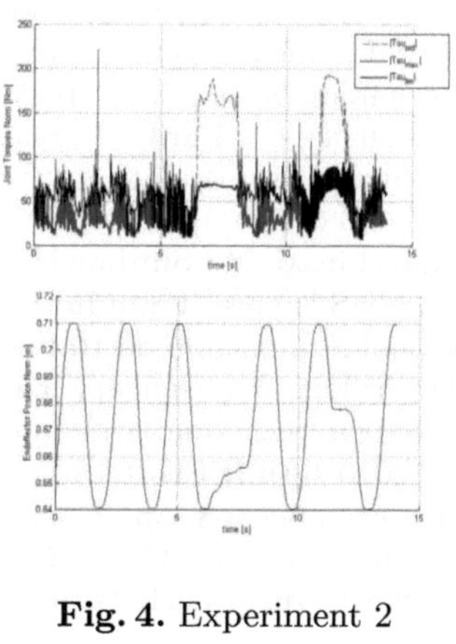

Fig. 4. Experiment 2

is reached and then begins to move away. See Fig. 3 for torque limitation (top) and motion (bottom) view of the first experiment. Measurements with the wrist joint 6-DOF force sensor show the forces under 150 N at all times. In the second test, the interaction behavior during arm motion has been tested (Fig. 4). The robot arm performs a position-controlled sinusoidal end-effector motion, as the human approaches the robot two times. Putting forces higher than 150 N on any point along the robot arm will slow and stop the robot. When the force is reduced, the robot continues the interrupted motion. Again, torques (top) and Cartesian position (bottom) trajectories indicate the expected behavior.

4 Conclusion

The presented robot control architecture allows the combination of position-based trajectory planning and torque limitation through external force estimation. It enhances industrial robots to become safe and highly flexible industrial human-robot interaction systems for collaborative workplace sharing.

Acknowledgment. This research was partially supported by EU IP-Project PISA (Flexible Assembly Systems Through Workplace-Sharing and Time-Sharing Human-machine Cooperation) focused on human-centered assembly concepts and technology (Proj. Nr. 026697-2) and by EU Project ECHORD-RODIN (Robust control of human-robot-environment dynamic interaction for natural stone carving) focused on human-centered processing concepts and technology (Proj. Nr. 231143-10041006).

References

1. Haddadin, S., Albu-Schäffer, A., De Luca, A., Hirzinger, G.: Collision Detection and reaction: A Contribution to Safe Physical Human-Robot Interaction. In: IEEE/RSJ Int. Conf. on Intelligent Robots and Systems (IROS 2008), Nice, France, pp. 3356–3363 (2008)
2. Oberer, S., Schraft, R.D.: Robot-Dummy Crash test for Robot Safety Assessment. In: Proceedings ICRA 2007, Rome, Italy, pp. 2934–2939 (2007)
3. Pervez, A., Ruy, J.: Safe physical human-robot interaction - past, present and future. Journal of Mechanical Science and Technology 22, 469–483 (2008)
4. Duchaine, V., Lauzier, N., Baril, M., Lacasse, M.-A., Gosselin, C.: A Flexible Robot Skin for Safe Physical Human Robot Interaction. In: Proceedings ICRA 2009, Kobe, Japan, pp. 3676–3681 (2009)
5. Krüger, J., Katschinski, V., Surdilovic, D., Schreck, G.: PISA: Next Generation of Flexible Assembly Systems - From Initial Ideas to Industrial Prototypes. In: Proc. of 41st International Symposium on RoboticsISR/ROBOTIK 2010, pp. 84–89 (2010)
6. Surdilovic, D., Yakut, Y., Nguyen, T.-M., Pham, X.B., Vick, A., Martin, R.M.: Compliance control with dual-arm humanoid robots: Design, planning and programming. In: 2010 10th IEEE-RAS International Conference on Humanoid Robots (Humanoids), December 6-8, pp. 275–281 (2010)
7. European Clearing House for Open Robotics Development: RODIN, `http://www.echord.info/wikis/website/rodin`

The Geminoid Reality

Evgenios Vlachos and Henrik Schärfe

Aalborg University, Department of Communication and Psychology,
Nyhavnsgade 14, 9000, Denmark
{evlachos,scharfe}@hum.aau.dk

Abstract. Our society is on the borderline of information era, experiencing a transition towards a robotic one. Humanoid and android robots are entering with a steady pace into our everyday lives taking up roles related to companionship, partnership, wellness, healthcare, and education among others. The fusion of information technology, ubiquitous computing, robotics, and android science has generated the Geminoid Reality. The Geminoid is a teleoperated, connected to a computer network, android robot that works as a duplicate of an existing person. A motion-capture system tracks facial expressions, and head movements of the operator, and transmits them to the robot, overriding at run-time the preprogrammed configurations of the robots actuators. The Geminoid Reality is combining the Visual Reality (users' and robot's point of view) with an Augmented one (operator's point of view) into a new kind of mixed reality involving physical embodiment, and representation, causing the ownership transfer, and blended presence phenomena.

Keywords: geminoid, android, human-robot interaction, reality, presence, teleoperation.

1 Geminoid Android Robots

Androids, due to their anthropomorphic design, are used to facilitate social interaction, and to study the human nature, while geminoids are used as research tools to examine how the presence, the appearance, the behavior, and the personality traits of a robot affects the communication with human partners [1]. The geminoid, coined from the term "geminus" meaning "twin" or "double", and the suffix "-oides" which indicates similarity, is an android robot designed, and developed to resemble an existing person (the Original), envisioned and manufactured by Prof. Hiroshi Ishiguro, ATR Intelligent Robotics, and Kokoro Inc. [1-2]. A geminoid is mimicking the external appearance (the artificial body is of similar proportion), and the facial characteristics of its Original (Fig. 1). Facial characteristics include permanent wrinkles, skin texture, skin coloration, skin pigmentation, bone structure, facial hair, hair coloration, and hair style. It is remotely controlled, with no intelligence of its own, but able to execute pre-programmed sequences of movements (subtle expressed motions such as breathing, blinking emulating the human autonomous system to maintain natural behavior), overridden at run-time by the conscious behavior controller driven by a

C. Stephanidis (Ed.): Posters, Part II, HCII 2013, CCIS 374, pp. 621–625, 2013.

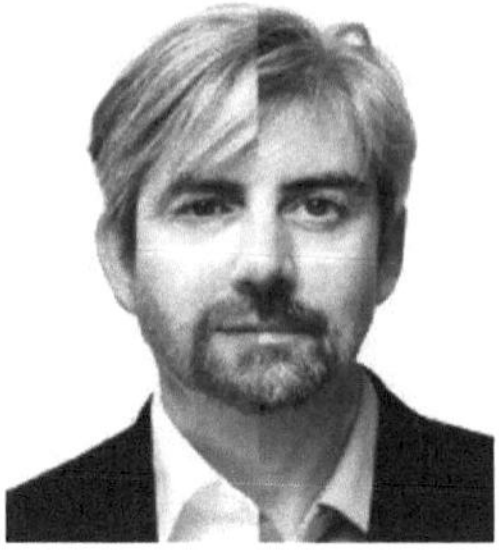

Fig. 1. The Geminoid|DK (left side) with its Original (right side)

motion-capture system that tracks the facial expressions, and head movements of the operator [3-4]. Movement is executed by means of pneumatic actuators inside the robot in all the geminoid versions (HI-1, HI-2, F, DK) [5]. The speech of the operator is also transmitted through the computer network of the geminoid to a speaker located either inside, or around the robot.

1.1 Entering the Realm of Geminoid Reality

While Augmented Reality refers to a real-time direct, or indirect view of a physical real-world environment enhanced with virtual computer-generated sensory [6], and Visual Reality to a constructive process formulated by evolution to guide adaptive behavior [7], the Geminoid Reality (GR) is combining them into a new kind of mixed reality that encompasses physical embodiment, and representation (Fig.2). Being present means readiness to engage, cope, and deal with the surrounding environment, but also ability to witness subjects, objects, and actions, while keeping a record of the witnessed events [8]. In GR, all the intentionality from the surrounding environment is being directed towards the android, but witnessed by the operator through a telepresence system. As long as the GR is in effect, the geminoid with its operator form a symbiont unity which creates a situation akin to mirror-touch synesthesia; a tactile hallucination triggered by observing touch to another person which enables the observer to simulate another's experience by activating the same brain areas [9 – 11]. The illusion of body *ownership transfer* felt by the operator, occurs due to the synchronization between the operation of the robot, and the visual feedback of seeing the geminoid's motion [12].

Apart from the operator, interactions with a geminoid affect also the users. The anthropomorphic appearance of the geminoid tricks the human mind by taking advantage of the same brain mechanisms that human beings use to understand other humans [13]. This conflict inside the human mind describes the notion of the *blended presence*,where the brain fails to categorize an agent that appears human, but moves mechanically. The selectivity of the human action perception system for the appearance and/or motion of a perceived agent was explored using functional magnetic resonance imaging repetition suppression, confirming the blended presence phenomenon [14].

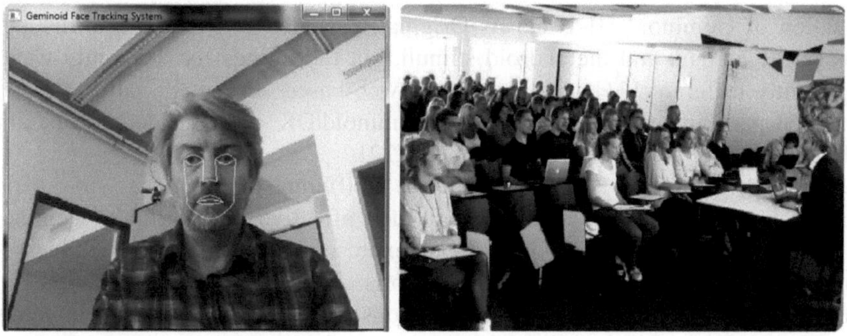

Fig. 2. Left: Augmented Reality (part of the operator's point of view). Right: Visual Reality (users' experience).

2 Interaction Scenarios and Report Evaluation Results

Despite the fact that the GR has been studied mainly inside laboratories, and research environments, its scope is to be gradually integrated into a form of Ubiquitous Intelligence, where technology is deployed in such way that it becomes an invisible part of the fabric of everyday life [15]. Placement of geminoids in real life scenarios enriches our knowledge on human-robot communication, our experience on practical implications, our database on recorded reactions of interaction partners, and our understanding on how the robot is perceived. Extending the use of GR in the real world, an observational field study on unscripted interactions between humans and the Geminoid HI – 1 was conducted in a public café in Linz, Austria, where 43 participants (out of 98), either mistook the robot for a human, or did not notice it at all, as it seemed to appear human-like [16]. Another instance, is when the Geminoid-F was used as an actor in a play, performing live on stage in theatres around the world [17]. The results indicated that androids might be better poetry reciting agents than humans, and that they can span their usage beyond a practical media interface. An experiment on how touch can be used as a way of inducing trust when interacting with an android was conducted in a typical office room, where the Geminoid|DK (in business attire dress code) was proposing a business deal to the participants [18]. Trust towards the robot was increasing when subjects were touching it before the business proposal. The Geminoid|DK also took up the role of a university lecturer and delivered a 45 minute lecture in front of 150 students at Aalborg University [19]. Overall, the robot was accepted as a lecturer, but during the lecture a change of perception regarding the geminoid has been observed. There were strong indicators that females had higher expectation concerning the geminoid's communication skills, raising an issue on the role of the gender of the robot. A noticeable detail was that several students constructed the impression that the lecturer was human, and maintained it till the end of the lecture.

A fact that all experiments share, is that at first sight, and from a distance it is difficult to tell the Original, and the geminoid apart [20]. In a questionnaire for the evaluation of Geminoid HI-1 and its Original, participants were able to distinguish between the human, and the android stimuli, but the ratings for likeability were not significantly different [21]. Additionally, a web-based survey for rating robots (40 robots-151 participants), claimed that the Geminoid|DK was considered to be among the highly likeable and less threatening ones [22].

Different geminoid versions present different limitations in expressing/mimicking/revealing emotions through their affective interface. The Geminoid-F was found to successfully produce facial expressions of Happiness, Sadness, and Neutral Face, but failed in expressing Surprise, Anger, and Fear [20]. Alike, the Geminoid|DK reproduced all six basic emotions, but Fear and Disgust [9]. Geminoid developers should cater to accommodate the need for more actuators around the areas of the nose, the mouth, and the eyes in future geminoid versions, for a more natural, and believable interaction.

3 Conclusion

The Geminoid Reality is a very recently conceived reality, with no formulated and pre-determined boundaries, still under development, since both the field of robotics is expanding, and we -as humans- have not yet unlocked the brain mechanisms that steer our thought, and action. To sum up, the main properties of the GR could be structured around the following two distinct phases towards the robot; ownership transfer from the perspective of the operator, and blended presence from the perspective of the interaction partner.

Whether, or not, the scenarios discussed in this paper will become applications is a matter left to be discovered in the imminent future. The teleoperated, semi-autonomous, portable facility of geminoids, paves the way for many potential uses, making them possible substitutes for clerks, for instance, that can be controlled by one human operator only when non-typical responses are required [2]. Today, we count very few geminoid robots, located in very few research laboratories around the world, scattered in different continents, facts that impose a very slow pace in the GR research in contrast to other kinds of reality.

References

1. Ishiguro, H., Nishio, S.: Building artificial humans to understand humans. Journal of Artificial Organs 10(3), 133–142 (2007)
2. Nishio, S., Ishiguro, H., Hagita, N.: Geminoid: Teleoperated Android of an Existing Person. In: de Pina Filho, A.C. (ed.) Humanoid Robots, New Developments, pp. 343–352. Intech (2007)
3. Sakamoto, D., Kanda, T., Ono, T., Ishiguro, H., Hagita, N.: Android as a telecommunication medium with a human-like presence. In: Proc. of the 2nd ACM/IEEE Int. Conf. on Human-Robot Interaction, pp. 193–200. IEEE Press (2007)
4. Nishio, S., Ishiguro, H., Anderson, M., Hagita, N.: Representing Personal Presence with a Teleoperated Android: A Case Study with Family. In: Proc. of the AAAI 2008 Spring Symposium on Emotion, Personality, and Social Behavior, pp. 96–103. AAAI (2007)

5. Hiroshi Ishiguro Laboratory, `http://www.geminoid.jp`
6. Carmigniani, J., Furht, B.: Augmented Reality: An Overview. In: Furht, B. (ed.) Handbook of Augmented Reality, vol. 1, pp. 3–46. Springer, LLC (2011)
7. Hoffman, D.D.: The Construction of Visual Reality. In: Blom, J.D., Sommer, I.E.C. (eds.) Hallucinations: Research and Practice, pp. 7–15. Springer, LLC (2012)
8. Turner, P.: An everyday account of witnessing. AI & Society: Special Issue: Witnessed Presence 27(1), 5–12 (2012)
9. Vlachos, E., Schärfe, H.: Android Emotions Revealed. In: Ge, S.S., Khatib, O., Cabibihan, J.-J., Simmons, R., Williams, M.-A. (eds.) ICSR 2012. LNCS, vol. 7621, pp. 56–65. Springer, Heidelberg (2012)
10. Blom, J.D., Sommer, I.E.C.: Hallucinations of Bodily Sensation. In: Blom, J.D., Sommer, I.E.C. (eds.) Hallucinations of Bodily Sensation, vol. 2, pp. 157–169. Springer US (2012)
11. Banissy, M.J., Ward, J.: Mirror-touch synesthesia is linked with empathy. Nature Neuroscience 10(7), 815–816 (2007)
12. Nishio, S., Watanabe, T., Ogawa, K., Ishiguro, H.: Body Ownership Transfer to Teleoperated Android Robot. In: Ge, S.S., Khatib, O., Cabibihan, J.-J., Simmons, R., Williams, M.-A. (eds.) ICSR 2012. LNCS, vol. 7621, pp. 398–407. Springer, Heidelberg (2012)
13. Gazzola, V., Rizzolatti, G., Wicker, B., Keysers, C.: The anthropomorphic brain: The mirror neuron system responds to human and robotic actions. NeuroImage 35(4), 1674–1684 (2007)
14. Saygin, A.P., Chaminade, T., Ishiguro, H., Driver, J., Frith, C.: The thing that should not be: predictive coding and the uncanny valley in perceiving human and humanoid robot actions. Soc. Cogn. Affect Neurosci. 7(4), 413–422 (2012)
15. Hsu, C.H.: Ubiquitous Intelligence and Computing: building smart environment in real and cyber space. J. of Amb. Intel. Human. Comp. 3(2), 83–85 (2012)
16. Pütten, A.M.V.D., Krämer, N.C., Becker-Asano, C., Ishiguro, H.: An android in the field. In: 6th ACM/IEEE Intl. Conf. on Human-Robot Interact, pp. 283–284. IEEE (2011)
17. Ogawa, K., Taura, K., Ishiguro, H.: Possibilities of Androids as Poetry-reciting Agent. In: The 21st IEEE International Symposium on Robot and Human Interactive Communication, pp. 565–570. IEEE (2012)
18. Dougherty, E.G., Scharfe, H.: Initial Formation of Trust: Designing an Interaction with Geminoid-DK to Promote a Positive Attitude for Cooperation. In: Mutlu, B., Bartneck, C., Ham, J., Evers, V., Kanda, T. (eds.) ICSR 2011. LNCS, vol. 7072, pp. 95–103. Springer, Heidelberg (2011)
19. Abildgaard, J.R., Scharfe, H.: A Geminoid as Lecturer. In: Ge, S.S., Khatib, O., Cabibihan, J.-J., Simmons, R., Williams, M.-A. (eds.) ICSR 2012. LNCS, vol. 7621, pp. 408–417. Springer, Heidelberg (2012)
20. Asano, C.B., Ishiguro, H.: Evaluating facial displays of emotion for the android robot Geminoid F. In: 2011 Work. on Affec. Comput. Intell. (WACI), pp. 1–8. IEEE Press (2011)
21. Bartneck, C., Kanda, T., Ishiguro, H., Hagita, N.: My Robotic Doppelgänger – A Critical Look at the Uncanny Valley. In: The 18th IEEE Intern. Symp. on Robot and Human Interactive Communication, pp. 269–276. IEEE Press (2009)
22. Pütten, A.M.V.D., Krämer, N.C.: A survey on robot appearances. In: 7th ACM/IEEE Intern. Conf. on Human-Robot Interact. (HRI 2012), pp. 267–268. IEEE Press (2012)

Remote Controller for Regression Test in the Robot Framework

Ziyuan Zhang[1], Haoran Guo[2], and Heng Wang[3]

[1] Peking University, School of Software and Microelectronics, China
zhangziyuan@pku.edu.cn
[2] Nanyang Technological University,
Wee Kim Wee School of Communication and Information, Singapore
hguo004@e.ntu.edu.sg
[3] Peking University, School of Electronics Engineering and Computer Science, China
hw@pku.edu.cn

Abstract. Robot framework is an open source efficient test automation framework. Regression test is an expensive but necessary maintenance activity on modified software. Although robot framework supports test suite and can generate straightforward test report and log. However, deployment of robot framework on various testers' computer is expensive and time-consuming. In addition, testers may only use the framework in specific project because they could focus on other test technology on other projects. It is also hard to manage test reports and logs because test work can take place in the same or different place at the same or different time under the label Computer Support Cooperative Work. In this paper, we design and implement a tool called Remote Controller to solve problems existed in the robot framework. To demonstrate the usability of the Remote Controller for research and design, we use Remote Controller to explore the cost saving in different projects: Enterprise Architecture and Relay loader.

Keywords: Remote Controller, Computer Supported Cooperative Work, Human-Computer Interaction.

1 Introduction

Regression testing is a major task of software maintenance and it accounts for more than one-third of its total costs [1].

Robot framework is an efficient test automation framework for regression testing. Because remote controller can provide very simple keywords to create user cases and straightforward test report and log, and its remote library interface enables distributed testing and implementing test libraries in any programming language [2].

Computer Supported Cooperative Work (CSCW) provides a lot of advantages including work together asynchronously without the concern of geographic restraints [3], and also the end-to-end support of communication, collaboration, and coordination tasks [4].

C. Stephanidis (Ed.): Posters, Part II, HCII 2013, CCIS 374, pp. 626–629, 2013.

And for regression test work, it can take place in the same or different place at the same or different time.

Shareholders with different backgrounds such as users, testers and DBAs need to execute test together or check the test reports and logs.

In this paper, we design and implement a tool called Remote Controller to help people communicate, collaborate and coordinate in the robot framework (Figure 1).

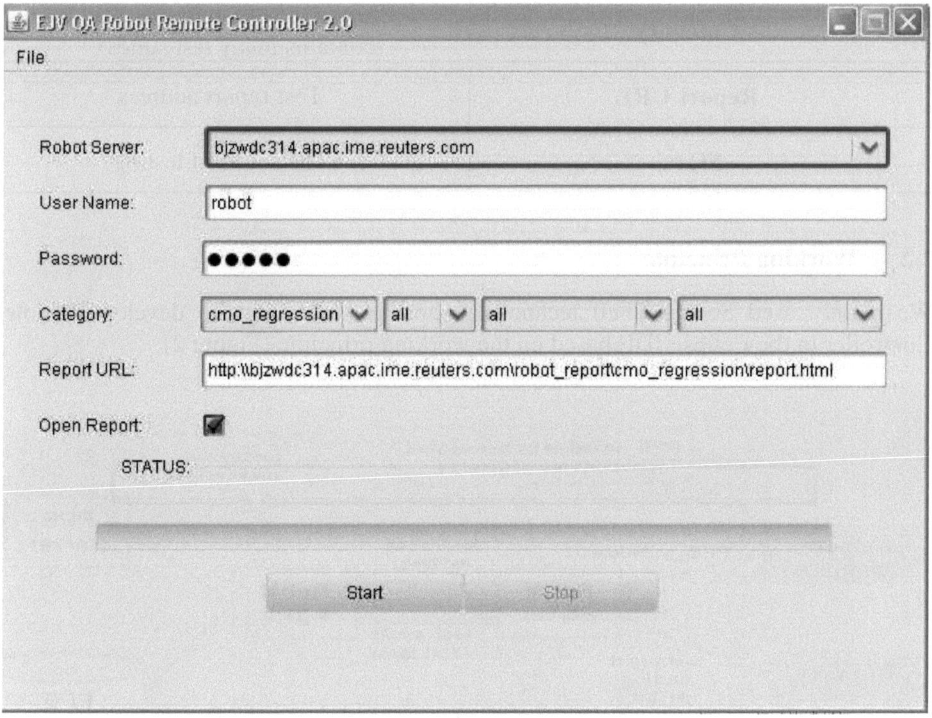

Fig. 1. Remote Controller

We use Remote Controller to explore if it can also bring about major cost savings to companies in many projects and allow employees to work at home by eliminating the need for travel, rented office space, parking, and electronic office equipment [5].

2 The Approach to the Research

2.1 Functions Design

We design the Remote Controller based on the Table 1.

Table 1. Details of Functions Degisn

Robot Server	Remote server, on which you want to execute the test
User Name	User name for the server
Password	Password of the user
Category	Choose the test suite (or a folder contains many test suites)
Report URL	Test report address
Status	The status of testing

2.2 Working Principle

We mainly used Secure Shell technology, apache technology to develop Remote Controller in the Eclipse IDE based on the working principle (Figure 2).

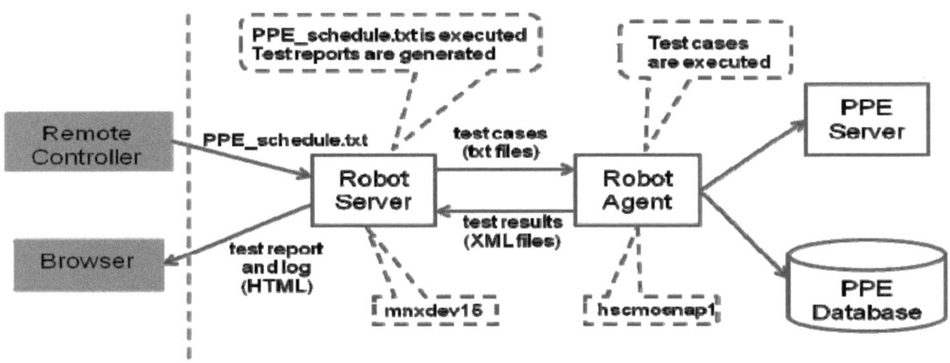

Fig. 2. Working Principle of the Remote Controller

Human-computer interaction design of Remote Controller is accessible to all testers. The operation of the Remote Controller is very easy but has following powerful features:

1. upload test suite to the remote server
2. execute test on the remote server
3. display the status of test
4. save test report and log in remote specified server path and check them locally
5. support both windows server and Linux server.

3 Preliminary Results

We use the Remote Controller in two regression test projects: Relay loader and Enterprise Architecture to explore the usability of the tool and the testers involved in two projects are 11 and 15.

We show that the there is an obvious change in the cost saving (Table 2).

- Depend on times of regression (N)
- Depend on count of web tools need to do regression test

Table 2. Cost Saving

Category	Regression Web Tool	Cost if not change	Cost after improved	Saving
Simplification	Relay Loader	3 Man Hr	4 mins	3 * N Man Hr N * 178 RMB
	Enterprise Architecture	4 Man Hr	6 mins	4 * N Man Hr N * 238 RMB

References

1. Tao, C., Li, B., Gao, J.: A Systematic State-Based Approach to Regression Testing of Component Software. Journal of Software 8(3), 560–571 (2013)
2. Google Project Hosting, https://code.google.com/p/robotframework/
3. González-Ibáñez, R., Haseki, M., Shah, C.: Understanding effects of time and proximity on collaboration: implications for technologies to support collaborative information seeking. In: Proceedings of the 2012 ACM Annual Conference Extended Abstracts on Human Factors in Computing Systems Extended Abstracts, pp. 1805–1810. ACM (2012)
4. Grudin, J., Poltrock, S.E.: Taxonomy and theory in Computer Supported Cooperative Work. In: Kozlowski, S.W.J. (ed.) The Oxford Handbook of Industrial and Organizational Psychology. Oxford University Press, New York (2012)
5. Wikipedia, http://en.wikipedia.org/wiki/Computer_supported_cooperative_work#cite_note-19

Part X
Smart Environments

Participate: Pervasive Computing for Environmental Campaigns

Alan Chamberlain[1], Dominic Price[1], Martin Flintham[1], Kevin Glover[1], Chris Greenhalgh[1], Steve Benford[1], Andy Gower[2], and Amanda Gower[2]

[1] University of Nottingham, Jubilee Campus, Wollaton Road, Nottingham, UK
firstname.lastname@nottingham.ac.uk
[2] BT (Adastral Park, Martlesham, Ipswich, Suffolk, UK
andy.gower@BT.com

Abstract. Participate was a three year collaboration between industry and academia to explore how mobile, Web and broadcast technologies could combine to deliver environmental campaigns. In a series of pilot projects, schools used mobile sensors to enhance science learning; visitors to an ecological attraction employed mobile phones to access and generate locative-media; and the public played a mobile phone game that challenged their environmental behaviours. Key elements of these were carried forward into an integrated trial in which participants were assigned a series of environmental missions as part of an overarching narrative that was delivered across mobile, broadcast and Web platforms. These experiences use a three-layered structure for campaigns that draw on experts, local groups and the general public, who engage through a combination of playful characterisation and social networking.

1 Introduction

This short paper aims to give a whistle-stop tour of the Participate project. At the turn of the 21st century we have become involved in a global debate about the nature and impact of climate change and our role as individuals and societies in managing this. To pursue this debate we must address three key challenges. We need to gather information about the environment on a greater scale than ever before, including scientific measurements, documentation of local conditions and accounts of people's behaviours [1]. We need to inform debate by conveying environmental knowledge in new ways that engage the widest possible audience. Ultimately, we will also need to persuade people to change their behaviour. Pervasive computing has the potential to play a unique and vital role in addressing these challenges. Networks of wireless sensors can gather data on an unprecedented scale, while millions of mobile camera phones can annotate scientific measurements with documentation of local environmental conditions [2][3]. Context-aware computing [4] can deliver environmental information in situ, engaging people at the most appropriate times and locations. Finally, a new generation of mobile experiences such as pervasive games that are interwoven with the patterns of daily life and our location may reach new audiences,

C. Stephanidis (Ed.): Posters, Part II, HCII 2013, CCIS 374, pp. 633–637, 2013.

encourage them to participate, and persuade people to reflect on and change their behaviours. In short, we believe that pervasive computing can ultimately engage millions of people in mass participation environmental campaigns, raising awareness of environmental issues, supporting education, activism and democracy [5], and delivering environmental data on a scale never before possible. The literature demonstrates the breadth and depth of the research, relating to the new and rapidly evolving fields of pervasive, persuasive computing and their application to environmental-behavioural change [6].

2 Participate

There is an established history spanning more than twenty years of 'big science' projects in the UK in which broadcasters encourage the nation to gather data that is then distilled and fed back though television programmes. For example, the BBC's annual Springwatch TV series harnesses the reach of television to recruit hundreds of thousands of people to record the first signs of spring in their gardens, each contributing to an evolving national map of climate change. The emergence of pervasive computing can greatly enhance such campaigns by enabling the public to document the world about them in far richer detail, while also delivering analysis to them in context, directly enhancing their understanding of a particular place or activity. Building on this tradition, Participate was a UK project that brought together broadcasters (BBC), telecommunications companies (BT), computing companies (Microsoft), artists (Blast Theory) and Universities (Nottingham) to explore the potential of pervasive computing to support widespread participation in environmental campaigns. Our collective aim was to explore how the convergence of mobile, online and broadcast media might enable a broad cross-section of the public to contribute to, as well as access, environmental information – on the move, in public places, at school and at home. We followed the approach of 'research in the wild' in which iterative public trials and observational studies of emerging technologies inform the generalisation of broader concepts and platforms. In the early stages of the design-cycle of the project we consulted with institutions such as the World Wildlife Fund and used information provided from the Energy Savings Trust in order to further understand the issues associated with behavioural change in regard to environmental issues. Throughout the design-cycle we also fed in the feedback that arose from the each of the trial stakeholders. We briefly discuss two of our first iterations that related complemented in different settings (Stories@Kew and Prof Tanda), while the second iteration drew these together into an integrated cross-platform campaign called Bicker Manor.

3 Stories@Kew

A way to engage people with environmental issues is through visitor attractions, which champion environmental themes. The Royal Botanical Gardens at Kew in London is one such attraction, combining a leading research centre working at the forefront of conserving plant life worldwide with a major public attraction set in 300 acres of parkland. This provided the setting for our second trial, in which we explored how visitors could use mobile phones to access and create location-based media. Stories@Kew invited members of the public to explore Kew Gardens and discover bundles of media virtually located at key Points of Interest (POIs) distributed throughout the park. On discovery of a POI participants were able to view professionally created editorial material as well as user-generated content (UGC) from previous visitors, after which they were asked a question and prompted to publish their own stories in return. Two systems were trialed. Our 'low tech' approach used a Nokia 6630 mobile phone, a physical map and signage placed at each POI location. Once a user had made their way to a POI using the provided map they keyed in the number displayed on the signage in order to access the relevant media. This system also used a third party GPRS media communications service provided by Shozu to upload user-generated videos to a specified email account that was monitored by the production team. Our 'high tech' used a Nokia N73 paired with a TomTom GPS receiver. Approximately 130 groups trialed Stories@Kew. Our observations, interviews and questionnaires revealed that both the editorial media and UGC engaged users. Although UGC was generally accessed less than the editorial content, participants were typically still able to recall a favourite user generated video clip. We found that being able to view others' content was an important part of the creative content generation process, with participants referencing others' videos before creating their own responses.

4 Professor Tanda

Our second early trial focused on engaging individuals as they went about their daily activities rather than in the specific context of a classroom or visitor attraction. We created a context-aware game for mobile phones called Prof. Tanda's Guess-A-Ware [7] that attempted to build a picture of the player's environmental behaviour over a period of several weeks, inviting them to reflect on or even change their daily routines and to understand what explicitly motivated people to participate in environmental campaigns such as this. Prof Tanda is a character that lives on a player's phone and interacts with them for just a few minutes each day, asking them to answer questions, perform a task or share an activity with nearby people. He will typically initiate contact once a day, although players are free to contact him more frequently if they wish. He is portrayed, in a cartoon style, as being entertainingly egocentric; a quirky character who combines serious questions with playful ones, is obviously well informed about the environment, and yet is not infallible and is shown to have somewhat suspect tastes. His aim was to entertain players while also informing and provoking them, but without being patronising or preachy. Sessions exist such as Prof Tanda instructs a player to measure the amount of water they consume when taking a shower. The key to activities such as this is delivering them in context; that is at those moments when players will be able to engage in them (e.g., at home in the early morning when they might be ready to take a shower). Consequently, the game also gathers context information to inform decisions about how to schedule activities for individual. The initial trial involved 30 players over two weeks, with feedback being gathered through questionnaires and system logs of interactions. In general, players reported enjoying their interactions with Prof Tanda, especially the use of humour and the way in which he engaged them in local activities: an aspect of the game that they would like to see expanded in future.

5 Bicker Manor

We carried forward the lessons we had previously learned into a final integrated trial called Bicker Manor whose goals were to: engage participants through narrative and character; encourage and direct them to undertake a wide variety of environmental activities, from casual information gathering to more significant experiments and interventions; and enable them to generate, contribute and share their own documentation of these activities. Bicker Manor was driven by an overarching narrative in which a fictitious family named 'the Bickers' provided the back-story for the experience and enabled players to share a common goal. Each member of the Bicker family had their own perspective on climate change. Michaela, the teenage daughter, guided participants into the experience and provided an overall and relatively neutral commentary on events, including showcasing the 'best of' user generated content. She introduced the campaign as a contest between her parents, Eve and Isambard, who offer directly contrasting lenses through which to view environmental issues. Initially, Michaela asks the public to "Pick a side. Will you pick my mum Eve with her green evangelist views or my Dad Isambard with his thrifty green sceptic ways? It's up to you to decide." When participants first sign-up to take part they are asked to choose either Eve or Isambard as their host character. Their choice directly influences their overall experience, as it affects the missions offered to them and the feedback they receive. At the heart of Bicker Manor are missions, the core unit of activity from which the narrative is built. Eve and Isambard set various missions that invite participants to engage in activities such as answering questions, taking photos or making videos. Daily Mini Missions maintain ongoing engagement through lightweight activities that can be completed almost immediately. In contrast, Mega Missions are set every four days or so and involve undertaking and documenting more significant challenges. Missions were delivered across three platforms: Web, mobile and Internet Protocol Television (IPTV) as shown in. The website was at the core of the experience and provided full functionality, enabling participants to respond to and complete all missions, view and rate user generated content, and manage their profile and friends lists. Participants were also encouraged to register their mobile phone, after which they could respond to missions via SMS and MMS, including uploading images and videos.

6 Conclusion

Participate's varied trials have demonstrated a multiplicity of approaches to public campaigns, environmental or otherwise, which might potentially involve many different kinds of participant and technology. Based on this experience, we propose a 'three layer' approach to structuring participation in such campaigns that focus upon the public, local groups and experts. We suggest that a successful environmental campaign needs to engage all three layers and develop synergistic relationships between them, as exemplified by our pilots. We have also explored various factors that might motivate these different participants to engage. Social interaction is clearly a great potential motivator, as seen in phenomenal spread of social networking applications such as Myspace or Facebook, YouTube and others over recent years, and reflected in our pilots through the popularity of sharing data and media with friends and groups.

Acknowledgments. This work was supported by the EPSRC and TSB. We would also like to thank the BBC, BT and Microsoft Research for their input into the project, and acknowledge the Challenge of Widespread Ubiquitous Computing EP/F03038X/1 for allowing us to expand upon our research into the project.

References

1. Burke, J.A., et al.: Participatory sensing. Presented at the World Sensor Web Workshop. ACM Sensys, Boulder (2006)
2. Honicky, R., et al.: N-smarts: networked suite of mobile atmospheric real-time sensors. Presented at the Proceedings of the Second ACM SIGCOMM Workshop on Networked Systems for Developing Regions, Seattle, WA, USA (2008)
3. Mainwaring, A., et al.: Wireless sensor networks for habitat monitoring. Presented at the Proceedings of the 1st ACM International Workshop on Wireless Sensor Networks and Applications, Atlanta, Georgia, USA (2002)
4. Schilit, B., et al.: Context-Aware Computing Applications. In: IEEE Workshop on Mobile Computing Systems and Applications, Santa Cruz, CA, US (1994)
5. Joki, A., et al.: Campaignr: A Framework for Participatory Data Collection on Mobile Phones (December 18, 2007), `http://repositories.cdlib.org/cens/wps/770`
6. Froehlich, J., et al.: The Design of Eco-feedback Technology. Presented at the ACM Conference on Human Factors in Computing Systems, Atlanta, GA, USA (2010)
7. Chamberlain, A., et al.: Professor Tanda: greener gaming & pervasive play. Presented at the Proceedings of the 2007 Conference on Designing for User Experiences – ACM DUX 2007, Chicago, Illinois (2007)

Changing Interactions to Reduce Energy Consumption: Specification of a Context-Aware System Centered on the Home Occupants' Concerns

Myriam Fréjus[1], Michele Dominici[2], Frédéric Weis[2], Germain Poizat[3], Julien Guibourdenche[4], and Bastien Pietropaoli[2]

[1] EDF Research & Development, Clamart, France
myriam.frejus@edf.fr
[2] INRIA/IRISA, Rennes, France
firstname.lastname@inria.fr
[3] University of Geneva, 40 Geneva, Switzerland
germain.poizat@unige.ch
[4] University of Lyon, Bron, France
guibourdenche@hotmail.com

Abstract. This paper presents the specification of a context-aware system dedicated to assist home occupants in their everyday life while reducing their energy consumption. The system behavior and the interaction are built upon the definition of "situation spaces" based on a prior definition of the contexts of activity from the point of view of each actor in the home, i.e. taking into account actors' concerns. The interaction specification appears to be a way to manage the discrepancy between users' concerns and the system context, which can reduce errors. To develop context-aware systems that can easily be appropriated and thus potentially "invisible," we believe it is essential to articulate choices about architecture and interaction with models of individual-collective activities built upon real-life observations.

Keywords: Context-aware computing, user-centered design, sustainability, ambient computing, interaction design.

1 Introduction

Our research lies at the intersection of ambient computing and sustainability research. It differs from approaches that seek to reduce energy consumption in the home by influencing people and changing their behavior. Instead, we are working to use context-aware computing to assist home occupants and reduce energy consumption without necessarily requiring intentional actions to achieve this goal. Harris and Cahill referred in [8] to context-aware power management.

Research in the social sciences indicates that energy consumption is not a behavior, but is rather the result of behaviors whose purpose is not generally related to energy savings. Individual activity at home is constituted of multiple lines of different

C. Stephanidis (Ed.): Posters, Part II, HCII 2013, CCIS 374, pp. 638–642, 2013.

concerns which structure the involvement in the activity [7]. However depending on conditions in which the activity occurs, the potential concerns relative to energy management may not be actualized and produce energy control actions. Thus we aim to design a technical system that will take over part of the responsibility for reducing energy consumption, contributing to build sustainable human-environment interactions, and especially sustainable situations; that is, both from householders' points of view (not affecting their activities) and from a sustainable perspective (saving energy).

However, designing context-aware systems to reduce energy consumption implies a prior definition of the contexts in which power management must be implemented in order to guarantee "relevant" actions from the system. According to Dey and Abowd [3], "a system is context-aware if it uses context to provide relevant information and/or services to the user, where relevancy depends on the user's task". This definition links the system actions to those of the user. But ambient computing marks a radical break regarding the user context that needs to be taken into account. The context is no longer the classic conception of machine use, as the "user" is quite likely to be interacting with a computer system while being engaged in a completely different activity. We believe that the design of context-aware systems must be based on a prior definition of the contexts of activity from the point of view of each actor in the home. However, activity models often show that human activity is very complex and that the underlying contexts are difficult to determine [7]. Yet from a system point of view, contexts must be defined by measurable values. If the system context and the human (subjective) context cannot be fully brought together, it is nevertheless vital to assess this discrepancy so that the system can respond in a relevant manner.

This discrepancy between human and machine contexts prevents the system from being fully automatic. However, direct interaction with the user must be limited so as not to be perceived as bothersome. This raises the question of how to strike a balance between automation and direct interaction. In the case of implementing systems for energy management, the system behavior should facilitate the action (ensure light and heating) and energy efficiency (no overuse), but without the need to be initiated by the users, who do not necessarily see themselves involved in interaction [4]. In such a situation, the dynamic transition between the different types of interaction is a key issue to promote invisible use, which allows users to focus on the objective of their activity. System invisibility is not necessarily physical disappearance or having an implicit nature. An invisible system refers to a system that has been appropriated and incorporated into daily practices [6].

2 Presentation of the Implemented System

Our approach required the constant articulation of competence in the fields of cognitive ergonomics and ambient computing. It was structured by a series of steps, presented in the following sections, each of which was instrumental in developing an initial prototype for the home.

2.1 Modeling Domestic Activities

To anticipate the design of future services and context-aware systems, we have developed a research program to analyze home activities in real-life situations and produce models useful for design over several years. Our analysis is based on an initial observation of domestic activities (continuous video recordings of activities, post-recording interviews), transcribed and processed in order to grasp the meaning each occupant gave to his or her own activity. Our results show the different characteristics of collective activities in domestic settings, with implications for the design of ubiquitous technologies, see for ex. [10], [7].

These studies also show that activity at home is constituted of multiple lines of different concerns. Inhabitants manage several activities at the same time with several underlying concerns, which take part in their individual context. For example, someone involved in cooking in the kitchen may also listen to a radio broadcast and be concerned by keeping an eye on a child, waiting for a phone call, and intend to watch a TV show later. A concern can be interrupted in favor of another and be reopened later (for ex. stop cooking to go to see the child, leaving the cooking activity "opened"). In this situation some appliances are still on without necessity (lights, radio) while others (stovetop) must not be necessarily turned off because the activity is paused and not closed.

We used our prior activity analysis to point out the relevant behavior of a context-aware system for typical situations (for ex. not turning off the stovetop but providing distant interaction to remotely take over the unattended stovetop). Then, during the specification phase, it was possible to link an action / non-action of the system with its identification of a situation on the basis of measured values from simple sensors.

2.2 Defining a Technical Architecture to Infer Human Actor's Involvement

We developed an architectural model likely to respond to our objectives and constraints [5]. This model was inspired by the four-layer architectural model suggested by Coutaz and al. [2]. In order to foster the acceptability and adoption of the system by real households, we imposed some constraints on the equipment (no wearable technologies, choice of sensor that minimize privacy concerns, no video cameras, no information about the identity of the occupants). The sensor data (pressure, motion, sound…) are first interpreted into a higher, domain-relevant concept, such as whether a room is occupied. This higher-level concept is called context. Contexts are then combined to infer the occurrence of situations, which are abstract states of affairs of interest to the applications.

The context and situation modeling and reasoning framework we adopted is called context spaces theory [9]. According to this theory, basic contextual information like the presence of a person or the status of an appliance is called a context attribute and is modeled as a dimension in multidimensional space. The values of context attributes are provided either by augmented appliances or as an outcome of sensor data fusion, performed using Belief Functions Theory (also known as Dempster-Shafer or evidence theory [11]). The situation spaces, which model real-life situations, are subspaces defined over regions of acceptable values of selected context attributes. For instance, the situation space "sleeping" can be modeled as the combination of the fact that a person is in a room and that he or she is seated or lying down. The occurrence of situation spaces, detected by reasoning on the runtime context attribute values, provides evidence of the involvement of an actor in some activity. We do not aim to model the reasons underlying the real-world situations. We instead model the particular conditions that solicit a particular action (for ex. regulating the heating). Thus, the same real-world situation can be modeled by different situation spaces and result in different behaviors from the system.

2.3 Defining Services and Designing Interaction

The activity analysis identified the actions that could be assigned to an adaptive ambient system either because they are a help to the flow of activities and/or because they are of interest from an energy point of view, for ex., turning the lights on/off automatically or providing a means to interact through existing interactive devices.

The discrepancy between the system knowledge and the inhabitants' concerns is taken into account during the definition of the system actions for each type of situation. Depending on the detected situation, three modes of contextual interaction are proposed as a way to manage the consequences of the discrepancy: incidental, direct, and direct-incidental.

Incidental interaction is implemented using established clues to automate certain actions: presences/absences, the occupability criterion (rooms near the scene of ongoing activities are considered as more likely to be occupied than others). Depending on the level of confidence attributed on these dimensions, it is possible for the system to act alone, after a time frame to be sure that the action has to be done. We also introduced "mid-level actions": switching off the TV screen but leaving the sound...

When the situation is considered undecidable or potentially dangerous, the system must let the user act. In our previous example, where a stovetop is left switched on while the user is in another room (situation space "monitor cooking"), there is no automatic switching off of the stovetop because it is impossible on the basis of the available information to decide between an oversight (i.e. a dangerous situation) and deliberate action (i.e. leaving a meal to simmer). A direct interaction is presented on the interactive devices in the rooms being occupied (uncertainty about who is the actor).

We also introduced the notion of direct-incidental interaction as a way to anticipate that two concerns might become concurrent, for ex. talking over the telephone while the radio is on. The system must let the users decide whether to mute the radio. It is indeed not possible to ask the user whether to turn off the radio and then allow him or her to answer the call. It is achieved by modifying the phone interface to provide a further action: answer the phone AND turn off the radio.

To these three forms of interaction provided by our script, we can add the direct non-contextual interaction. The user is free to put the entire home, certain rooms, or certain appliances into "auto" mode: this mode means that actions to turn appliances on or off will be performed automatically [10].

2.4 Building Sustainable Situations

We implemented and experimented our distributed architecture, where contextual information is processed by several entities in a collaborative fashion. The system functionalities (automatic actions, provision of information, interaction with users) are carried out by distributed devices and augmented appliances. Every device and augmented appliance runs an implementation of context spaces theory [1] and the resulting functionalities. For this reason, the devices are designed to self-operate in a situation-aware manner, minimizing their energy consumption while preserving user comfort.

3 Contributions and Perspectives

This first implementation was made for a set of situations extracted from real life. We succeeded in taking into account real collective activity and combining criteria to assist human activity with criteria to reduce energy consumption. However, we now need to consolidate the system and widen the situations to test it in real situations and assess the achievement of its appropriability and invisibility.

References

1. Boytsov, A., Zaslavsky, A.: ECSTRA – Distributed Context Reasoning Framework for Pervasive Computing Systems. In: Balandin, S., Koucheryavy, Y., Hu, H. (eds.) NEW2AN 2011 and ruSMART 2011. LNCS, vol. 6869, pp. 1–13. Springer, Heidelberg (2011)
2. Coutaz, J., Crowley, J.L., Dobson, S., Garlan, D.: Context is key. Commun. ACM 48, 49–53 (2005)
3. Dey, A.K., Abowd, G.D.: Towards a better understanding of context and context-awareness. In: Gellersen, H.-W. (ed.) HUC 1999. LNCS, vol. 1707, pp. 304–307. Springer, Heidelberg (1999)
4. Dix, A.: Beyond intention - pushing boundaries with incidental interaction. In: Conf. Building Bridges: Interdisciplinary Context-Sensitive Computing (2002)
5. Dominici, M., Fréjus, M., Guibourdenche, J., Pietropaoli, B., Weis, F.: Towards a System Architecture for Recognizing Domestic Activity by Leveraging a Naturalistic Human Activity Model. In: ICAPS 2011 « GAPRec » Workshop (2011)
6. Dourish, P.: What we talk about when we talk about context. Personal and Ubiquitous Computing 8(1), 19–30 (2004)
7. Fréjus, M., Guibourdenche, J.: Analysing domestic activity to reduce household energy consumption. Work 41, 539–548 (2012)
8. Harris, C., Cahill, V.: Exploiting User Behaviour for Context-Aware Power Management. In: Proc. Wireless and Mobile Computing, Networking And Comm., vol. 4, pp. 122–130 (2005)
9. Padovitz, A., Zaslavsky, A., Loke, S.W.: A Unifying Model for Representing and Reasoning About Context under Uncertainty. In: Proc. IPMU (2006)
10. Poizat, G., Fréjus, M., Haradji, Y.: Ergonomics at home: Contribution to the design of a smart home lighting Service. In: Proc. AHFE, Advances in the Human Side of Service Engineering. CRC Press (2012)
11. Shafer, G.: A Mathematical Theory of Evidence. Princeton University Press, Princeton (1976)

Designing of Face Image Processing Technique for Sorting Out Japanese Raccoons Form Raccoons

Tadasuke Furuya[1], Yayoi Kaneko[2], Hiroaki Ishii[2], and Takafumi Saito[2]

[1] Tokyo University of Marine Science and Technology
tfuruya@kaiyodai.ac.jp
[2] Tokyo University of Agriculture and Technology
txsaito@cc.tuat.ac.jp

Abstract. To observe mode of life of wild animals, it needs to research individual animal continually. We have to capture these animals temporarily. We need to capture them safely, of course, without hurting them. In general, we make use of traps and capture wild animals. Automation and remote-control operation which monitor traps are needed to reduce costs such as labor costs related to capture for long periods of time. For this reason we developed new type of traps that is possible of remote monitoring and remote operation over the network. Furthermore, we try to recognize face image toward automatic discrimination. In this study, we explain about preprocessing that face recognition is needed.

Keywords: animal trap, mobile telephone, non-photo realistic.

1 Introduction

To observe mode of life of wild animals, it needs to research individual animal continually. We observe mode of life of Japanese raccoons and raccoons at the present day. Therefore, we have to capture these animals temporarily. We need to capture them safely, of course, without hurting them. In general, we make use of traps and capture wild animals. However, there are roughly five problems about the capture by this trap.

These are 1)capture of error, 2)well-being of captive animals, 3)security of workers, 4)misclassification of captive animals, 5)high cost related to maintenance of traps. Recently, utilization of traps which have an effect of preventing capture of error, for example, egg traps and traps with a trigger of preventing by catch is carried forward. Automation and remote-control operation which monitor traps are needed to reduce costs such as labor costs related to capture for long periods of time.

2 Trap

In this study, we developed new type of traps (Fig.1) that is possible of remote monitoring and remote operation over the network.

C. Stephanidis (Ed.): Posters, Part II, HCII 2013, CCIS 374, pp. 643–646, 2013.

This trap carries communications device (Fig.2), mobile network, IP camera and remote door open system. We operate from browsing software like general pc and cellular phone over the network and take images in the trap. We can also monitor and remote-control the door of the trap open. After opening the door, it is possible to reset the trigger (Fig.3).

We indicate specifications of controlled box. We set cages at distant place and check connection of networks. When animals enter the cages, we receive notice by twitter. We check images of our cellular phone, then we open the cages if we capture animals excepting for raccoons. It is often difficult for distinguishing animals for the reason that captured images are small or are not bright etc. Also, we sometimes cannot send high-quality images in succession for the reason of communications line velocity or camera memory shortage. So, we generate images that humans can understand shot animals in a short time on condition that there are a small number of images, contents are not recognized and brightness is not controlled. Furthermore, a system that automatically recognize what kind of animal it is among pictures of animal's faces and automatically open cages is expected. It is difficult for us to recognize faces of animals shot outside. Then, in this study, we consider preprocessing toward recognition.

The trap makes us possible to detect captured animals at an early date, deal with the matter appropriately and prevent them from injuries and weakness. We can also simultaneously monitor several traps in a remote location and decrease frequency of going in for a look-around. Therefore, it leads to cost reduction of labor costs. In addition to this, it is possible for a few specialists to monitor several regions and several traps at one time. Then, they can discriminate among captured animals. In the end, the trap leads to the prevention of killing captured individuals by mistake.

Moreover, if the starting time we operate the traps can be shorten, wild animals are less affected by the stress.

To realize this, it is needed to the equipment which is classified faces of animals and automatically let go of animals that we don't want to observe. In this study, we consider the method of image processing related to distinguish Japanese raccoons from raccoons.

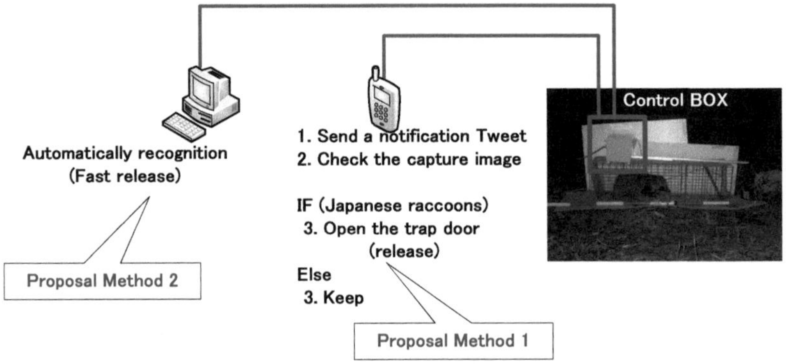

Fig. 1. Trap system

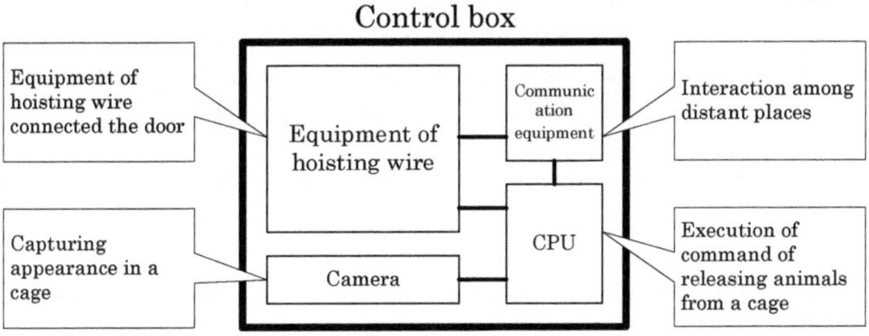

Fig. 2. Control Box

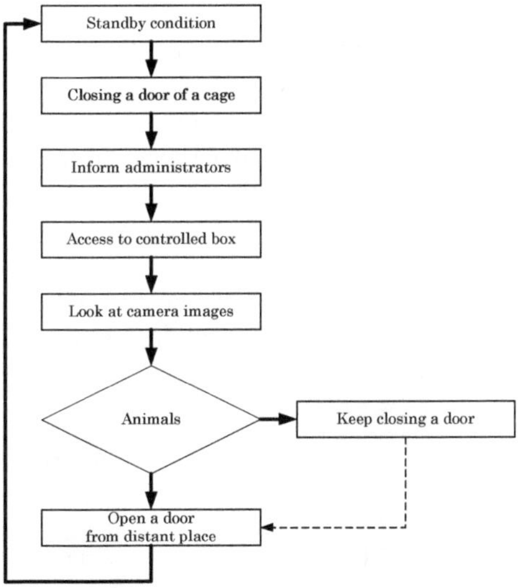

Fig. 3. System Flow

3 Proposed Method

It is difficult to extract a part of feature from faces of animals covered with fur. The images pictured outside aren't also available images to judge animals sufficiently. Under the conditions, it is needed to emphatically display the figure of faces. Generally, space filter and concentration conversion are often utilized. In this method, though processing speed to combine with easy image processing is fast, it is difficult to express the images sophisticatedly due to manipulate all of the images uniformly. So, we consider examine the environment for the usage of the trap, and examine the method independent of lighting condition without interactive operation.

It is hard to use color information of shooting images because the animals made the color of their fur change with the seasons. In addition it is difficult to judge whether a part of shooting images is pattern or shadow. Then, we make rough texture information and images we can recognize the direction of their fur.

In this study, we attempt to emphasize distinctive line of the animals through the use of multi scale analysis. By combining with several variously-sized Gaussian filters, we do frequency decomposition and recombine weight for each band-pass images, then we control systematic level of detail at each band.

1. Generation of gray-scale images from captured images(Fig.2,5) and normalization brightness value
2. Generation of different scale of smoothing images
3. Acquisition of band images from difference of neighboring scale of smoothing images
4. Addition of adequate bias value
5. Mapping on adequate brightness coverage from obtained brightness value

In this method, we generate the composite images that leave quite characteristic of the animals clearly and detail characteristic of them. At this time, we make out two types of images that change the rule of weight. We read the features of Japanese raccoons and raccoons through these two types of images. Generally speaking, raccoons contain a black line between their eyebrows, on the other hand, Japanese raccoons don't contain that. The verge of raccoon's ears also is white, but that of Japanese raccoon's ears is black. From an examination of image processing, we can understand their characteristics which are displayed from the composite images. We can also obtain the stable consequence without depending on lighting conditions.

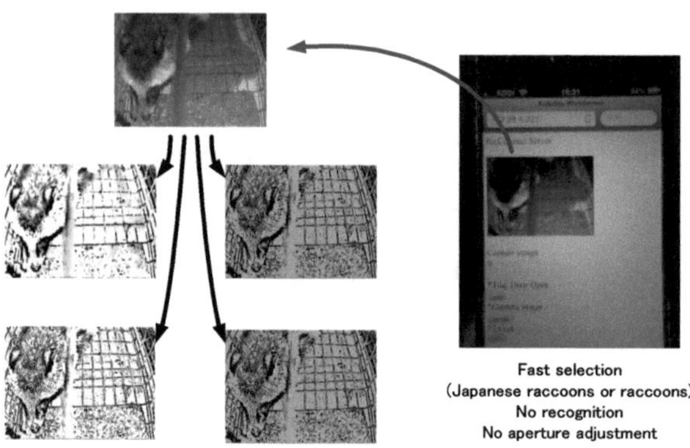

Fig. 4. Cellular phone screen

4 Conclusion

For the future, we try to automatically select face of raccoons and that of Japanese raccoons by extracting the features of their eyes, nose and mouth from images based on this method or by mapping on the characteristic space.

Infoscope: A Mobile Device Supporting Exploratory and Playful Knowledge Discovery in Physical Environments

Dimitris Grammenos

Institute of Computer Science, Foundation for Research and Technology – Hellas (FORTH), N. Plastira 100, Vassilika Vouton, GR-70013 Heraklion, Crete, Greece
gramenos@ics.forth.gr

Abstract. Infoscope is a novel mobile device that can support knowledge discovery and exploratory playing in physical environments. More specifically, Infoscope utilizes RFID technology to provide audio guiding and localized question / answer games and employs wireless communication technologies to exchange information about its user's interests with computer platforms in order to present through them related supplementary multimedia information. The device comes with two accompanying software components: one for editing / updating its contents, and one running on personal computers for providing supplementary multimedia information. Infoscope has been evaluated and tested as a museum guide and as a knowledge discovery toy for toddlers.

Keywords: Interactive museum guides, knowledge discovery toys, RFID device, Ambient Intelligence.

1 Introduction

The development of small-sized, low-cost RFID (Radio Frequency Identification) readers gave rise to their broad spread and use in combination with various types of mobile devices. RFID technology is currently used for supporting a wide range of applications, ranging from inventory management systems to museum guides and smart toys. RFID readers usually come as add-ons for personal computers, laptops and mobile devices, but a more recent technological trend dictates the integration of NFC (Near Field Communication) technology, which builds upon and extends earlier RFID systems, to smartphones. Additionally, there are several specialized mobile devices comprising RFID reading capabilities, which are mainly targeted to asset management, thus essentially complementing or replacing barcode scanners.

In practice, RFID technology constitutes a very efficient and cost-effective means for building interactive context-aware tools that support "physical browsing" [1], effectively allowing users to easily identify and retrieve digital information through physical objects and places. Two application domains where physical browsing is highly useful and can have considerable impact are: (a) electronic guides for museums and exhibition areas [e.g., 2; 7; 10]; and (b) mobile learning (e.g, [8]). In both domains, R&D efforts related to "physical browsing" can be broadly classified in two categories according to the technological approach followed:

C. Stephanidis (Ed.): Posters, Part II, HCII 2013, CCIS 374, pp. 647–651, 2013.

1. Software applications installed on general-purpose mobile computing platforms (e.g., mobile phones, PDAs, tablets); e.g. [2; 5; 7; 10].
2. Specialized devices that, following the Tangible User Interfaces paradigm [6], are explicitly designed for the task at hand; e.g. [9; 10].

Some of the disadvantages of the first category include that: (a) since the devices are not optimized for the task, they often suffer from several ergonomic and usability problems; (b) unless special precautions are taken, their users may (intentionally or not) gain access to basic device functionality (and e.g., become lost, or even alter its contents); (c) if RFID reader components are not seamlessly integrated, they can easily become detached, lost or stolen. The main disadvantage of the second category is that existing systems are mostly research prototypes offering no particular precautions or tools regarding their day to day use in a real setting (e.g., power consumption considerations, power charging procedure) or content management (e.g., adding, updating, editing). Up to now, none of the existing systems in both categories allows its users to collect information that can be browsed later on.

In addition to the above, mainly in the domain of museum guides, there has been a long-lasting "modality debate" between those supporting audio-only information provision and those opting for augmentation though multimedia, on the basis of a possible antagonism between the actual exhibits and the digital information [4; 5]. On the one hand, audio has the advantage of allowing users to look at objects while listening to description without making visual demands on their attention and not forcing them to context-switch between looking at the device and the location [11]. Furthermore, multimedia guides offer multiple choices raising problems of use, dividing the users according to their skill with portable devices [3]. On the other hand, multimedia guides can offer much richer and stimulating information, even overlaid on the real environment (e.g., augmented-reality approach [4]).

2 Infoscope

Infoscope is a wireless mobile device that can read, transmit and reproduce digital information. Infoscope integrates RFID reading capabilities and can play related

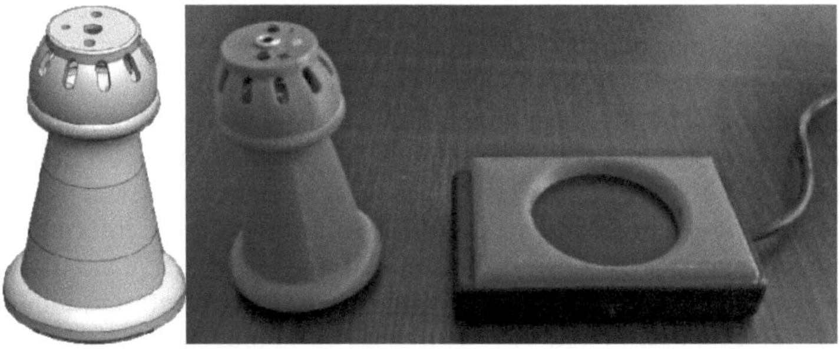

Fig. 1. Left: Infoscope industrial design (OBI industrial design patent 6003410) Right: Fully working prototype and docking station

audio information which can be adapted to its user's profile (e.g., language, age, interests). The device is embedded in an ergonomically-designed shell (Fig. 1) the industrial design of which has already been patented by the Hellenic Industrial Property Organization, while the related invention patent is currently pending.

The outer shell of the device is modeled after the shape of the earphone of antique phones. On its top side there are two buttons which are used for adjusting the audio level, a standard 3.5mm headphone jack socket and a color led providing visual feedback, e.g., when audio is playing there is a green flashing light, and when the battery level is critically low there is a constant red light. The device also integrates a small speaker allowing headphone-free use (e.g., when multiple users are sharing it). A strap can be easily adjusted around the "neck" of the device, so that it can be securely fastened around the arm or neck of its user.

Infoscope is extremely easy to use, as it mimics the use of a typical doctor's stethoscope. When a user is interested into a specific item, all she has to do is to put the device over a related RFID tag in order to listen to a corresponding audio description. Additionally, by "listening to" appropriate tags (see Fig. 2), the user can adapt the audio descriptions to her personal profile traits (e.g., language, age group. interests). RFID tags are inexpensive, highly durable and come in various shapes and sizes, allowing them to be easily integrated in diverse environments and even on (or inside) most objects (e.g., books, furniture, devices, toys). Beyond localized information presentation, Infoscope supports exploratory gaming in physical environments through question / answer games, where a tag is used to trigger a question (which is adapted to the user's profile) that has to be answered by "listening to" the tag of the corresponding place / item.

Infoscope can keep track of the RFID tags detected in each session, the order and number of times that each one was read, as well as of the answers given to the "question" tags. All this information is wirelessly transferred to a docking station, which is also used for charging the device (Fig. 3 left). The docking station communicates with an interactive application, which is installed at its host computer and can present user-profile-adapted multimedia material related to the tags read by the device, as well as the game's score and detailed information about each user's answer. Thus, this approach can provide a novel hybrid solution to the "modality debate" mentioned in the previous section.

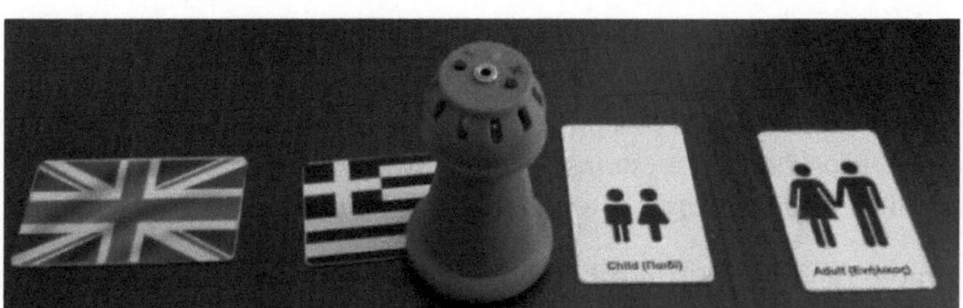

Fig. 2. Setting the user's profile by "listening to" appropriately marked RFID tags

Setting up a space supporting knowledge exploration through Infoscope is extremely easy, fast and does not require any type of physical intervention. All it takes is to just (temporarily or permanently) attach a number of RFID tags in appropriate places. Another nice feature is that there can be multiple tags referring to the same piece of information, thus allowing access to it through diverse locations (e.g., at different heights for adults and children, or people in wheelchairs, replicated tags for crowded points of interest). New tags can be easily added to the system using a visual interface (Fig. 3 right) which supports the management and editing of the actions and profile-adaptable information triggered by it.

Infoscope can be used in various application domains where location-based knowledge discovery is needed. Up to now three "generations" of fully functional prototypes have been created and the fourth is currently under way. Each successive prototype builds upon its predecessor, improving it in terms of usability, functional, and technical characteristics, based on the results of experimental use, evaluation and testing with representative users in two application domains: (a) museum guides and (b) knowledge discovery toys for toddlers and young children.

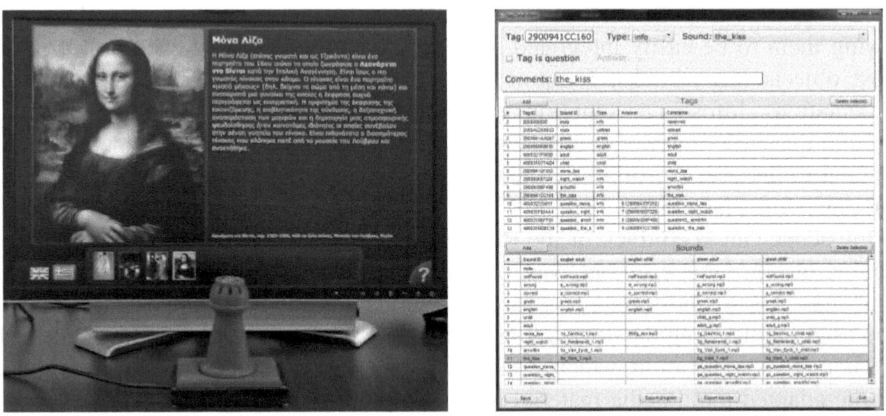

Fig. 3. (left) Docking Infoscope to its station for retrieving multimedia information. (*right*) Content editing software.

3 Conclusions

Infoscope constitutes a novel approach in the domain of mobile location-based retrieval and presentation systems, which overcomes shortcomings of previous approaches, also offering some new capabilities. Its main advantages include:

- Very simple (and playful) use by people of all ages, not requiring any experience or familiarity with computer technologies.
- Ability to retrieve information adapted to the user's profile.
- Easy and fast installation in any space, without any physical interventions.
- Does not distract the user's attention away from the objects of interest.

- "Remembers" which items were accessed by the user, and in cooperation with a personal computer can provide additional information.
- Small, lightweight, highly durable device.
- Innovative, ergonomic and functional design.
- Very low power consumption levels.
- Easy editing, update and extension of its content.
- Ability to change the shape of its shell, so that it fits the aesthetics and ambience of the environment where it is being used.
- Low production cost.

Up to now, the experimental use of a fully functional prototype for supporting knowledge-discovery tasks in various settings with representative end-users of various ages has shown that Infoscope has the potential to claim its own ground in the dynamically expanding universe of everyday mobile devices.

Acknowledgments. This work has been supported by the FORTH-ICS RTD Programme "Ambient Intelligence and Smart Environments". Special thanks to Athanasios Toutountzis and Nikolaos Pateromichelakis for their contribution to the development of the Infoscope prototypes.

References

1. Ailisto, H., Plomp, J., Pohjanheimo, L., Strömmer, E.: A Physical Selection Paradigm for Ubiquitous Computing. In: Aarts, E., Collier, R.W., van Loenen, E., de Ruyter, B. (eds.) EUSAI 2003. LNCS, vol. 2875, pp. 372–383. Springer, Heidelberg (2003)
2. Aoki, P.M., Grinter, R.E., Hurst, A., Szymanski, M.H., Thornton, J.D., Woodruff, A.: Sotto voce: exploring the interplay of conversation and mobile audio spaces. In: CHI, pp. 431–438 (2002)
3. Barbieri, G., Celentano, A., Orsini, R., Pittarello, F.: Understanding Art Exhibitions: From Audioguides To Multimedia Companions. In: Int. Conf. on Distributed Multimedia Systems, pp. 250–255 (2009)
4. Damala, A., Cubaud, P., Bationo, A., Houlier, P., Marchal, I.: Bridging the Gap between the Digital and the Physical: Design and Evaluation of a Mobile Augmented Reality Guide for the Museum Visit. In: DIMEA, pp. 120–127 (2008)
5. Ghiani, G., Paternò, F., Santoro, C., Spano, L.D.: UbiCicero: A location-aware, multi-device museum guide. Interacting with Computers, 288–303 (2009)
6. Ishii, H., Ullmer, B.: Tangible Bits: Towards Seamless Interfaces between People, Bits and Atoms. In: CHI, pp. 234–241 (1997)
7. Mäntyjärvi, J., Paternò, F., Salvador, Z., Santoro, C.: Scan and tilt: towards natural interaction for mobile museum guides. In: Mobile HCI, pp. 191–194 (2006)
8. Sánchez, I., Cortés, M., Riekki, J., Oja, M.: NFC-based interactive learning environments for children. In: IDC, pp. 205–208 (2011)
9. Tanenbaum, K., Tanenbaum, J., Antle, A.N., Bizzocchi, J., El-Nasr, M.S., Hatala, M.: Experiencing the reading glove. In: Tangible and Embedded Interaction, pp. 137–144 (2011)
10. Wakkary, R., Hatala, M.: Situated play in a tangible interface and adaptive audio museum guide. Personal and Ubiquitous Computing, 171–191 (2007)
11. Woodruff, A., Aoki, P.M., Hurst, A., Szymanski, M.H.: Electronic Guidebooks and Visitor Attention. In: ICHIM (1), pp. 437–454 (2001)

Spot-Light: Multimodal Projection Mapping on Food

Yui Kita[1] and Jun Rekimoto[1,2]

[1] Interfaculty Initiative in Information Studies, The University of Tokyo, 7-3-1 Hongo, Bunkyo-ku Tokyo, 113-0033 Japan

[2] Sony Computer Science Laboratories, Inc. 3-14-13 Higashigotanda, Shinagawa-ku Tokyo, 141-0022 Japan

yuikita21@gmail.com, rekimoto@acm.org

Abstract. Spot-Light is a projection mapping system for foods that enriches dishes by projecting images or sounds on foods. Tastes of foods are constructed not only with simple gustation, but also with appearances and sounds. For better appearances, ordinary cooking methods such as food coloring agents or crunching sounds of pie contribute to modify these food properties. However, it is not possible to purely modify them because all ingredients are inevitable from chemical interruptions into the original food. Our system enhances these properties by visual and sound projection with a RGB camera, a depth camera, a parametric speaker and a projector.

Keywords: Food, Projection Mapping, Kitchen.

1 Introduction

1.1 Cross-Modality on Dinning

Appearances and sounds are important on a dinning experience as well as gustation. For example, some soft drinks provide various flavors only by visual difference although they contains mostly same ingredients. Professional chefs often use extra colors in recipes to modify the food appearances. For example, a recipe uses paprika's red as an additional color when using apple mint: the red color reminds guests the apple flavor which complements weak aroma of the apple mint. Thus, our resulting gustation is effected by prior perceptions (the effect is widely studied as cross-modality [1]). This suggests that modifications on appearances and sounds are effective to enrich the original dish.

2 Spot-Light

Spot-Light is a system that enhances such modalities. The system is in the shape of a desk light. For multimodal projections, a RGB camera, a depth camera, a parametric speaker and a projector are attached on the head part of the system. There are three functions in this system. The first function is to emphasize the surface color of the dish (for example, the saturation of green salad or browning of steaks). It uses a RGB

C. Stephanidis (Ed.): Posters, Part II, HCII 2013, CCIS 374, pp. 652–655, 2013.

camera and a depth camera for a precise projection mapping. The second function is to emphasize the sounds of the dish (for example, the crisply sound of baked pies or sounds of breaking a caramel of crème brûlée) so that it reminds guests extra rich textures of food. The third function is to project additional animations (for example, melting butters or surface shines).

We describe details of these functions and potential functions below.

2.1 Appearance Augmentation for Food Coloring

Chefs create better perceptions for foods by designing the food surface. As we mentioned above, the designing of the appearance is one of the designing process of gustation because the visual perception largely effects to the gustatory sensation.

Coloring is the basic of visual designing of food. The ordinary method to modify the color is to use natural or artificial colorings. However, there are some health risks when using these colorings. In addition, there are also limitations on their effects because they contain chemical materials that unexpectedly affect the original taste of food itself.

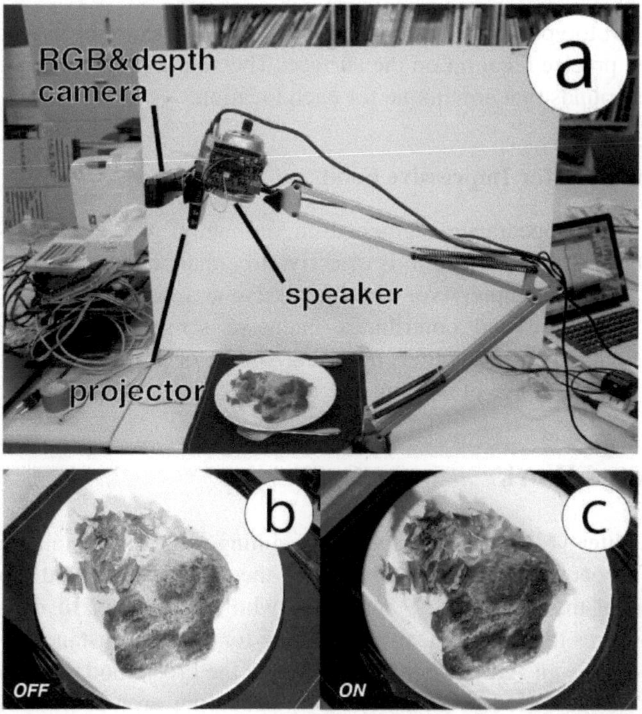

Fig. 1. Spot-Light consists of devices for multimodal projection mappings on the head part of a desk light (a). b and c shows the comparison of food's appearance without appearance augmentations (b) and with augmentations (c). The system first capture the RGB and depth image of the dish, and projects images that was processed so that it maximize the parts that effects positive gustation (for example, the saturation of green salad or browning of steaks).

Spot-Light captures a RGB image of the dish, and projects modified images on it after processing the image so that it maximize the food's appearances. This function enables us to coloring the food without taking the heal risk, or changes of the original tastes. In addition, the system creates precise projections by using the depth camera in addition to the RGB camera: the depth information helps to provide warp-free projections. The precise projection mapping minimizes the artificial impression that results in a negative impression of food.

2.2 Sound Augmentation for Food Texture

Sounds also effect the gustation. Charles Spence [2] found that participants feel potato chips crisper when processed noise was presented while eating. Chewing jockey [3] is another project that enriches eating by giving additional chewing sounds while eating.

Spot-Light creates sounds of food such as breaking sounds of baked crispy pie or caramel of crème brûlée. To realize natural sound effects, we used a parametric speaker. The speaker can create sounds from a particular location of a surface with ultrasonic waves.

Our first prototype senses cutting gestures with a electrode and add extra crispy sounds to the precise location on the surface. The sound projection is programmed so that it makes sounds that are unique for each location.

2.3 Animations for Impressive Food

In addition to the appearance augmentation, animation projections are also provided. While the static image projection is effective to enhance the basis of the appearance, animations are more impressive. The impressiveness helps the guests to relate their memory to gustation and contributes intensive sensation. The system generates animations such as melting butter, up going smoke or surface shines that remind the guests a richer experience of dinning.

3 Related Work

DinningPresenter [4] projects images on a dining table. It contains a camera and a projector. The camera captures the image of the dinning table and projects image on it. The focus of this project is to enrich the whole experience of dinning. It projects colors and images to promote healthier dinning for kids, for instance.

Meta-Cookie is an AR system that leverages the cross-modality to enhance foods. It modifies the gustation or satisfaction by providing aromas or modified shape of cookie with an AR environment. Although Meta-Cookie is effective way to modify our perceptions, it is not practical because of large devices required for the AR environment.

4 Conclusion

In this paper, we propose Spot-Light which enriches dishes by visual and sound projection mapping. This system is in the desk light shape with devices attached on the head part of it. The device includes a RGB camera, a depth camera, a parametric a speaker and a projector.

The system contains three functions. The first function is to capture the surface of food such as the brown area of steaks and projects extra visuals after processing the captured image so that it enriches the appearance. This function is supported by depth image captured by the depth camera, which helps a precise projection mapping that is important to eliminate the negative artificial impressive often occurs in simple projection mappings.

The second function is augmentations for the sound of food. The system adds sounds such as crispy sounds for baked pie when a knife touched on it. A parametric speaker is used to create sound on the surface.

The third function is animation projection. Animations such as melting butter on steaks are projected. The animation helps the guests to imagine gustation and helps intensive sensations.

By utilizing RGB and depth image, the system can project various properties on foods. For example, Spot-Light can be a real-time baking machine by attaching a laser.

Fukuchi [6] et al. used a laser for the use of baking the surface of food. They first captured the surface of the food and baked intended parts by processing the captured image. This suggests that Spot-Light can realize a real-time baking function with a laser.

References

1. Simner, J., Cuskley, C., Kirby, S.: What sound does that taste? Cross-modal mappings across gustation and audition. Perception 39(4), 553 (2010)
2. Zampini, M., Spence, C.: The role of auditory cues in modulating the perceived crispness and staleness of potato chips. Journal of Sensory Science 19, 347–363 (2004)
3. Koizumi, N., Tanaka, H., Uema, Y., Inami, M.: Chewing jockey: augmented food texture by using sound based on the cross-modal effect. In: Proceedings of the 8th International Conference on Advances in Computer Entertainment Technology, ACE 2011 (2011)
4. Mori, M., et al.: Dining Presenter: Augmented Reality system for a dining tabletop. In: Ajunct Proceedings of Ubicomp, pp. 168–169 (2009)
5. Narumi, T.: Meta cookie. In: ACM SIGGRAPH 2010 Posters. ACM (2010)
6. Fukuchi, K., et al.: Laser cooking: a novel culinary technique for dry heating using a laser cutter and vision technology. In: Proceedings of the ACM Multimedia 2012 Workshop on Multimedia for Cooking and Eating Activities. ACM (2012)

A Study of Properties and Services of a Smart Home for the Elderly

Sun Jung Lee, Hyo Chang Kim, Sang Min Ko, and Yong Gu Ji

Department of Information & Industrial Engineering, University of Yonsei, Seoul, 120-749
{sunjung,huychag1,sangminko,yongguji}@yonsei.ac.kr

Abstract. Republic of Korea is expected to enter into a super-aged society. Therefore, the needs of studying improved services and policies which support the quality of life, health, and comfortable living condition of the elderly are likely to increase. This study suggested a research direction of necessary properties and services for a smart home by analyzing existing studies to support the life of the elderly. Through investigation and analysis of studies of smart home and the elderly, we identified problems and implications of current smart home related studies.

Keywords: Smart Home, Smart Home Service, Elderly, Ergonomics.

1 Introduction

According to the standards of UN, a country is considered as a super-aged society if the percentage of population aged over 65 is more than 20 percent. Korean aging population is expected to go over 20% by the end of 2026 and heading towards a super-aging society [7]. With rapid aging of Korean society, a peaceful life for the elderly is becoming more important issue. The elderly people spend most of their time in their home because their range of activity is limited according to their body capability. Therefore, it is an important issue that how much the living space can support the elderlies' independent lives [14]. To support a peaceful life for the elderly, this study focused on studying services and properties of smart home.

Smart home means high quality life supporting technology which connects home appliances together by naturally interacting with humans. Smart home is based on wired/wireless communication and digital information appliance. It provides any time accessible ubiquitous environment using home networking and network accessible home appliances. Therefore, smart home means intelligent living environment aiming for 'intelligent living space, environment friendly life, and recreation of quality of life' [3]. As consuming high quality contents is becoming more common these days and the number of network accessible home appliances is increasing, smart home services are extending its range to home entertainment, home controlling, healthcare and more. Development of IT technology and info-communication increased possibility of supporting studies for smart home based on connected home appliances as well as possibility of supporting living conditions of the elderly using smart home

C. Stephanidis (Ed.): Posters, Part II, HCII 2013, CCIS 374, pp. 656–660, 2013.

technologies. More studies about building smart home which fit in the properties and living conditions of the elderly to support the elderly's comfortable living conditions and their actual lives are needed.

2 Related Work

To analyze existing smart home related studies and services 1) we studied actual conditions and trends of existing studies of smart homes related to individual foreign countries and 2) we investigated actual technologies and services of domestic smart homes.

2.1 Trends and Related Work of Smart Home

About 440 thousands of smart homes are estimated to be built around the world, and it is expected to increase to 5,380 thousands of smart homes by the year of 2015 [5]. Since 1991, America is concentrating on developing technologies such as interface technology which connects humans with computers according to "Networking and IT R&D; NITRD". America is interested in developing smart devices which can provide services according to individual user's properties and needs by focusing on developing applications and devices using computing technologies. Japan is running a smart home project cooperated by Toyota Motors Corporation and Toyota city. They have house type for their smart home, and they are planning to apply IT technology to the whole city [6]. Netherlands is trying to expand green home field to minimize the CO2 emission. Unlike other countries, Netherlands is approaching to smart home in the perspective of welfare and they provide many designs for the elderly, the disabled, and the weak [8, 15-16]. Australia is running a government driven business named 'Climate Smart Home', so anyone can volunteer for the project. Most of their smart home field is focused on smart grid [1].

Table 1. Summary of studies related to smart home

Categories		Subject
Technology Centered Studies	Smart Home Concept	A study of smart home standards and suggestion of smart home guidelines [9, 13].
	Application of Smart Home Technology	A study of related technologies which can be applied to smart home related services and system construction of smart home [12, 17].
User Centered Studies	User Analysis	A study of predicting and analyzing behavior patterns of smart home service users [4, 10, 18].
	Usability and Technology Evaluation	A usability test of particular smart home service and technology [2, 11].

In this study, we collected and analyzed studies of smart home as shown in the Table 1. Smart home related studies can be divided into 1) technology centered studies which study smart homes theoretically and studies which construct systems

2) user centered studies which study behavior patterns of smart home users and studies which conduct a usability test of particular smart home services and technologies.

2.2 Trends and Related Technology of Smart Home

Smart homes in Republic of Korea provide home platform technology which allows home networking service, home networking technology which allows access to information appliances by using wired and wireless internet, intelligent information electronic appliance technology which allows convergence information appliances to provide customized service, and green home technology which minimizes emission of CO_2 and energy consumption in residential area (Table 2). We investigated smart home services and technologies in Republic of Korea. Major construction companies in Republic of Korea adopt smart home service in their new apartments. The companies concentrate on smart grid services which can remote control home appliances in home. For example, 80% of smart home in Jeju island in Republic of Korea concentrated on energy saving and smart grid services. Therefore, we could conclude that smart homes in Republic of Korea have many services related to energy.

Table 2. Summary of technologies related to smart home in Republic of Korea

Categories	Explanation	Related Technology
Home Platform	A technology that allows emotional home networking services based on external network and home convergence contents	• Home server / Gateway • Apartment complex server linkage • Home device architecture
Home Networking	A technology that allows access to information appliances by mixing wired internet and wireless internet at any time	• Wired home networking • Wireless home networking • Wired/ Wireless linkage technology
Intelligent Information Electronic Appliance	A technology that allows convergence information appliances to provide customized services by recognizing its surrounding using sensors	• Information appliances • Home sensors • Realistic home theater • UI and interaction technology
Green Home	A technology which minimizes the emission of CO_2 and energy consumption in a residential area	• Green home energy management • Smart grid linkage • Green home environment management

Properties of services and technologies applied to smart homes in Republic of Korea are as follow. Smart home companies in Republic of Korea provide a service which identifies individual resident by their own identification card to secure the home. The companies also provide a service which allows the residents to remote control their home appliances by their smart devices as well as a service which allows the residents to check their home information and remote control their home appliances by their smart living information appliances. As we can see above, current problem of smart home in Republic of Korea is that their smart home services and technologies are depend too much on construction companies and smart home related companies not on actual residents. Therefore, ergonomic approach to smart home is essential and urgent in Republic of Korea.

3 Issues on Smart Home for the Elderly

Other countries with the better growth in smart home field than Republic of Korea are studying to develop various smart home service models considering their residence characteristics and the elderly. However, there are lack of studies about residence characteristics and the elderly in Republic of Korea, and those studies are limited to technical realization and service presentation. Furthermore, the construction companies strongly depend on other countries' cases when they develop new smart home services. When comparing to other countries' study cases, smart home studies for the elderly are insufficient in Republic of Korea. The elderly people spend most of their time in their home and have limited body capability. Therefore, future studies should focus on smart home studies that can support the elderly living in Republic of Korea that have physical limitations, cognitive ability limitations, and low technology acceptance. Indigenous smart home in the Republic of Korea should be studied considering cultural differences and living properties of the elderly.

Acknowledgements. This work was supported by Basic Science Research Program through the National Research Foundation of Korea (NRF) funded by the Ministry of Education, Science and Technology (MEST) (2012R1A1A2006949).

References

1. Tools of Change: Queensland's Climatesmart Home Service (2012)
2. Demiris, G., Skubic, M., Rantz, M., Keller, J., Aud, M., Hensel, B., He, Z.: Smart Home Sensors for the Elderly: A Model for Participatory Formative Evaluation. In: The IEEE EMBS International Special Topic Conference on Information Technology in Biomedicine (2006)
3. Lee, G.-W., Shin, Y.-R., Lee, S.-J., Park, J.-Y., Huh, E.-N., Koh, S.-K.: Design of Interoperable Interface for Smarthome Service between Home Gateway and Home Cloud. Korean Society for Internet Information, 141–142 (2011)
4. Hung, Y.-S., Chen, K.-L.B., Yang, C.-T., Deng, G.-F.: Web Usage Mining for Analysing Elder Self-Care Behavior Patterns. Expert Systems with Applications 40(2), 775–783 (2013)
5. Berg Insight.: Smart Homes and Home Automation (2011)
6. Kaikan, K.: Future City Model Projects (2011)

7. Kang Kyung, W., Jeong, T.K., Woo, K.K.: Reconsideration the Relationship between the Rapid Aging of the Societies and the Older Driver"S Traffic Accidents. Journal of the Korean Society of Civil Engineers 27(1D), 19–26 (2007)
8. Kyoung, B.E.: A Study on the Smart Home Focused on the Change of Housing Space. Journal of the Korean Institute of Spatial Design 3(2), 49–59 (2008)
9. Soon Jae, L., Ra Arh, K., Yong Hwan, P.: Comparative Analysis of Healthcare Smart Home Guidelines for the Elderly. Architectural Institute of Korea 31, 163–164 (2011)
10. Lee, H., Park, S.J., Kim, M.J., Jung, J.Y., Kim, J.T.: Deducing Behavioural Patterns of Elderly People to Improve Smart Home Services. In: 6th International Symposium on Sustainable Healthy Buildings, Seoul, Korea (2012)
11. Portet, F., Vacher, M., Golanski, C., Roux, C., Meillon, B.: Design and Evaluation of a Smart Home Voice Interface for the Elderly: Acceptability and Objection Aspects. Personal and Ubiquitous Computing 17(1), 127–144 (2013)
12. Raad, M.W., Yang, L.T.: A Ubiquitous Smart Home for Elderly. Information Systems Frontiers 11(5), 529–536 (2009)
13. Shim, S.-G., Park, H.-J., Park, J.-H.: Status and Strategies of Standardization in Smart Home. Communications of the Korea Information Science Society 30(8), 19–25 (2012)
14. Shin, Y.S.: A Study of Home Concept for Homelike Elderly Housing Facility Design. International Journal of Human Ecology 39(12), 141–158 (2001)
15. Sponselee, A.-M., Schouten, B., Bouwhuis, D., Willems, C.: Smart Home Technology for the Elderly: Perceptions of Multidisciplinary Stakeholders. In: Mühlhäuser, M., Ferscha, A., Aitenbichler, E. (eds.) Constructing Ambient Intelligence, vol. 11, pp. 314–326. Springer, Heidelberg (2008)
16. Šťáhlavský, R.: Amsterdam Smart City Project (2011)
17. Shin, Y.-R., Lee, G.-W., Lee, S.-J., Park, J.-Y., Huh, E.-N., Eom, B.-Y.: Design of Personal Information Management System for Personalized Service on Cloud. Korean Society For Internet Information, 145–146 (2011)
18. Zhang, J.-G., Ishikawa-Takata, K., Kazuko, I.-T., Hideo, Y., Toshiki, O.: Is a Type a Behavior Pattern Associated with Falling among the Community-Dwelling Elderly? Archives of Gerontology and Geriatrics 38(2), 145–152 (2004)

A Novel Layer-Scanning Method for Improving Real-Time People Counting

Daw-Tung Lin and Dong-Han Jhuang

Department of Computer Science and Information Engineering,
No.151, University Rd., Sansia Dist., New Taipei City 23741, Taiwan (R.O.C.)
dalton@mail.ntpu.edu.tw, s49885046@webmail.ntpu.edu.tw

Abstract. People counting is an important subject for various applications and analyses. This paper proposes a novel method for counting the number of targets by using the layer scanning of depth information provided by the Kinect® sensor. The steps of this method include constructing a depth image background model, deriving foreground depth map, filtering the noise, classifying the targets, and screening the area of targets with layer scanning to calculate the number of targets by determining the highest position of the respective targets, tracking and analyzing the objects, and counting the number of the objects. Moreover, the dynamic number of targets is calculated using a tracking algorithm. The proposed system is beneficial in automatic, effective, and precise calculation of the number of targets in a specific area. Furthermore, the technique of the present method is not affected by the changes of the ambient light which can effectively reduce the interference of the background.

Keywords: People counting, Kinect®, depth information, layer scanning, object tracking.

1 Introduction

Calculating the number of the objects within a certain regional space is important to manage the objects. Although infrared rays and ultrasonic sensors have been used for people counting, no perfect solution can overcome crowded and occluded situations. Several methods have been proposed to count passersby in several indoor spaces with a mounted overhead camera. Masoud and Papanikolopoulos [1] implemented a blob-tracking method that can alleviate several occlusions or overlapping conditions. Chen [2] implemented a useful method on solving the merge-split problem when tracking people. The purpose of [3] and [4] was to solve the crowd-counting issue by using various methods. Chen et al. [5] expanded the field of counting people to a more applicable level. Antic et al. [6] used the K-means algorithm to analyze the number of passing people. Lu et al. [7] have applied the Kinect® sensor to track people. In order to overcome the disadvantage of the various instruments in the prior art, this work uses a Kinect® infrared depth sensor and supplemented by the detection method to provide a real-time layer scanning method to enhance the accuracy of the counting objects.

C. Stephanidis (Ed.): Posters, Part II, HCII 2013, CCIS 374, pp. 661–665, 2013.

2 System Architecture

The proposed people-counting system uses a Kinect® sensor mounted on a ceiling to allow the sensor to capture the downward-vertical viewing field. Figure 1(a) shows the scenario of the system setup and application. The scene has incoming and outgoing pedestrians, and they are detected and tracked when they enter the viewing region. Figure 1(b) shows the complete flowchart of the proposed procedure and implementation, which comprises three parts: depth image background modeling, the layer-scanning method, and objects analysis and counting. The first N depth frames are averaged for use as the main background for the image subtraction step in layer-scanning.

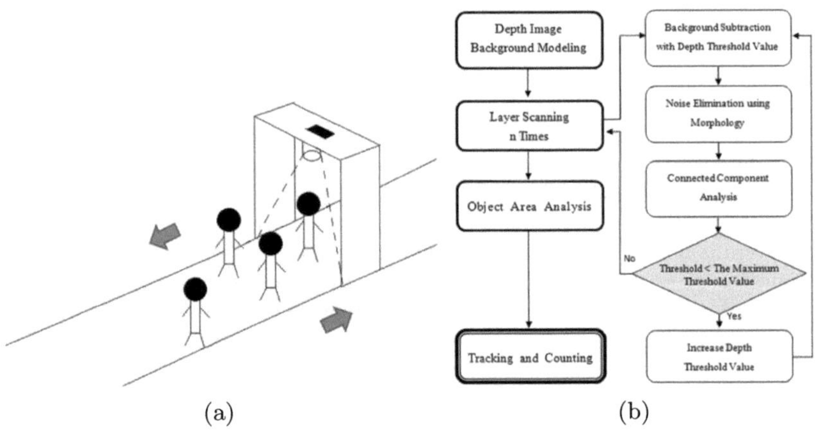

Fig. 1. (a) The people counting scenario; (b) The complete system flowchart

3 Proposed Layer Scanning Algorithm

3.1 Depth Background Subtraction and Value of Interest(VOI) Foreground Extraction

In contrast to the ordinary method of background subtraction, the image that is analyzed in this study is a depth image. Background subtraction is employed to derive a foreground object which means shooting a (N+1)th frame where objects appears and comparing with the background map constructed in the previous N frames as illustrated in Section 2. The background will be updated periodically. After setting this value according to our interests (value of interest (VOI)), the appropriate foreground was obtained after background subtraction. Next, morphological opening and closing operations followed by connected component analysis were applied to remove the noise and obtain a smoother foreground for post-estimation.

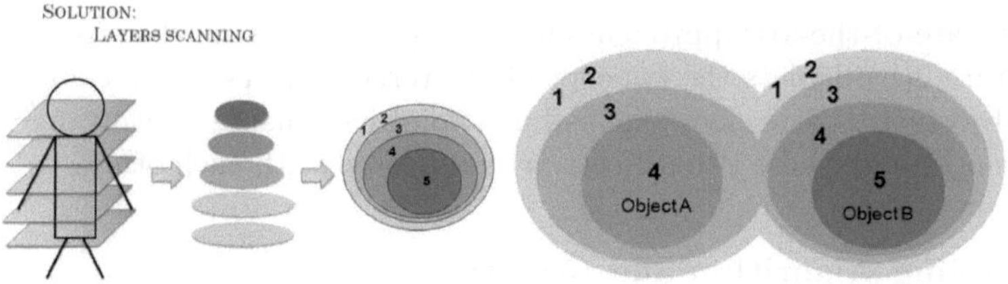

(a) (b)

Fig. 2. (a) Layer-scanning concept diagram; (b) Cluttered objects separation using layer-scanning method with different depth range layer labels

3.2 Layer-Scanning Algorithm

Figure 2(a) shows the fundamental concept of this method. Because the direction of the proposed sensor is vertically downward, the shapes of the pedestrians in the scene are similar to ellipses. The area of projection of the upper portion of a person is normally smaller compared to the lower one; thus, if when comparing and stacking the areas of every layer from low to high, the top portion of each object can be estimated. Algorithm 1 shows the pseudo-code of the proposed layer scanning method.

Algorithm 1. Layer-scanning

```
initialization value of interest(VOI) depth threshold
while VOI threshold does not reach limit value do
    background subtraction
    morphology(opening and closing)
    connected component analysis
    copy processed object area and provide new label mark to the object area
    if VOI depth threshold is less than limit value then
        increase VOI depth threshold by one layer value
    end if
end while
```

3.3 Object Area Analysis and Cluttered Objects Separation

An area range condition was set to eliminate the smashed area based on $A_1 \cap A_2 \cap A_3 \cap \cdots \cap A_n = result$, where $low\_area\_value < A_i < high\_area\_value$, $0 < i \leq n$. Generally, a first loop scanned by the first scan is shown in Fig. 2(a) labeled by 1. The range 1 is the depth range of the knee to the foot of a human, the foreground depth map thereof has a lighter grayscale value. Superposing the obtained foreground depth maps respectively, and removing the discrepant area to obtain a highest height portion, thereby determining the highest position of the object is the range n. Furthermore, the cluttered objects can be correctly separated by identifying the above mentioned highest portion of the objects using different depth range layer-scanning. Therefore, the proposed method is superior to the other state-of-the-art approaches in the aspect of solving the crowd-counting issue. Figure 2(b) depicts the concept of cluttered objects separation. The foreground objects are correctly identified as two objects using depth range labels 4 and 5, even-though these two objects are connected with each other.

3.4 Tracking Algorithm and Counting

After using the proposed layer scanning method, each frame may possess candidate moving objects. The objects adjacent to each other are reclassified to obtain the number of the objects. The tracking in this study may fulfilled by comparing the foreground depth map in consecutive video frames and selecting the shortest distance for pairing. Furthermore, the vector of each object can be estimated by calculating the difference in the coordinates of an object. Thereafter, the vector information can be used to identify whether an object is moving upward or downward.

4 Experimental Results and Discussion

The proposed real-time people-counting system was implemented to operate at approximately 30 FPS. The sensor is set approximately 3 m above the floor. All of the experiments were performed in real-time. Several conditions of the experiments are shown in Fig. 3, including normal speed walking, fast moving, bi-directional moving, several people walking closely, etc.. The proposed people-counting system can, on average, count people with an accuracy of 96.11% in the range of 50 to 200 cm. Table 1 presents the results of the experiments. Figure 3(c) shows the situation of false counting caused by an object of a pedestrian has the same depth value as the pedestrian. To solve this issue, the feature value

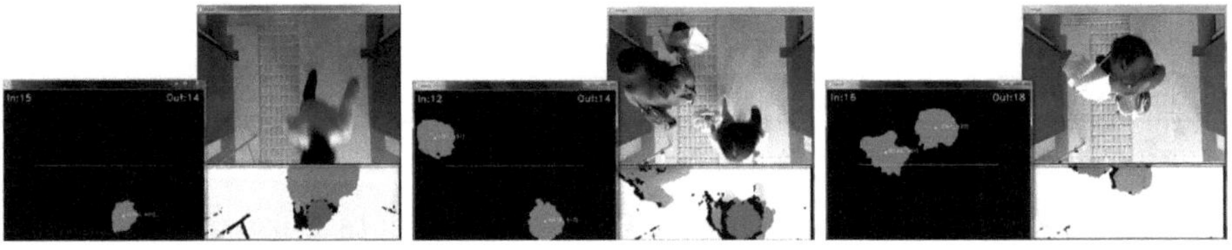

(a) (b) (c)

Fig. 3. (a) One fast moving person test; (b) Two people walking in bi-directional way; (c) False count condition

Table 1. Experimental results

Test	In	Out	Correct In	Correct Out	Accuracy
1	57	38	55	37	96.93%
2	103	125	99	123	97.25%
3	223	195	211	187	95.24%

regarding shape can be integrated into the system or the color histogram can be used to determine more accurately if an object is human. Moreover, the fast-moving objects and sudden switching on and off of the light test indicated that both of these conditions do not influence the people-counting result.

5 Conclusions

This paper proposed a novel method for counting the number of the targets using the layer scanning method based on the depth information provided by Kinect® sensor. The steps of this method includes constructing a depth image background model, filtering the noise of foreground frame and classifying the targets, and screening the area of targets based on layer scanning to calculate the number of targets by determining the highest positions of the respective targets. The depth data and proposed algorithm were used to view the top region of each object with the Kinect® sensor; thus, each object was tracked correctly, despite their lower portions being connected and the highest portions not being connected. In addition, the dynamic numbers of targets are calculated using tracking algorithm. The proposed people-counting system can, on average, estimate people with an accuracy of 96.11% in the range of 50 to 200 cm. The results were not influenced by changes in lighting condition, except when exposed to sunlight or other strong luminaries according to the experimental results.

References

[1] Masoud, O., Papanikolopoulos, N.P.: A Novel Method for Tracking and Counting Pedestrians in Real-time using a Single Camera. IEEE Transactions on Vehicular Technology 50(5), 1267–1278 (2001)
[2] Chen, T., Chen, T., Chen, Z.: An Intelligent People-Flow Counting Method for Passing through a Gate. In: IEEE Conference on Robotics, Automation and Mechatronics, pp. 1–6 (2006)
[3] Conte, D., Foggia, P., Percannella, G., Tufano, F., Vento, M.: A Method for Counting People in Crowded Scenes. In: IEEE International Conference on Advanced Video and Signal Based Surveillance, Washington, USA, pp. 225–232 (2010)
[4] Chen, F., Zhang, E.: A Fast and Robust People Counting Method in Video Surveillance. In: IEEE International Conference on Computational Intelligence and Security, pp. 339–343 (2007)
[5] Chen, C.H., Chang, Y.C., Chen, T.Y., Wang, D.J.: People Counting System for Getting In/Out of a Bus Based on Video Processing. In: IEEE Conference on Intelligent Systems Design, vol. 3, pp. 565–569 (2008)
[6] Antic, B., Letic, D., Culibrk, D., Crnojevic, V.: K-means Based Segmentation for Real-time Zenithal People Counting. In: IEEE International Conference on Pattern Recognition (2009)
[7] Lu, X., Chen, C.-C., Aggarwal, J.K.: Human Detection using Depth Information by Kinect. In: IEEE Computer Society Conference on Computer Vision and Pattern Recognition Workshops (CVPRW), pp. 15–22 (2011)

iEat: An Interactive Table for Restaurant Customers' Experience Enhancement

George Margetis[1], Dimitris Grammenos[1], Xenophon Zabulis[1], and Constantine Stephanidis[1,2]

[1] Foundation for Research and Technology – HELLAS, Institute for Computer Science (FORTH – ICS)
[2] Computer Science Department, University of Crete
{gmarget,gramenos,zabulis,cs}@ics.forth.gr

Abstract. An active field of research today is the technological enrichment of everyday activities using augmented reality and ambient intelligence technologies. To this end, augmenting dinner tables is a challenging task, requiring a high-quality user experience unobtrusively supporting and enhancing the user's main goal: eating and socializing. This work presents an augmented restaurant table, facilitating customers' ordering and enhancing their experience through entertainment and socialization features, as well as through interaction with physical objects placed upon the table surface.

Keywords: augmented reality, ambient intelligence, interactive tabletop.

1 Introduction

The emergence of augmented reality and ambient intelligence has motivated several research efforts to pursue the technological enrichment of everyday life activities, mainly in the areas of home, workplace, health and education. Lately, however, the areas of socialization, communication and entertainment have gained increased interest for multimodal and ubiquitous interaction towards enhancing common activities such as dining.

To this end, initiatives that aim to entertain and foster human communication and socialization through dining have already appeared as commercial solutions. For instance, the Inamo and Touche Diner restaurants [1, 2] try to provide technology enhanced entertainment and socializing during dinner.

This work presents an innovative smart restaurant table, named iEat that aims to enhance restaurant customers' experience in terms of entertainment, socialization, food selection and ordering, providing the users with natural interaction with the table itself, as well as with physical objects placed upon its surface.

2 Related Work

The concept of augmenting dinner tables is challenging, mainly due to the fact that the interactive features of the table should not overwhelm the user's main goal, eating

C. Stephanidis (Ed.): Posters, Part II, HCII 2013, CCIS 374, pp. 666–670, 2013.

and socializing with other diners. Nevertheless, the idea of providing new types of interaction and facilities for this everyday human habit has led to numerous approaches. For example, Dinner Party [3] provides entertaining interaction between a person dining on a table and objects placed on top of it. The user can move these objects casting virtual shadows on the tabletop while animated creatures which were initially hiding in these shadows eventually appear. Another example is Neon Racer [4], a multi-user augmented reality racing game that can be played on a tabletop setting, providing social interaction in open environments. Food Media [5] aims to engage people dining at different locations into social communication and entertainment, supporting an integrated teleconference system, movement of partner's dishes remotely, display of various information, graphics or slow-rate animations through controlled color changing on the tablecloth and transmission of remotely designed patterns or messages using real edible food. A similar approach presented in [6] aims to support remote guests in experiencing a sense of togetherness, playfulness and sharing in a dinner party.

The work presented here discusses an augmented restaurant table facilitating the dinner process and fostering socialization and communication of the diners. It provides alternative types of natural interaction through the use of infrared lightpens based on the work presented in [7], as well as through the positioning and movement of existing plates on the table surface, supporting thus a large degree of interaction freedom to the users.

3 The iEat Table

An experimental installation of the iEat system is illustrated in Fig. 1 (left) comprising a white surfaced restaurant table for two persons (90 cm x 80 cm), an Intel Core 2 Duo PC, a HD ready projector lying above the table, as well as a high definition infrared camera and a Microsoft Kinect sensor, both placed adjacent to the projector overlooking the table surface. The high definition camera tracks light sources in the infrared spectrum as in [7]. The Kinect is employed in tracking plates

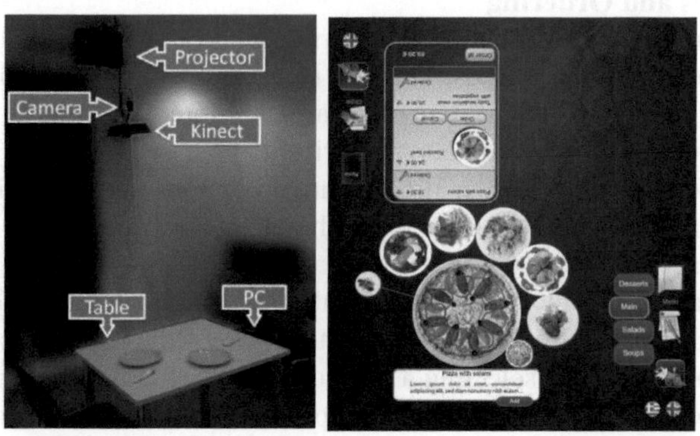

Fig. 1. Left: Experimental installation of the iEat table. Right: UI layout.

on the table, which is achieved by analyzing the depth image and detecting plates through their circular height patterns.

Currently, user interaction is supported through moving / placing the plates on the table as well as through infrared lightpens, which are stylus-shaped, LED-based, infrared light (IR) emitters. The infrared lightpens emit light only when they touch the table surface, providing the following interaction gestures: (a) Click: Touch the table surface and instantly raise lightpen (abstaining from any lateral motion); (b) Down: Touch the table surface; (c) Up: Raise the lightpen above the table surface; (d) Move: Move the lightpen while touching the table surface.

3.1 User Interaction

The main objective of the iEat table is to augment restaurant customers' experience beyond standard activities performed at restaurants (i.e., reading the menu, ordering, chatting and eating) towards new levels of entertainment and communication. To this end, the iEat table provides a diversity of technology augmented facilities such as ordering, playing, decorating the table surface and communicating.

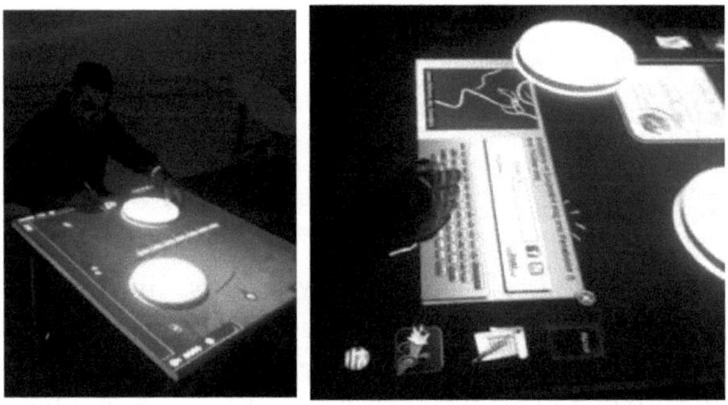

Fig. 2. Left: Playing games using plates and lightpen. Right: posting doodles and sketches to Facebook and Twitter.

Selecting Dishes and Ordering

The iEat system integrates an intuitive ordering facility enabling customers not only to find and order restaurant dishes, but also to get a preview of the dish that will be served. Fig. 1 (right) depicts the iEat ordering User Interface, which mainly consists of three components: (a) basic menu categories, (b) list of dishes and dish details for the selected category and (c) order list. The menu options and order list are placed at the customer's right hand side, while the dish details are projected upon and laterally an empty plate near the customer.

In more details, customers can explore the restaurant menu, by clicking on the main navigation menu button and then selecting one of the categories that have been expanded just next to it. By selecting a category, the iEat table displays thumbnails of the selected category's dishes around the empty dish which is nearest to the customer. If a customer clicks on a thumbnail, a larger photo is displayed on the surface of the dish, accompanied by additional details regarding for example its ingredients, nutrition facts, etc. The option for ordering the plate is also readily available for selection.

Furthermore, a customer is able to review the dishes in the order list and place the order. The order list summarizes all the dishes that have been added by the two diners, providing facilities for removing a dish from the list, view more details for a particular dish, order a specific dish and order all the dishes in the list. The iEat system provides an API for intercommunicating with restaurant ordering software, allowing its trouble-free installation and interoperation with systems already used in restaurants.

Playing

Aiming to entertain the diners while waiting for the dishes to be served, the iEat table features interactive games played using the empty plates and the lightpens. In the current prototype, a breakout type game has been developed (**Fig. 2**, left). The goal of each player is to hit as many tiles as possible, using the cannonballs launched by a cannon lying in front of the player. Moreover, players get more points if they manage to place their cannonballs to a particular opponent's territory. The aiming direction of the cannon is determined by the players moving their lightpens to the left or to the right in front of their cannons. Cannonballs can be repelled using plates as shields (in order to screen the opponent's cannonballs). Forthcoming versions of the iEat table will support additional games, accommodating a variety of potential player preferences.

Decorating and Communicating

Additionally, the iEat table supports facilities for decorating the table surface, through a library of alternative virtual backgrounds (tablecloths), as well as highly customizable drawing toolset (allowing users for example to select brush size and color, undo and redo action, etc.). Drawing and doodling is facilitated through the use of lightpens. Furthermore, users are able to post their drawings to their Facebook and Twitter accounts, sharing thus their experience with friends and followers (**Fig. 2** right).

4 Formative Evaluation

The current iEat table prototype has been evaluated by four usability experts following the heuristic evaluation method [8]. In summary, sixteen usability problems were found, most of which were rated as aesthetic or minor. Two problems that were rated as major were the following: (i) the user cannot easily find out about the drawing options menu, since it is not included in the main navigation menu and it is displayed only if the users perform a click to a non-interactive table area, and (ii) if the dishes list contains more than seven items, the leftmost and rightmost dishes are displayed smaller in order to indicate that by selecting them the dishes carousel will rotate, however this will be difficult for users to find out. Furthermore, the evaluation also resulted in a list of the most interesting and usable system features, including among others the plates' interaction facilities, the overall look and feel of the application, as well as its sociability features.

5 Conclusions and Future Work

This work has presented an interactive restaurant table aiming not only to support ordering at the restaurant, but also to enhance customers' socializing and entertainment. The table features innovative interaction facilities, using the empty plates placed on the table and lightpens. The initial prototype of the iEat table has been evaluated by usability experts, having identified the strengths and weaknesses of the current implementation. Future work will address the usability problems that were found and will enrich the existing content, by adding beverages' information and additional entertainment games. Furthermore, user-based tests will be carried out aiming to assess diners' overall user experience.

Acknowlegdments. This work is supported by the FORTH-ICS internal 'Ambient Intelligence' RTD Programme.

References

1. Inamo restaurant, Soho, London - interactive oriental fusion restaurant and bar, `http://www.inamo-restaurant.com/`
2. Touche - Touch Table Diner Bar, `http://www.touchediner.com/`
3. Nam, H.Y., DiSalvo, C., Do, E.Y.L., Mendenhall, S.: Dinner Party sociable interfaces in a tabletop art project. In: First International Conference on Intelligent Interactive Technologies and Multimedia, pp. 306–310. ACM (2010)
4. Litzlbauer, W., Stuppacher, I., Waldner, M., Weilguny, M.: Neon Racer: Augmented Gaming. In: 10th Central European Seminar on Computer Graphics, CESCG (2006)
5. Wei, J., Wang, X., Tache, R., Peiris, R.L., Choi, Y., Halupka, V., Cheok, A.D.: Food Media: exploring interactive entertainment over telepresent dinner. In: 8th International Conference on Advances in Computer Entertainment Technology, p. 26. ACM (2011)
6. Barden, P., Comber, R., Green, D., Jackson, D., Ladha, C., Bartindale, T., Olivier, P.: Telematic dinner party: designing for togetherness through play and performance. In: Designing Interactive Systems Conference, pp. 38–47. ACM (2012)
7. Margetis, G., Ntelidakis, A., Zabulis, X., Ntoa, S., Koutlemanis, P., Stephanidis, C.: Augmenting physical books towards education enhancement. In: Workshop on User-Centred Computer Vision, in Conjunction with Workshop on the Applications of Computer Vision 2013, Florida (2013)
8. Nielsen, J., Molich, R.: Heuristic evaluation of user interfaces. In: SIGCHI Conference on Human Factors in Computing Systems: Empowering People, pp. 249–256. ACM (1990)

My Mirror- A Tool to Support Self-awareness

Afarin Pirzadeh[1], Reecha Bharali[1], and Terri Wada[2]

[1] Indiana University School of Informatics, IUPUI
{apirzade,rbharali}@iupui.edu
[2] Herron School of Art and Design, IUPUI
tawada@umail.iu.edu

Abstract. Studying different aspects of self such as self-awareness and self-reflection in the area of HCI is still growing. In this study we focus on the mirror as one of the main sources of self-information. We present a process of design research that we conducted to redesign the mirror and develop a low fidelity prototype of *My Mirror*, a tool to support self-awareness by triggering individuals' inner-speech.

Keywords: Design Research, Prototyping, Self-awareness, Self-talk, Inner-speech, Self-knowledge.

1 Introduction

Self-awareness occurs when one takes oneself as the object of one's own attention and actively identifies processes, and stores information about self [1]. One becomes self-aware through engaging in self-talk [2]. Self-talk or inner speech makes one be able to verbally identify, process and store self-information [3]. The mirror is one of the main physical devices that may trigger inner-speech as one gets exposed to it and can be used as a source of self-information [3]. In this study, we redesigned the mirror, through the use of design research methods, in order to trigger individuals' inner-speech and facilitate the process of gaining self-information that may eventually lead to self-reflection and improving self-knowledge. In this paper, we first provide a short background on self-awareness and technologies that support self-talk and self-reflection; then we present the user-centered design process that we conducted to develop a low fidelity prototype of *My Mirror* as a tool to support self-awareness and self-reflection. Finally, we discuss the results of our usability test and conclude with a final discussion and future works.

2 Background

Mirror is one of the more common physical stimuli that is likely to trigger self-talk when one gets exposed to it [3]; for example "I look very good today!" or "I am so huge!" Exposing to a mirror and engaging in self-talk can lead to self-information collection, reflection and eventually self-knowledge improvement. One's level of

C. Stephanidis (Ed.): Posters, Part II, HCII 2013, CCIS 374, pp. 671–675, 2013.

self-knowledge depends on the frequency, quantity and quality of self-information that one gains through this process [4].

Currently, personal informatics and designing systems to support self-awareness and improve self-reflection is growing. However, focus on physical stimuli to trigger self-reflection has received limited attention in this area.

In their studies, Andrés del Valle and Opalach [5] present their design process of the persuasive mirror, a tool to visualize continuous feedback on the behavioral data of users and support them in reaching their personal goals. However, our study takes a holistic view on different usages of a mirror and the user-centered design process of developing *My Mirror*, as a tool to provide different self-information for users, support self-reflection, and persuade them to engage in a positive self-talk.

3 Data Analysis

We conducted semi-structured interviews and a diary study to identify and state the main problem, establish the requirements, and develop our design concepts.

3.1 Interview Analysis

Semi-structured interviews were conducted with eight participants, five females and three males, within an age range of 22-30 and the mean of 26.4 years. We started interviews with simple questions that centered around participants use of mirrors, including how often and why participants interacted with this object and how it might trigger self-talk and help them gain self-information. We probed participants to tell us more until no relevant information was forthcoming.

Based on the result of interview analysis, we identified that the mirror triggers participants' self-talk and provides them with self-information, which eventually may affect their feelings and mood. However, different factors such as personality traits, mood, self-esteem, or available time mediate this process. This result helped us to finalize the focus of our project on the following problem statement: "How can we redesign a mirror to provide self-information that users need and trigger positive self-talk while they are exposed to this object?"

3.2 Diary Study Analysis

A diary study was used as the second method of data analysis to gather information and establish requirements for the problem statement identified above. To carry out this research method, we had eight participants, all were students, four female and four males with an age range of 23-28 and a mean of 24.1 years. Each participant was asked to record their answers to a set of questions immediately following any exposure to a mirror during one full day. The following are some of the questions that were asked: What time/why/where did you get exposed to the mirror? How were you feeling before/after seeing yourself in the mirror?

An affinity diagram was used to analyze the data collected in this stage and enabled the identification of three themes: physical appearance, self-encouragement or positive self-talk, and fun.

Physical Appearance

Participants reported that they check their physical appearance, such as weight, skin, or their outfits in the mirror. For example, participants documented saying the following, "I checked if my skin got better than yesterday," "I brushed my teeth and made sure my teeth are clean."

Self-encouragement and Positive Self-talk

Participants also reported that they sometimes encourage themselves and enhance their self-confidence in front of the mirror. For example, a couple participants said, "Sometimes when I have a talk at school, I encourage myself in the mirror before that!" "I enjoy seeing myself in the mirror specially when I look good in a nice outfit."

Fun

Having fun is the third category identified from data in this stage. Participants reported that they sometime entertain themselves in the mirror. For example, one participant said, "I was bored and the music was on, so I started singing and dancing in front of the mirror."

4 Prototyping

In this section we focus on the design process and explain how understanding the users based on the literature review, interview analysis, and diary study inspired us to develop a low fidelity prototype of *My Mirror.* This tool provides the user with required self-information, supports positive self-talk positive and attempts to elicit a positive mood. We discuss our design strategies based on three design concepts we identified from our data analysis in the previous section.

4.1 Physical Appearance

My Mirror provides users with their basic appearance information such as weight, size, and skin conditions. Users can also track their information in the specific time frames of a week, month and year. They can also get some health suggestions and recommendations based on their information. (Fig. 1.)

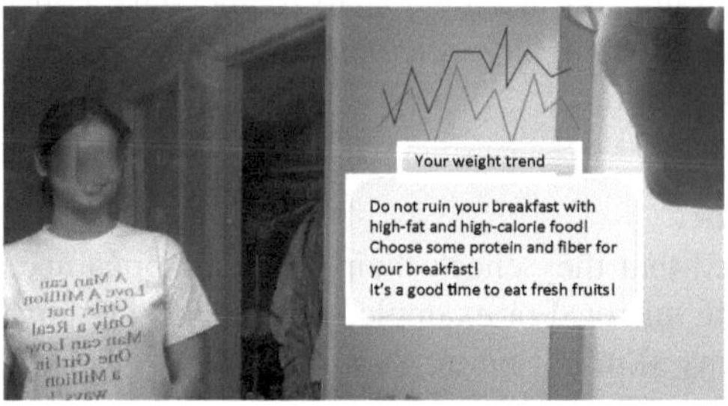

Fig. 1. Providing self-information, health recommendation, and self-encouragement

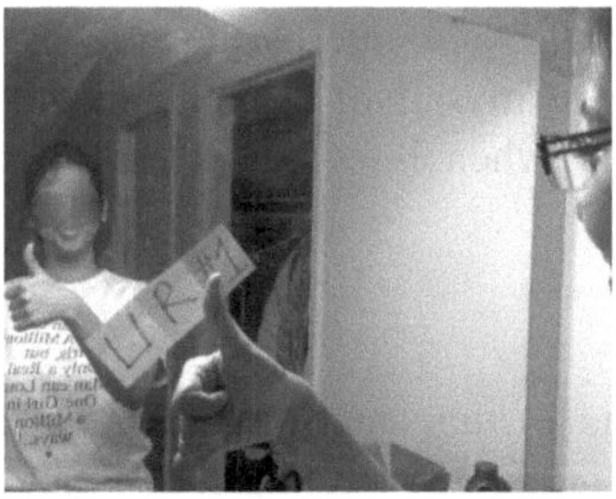

Fig. 2. Supporting positive self-talk

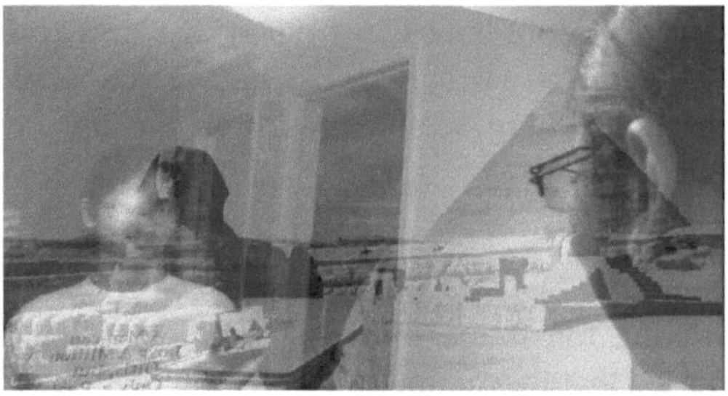

Fig. 3. Supporting entertainment

4.2 Self-encouragement and Positive Self-talk

We also explored different designed ideas to trigger positive self-talk and self-encouragement. Any improvement of users in different aspects of physical appearance would be encouraged by positive statements on the mirror to increase users' self-confidence. *My Mirror* also encourages users to follow different health recommendations that it provides for users. Participants also reported that they enjoyed getting engaged in a positive self-talk while seeing themselves in the mirror. To address this requirement, we designed a game in which we provide users with different positive emoticons, words and symbols and they can make positive statements describing themselves. *My Mirror* also provides users with self-motivating statements (e.g. "you are …") and users need to fill in the blank from limited number of positive words (e.g. "cool, kind, nice, or awesome). (Fig. 2.)

4.3 Fun

To address the desire for fun, *My Mirror* also supports users' entertainment needs. Participants reported that they sometime sing and dance in front of the mirror. My mirror can detect the song which users start singing and provide an audio or video of the singer on the mirror so that users can sing, dance, and have fun. Changing the environment is another strategy that My Mirror applies to entertain users (Fig. 3.).

For example, a user can hold up a picture of the desired environment, graphics, or shade and My Mirror would reflect that picture by changing its background based on the image.

5 User Evaluation and Conclusion

Usability evaluation was conducted with five users. Users were provided with instructions to interact with the low fidelity prototype through three main scenarios and five tasks. Tasks included exploring different physical self-information, playing around with different games and practices for positive self-talk, and having fun by singing, dancing, and changing the background. Results of the usability tests were positive about the use of My Mirror as a tool to support positive self-talk and provide relevant self-information. However, participants reported difficulties in interacting with low fidelity prototype. They also reported privacy issues being that it was challenging for them to express their actual feeling in front of the mirror in the presence of a usability expert.

To conclude, this study was more focused on exploring design ideas to redesign the mirror as one of the main sources of self-information. The plan for future studies is to develop a high fidelity prototype that users can interact with in a personal context, without the presence of a usability expert during a long period of time and to evaluate whether this tool can help users improve their self-knowledge in the long term.

References

1. Duval, S., Wicklund, R.A.: A theory of objective self-awareness. Academic Press, New York (1972)
2. Morin, A.: Self-talk and self-awareness: On the nature of the relation. The Journal of Mind and Behavior 14(3), 223–234 (1993)
3. Morin, A.: A neurocognitive and socioecological model of self-awareness. Genetic, Social, and General Psychology Monographs 130(3), 197–222 (2004)
4. Morin, A.: Levels of consciousness and self-awareness: A comparison and integration of various neurocognitive views. Consciousness and Cognition 15(2), 358–371 (2006)
5. Andrés del Valle, A.C., Opalach, A.: The persuasive mirror: computerized persuasion for healthy living. In: Proceedings of the 11th International Conference on Human-Computer Interaction (2005)

Relationship Analysis between the Child's Behaviors Patterns and Sense of Anxiety

Ayako Sasase[1] and Toshikazu Kato[2]

[1] Industrial and Systems Engineering, Graduate School of Science and Engineering, Chuo University, 1-13-27 Kasuga, Bunkyo-ku, Tokyo, 112-8551, Japan
a12.d45w@g.chuo-u.ac.jp
[2] Chuo University, 1-13-27 Kasuga, Bunkyo-ku, Tokyo, 112-8551, Japan
kato@indsys.chuo-u.ac.jp

Abstract. This study aims to provide an information assistance mechanism which estimates the child's state of emotion. This paper shows relationship between child behavior patterns and sense of anxiety. We assumed a typical situation; a mother is working at home without caring her child and the child is playing alone near the mother. We assumed that looking at his mother is a reflection of anxiety in the situation. Therefore, we have examined the number of times of looking at his mother. We could observe monolog behaviors in peace of emotion, while speaking to his mother, frequent moving around, and frequent change of behaviors in sense of anxiety. We also found distance between the child and his mother is important for peace of emotion because the anxiety is dissolved by sitting near his mother in his hand distance.

Keywords: behavior, anxiety, child, mother, communication.

1 Introduction

The progress of women's participation in the society is one of the reasons of reducing tight communication between a mother and a child. To attain rich communication in a short period, it is necessary for the mother to know the child's state of emotion.

This study aims to provide an information assistance mechanism to estimate the child's state of emotion through physical observation of child's behavior patterns.

It is necessary for us to reveal that relation the child's state of emotion and behaviors to realize this mechanism. Psychological studies show that some specific behaviors patterns of a child reflect state of emotion [1][2].

However they are fragmentary, they don't consider connections with behaviors.

We think observation of successively behaviors is important because the behaviors have some meanings.

The purpose of this study is to reveal that relation the child's state of emotion and successively behaviors to realize this mechanism.

This time the state of emotion is "anxiety". Prior research says that looking at his mother is a reflection of anxiety in the situation.

C. Stephanidis (Ed.): Posters, Part II, HCII 2013, CCIS 374, pp. 676–680, 2013.

Therefore, we have examined the number of times of looking at his mother in half an hour on the hypothesis that there is relation between the number of looking at his mother and sense of anxiety.

2 Experimental (Materials and Method)

We have assumed a typical situation; a mother is working at home without caring her child and the child is playing alone near the mother.

A. Observation the child's behaviors in the situation
B. Analysis a change of anxiety
C. Reveal relations the child's sense of anxiety and successively behaviors

1. Observation the child's behaviors in the situation

In our current experiment system, we adopted a video camera located at the corner of a room to monitor the behaviors of the mother and child in half an hour. The child is a boy, three years old. Mother solves calculation to make busy situation during the experiment. We ask mother to say to play with a toy himself to the child.

2. Analysis a change of anxiety

After recording, we check the video with mother to find child's change of anxiety. He can't answer own state therefore we regard his mother' answer as collect. Mother answers his state of emotion. We regard "be worrying" and "want her attention" as child's sense of anxiety.

3. Reveal relations the child's sense of anxiety and successively behaviors

We analyze a time series of kind of behaviors, reveal the behaviors reflex anxiety by compare the behaviors and anxiety.

3 Results and Discussions

Most behaviors are listed below.

- speaking to himself
- speaking to his mother
- looking at his mother's face (Looking)
- moving around his mother (Moving)

Figure 1 shows four behaviors and sense of anxiety.We regard "Looking and Moving" as "check mother".

Fig.1 shows that anxiety increased after moving around his mother and speaking to his mother. Therefore the child can't be satisfied his mother's how to contact. In first half, the child has more sense of anxiety. After he moves next to mother in 13 minutes later, sense of anxiety decreased. We found that moving around had stopped after moving to mother side, which suggests the anxiety is dissolved by sitting near his mother in his hand distance. We performed t-test about "moving, looking and speaking himself". In conclusion, they have deference between before sitting next to his mother and after. (1%, 0.9%, 0.4%)

- Speaking himself
  Frequency of speaking himself increased after sitting next to his mother. It suggests sitting next to his mother give the child peace of emotion.
- Moving
  The child sat next to his mother after moving around his mother. After that, he was in peace of emotion. It suggests distance between the child and his mother is important for peace of emotion.
- Looking
  Frequency increased after sitting next to his mother. We consider that looking has 2 means; to find her and to check whether it is looking him.
  We assumed that to find her is "looking and approach", and to check it is "looking and play".
  This time looking is "looking and play" because the child sat close to mother. However looking suggests the child in peace of emotion, it can't conclude when more 30 minutes later. Therefore we cannot be determined that looking reflects sense of anxiety, it is important to observe looking with behaviors after looking at his mother.

We could observe monolog behaviors in peace of emotion, while speaking to his mother, moving around his mother and frequent change of distance between the child and his mother in sense of anxiety. Importance of Observation about looking is not only that behaviors but also behaviors after looking.

More than that, we considered distance between the child and his mother is important. Actually, sense of anxiety decreased after sitting next to his mother.

That the child is close to his mother is more in peace of emotion than the child looks his mother's face.

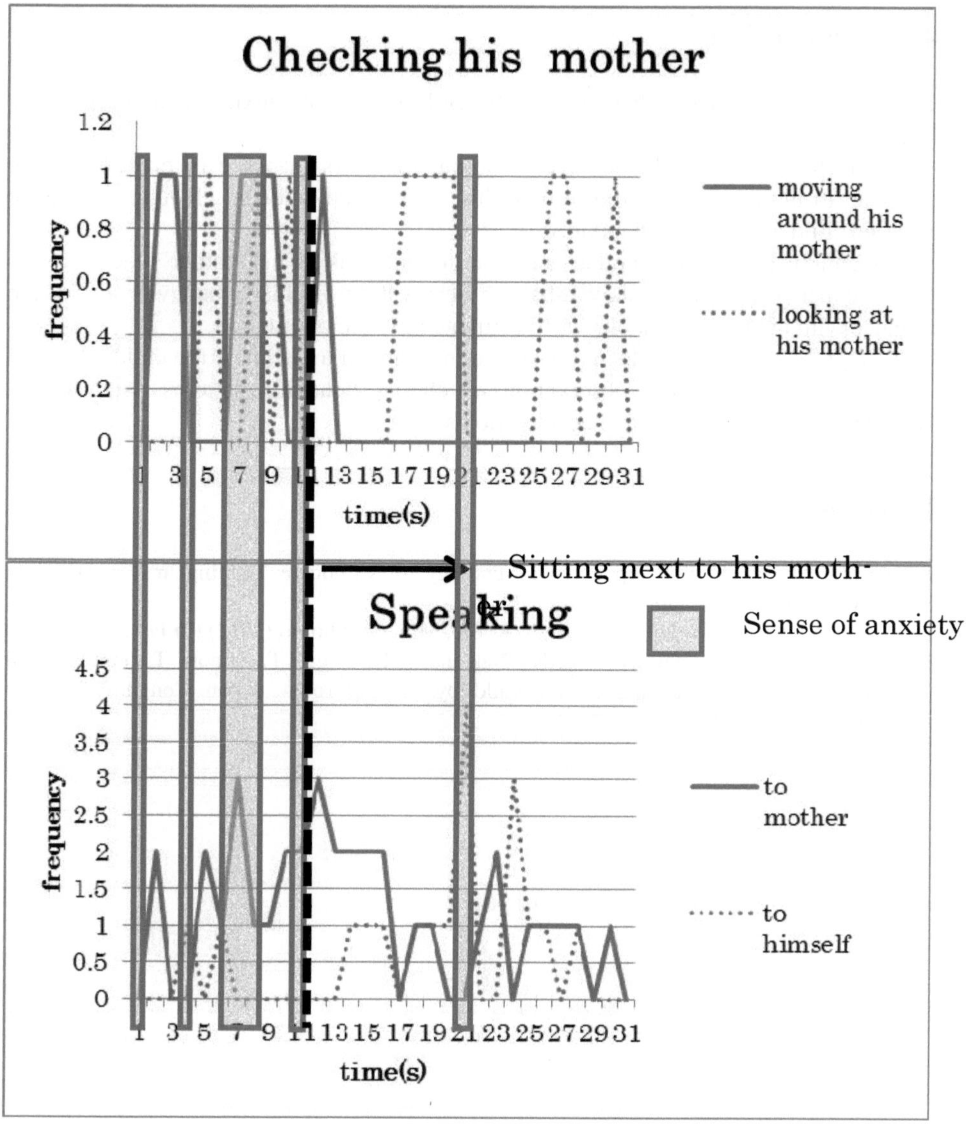

Fig. 1. Relation of check mother, Speaking and anxiety

4 Conclusion

This study aims to show that relation the child's sense of anxiety and successively behaviors.

In conclusion, we could observe monolog behaviors in peace of emotion, while speaking to his mother, moving around his mother and frequent change of distance between child and mother in anxiety.

The child is close to his mother is important than looking his mother's face.

Our experimental result shows that the observation of child's behavior and of the distance with his mother enables us to estimate his state of emotion.

It suggests we can provide an assistance mechanism to estimate the child's state of emotion through physical observation of child's behavior patterns using room-embedded Kinect and wearable acceleration sensors.

References

1. Fujisaki, M., et al.: Developmental Psychology for Childcare Training, rev. ed. (Tokyo, Shinyosya) (2007) (in Japanese)
2. Uchida, N.: Infant Psychology, rev. ed. (Kyoto, Minerva-Shobo) (2012) (in Japanese)
3. Iwasaki, A., Shimotomai, T., Abe, K., Nakamura, T., Nagai, T., Omori, T.: Fundamental study of personality estimation for child by playing robot. Japan Congnitive Sience Society (29), 1–10 (2012)

Designing a Technology–Augmented School Desk for the Future Classroom

Calliope Savvaki[1], Asterios Leonidis[1], George Paparoulis[1], Margherita Antona[1], and Constantine Stephanidis[1,2]

[1] Foundation for Research and Technology – Hellas (FORTH) - Institute of Computer Science
N. Plastira 100, Vassilika Vouton, GR-700 13 Heraklion, Crete, Greece
[2] University of Crete, Department of Computer Science, Heraklion, Crete, Greece
{calliope,leonidis,groulis,antona,cs}@ics.forth.gr

Abstract. Technological advancements and contemporary learning theories dictate the need for redesigning the school environment to emded technology in a seamless way. This paper describes an approach towards the development and modernization of the future classroom, by redesigning the student desk. A technology-augemented desk was designed following an iterative approach, leading to the creation and evaluation of several alternative solutions.

Keywords: school desk, future classroom, smart classroom, ambient intelligence.

1 Introduction

Information and Communication Technologies have been attributed with the potential to change and restructure the educational process, while a lot of studies have been devoted to discussing their role and uses in education. For example, ICTs have been claimed to improve the quality of education by motivating students to learn, facilitating the acquisition of basic skills and fostering inquiry and exploration [1].

Regarding the learning process, ICT can enable new ways of teaching and learning, moving away from the traditional teacher-centered pedagogy towards the direction of learner-centered approaches, by promoting active and collaborative learning [2]. This approach is supported by the constructivist theory, according to which technology takes a special place as a powerful tool for children's learning by doing, while it constitutes an integral component of the curriculum, a chameleon-like tool that can be used with almost any content [3]. On the other hand, in most contemporary learning theories, emphasis has been given to co-operative and social learning, as well as to the construction of knowledge from the students themselves [4].

As a result, the school environment needs to be reshaped in order to address the aforementioned needs by: (i) redesigning the learning spaces themselves, (ii) redesigning furniture and introducing technology-enhanced objects that facilitate learning and (iii) supporting knowledge-based communities in virtual and physical learning spaces [4]. This paper describes an approach towards the development and

C. Stephanidis (Ed.): Posters, Part II, HCII 2013, CCIS 374, pp. 681–685, 2013.

modernization of the future classroom for the improvement of the educational process, by redesigning the most essential classroom artifact, the student desk.

From a technology perspective, and in accordance with current learning theories, the notion of smart classroom has become prevalent in the past decade [5], supporting new means of interaction such as interactive whiteboards, touch screens, smartphones and tablet PCs. An initial approach towards investigating the role of technologies in the educational context and in the smart classroom environment was presented in [6], suggesting among others an augmented school desk. Evaluation of the first school desk prototype indicated that children were interested, and in some cases enthusiastic, about having such an artifact in their classroom; however, they expressed interest in a more aesthetically pleasant appearance of the desk [6]. Further to this initial evaluation, informal interviews conducted with target users of the desk indicated the overall "look and feel" as a key factor for acceptance of technologically enhanced artifacts in the classroom.

As a result, besides the high-level goals motivating the design of this new artifact, additional objectives deriving from the lessons learned from the first prototype, were to:

- preserve the traditional functionality of the school desk, allowing students to use typical school equipment, such as books, pencils, etc.
- embed technological devices, such as a multi-touch widescreen personal computer, headphones, keyboard, and a depth camera
- hide the technological complexity, by seamlessly embedding the equipment in the furniture
- create an appealing, easy-to-use and vandal-proof artifact.

The next sections describe in details the design of the proposed future classroom student desk by describing the design method that was applied (section 2), presenting the artifact itself (section 3) and providing a discussion and future directions (section 4).

2 Design Method

An iterative design approach was followed, driven by studying the target users and the intended context of use. Based on the design requirements, various solutions were proposed through the method of brainstorming, which were then combined in the creation of several concept mockups. These mockups have been evaluated in discussion groups, concluding with the design of a final desk concept.

Research regarding the users focused on their individual characteristics and preferences, their relation with technology, and the cognitive process behind the learning experience. An important parameter of an ergonomically designed desk, and therefore of this study, was the anthropometry attributes of young students, as they change across the various ages from primary school children to teenagers and young adults.

The context in which the artifact will be used is another important design parameter. Under this perspective, several learning theories and classroom arrangements have been studied, focusing on innovative proposals, aiming to support the major drives of change in education in the near future, such as [7]: developments in education dictated by the need to spread the expertise of the most able teachers more widely, and the need to stimulate children to achieve more; changes in the organization of the classroom environment – to enable, for example, a range of group sizes to be taught effectively in one space; developments in ICT; as well as the need for flexibility and adaptability. Furthermore, the most common currently used classroom layouts and the role of each one in the learning process have also been taken into account.

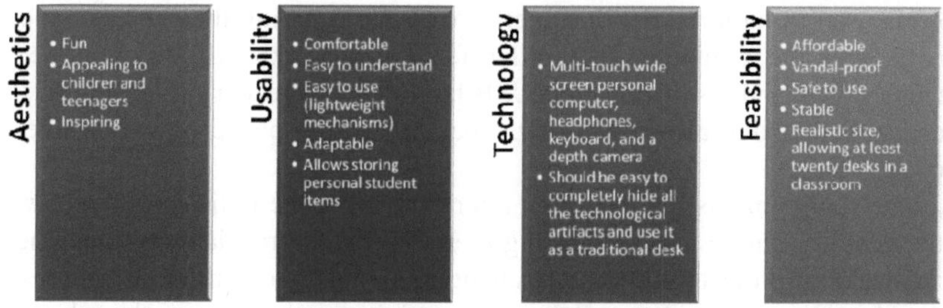

Fig. 1. Future school desk design requirements

Additionally, the artifact itself and its role as a personal object in a public environment have been considered. As a result, the student desk should function both as a personal space (e.g., for reading, or taking a test) and as a collaborative space for classmates' cooperation and ideas exchange.

The above research resulted in a set of design requirements that should be satisfied by the student desk, structured around four main categories, as shown in Fig. 1.

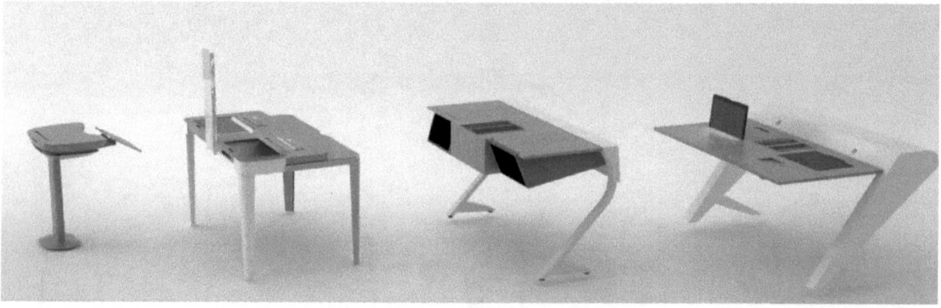

Fig. 2. Alternative desk concepts

Based on the design requirements, several solutions ranging from tablet-based to back-projected implementations have been proposed and evaluated following an iterative approach (see Fig. 2). Each design alternative has been evaluated by discussion groups involving an industrial designer, three software engineers and three interaction designers. The evaluation and redesign process led to the refinement of the initial requirements, based on which a final desk concept has been developed.

3 The Proposed School Desk

The result of the aforementioned research and iterative process was the design of a technology-augmented desk, as shown in Fig. 3, appropriate for use in the context of a smart classroom. The desk features a 24-inches wide all-in-one computer embedded in a rotatable steel frame covered with white-lacquered oak wood. The frame can be tilted from 0° to 180° using the available handles, to reveal a typical desk surface and facilitate paper-based activities, while when folded away its back becomes an ideal projection surface. On its top left corner, a steel pillar covered with white-lacquered oak wood is used to mount a depth camera. Apart from hiding the cables connecting the camera with the computer, the pillar features a corkboard that can be used for attaching notes, and a self-powered USB hub and card reader on its side to facilitate connection of external devices (e.g., memory cards, pen drives, portable hard drives, etc.).

One of the requirements that occurred after evaluating the initial prototypes was to design the desk for single use, facilitating therefore the appropriate rearrangement of classroom desks in order to address the changing demands of different teaching scenarios. For instance, given that collaborative activities can enhance the educational process [8], two adjacent desks can be connected to create a larger interactive workspace and promote teamwork.

Finally, the desk offers various practical and convenient solutions regarding daily activities that convey additional contextual information as well. In more details, the desk: (i) incorporates a mesh storage below the desk's surface to hold books and other personal belongings, (ii) integrates a steel hook equipped with a force sensor to detect the presence of the student's backpack, and (iii) embeds distance sensors in its front- and back- facing sides to detect students' presence, and pressure sensors to detect reckless behaviors (e.g., a student is sitting on the screen).

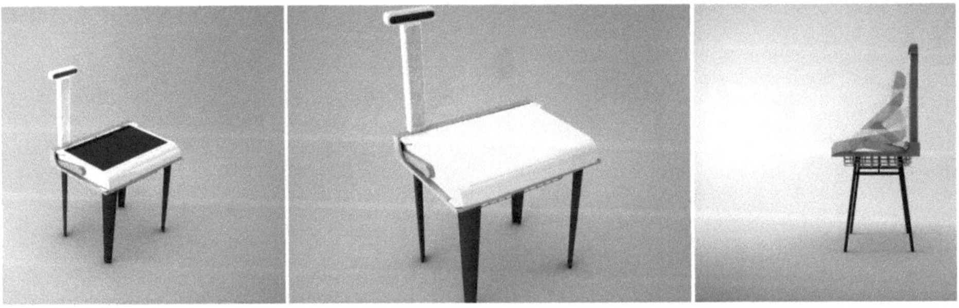

Fig. 3. Alternative views of the proposed desk

4 Discussion

This paper has described the iterative approach that was followed in the design of a technology-augmented student desk. In summary, the desk features attractive aesthetics and has successfully addressed the issue of technology integration in terms of size and design. The desk will be built of MDF wood and oak wood, with few metallic and stainless steel parts, which is a low cost solution. As a result, the proposed student desk can be easily introduced in existing classrooms, while it can also effectively address the requirements of future classrooms.

Future work will aim to improve the ergonomics of the proposed artifact regarding the screen rotation mechanism, which may be difficult for primary school students to handle. To this end, a prototype of the desk will be constructed and evaluated with school children of various ages.

Acknowledgements. This work is supported by the ICS-FORTH internal RTD Programme "Ambient Intelligence".

References

1. Haddad, W.D., Jurich, S.: ICT for Education: Potential and Potency. In: Haddad, W., Drexler, A. (eds.) Technologies for Education: Potentials, Parameters, and Prospects, pp. 34–37. Academy for EducationalDevelopment and Paris: UNESCO, Washington (2002)
2. Tinio, V.L.: ICT in Education. e-Primers for the Information Economy, Society, and Polity Series, e-ASEAN Task Force Secretariat, UNDP-APDIP (2003), http://www.apdip.net/publications/iespprimers/ICTinEducation.pdf (retrieved on March 26, 2013)
3. Strommen, E.F., Lincoln, B.: Constructivism, technology, and the future of classroom learning. Education and Urban Society 24(4), 466–476 (1992)
4. Mäkitalo-Siegl, K., Zottmann, J., Kaplan, F., Fischer, F.: Classroom of the future. Orchestrating Collaborative Space. Sense Publishers, Rotterdam (2010)
5. Xu, P., Han, G., Li, W., Wu, Z., Zhou, M.: Towards Intelligent Interaction in Classroom. In: Stephanidis, C. (ed.) UAHCI 2009, Part III. LNCS, vol. 5616, pp. 150–156. Springer, Heidelberg (2009)
6. Antona, M., Margetis, G., Ntoa, S., Leonidis, A., Korozi, M., Paparoulis, G., Stephanidis, C.: Ambient Intelligence in the classroom: an augmented school desk. In: Karwowski, W., Salvendy, G. (eds.) Proceedings of the 2010 AHFE International Conference (3rd International Conference on Applied Human Factors and Ergonomics), Miami, Florida, USA, July 17-20. [CD-ROM]. USA Publishing (2010) ISBN: 978-0-9796435-4-5
7. Britain, G.: Department for Education and Skills, corp creator (2002), Classrooms of the future: innovative designs for schools, http://dera.ioe.ac.uk/8640/1/classrooms_of_the_future.pdf (retrieved on March 26, 2013)
8. Prince, M.: Does Active Learning Work? A Review of the Research. Journal of Engineering Education 93, 223–231 (2004)

Automatic GUI Generation for Home Electric Appliances by Remote Controller on Ad-Hoc Wireless Communication

Hiroki Sawada and Tomohiro Hase

Ryukoku University
Seta, Otsu 520-2194 Shiga, Japan
hase@rins.ryukoku.ac.jp

Abstract. A majority of home electric appliances are now remotely operable with remote controllers. Users therefore need to operate a wide variety of remote controllers with designs that vary by model and by manufacturer. Also, along with the sophistication and functionality of the appliances, these remote controllers are each provided with an increased number of operation buttons. This makes it more difficult for users to find the correct button from the many buttons. Further, a television set, for example, is commonly used combined with other appliances. Users are then required to manipulate remote controllers for several appliances in the correct order, while thinking about the necessary procedure.

Keywords: remote, operate, Ad-Hoc, Wireless, Communication.

1 Introduction

In recent years, many household electric appliances have become remotely operable by using an infrared remote controller, thus increasing in usability. However, due to the increased number of household electric appliances in a house, users have to operate remote controllers of various designs, each different by model and by manufacturer. Further, a number of operation buttons laid on a remote controller has been increasing as more functions are added to household electric appliances, making it even more difficult for users to find a target button. As every house has as many remote controllers as the number of electric appliances it owns, finding the correct remote controller and appropriately using it are quite troublesome. Meanwhile, it is also difficult for users to get hold of the current operating and use statuses of all the electric appliances in a house. With the aim of addressing these problems, we propose a new GUI design in this paper.

2 Objectives of This Study and Proposed System

The objectives of this study include unifying operation buttons and designs of remote controllers so that the number of operation buttons is minimized for users. Further, it

C. Stephanidis (Ed.): Posters, Part II, HCII 2013, CCIS 374, pp. 686–690, 2013.

is desirable that users can get hold of the behavioral information of their household electric appliances on the remote controller.

To address these objectives, this study proposes the following two systems:

First, with the aim of unifying operation buttons and designs of remote controllers, physical buttons are changed to a graphical UI (GUI) screen. Next, by enabling to reflect the behavioral and locational information of the electric appliances on the remote controller GUI by means of ZigBee as the ad-hoc wireless communication standard, the minimum required number of buttons are displayed for the electric appliance that is located closest to the user so that the user can get its operating status.

3 Experimental Device

With the aim to verify effectiveness of this proposal, a ZigBee module was installed on the T-Engine of the embedded system development equipment mounted with an LCD, which was assumed to serve as a remote controller with the ad-hoc wireless communication functions. Three units of ZigBee terminals that were assumed as household electric appliances were located in a laboratory. The ZigBee module combined with the remote controller served as the coordinator, around which a network was established. The other three units are routers through which communication of other appliances can pass. Figure 1 shows an external appearance of the experimental unit.

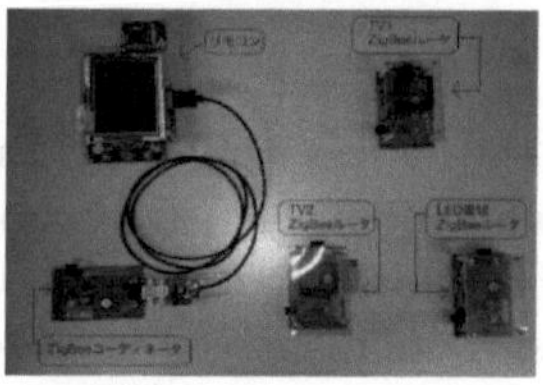

Fig. 1. Experimental units actually used

4 Experimental Method

The effectiveness of this experimental system was verified. First, we confirmed whether or not the icons for the appliance that was located closest to the remote controller were properly displayed. We also confirmed, by touching the icons, whether or not the operation screen of the corresponding remote controller was successfully displayed in the unified design. Next, moving around in the laboratory room, carrying the remote controller, we confirmed whether or not the icon display for each appliance also sequentially changed in a responsive manner. Further, when the electric appliances that were used combined with each other were located close to the remote controller, it was confirmed whether or not the operation GUIs for these electric appliances were also displayed in a combined form. Finally, by switching ON/OFF the terminals, we confirmed whether or not the behavioral information display changes and the power LED of the ZigBee module flashed. Figure 2 shows the diagram of the experimental method.

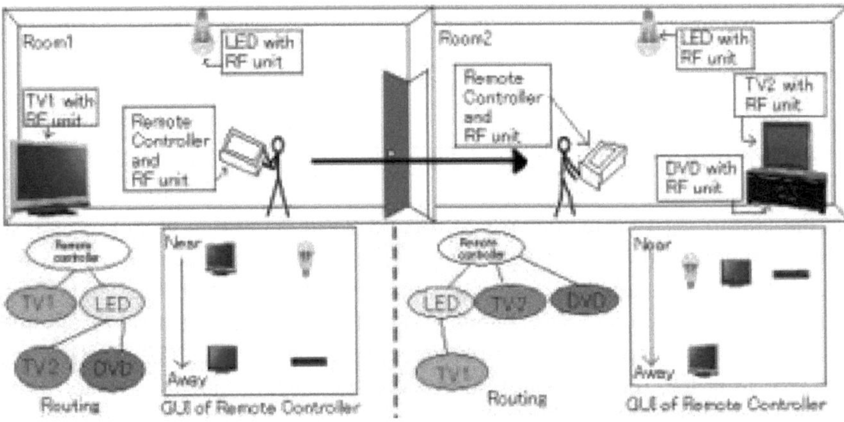

Fig. 2. Experimental method

5 Result

As the result of the experiment, it was confirmed that the operation status and the operation screen of the remote controller were correctly displayed. It was also confirmed that, even when the remote controller was moved to different places, the icons of the electric appliances were displayed in the order where those closest to the remote controller were preferentially laid out. When the electric appliances that were used combined with each other were located close to the remote controller, the operation GUIs of the remote controller were displayed correctly combined.

Next, with the electric appliances switched ON/OFF on the remote controller, the operation status display was also changed. Finally, it was confirmed by lighting-up of LED of the ZigBee module that the electric appliances were operable. Figure 3 shows

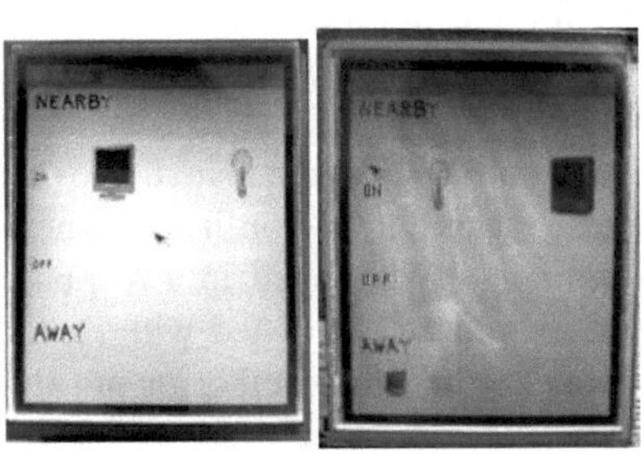

Fig. 3. Change in icon layout

a change in the icon layout and Figure 4 shows a change in the remote controller operation GUI from the one for general use to another for combined use. Figure 5 shows flashing of the ZigBee module LED.

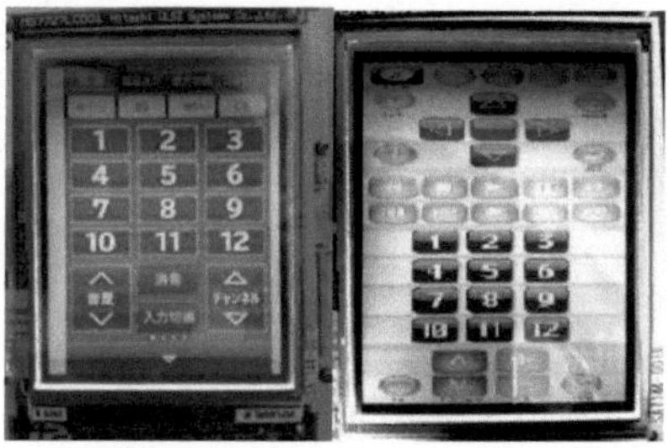

Fig. 4. Remote controller GUI displayed on T-Engine LCD

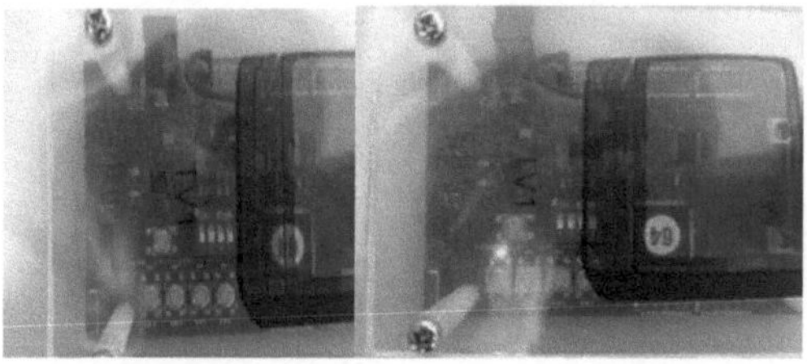

Fig. 5. Flashing of ZigBee module LED

6 Conclusion

This paper described automatic configuration of remote controller GUI and operation of household electric appliances by using ad-hoc wireless communication. In this paper, we proposed the method to display the minimum required number of operation buttons for users on the remote controller GUI screen of touch-panel type LCD that is designed common to various electric appliances. Further proposed was a system that can used to confirm, on a remote controller, the behavioral information of each appliance. In order to realize these proposals, by means of ad-hoc wireless communication, we gathered information of the household electric appliances on the remote controller. Then, we built an experimental device for the experiment. As a result of the experiment, the targeted objectives were achieved.

References

1. Digital Living Network Alliance "A Digital World Designed", http://www.dlna.org/home
2. ZigBeeSIG-J, "about_ZigBee", http://www.zbsigj.org/about_zigbee
3. Linux/M32R Home Page, http://www.linux-m32r.org/index_jpn.html
4. Matsuda, M., Nonaka, T., Nakata, T., Hase, T.: Dynamic Display Method In User Interface Based on Routing Information on AD-HOC Wireless Communication. In: Proc. ICCE 2007, Las Vegas, USA (January 2007)

CLIM: An Interactive Tabletop for Landscape Modeling

Matthew Swarts, Paula Gomez, Pedro Soza, Jonathan Shaw,
James MacDaniel, and David Moore

Imagine Lab, College of Architecture, Georgia Institute of Technology, USA
{matthew.swarts,jonathan.shaw}@coa.gatech.edu,
{paulagomez,pedro.soza,jmacdaniel3,dmoore38}@gatech.edu

Abstract. In this paper we describe our development of an interactive touch tabletop user interface for a landscape design tool. The user interface provides a view of the data, which combines the affordances of a multi-touch tabletop display with a vertical screen for real-time feedback. While the table metaphor fits well with the concepts of a top down view of land-scape, approachable from any direction, the board metaphor provides a clear, shared orientation for reading output charts. We also present a data model for landscape projects, which provides a knowledge-based approach to design decision making. We discuss the sourcing of the datasets that drive our landscape model.

Keywords: Interactive Tabletop, Landscape Design, Knowledge-based Design, Touch User Interface, Campus Information Modeling.

1 Introduction

Decision-making for campus landscape planning may take several months, as it requires a negotiation among various professionals, converging on a wide range of knowledge, ideas and goals into one concise plan. Within the scope of an intermediate landscape planning scale, we propose a landscape design tool that provides relevant information and real-time feedback during collaborative design-decision-making sessions. Our goals are to 1) to facilitate collaboration among experts by providing a tool that includes the professional knowledge of landscape design and real-time evaluations and 2) to document the decision-making processes allowing storage and retrieval of alternative design proposals. This paper is focused on describing how the landscape knowledge embedded into the model becomes activated by the user interface (UI) design. 'Campus Landscape Information Modeling' (CLIM) facilitates collaboration and rapid design development by addressing important quantitative and qualitative questions to evaluate design proposals and save alternative scenarios (sequence of projects) to compare over time. CLIM visually presents raster-based land use and vector-based landscape elements. Visual information is rendered into a large table to display, representing an aerial view of campus, and a vertical dashboard display networked with informative charts that update in real-time (Figure1a). Multi touch interaction facilitates collaborative user interaction with the visual model [1] providing access to elements' attributes (e.g. tree age, canopy radius) and information about

C. Stephanidis (Ed.): Posters, Part II, HCII 2013, CCIS 374, pp. 691–695, 2013.

land use type that impacts landscape decision-making. Shared visualization allows stakeholders to more readily understand the issues surrounding the existing landscape and proposed designs.

2 Related Work

A handful of tools have previously been developed to address collaboration, participation, and more natural methods of user interaction with landscape design. LANDISVIEW is a visualization tool for single landscape modeling [2], which uses a raster-based model that simulates and visualizes forest changes. SELES is a tool that allows "rapid model prototyping and modification," supporting collaborative landscape analysis [3]. Interaction with larger scale maps have also been explored for collaboration using gestures[4]. Other approaches propose stakeholder mutual understanding through virtual reality, demonstrating a clear interest for a "greater dimensionality representation" [5]. Additionally, tangible user interfaces for manipulating terrain data and visualizing analysis have utilized physical objects to better mimic traditional physical interaction methods[6, 7]. Smart Plan, by Sasaki Associates, uses a dual surface tool –table and board– that enables collaboration among planners and designers, providing physical, financial, and environmental feedback at any time of the planning phase. "Smart Plan helps clients visualize and quantify the trade-offs inherent in these choices" [8], however, it is not interactive. Complementary to the presented work, CLIM is a multi-dimensional tool that provides interaction among a group users, allowing them to access the model, information, and knowledge during individual or collaborative planning sessions. CLIM includes a multiple project-scenario structure, multiple representations of information and knowledge, touch table interaction, and board information views.

3 Sources of Landscape Knowledge

To support the contributions mentioned above, what is the specific landscape de-sign knowledge to be embedded into the tool that supports? In this project, we have included four fundamental sources of landscape knowledge: Postsecondary Education Facilities Inventory and Classification Manual (FICM)[9], Landscape Master Plan document (CMPU) [10], City planning workshops, and interviews with experts.

Facilities Inventory and Classification Manual, FICM. FICM by The National Center for Education Statistics (NCES), is used by institutions to evaluate the current space and plan for future space needs in both, building and landscape levels[9]. FICM describes what is included in building and landscape inventories; defines area measurements, space use types, and building data such as ownership, costs, and condition. It also includes functional categories, and space, land, and element types. Based on this manual, we created an infrastructure for spatial classification that helps us to construct the conceptual model of the tool. Additionally, evaluation methods derived from this manual–such as gross areas, cost, condition status, and maintenance cost– combine specific landscape knowledge and User Interface and Interaction design (Figure 1a).

Georgia Tech Landscape Master Plan, CMPU. The landscape master plan for Georgia Institute of Technology (GT) is an online document that consists of a Master plan map and a master plan report (2011), containing a compilation of design guidelines and practices for developing campus landscape. Its goal is to achieve a "livable, sustainable and beautiful campus"[10]. Some examples of the recommendations we have incorporated into our model are: Water Standards (Storm water management, Water courses), Vegetation Guidelines (Tree types, Tree replacement, Irrigation systems), and Hardscape guidelines (circulation types, pavement types, bicycle facilities, outdoor lighting). For example, one specific goal is to "increase total tree canopy coverage of the campus to 50% or more."

Urban Planning Workshops. Several Northside Avenue landscape projects developed in an urban planning studio at GT served as guidelines for the types of issues involved in urban planning decisions, which is similar in scale to campus scale landscape planning. The information that emerged from these projects is, for example, pedestrian movement and transportation systems and how they map to street sections, including sidewalks, street trees, bike crossing, and signalize. By studying the expert understanding of the problems reflected into the proposals, we came incorporated the concept of parametric street sections and a new measurement for distances: minutes' walk.

Interviews. We held two structured and unstructured interviews to collect expert knowledge. One was a conversation with an expert landscape designer from the unit of Capital Planning and Space Management (CPSM) at GT. The other was with a landscape and urban design student. Our goal was to understand and extract the primary knowledge users would expect to be embedded in CLIM. As a result of these interviews, we included new element types not considered in the current landscape planning manuals, and gained a new understanding of systems with the desire for an end-point element representation. For example, street lighting and recycling bins are considered end elements of a larger process network for energy and waste management. We decided to expand the system that currently represents visual perceivable elements to visualize more abstract process networks as well.

4 Landscape Representation

All relevant information about landscape areas, elements, and their dynamics, as well as the knowledge coming from experts, were translated into the 'Campus Land-scape Information Model' to be accessible through the touch table user interface.

Landscape Model. The purpose of our model is to organize frameworks for data and knowledge, for comparison across systems, and for exploration and understanding of implications. So far, CLIM includes two fundamental models: Land use and tree inventory, which are translated into raster representations and vector point representations respectively. For the land use raster model, we created a scale map of the GT campus in a vector format. By referencing existing planning documents, satellite imagery, and observation of land use, we constructed a colored vector file, corresponding to 29 land use types defined in CMPU. For the campus tree inventory data, which has more than 11,000 trees, includes information about tree location, height, canopy, species, and condition among others. These models provide a way to answer specific questions by putting experts together with the model information. As an example, users can propose an irrigation system and see how it fits into the scope of the whole system, and how it might impact tree development over time.

User Interface and Interaction Design. In order to support collaboration among experts using real-time visualization and feedback, we designed a two large-screen display interface [4], combining the table and board metaphors. The table metaphor provides support for group collaboration due to its physical characteristics, such as size, orientation and height [11]. It is based on map visualization, accessible through touch interaction. The board metaphor renders feedback for collaborative design decision-making [12]. The physical separation between the touch table's interactive model and the board's dashboard is the main divider for overall layout organization. On the touch table, a raster model and the icons to interact with it are displayed, such as land type selection-and-painting and tree type selection-and-planting. A dashboard composed of graphs and counters organized by budget and cost, performance, project scenarios comparison, land type percentage areas, and elements counters is displayed on the vertical board (Figure 1a). The combination of the selected metaphors integrates the various views of the landscape model to provide a more instinctive comprehension and interaction of the information (Figure 1b).

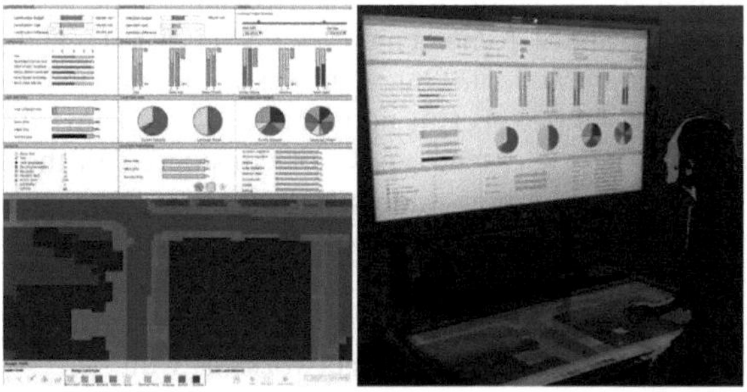

Fig. 1. a: Board screen displaying dashboard vertically aligned with table screen displaying the raster model of a section of the campus. b: User interaction with the touch table and dashboard.

Landscape knowledge was translated into the user interface and interaction at three levels: graphic elements, screen layout, and physical organization. The graphic representation provides visually accessible information and knowledge of the entities. The layout of the graphic elements is around the border in the table view and it more grid-based for the output charts on the board. For the physical organization, the table metaphor matches the 2D aerial view of campus land use types. The table is visually accessible from any angle in a top-view perspective, providing a gravity-based orientation. The touch capability allows users to directly interact and modify the view, one of the primary goals of the tool. The vertical dashboard is primarily designed to provide a shared orientation, allowing users to view real-time feedback based on their changes to the table view. The dashboard, which primarily consists of outputs indicating absolute and relative counts of change elements, provides a clear orientation for everyone to read without having to stand in an awkward posture.

5 Case Study Walkthrough

To revise CLIM functionality and user interface design for information and knowledge accessibility, we walked through the West Campus project, a landscape and building project that has a budget, schedule, and goals of increasing the number of beds, parking spots, and green areas. While we are about to begin more systematic user testing, we are using this project as a walkthrough for a real scenario. We found that the knowledge and information represented for planning is accessible through the touch table and board user interface.

Acknowledgements. We would like to thank Professor of Practice Michael Dobbins and the students in his course for providing access to real project scenarios to complement our approach.

References

1. Sims, R.: Interactivity: A forgotten art? Computers in Human Behavior 13, 157–180 (1997)
2. Birt, A.G., Xi, W., Coulson, R.N.: LANDISVIEW: A visualization tool for landscape modelling. Environmental Modelling & Software 24, 1339–1341 (2009)
3. Fall, A., Daust, D., Morgan, D.G.: A framework and software tool to support collaborative landscape analysis: fitting square pegs into square holes. Trans. in GIS 5, 67–86 (2001)
4. MacEachren, A.M., Cai, G., Brewer, I., Chen, J.: Supporting Map-based Geocollaboration Through Natural Interfaces to Large-Screen Displays. Cartographic Perspectives, 16–34 (2006)
5. Ball, J., Capanni, N., Watt, S.: Virtual reality for mutual understanding in landscape planning. Development 2 (2005)
6. Piper, B., Ratti, C., Ishii, H.: Illuminating Clay: A 3-D Tangible Interface for Landscape Analysis, pp. 355–517. Association for Computing Machinery, New York (Year)
7. Underkoffler, J., Ishii, H.: Urp: A Luminous-Tangible Workbench for Urban Planning and Design, pp. 386–393. ACM Press, United States (Year)
8. Sasaki Associates, Inc., `http://www.sasaki.com/project/272/smartplan/`
9. Korb, R.: National Working Group on Postsecondary Facilities Kreon L. Cyros (2006)
10. Georgia Institute of Technology, `http://www.space.gatech.edu/landscapeplan/`
11. Reilly, D., Voida, S., McKeon, M., Le Dantec, C., Bunde-Pedersen, J., Edwards, K., Mynatt, E.D., Mazalek, A.: Space Matters: Physical-Digital and Physical-Virtual Codesign in inSpace. IEEE Pervasive Computing 9, 54–63 (2010)
12. Ishii, H., Kobayashi, M., Bauersbeld, P., Bennet, J., Lynch, G.: ClearBoard: a seamless medium for shared drawing and conversation with eye contact. In: CHI 1992 Conf. Proc. ACM Conf. on Human Factors in Computing Systems. Striking a Balance, ACM Press (1992)

Part XI
Virtual and Mixed Environments

CamouLED: Real-Time Generation of Pixel Pattern for Camouflage

Woon Jung Cho[1], Hye-Kyoung Seo[2], Hannah Kim[1], Jiyeun Lee[1], Dong-Hyun Kang[2], Min-Ki Kim[2], and Kwang-Hee Han[1,*]

[1] Cognitive Engineering Lab. Department of Psychology, Yonsei University, Korea
{chrischo,khan}@yonsei.ac.kr, trinityhkim@gmail.com, amethystljy@naver.com

[2] Department of Mechanical Engineering, Yonsei University, Korea
{cine5,kangtong13,alsike00}@yonsei.ac.kr

Abstract. This study has developed CamouLED, which is a real-time patterning technique for active camouflage, using light emitting diodes (LED). Once a CMOS camera receives a background image, camouflage patterns are generated real-time by the patterning program. The major strategies for color combination include Average, Main and Mosaic. Two arrangement types (Arrange, Random) control background properties and distribution of pixels to generate patterns. The generated patterns are then displayed on an 8 x 8 LED matrix. The system provides over 85% of color consistency between the inputted and outputted colors. Future researches should concentrate on improving the fine details of the real-time patterning program as well as the LED controlling technique for better adaptive camouflage.

Keywords: active camouflage, visual stealth, camouflage patterning algorithm, adaptive pattern, real-time patterning.

1 Introduction

Camouflage or concealment concerns avoiding detection and preventing recogni-tion. This is highly affected by various factors such as season and surrounding environment [2]. Especially in today's combats, there is a growing need for new combat uniforms, as well as military strategies and weapons that have effective camouflage ability, known as active visual stealth.

Therefore, this study has developed a real-time patterning technique named CamouLED. Given a real scene, the patterning program previously invented by the authors [1] could generate only one type of camouflage pattern. Since then, improvements have been made to the program, and it is now able to generate six types of camouflage patterns. CamouLED attempts to take one step further, by using light emitting diodes (LED). A camera attached to the system reads the surrounding environment and an LED display dynamically changes its color pattern accordingly. The patterning program controls the displayed color patterns.

* Corresponding author.

C. Stephanidis (Ed.): Posters, Part II, HCII 2013, CCIS 374, pp. 699–703, 2013.

2 Development of an Automatic Patterning Program

2.1 Color Strategies for Camouflage

In order to develop an algorithm for generating camouflage patterns, we have reviewed visual camouflage researches and devised several color combination strategies. Their effectiveness was then assessed via a photo simulation experiment. Three color combination and two digital pattern arrangement strategies were selected. Each one of them is described below (Fig. 1):

2.1.1 Color Combination Strategies

- Average: The entire background image is divided into a 3 x 3 grid. The average color of the target grid that contains the camouflaged pattern is used to generate a suitable pattern. Once a reference color is selected, its tone is adjusted according to its luminance to produce four colors that constitute the camouflage pattern. The colors are assigned to a specific location according to their familiarity to the target area.
- Main: Main color is the color that has the highest frequency in the entire background. Four colors with the highest frequency are selected, and they are arranged according to their frequency and the proportion of the area they occupy within the target area.
- Mosaic: A selected area is divided into units and the average color of the target unit is allocated.

2.1.2 Pattern Arrangement Strategies

- Arranged distribution: Original location of the pixels is preserved when a camouflage pattern is applied. Thus the edges of the object in the scene are identifiable.
- Random distribution: Original location of the pixels is ignored; they are randomly distributed. Thus the edges are disrupted.

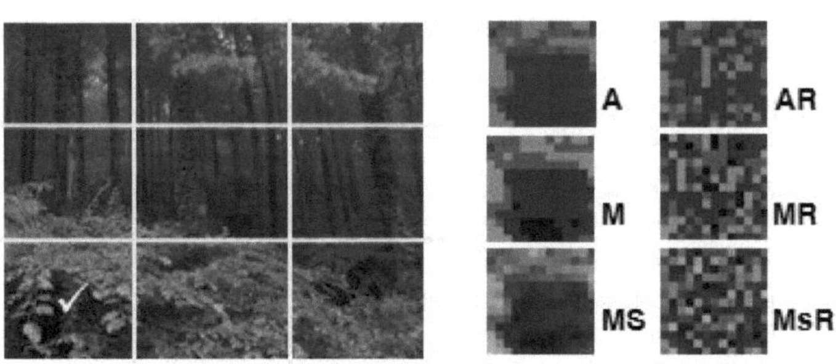

Fig. 1. Sample patterns for each strategy

2.2 Automatic Patterning Program

Based on the pattern algorithms, a program that automatically generates pattern-stimuli under dynamic backgrounds was created. This allows easier generation of pixel-dot patterns for various backgrounds based on quantitative descriptions of background features, including color information. The program contains total six strategies, as each color combination strategy (Average, Main, Mosaic) can adopt two pattern arrangement strategies (Arranged, Random).

Also included in the program are pattern strategy preset and parameter (target size, array size, number of colors, seed size, threshold) control functions. It also allows preloading a background image, defining a target area, extracting camouflage colors and creating and saving pattern strategies. Thus once an image is loaded and the pattern strategy is determined, the program extracts camouflage colors according to the selected strategy and distributes them to create a digital pattern.

3 CamouLED: Real-Time Patterning for Camouflage

The camouflage patterns generated from the program were implemented on an 8 x 8 LED display. Several studies have discussed the effectiveness of lights as a means of active stealth. For example, in the project codename Yehudi, the US Navy used lights instead of colors to blend their aircraft into the sky background. Camouflage color was not of a concern, as the airplane would be a black dot against the sky. However, adjusting the light intensity to match that of the sky succeeded in making it less visible [3]. It is from this point that the current study attempted to implement the camouflage pattern on the LED display (Fig. 2).

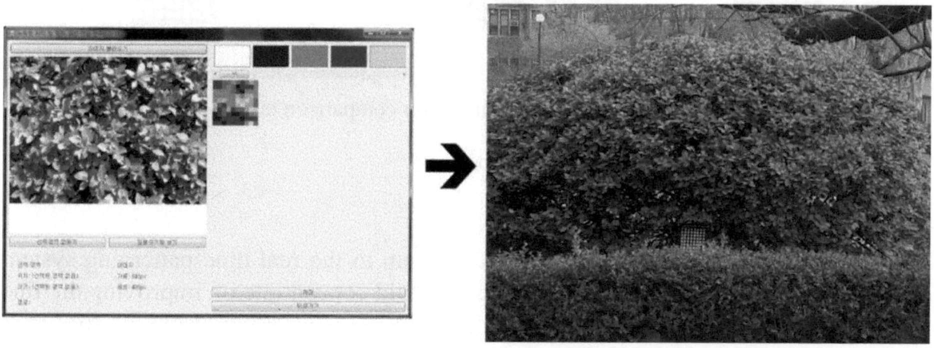

Fig. 2. Overview of CamouLED

As an input device, CamouLED uses a CMOS camera to read the background scene (Fig. 3). Once an image is received through the camera via a CCD image sensor, it is processed by the patterning algorithm. The processed digital signal is then converted into an analog signal and sent over to the LED display. A color comparison test showed that the system provides over 85% of color concordance between the inputted and outputted colors (Fig. 4).

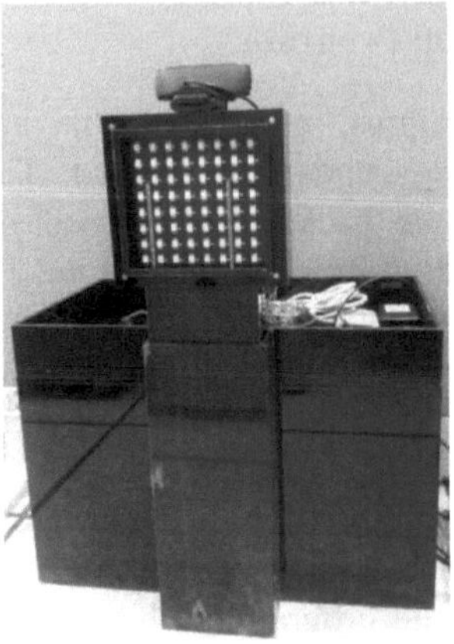

Fig. 3. CamouLED hardware

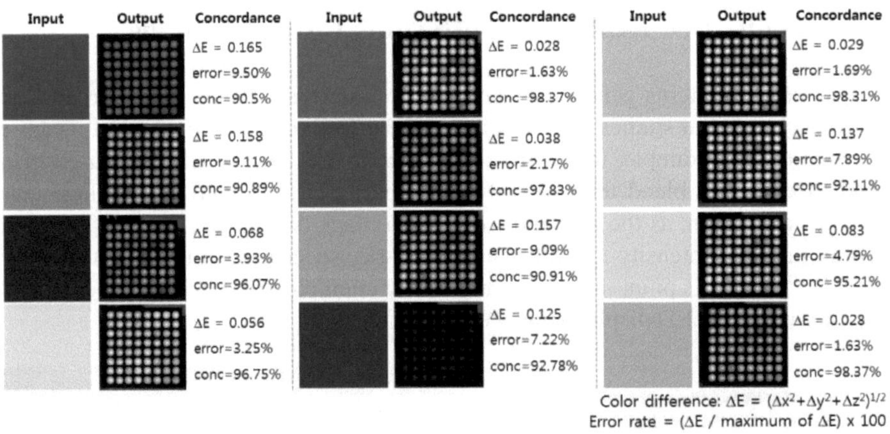

Fig. 4. Results from the color comparison test

4 Conclusion

The present study applied the patterning program to the real-time patterning system that uses an LED display. Future researches should concentrate on improving the fine details of the patterning program as well as the LED controlling technique for better adaptive camouflage. In addition, optical fibers are receiving much attention as a means of visual camouflage. Thus, the use of optical fibers instead of an LED display would broaden the system's application and use.

Acknowledgement. This work has been supported by the Low Observable Technology Research Center program of Defense Acquisition Administration and Agency for Defense Development.

References

1. Cho, W.J., Ahn, W., Kim, M.S., Park, J., Kim, S., Han, K.-H.: Making pixel patterns automatically for camouflage-Using color information from their background. In: Stephanidis, C. (ed.) Posters, Part II, HCII 2011. CCIS, vol. 174, pp. 98–101. Springer, Heidelberg (2011)
2. Friskovec, M., Gabrijelcic, H., Simoncic, B.: Design and Evaluation of a Camouflage pattern for the Slovenian Urban Environment. Journal of Imaging Science and Technology 54(2) (2010)
3. Barrett, R.: Hypermanoeuvrability and visual cloaking: new adaptive aerostructures technologies for UAVs. Aeronautical Journal 114(1156) (2010)

Cloth Handling in Virtual Space

Shigeru Inui[1], Yuko Mesuda[2], and Yosuke Horiba[1]

[1] Faculty of Fiber Science and Technology Division, Shinshu University,
3-15-1 Tokida, Ueda City, Nagano 386-8567 Japan
[2] Graduate School of Science and Technology, Shinshu University,
3-15-1 Tokida, Ueda City, Nagano 386-8567 Japan
{inui,12st115c,horiba}@shinshu-u.ac.jp

Abstract. Cloth is used for design and production of clothing and virtualization of cloth is beneficial. In this study cloth handling is virtualized. Cloth is mechanically formulated and modeled. The motion of the position of human hand in the real world is captured using Kinect that is a sensor of game-machine. The motion of the position of human hand to the cloth model and handling of cloth is simulated in the virtual world. Handled cloth interferes with other object in the virtual space because collision detection and reaction are defined for the cloth model. Three-dimensional shape of hand is extracted from the depth image of Kinect and the motion of the shape of the hand in the virtual space is displayed.

Keywords: Cloth Handling, Simulation, Kinect.

1 Introduction

In the real world, cloth is touched and handled in the process of apparel design or production. Designer touch cloth to determine which cloth is suitable for designed clothing. Cloth is also touched and handled to design or make clothing. “Draping ” is one of the methods to make clothing pattern. While making a garment, cloth is pinned, cut away, and marked. If the pinned cloth matches the designer's ideas, dress patterns are made from the marked cloth. However, Draping is a costly, troublesome, time-consuming task. Although draping better enables garments to be made that reflect the designer’s vision and better fit the wearer’s shape, the time the process takes can be long and expensive. With today’s information and communication technology, virtualized draping reduces time and cost, as well as enabling mass customization from remote places.

Some systems for making dress patterns in virtual space have been developed. It is important to develop techniques for real-time virtual draping because this has certain advantages, one being the sensation that the real-time operations offer more realism than other methods. The position to pin or cut is not determined in advance while cloth is manipulated. The position of cuts or starting point of pinning can be decided interactively through automated program interface protocols. If the shape of the cloth can be calculated from its mechanical properties in real-time, it then becomes possible to manipulate the cloth and watch how the shape of the cloth changes.

C. Stephanidis (Ed.): Posters, Part II, HCII 2013, CCIS 374, pp. 704–707, 2013.

Real-time simulation of cloth handling has also been conducted. Dummy is dressed in simulation by handling garment patterns [1]. Cloth is pinned on a doll by marking the cloth and the doll, then the pinned cloth can be moved [2]. In these studies, mouse is used to manipulate cloth although the feeling differs from actual cloth handling. Handling by gesturing would be more realistic than mouse manipulations. In addition, most of the time the methods are able to perform only one manipulation.

We proposed a method in which controlling cloth handling follows the hand gestures in the real world. However, manipulating cloth is not all that cloth handling entails. Other manipulations, such as choosing fabrics, attaching and releasing cloth, are also needed. Among those operations, cloth cutting is also included.

2 Cloth Handling

In the handling of the cloth model, the model in virtual space is moved according to the motion of hand in the real world. The cloth model follows the motion of hands in the real world in the handling in this model.

Kinect (Micorsoft) is utilized for a sensor to detect human motion for our study. It is a game-machine sensor that controls game software through body motion or voice inputs without the need of a controller. A software program designed for human-motion capture and in particular hand gesturing can be utilized for Kinect. Three-dimensional coordinates of various parts of the body are tracked. In adapting to cloth handling, hand coordinates and hand gestures can be obtained by Kinect.

For simulation, cloth has to be formulated as a model. The cloth model here is based on a two-dimension lattice of particle-spring nodes. This model consists of particles arranged on grid with springs connecting nearest and next-to-nearest particles. Thus, a particle is connected by springs to eight others to represent the forces of fabric's warp, weft, and bias directions. Given masses and spring constants, the modeling of the dynamic response of cloth is calculated using the leap-frog method in the numerical integration of the discretized equation of motion [3-5]. Gravitational force and spring forces are applied to each particle. For each iteration in the numerical integration, the position of each particle in the next step is calculated from the present position of each particle and the forces applied to each particle.

In the virtual space, collision detection and reaction are defined between cloth and objects, such as a dress dummy, created in the computational domain. A virtual object consists of point cloud. Collision detection [3-5] involves calculating the distance between each particle in the cloth model and object. If the shortest distance is smaller than a predefined constant, collision between cloth model and object is signaled. If collision is detected, a repulsive force is applied to the colliding particle in the cloth model.

3 Results and Discussions

Handling of cloth in the virtual space was tried with the model described above. BacBook Pro (Core i7 2.4GHz, GeForce 650M (GPGPU is utilized), Windows 8,

VisualStudio 2010) was used for the simulation. As an example, it was virtualized to handle a cloth by picking up two corers of a square cloth. For this simulation, to detect the position of hand and to apply the position to two corners of a cloth are needed.

Motion of both hands is captured by Kinect which is originally designed for a sensor of game-machine. A camera to take images and a sensor to capture depth are equipped, and the depth for each pixel of depth image can be acquired. It also has a function designed to extract the coordinate of skeletal joints form the depth image. The coordinate of the left and right hand skeletal joints are tracked form all the joints in real-time.

The virtual cloth model follows the motion of both hands in the real world. The cloth consists of 10 by 10 nodes. The left-hand coordinate is given to the particle at the upper left edge of the cloth, and that of the right hand to the particle at the upper right edge. Subsequently, numerical integration, performed after a predefined time interval, calculates the motion of the cloth.

Figure 1. shows the results of the simulation. In the figures, vertical cloth and horizontal plate are shown. The position of the plate is fixed, and collision detection and reaction are defined between the cloth and the plate. In the right side figure, the lower half of the cloth is laid on the plate. It was succeeded to handle the virtual cloth in real-time. The density of the nodes for the cloth and the plate has to be tuned because it is observed that sometimes a part of the cloth goes through the plate.

The dynamic shape of hand in the real world is recognized and reproduced in the virtual space. The coordinate of the right hand skeletal joint is picked up form all the joints to detect the motion of hand. A domain that contains the right hand is set, and the depth image points that are included in the three-dimensional domain are picked up. Approximate three-dimensional shape of the right hand can be recognized and extracted by the method. As this is processed in real time, the movement of three-dimensional shape of the right hand can be extracted in real time. Figure. 2 shows the results of extraction, rock, scissors and paper of right hand respectively. It was succeeded to reproduce dynamic three-dimensional shape of the right hand in the virtual space in real-time. It is expected to react the shape of the virtual cloth according to the motion of the fingers of the right hand.

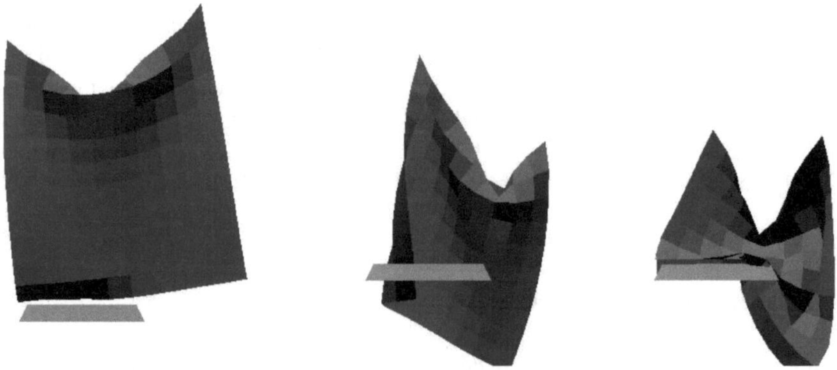

Fig. 1. The results of real-time cloth handling simulation

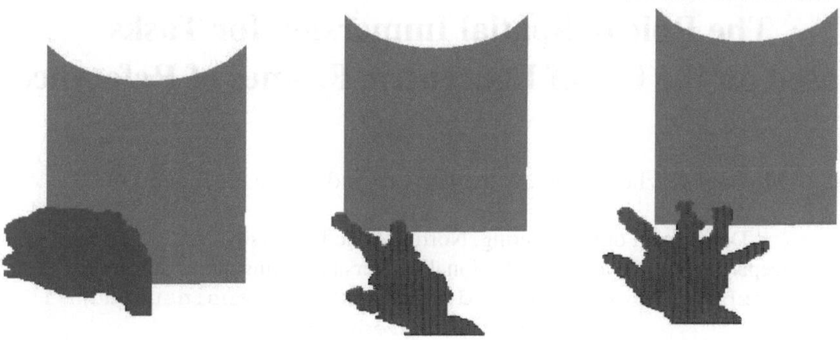

Fig. 2. The results of extraction of the shape of the right hand in the shape of rock, scissors and paper

Acknowledgments. This work was partly supported by Grants-in-Aid for Scientific Research (No. 23240100, 24220012) from the Ministry of Education, Science, Sports and Culture and Grants for Excellent Graduate Schools, MEXT, Japan.

References

1. Meng, Y., Mok, P.Y., Jin, X.: Interactive virtual try-on clothing design systems. Computer-Aided Design 42, 310–321 (2010)
2. May, P., Ehrlich, H.C., Steinke, T., Igarashi, T., Hughes, J.F.: Clothing Manipulation, UIST and I3D Reprise session. In: ACM SIGGRAPH 2003, p. 697 (2003)
3. Fuhmann, A., Gros, C., Luckas, V.: Interactive animation of cloth including self collision detection. In: Proc. WSCG, pp. 141–148 (2003)
4. Fuhmann, A., Sobottka, G., Gros, C.: Distance fields for rapid collision detection in physically based modeling. In: Proc. Graphi. Con., pp. 58–65 (2003)
5. Harada, T., Koshizuka, S.: Real-time collision computation between cloth and highly-tessellated models. Transaction of Information Processing Society of Japan 48, 1829–1837 (2007)

The Role of Spatial Immersion for Tasks Based on the Use of Egocentric Frames of Reference

Michael Kozhevnikov[1], Dana Hayes[1], and Maria Kozhevnikov[2]

[1] Department of Engineering, Norfolk State University, VA, USA
[2] Department of Psychology, National University of Singapore, Singapore
mkozhevnikov@nsu.edu, d.m.hayes@spartans.nsu.edu,
psymaria@nus.edu.sg

Abstract. The focus of the current study was to understand which aspects of 3D immersive virtual reality are particularly useful for tasks based on the use of egocentric frames of reference. Twenty-two undergraduate students learned relative motion concepts in an interactive virtual reality simulation, either in an immersive virtual environment (IVE) or non-immersive desktop virtual environment (DVE). Our results show that the IVE group improved more significantly than the DVE group on solving relative motion problems after training in the simulations. The students' improvement from the pre- to post- problem solving test revealed that, through correlation analysis and rating different scales of presence, only spatial immersion scale showed a significant correlation which favored the IVE. This result supports our hypothesis that egocentric encoding of the scene in IVE is beneficial for tasks based on the use of egocentric frames of reference.

Keywords: Immersivity, Virtual Reality, Relative motion.

1 Introduction

Recently, as an alternative to traditional 2D displays, more realistic non-immersive 3D displays (e.g., using stereoscopic glasses) and immersive 3D virtual environments are being applied to a variety of human-computer interface domains and being used as a new, more ecologically valid research tool [1-3]. Although these 3D environments are richer with object and spatial information and more appealing to the user, research has so far provided conflicting evidence regarding its effectiveness in learning and task performance [4-5]. For example, for some tasks, such as collision avoidance, the 3D displays were found to be beneficial over 2D [5], whereas other researchers reported lower efficiency of 3D over 2D displays [6], as well as more difficulties in performing fine motor tasks in virtual environments as compared to real world environments [7]. In order to resolve these conflicting findings and determine the relative value of 3D immersive environments for real-world applications versus 3D non-immersive and more traditional 2D displays, more systematic examination of human performance of a variety of visual-spatial tasks in these environments is needed. The focus of the current study is to understand which unique features of an immersive

C. Stephanidis (Ed.): Posters, Part II, HCII 2013, CCIS 374, pp. 708–712, 2013.

virtual reality environment are useful for tasks based on the use of egocentric frames of reference.

2 Method and Activities

2.1 Participants and Assessment Materials

Twenty two undergraduate and graduate students majoring in different disciplines (engineering, computer science, information technology, and social sciences) from Norfolk State University (VA, USA) and George Mason University (VA, USA) participated in the study. Participants were randomly assigned to either immersive virtual environment (IVE) or desktop virtual environment (DVE) conditions. There were 14 students assigned to IVE conditions and 8 students assigned to DVE conditions.

First, participants were pre-tested with the Relative Motion Problem Solving Questionnaire (RMPSQ). The RMPSQ included 8 one-dimensional and 2 two-dimensional relative motion problems. The internal reliability of the questionnaire (alpha Cronbach) is 0.70. After pre-tests, all the participants were exposed to either IVE or DVE virtual simulations on relative motion. The activities in the relative motion simulations generally lasted for 30 - 40 minutes. The students were videotaped during their activities in the virtual simulation. Their videotapes were transcribed and analyzed. After completing these activities, all of the participants were post-tested on the same RMPSQ physics questionnaire that was administered in the pre-test. Finally, all of the participants were given a self-report Presence Questionnaire (PQ: [8]) that measures the extent of the user's subjective sense of "being" in a virtual environment. We tailored the latest version of the PQ (version 4.0) for the purpose of our research. The internal reliability (alpha Cronbach) of the PQ is 0.81.

2.2 Relative Motion Simulation Activities

Both simulations, in IVE and DVE, included the same activities with five levels of increasing complexity. In the IVE environment, the activities were presented to the participants through an nVisor SX60 (by Nvis Inc) Head Mounted Display (HMD). The HMD has a 44" horizontal by 34" vertical field of view (FOV) with a display resolution of 1280 x 1024. Sensors on the HMD enabled real-time simulation in which any movement of the subject's head immediately caused a corresponding change to the image rendered in the HMD. The participant's head position was tracked by 4 cameras located in each corner of the experimental room and responsive to an infrared light source mounted on the top of the HMD. The rotation of the user's head was captured by a digital compass mounted on the back of the HMD. The participant was able to interact with the immersive virtual simulation (i.e., to send different commands) by using a handheld wireless remote control. For DVE condition, the students observed the simulation while looking at a conventional 2D display, and they were able to interact with the simulations using a computer mouse.

Both IVE and DVE activities were based on the same simulation module featuring either two air tracks, with one glider on each track (laboratory setting) or two human avatars (realistic setting), as shown in Figure 1. The module is comprised of virtual activities with five levels of increasing complexity. In the first three levels, the air tracks were aligned parallel to each other, so that students could predict and observe one-dimensional relative motion. In levels 4 and 5, the air tracks were set up at a 90-degree angle, so that students could observe and predict two-dimensional relative motion. Except for the first level, each level includes an observational mode in which students observe the motion of two gliders from a laboratory frame of reference, a prediction mode in which students are asked to predict the velocity of one of the gliders in the frame of reference of the other glider, and a verification mode in which the students could observe the motion of one of the gliders while virtually riding on the other glider.

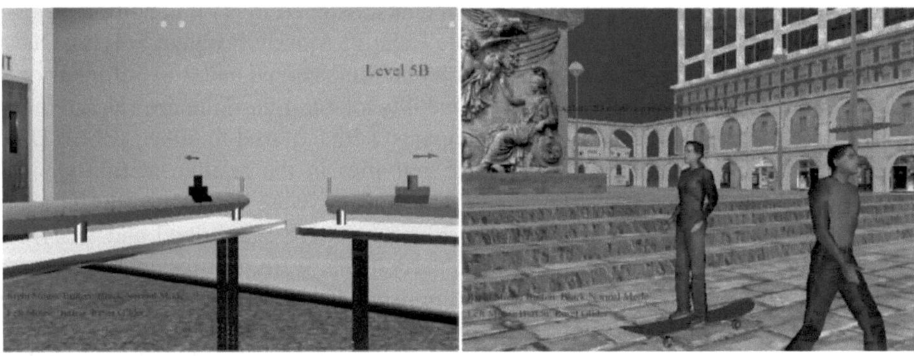

Fig. 1. A screenshot from the virtual simulations on two-dimensional relative motion: virtual laboratory setting featuring two air tracks and two gliders (left), and realistic mode (virtual city) featuring two human avatars (right)

Students could make turns and watch the scene from different perspectives as well as switch between moving and stationary frames of reference. Arrows indicating predicted and actual relative velocities that were attached to the gliders offered feedback for the students. Students could also switch back and forth between a realistic and an impoverished "dark mode" in the virtual lab, in which only the two moving gliders and their relative velocity arrows were visible, to enhance the feeling that the moving glider (avatar) was a new frame of reference.

3 Results

3.1 RMPSQ

We conducted a 2X2 MIXED ANOVA analysis with time (pre-RMPSQ and post-RMPSQ) as a within-subject variable and learning environment (DVE and IVE) as a between subject variable. The analysis revealed that all the participants significantly improved their performance on RMPSQ from the pre- to post-test: $F(1,20) = 23.774$, $p < 0.001$. The effect of environment was significant, $F(1,20) = 5.94$, $p = 0.02$ as well as the effect of interaction between time and environment, $F(1,20) = 8.94$, $p = 0.03$. Follow-up ANOVAs indicated that while there was no significant difference between these two groups on pre-test [$M_{IVE} = 2.92$ (SD = 1.94), $M_{DVE} = 2.12$ (SD = 1.35); $F(1,21) = 1.06$, $p = 0.31$], the difference on the post-test was significant [$M_{IVE} = 5.92$ (SD = 2.16), $M_{DVE} = 3.25$ (SD = 1.58); $F(1,21) = 9.31$, $p = 0.006$], so that students in immersive conditions outperformed those in the desktop condition on the post-test.

3.2 Presence Questionnaire

Based on Witmer's et al [8] four-factor model of the PQ obtained as a result of principle component analyses, we assigned the items of the PQ (modified version 4.0) to the following scales:

- *Involvement/control* - relates to the perceived ability to control virtual environment (VE) events, responsiveness of the VE to the user-initiated actions, and overall involvement in the VE experience;
- *Visual Fidelity* – relates to the degree to which the VE configuration permits active search or survey of objects in the VE using vision;
- *Interface Quality* – relates to perceived quality of the VE interface and the extent to which it does not interfere with activities in the VE;
- *Adaptation* – relates to how quickly the user adjusts to/feels immersed into the VE experience;
- *Psychological Immersion* – relates to the perceived proficiency of interacting with and operating in the VE;
- *Spatial Immersion* - relates to the extent to which the user feels part of the virtual environment being surrounded by the virtual objects ("looking out") rather than looking on the scene from the outside ("looking in").

First we correlated students' improvement from pre- to post-RMPSQ (computed as differences between students; scores on post- and pre-RMPSQ) with their ratings of different types of presence. We found a significant correlation between improvement on RMPSQ and students rating on adaptation scale of the presence questionnaire ($r = 0.47$, $p = 0.027$) as well as marginal correlation between improvement on RMPSQ and spatial immersion scale ($r = 0.390$, $p = 0.07$). All other correlations were non-significant. Interestingly, there was no correlation between students' improvement and their ratings on psychological immersion scale ($r = 0.041$, $p = 0.85$).

To compare how individuals in IVE and DVE conditions rated different types of presence in these learning environments, we conducted One-way ANOVAs with learning environment (DVE vs. IVE) as a predictor and their ratings on different types of presence as criterion variables. We found a significant difference between participants' rating of spatial immersion in IVE and DVE environments ($p = 0.04$) so that those in IVE condition rate spatial immersion higher than those in DVE condition; and a marginal difference between participants' rating of interface quality of IVE vs. DVE environments ($p=0.08$) in the favor of IVE environment. No difference in participants' rating was found for other presence scales.

4 Conclusion

Our results show that the IVE group improved more significantly than the DVE group on solving relative motion problems after training in the simulations. Our correlation analysis of the students' improvement from pre- to post- problem solving test with their ratings of different scales of presence revealed that only *spatial immersion scale* showed a significant correlation and it favored the IVE environment. The spatial immersion scale relates to the extent to which the user finds the VE perceptually convincing: looking out as if they are a part of the virtual environment being surrounded by virtual objects, rather than looking in on the scene from the outside. This result supports our hypothesis that egocentric encoding of the scene in IVE is beneficial for tasks based on the use of egocentric frames of reference.

Acknowledgment. This research has been supported in part by US National Science Foundation grant EEC-0935006.

References

1. Lee, J.H., Ku, J., Kim, K., Kim, B., Kim, I.Y., Yang, B.-H., Kim, S.H., Wiederhold, B.K., Wiederhold, M.D., Park, D.-W., Lim, Y., Kim, S.I.: Experimental Application of Virtual Reality for Nicotine Craving through Cue Exposure. Cyber Psychology & Behavior 6(3), 275–280 (2003)
2. Lo Priore, C., Castelnuovo, G., Liccione, D.: Experience with V-STORE: considerations on presence in virtual environments for effective neuropsychological rehabilitation of executive functions. Cyber Psychology & Behavior 6(3), 281–287 (2003)
3. Lee, J.-H., Lim, Y., Wiederhold, B.K., Graham, S.J.: A Functional Magnetic Resonance Imaging (fMRI) Study of Cue-Induced Smoking Craving in Virtual Environments. Applied Psychophysiology and Biofeedback 30(3), 195–204 (2005)
4. Haskell, I., Wickens, C.: Two- and three-dimensional displays for aviation: A theoretical and empirical comparison. International Journal of Aviation Psychology 3(2), 87–109 (1993)
5. Van Orden, K., Broyles, J.: Visuospatial task performance as a function of two- and three-dimensional display presentation techniques. Displays 21, 17–24 (2000)
6. Hollands, J.G., Pierce, B.J., Magee, L.: Displaying information in two and three dimensions. International Journal of Cognitive Ergonomics 2, 307–320 (1998)
7. Arnold, P., Farrell, M.J., Pettifer, S., West, A.J.: Performance of a skilled motor task in virtual and real environments. Ergonomics 45, 348–361 (2002)
8. Witmer, B.G., Jerome, C.J., Singer, M.J.: The factor structure of the presence questionnaire. Presence 14(3), 298–312 (2005)

What Does the HUD Tell Us?: The Heads Up Display as a Meta-communication in Videogames

Stein C. Llanos

Norwegian School of Information Technology
steinllanos@nith.no

Abstract. How important is the overlay interface, or Heads Up Display (HUD) to the identification of games for videogame players? In order to investigate this issue I created an on-line survey where respondents were asked to identify games by genre based on screenshots of the game with and without HUD. While the data indicate that the presence of the HUD increases the overall number of correct categorizations of the games and the respondents' confidence in their anwers, the effect is much smaller than anticipated relative to other cues such as camera position and avatar placement.

Keywords: Entertainment, Immersion, Embodiment, Video Games.

1 Introduction

The "Heads Up Display", or HUD, first appeared in the late 1950's as an information display technology projecting information on the windscreen of a fighter airplane, allowing pilots to receive information while keeping their attention focused on their surroundings (Shneiderman, 1998). The advantages of the concept soon became obvious beyond this narrow military application, and the principles involved have since been applied in a range of areas, from commercial airlines to industrial simulations.

Videogames quickly embraced the HUD. Presenting system information on a separate layer allow designers to give players an insight into the intricate inner machinations of more complex systems and virtual worlds (Jørgensen, forthcoming). As games moved beyond representations that could be contained on a single-screen the HUD played an essential role in helping players orient themselves as the screen became a window into increasingly complex environments.

1.1 The HUD Controversy

Over the years the type and quantity of the system information displayed has varied depending on a number of factors. Peter Jackson's King Kong (Ubisoft Montpellier, 2005) has no HUD at all, whereas in Championship Manager (Domark Group Ltd., 1992), and many of its sequels, the system information takes over the entirety of the display area, leaving the players to imagine the world behind the numbers on the

C. Stephanidis (Ed.): Posters, Part II, HCII 2013, CCIS 374, pp. 713–717, 2013.

screen. Still, for all its utility, some game developers are not happy with the HUD, and would rather purge it from their games altogether. In 2006 Greg Wilson published his article "Off with their HUDs" on Gamasutra (Wilson, 2006), where he claims that a traditional HUD is in the way of an "immersive experience.

According to my personal experience, which is corroborated by Kristine Jørgensen (forthcoming), to the trained eye the HUD is one of the most informative and succinct ways to communicate what a game is all about and situate the game in a genre.

My hypotesis is then that most players can instantly recognize the principal interactions afforded by a game after a glance at the screen output or a screenshot of actual gameplay, and that the HUD plays an instrumental role in this process.

2 Survey Design

The survey consists of two main parts. The first collects demographic data on the respondents, including factors such as age, gender and game-playing habits. In the second part the respondents are asked to categorize games by genres based on screenshots representative of each game's core gameplay, first with, then without, a HUD. For each screenshot they are also asked to indicate how confident they are in their answer and whether they recognized and/or had played the title in quesion.

2.1 Access Points

The survey was created in SurveyMonkey, using Facebook and a link on the "videogaming open" forum on RPG.net as my two access points. Facebook in particular was a fruitful source of respondents, with several people re-posting the link to the survey on gaming forums. I had planned to roll out more access points gradually, but as it turned out these two sources alone produced enough respondents for my purposes. Having limited experience with quantitative studies, I was content with around 100 answers, which would give me a 90% level of confidence, given a random sample.

2.2 Sampling Bias

The chosen access points introduce a strong sampling bias, however. As with all on-line surveys there is a largely unavoidable self-selection bias. Fortunately the demographic data from the first part of the survey is quite helpful when it comes to establishing in what ways my sample differs from more comprehensives studies of the game playing public. When interpreting the findings of the survey it is important to keep in mind that the study uses a limited sample that seems to be skewed towards more mature players with an affinity for Role-Playing Games and an aversion for sports games.

2.3 Attrition

The response data include 173 completed surveys and 36 incomplete surveys. 7 respondents only provided gender and age data, and after that there is a steady drop-out rate. As the survey design is based on comparison between screenshots with and without HUD, I have only used completed surveys in the final analysis.

2.4 Selection of Genres

For the purpose of this particular study game genres serve as shorthand for groups of interactions that typically occur together. Some fidelity is certainly lost through the 15 genres I have presented to my respondents, and while the genres might make the survey a bit harder for the non-gamers, it is intended to make the process faster for the majority of my respondents.

The genres were selected with the intention that they be familiar or intuitive to the majority of the respondents, represent sufficient breadth for the categorization to not be trivial and to represent a breadth of social contexts of play. I have assigned each game to two genres, based on the publisher's own categorizations of the games.

3 Data Analysis

When analyzing the data I grouped the HUD/No HUD pairs and looked at the number of correct categorizations and the increase in confidence in the answers.

3.1 Effect on Categorization of Games

In the table below I have counted all the right answers for each game, with and without HUD present. I have counted an answer as correct as long as at least one of the two genres assigned to the game are present in the respondent's answer.

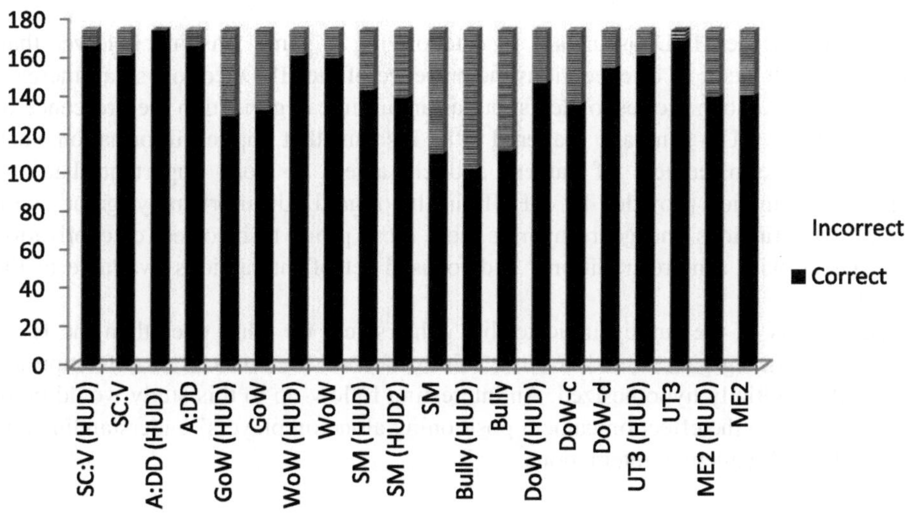

Fig. 1. Impact of HUD on categorization

3.2 Effect on Respondent Confidence

With ordinal data and a subjective scale I am limited in what operations I can perform on this data. What is immediately evident from the graph, however, is that the presence of the HUD increases respondent genre confidence for the majority of the studied games.

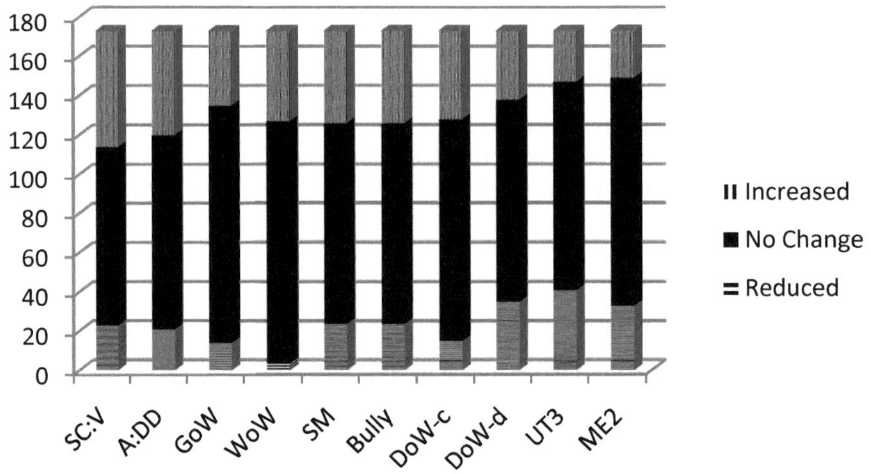

Fig. 2. Impact of HUD on respondent confidence levels

4 Conclusion

The effect of the HUD as an aid to categorizing a game was much lower than expected. with a couple of exceptions the presence of the HUD led to a small increase in confidence among the respondents, but as an aid in categorization the prescence or absence of the HUD generally mattered little. It seems that implicit information, such as the relative placement of camera and characters is more important than the explicit information provided by a HUD in this regard. Unsurprisingly, games with complex interactions and genre hybrids were more prone to incorrect categorization than games with a more traditional and focused set of interactions available to the player.

The results of the survey indicate that gamers rely on other cues than the HUD when categorizing games, and are less able to decode the nuances of contemproary HUDs than initially hypothesized. An interesting follow-up to this study would be to try to determine the effect on camera positioning alone on players' understanding and expectation of gameplay interactions.

References

1. Domark Group Ltd. Championship Manager. Domark Software Ltd. (1992)
2. Jørgensen, K.: Between the Game System and the Fictional World. A Study of Computer Game Interfaces. Games and Culture. A Journal of Interactive Media (forthcoming)
3. Shneiderman, B.: Designing the User Interface. Strategies for Effective Human- Computer Interaction, 3rd edn. Addison Wesley Longman, Reading (1998)
4. Ubisoft Montpellier, Peter Jackson's King Kong (Xbox 360) Ubisoft (2005)
5. Wilson, G.: Off With Their HUDs! Rethinking the Heads-Up Display in Console Game Design. In: Gamasutra, Feature (February 3, 2006), http://www.gamasutra.com/features/20060203/wilson_01.shtml

Interactive Stereoscopic Authoring in MR-Based Pre-visualization for 3D Filmmaking

Shohei Mori, Fumihisa Shibata, Asako Kimura, and Hideyuki Tamura

Graduate School of Information Science and Engineering, Ritsumeikan University
1-1-1 Noji-Higashi, Kusatsu, Shiga, 525-8577, Japan
mori@rm.is.ritsumei.ac.jp

Abstract. This paper presents a mixed reality (MR) based system for on-set pre-visualization (PreViz) of stereoscopic 3D (S3D) films. PreViz refers to simple computer-generated shots created in the preproduction phase (before shooting). In terms of stereography, this preparation enables stereographers to design S3D effects on the screen and camera-work using rather cheap computer graphics (CG). However, how a scene actually looks like in S3D are unknown until the production phase on-site. Therefore, we propose a system, which enables users to visualize expected results in the preproduction phase instead of the usual production phase.

Keywords: Mixed Reality, Stereoscopic 3D, Filmmaking, Camera Registration.

1 Introduction

Pre-Visualization (PreViz) occupies one of the most important positions in the film industry as the process becomes more complicated. PreViz refers to the rough CG-animated movie created in the early stage of filmmaking to visualize scenes before the actual filming. Such planning is regarded to be important especially for live action shooting in stereoscopic 3D (S3D). However, the actual looks of the scenes are still unknown until the production phase on-site.

To solve this problem, we proposed a mixed reality (MR) based PreViz system named S3D MR-PreViz [1], which is based on its former self, MR-PreViz [2]. The system superimposes CG-animated characters onto scenes from a cinematographic stereo camera (stereo rig (Fig. 1)) and displays it in S3D (Fig. 2). One of the important requirements of this system is to accomplish camera registration as quickly as possible because venue and labor cost are incurred at all time during preparation such as 3D reconstruction and feature description.

On the assumption that camerawork is roughly determined before shooting, we developed a feature point-based camera tracking method named rehearsal path method to improve speed of offline setup and robustness of realtime camera tracking. Furthermore, in this paper, we propose to integrate the setup into the realtime camera tracking using some additional assumption of stereo rig and S3D cinematography for improving system interactivity.

C. Stephanidis (Ed.): Posters, Part II, HCII 2013, CCIS 374, pp. 718–722, 2013.

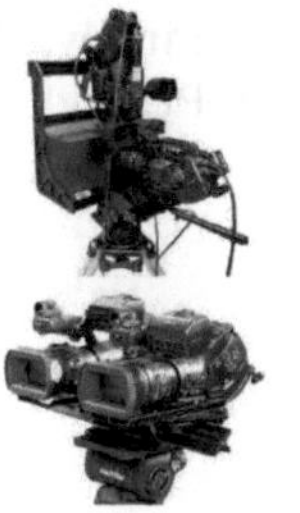

Fig. 1. Stereo rigs (Top: Beamsplitter rig. Bottom: Parallel rig)

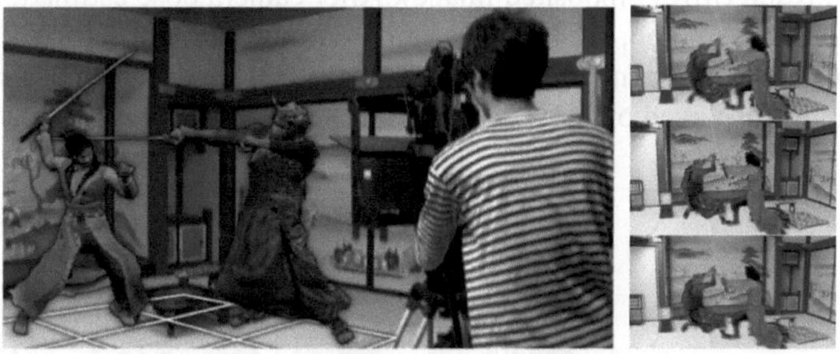

Fig. 2. Image of on-set S3D MR-PreViz. Left: CG-animated characters are superimposed in realtime and it enables stereographers to confirm the results in the early stage. Right: Results of disparity adjustment in S3D MR-PreViz system.

2 Related Work

Koppal *et al.* [3] proposed a view-centric editor for disparity adjustment in S3D shooting. It enables a user to change S3D effects virtually (increase or decrease depth of the scene by changing the disparity of a scene) based on their mathematical framework. While this tool provides users a way to edit captured stereo image sequences on a PC with GUI, the aim of our study is to develop a PreViz system.

Regarding stereo camera registration, we propose an approach for realtime 3D matchmoving without any prior knowledge. Existing approaches suffered from computational speed mainly due to trying to widen the range of applicability and using computationally expensive image feature descriptors for improving robustness [4, 5]. Our approach to the problem is to limit the range of application, to simplify the feature description based on the setup of the stereo rig used for filming, and to actively use multi-core processing. We also assume that a camerawork is roughly determined in advance and our camera passes close to the path repeatedly for improving the robustness.

3 S3D MR-PreViz System

3.1 System Configuration

The proposed system is composed of a stereo rig, 3D displays, and a workstation (Fig. 3). We assume that the stereo rig is calibrated in advance using [1]. First, two 1280x720 (720p/30) YUV video streams are sent to the workstation from two cameras (Sony PMW-EX3) in the stereo rig (Nac 3D rig II). The input video stream is captured by Blackmagic DeckLink HD Extreme 3D+, a video capture card installed in the workstation. The proposed system uses HD SDI as input interface. Second, input video streams are converted into a grayscale and RGB stereo images using GPGPU [1]. The former is used for vision-based camera tracking and the latter is used for the final result (MR composited image). After camera pose estimation, which is described in the later section, CGI is superimposed onto the left and right images. Finally, the two images are converted into one of the S3D video format using GPGPU and the result is displayed on a 3D display (JVC GD-463D10).

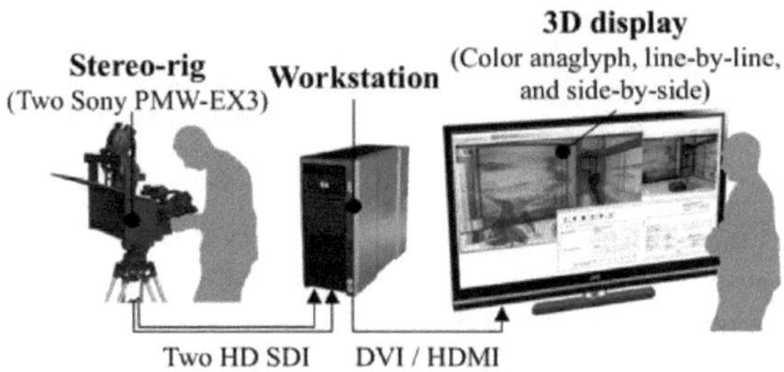

Fig. 3. System configuration

3.2 Procedures of S3D MR-PreViz Shooting

S3D MR-PreViz shooting is done as follows.

(1) Setting up the stereo rig: Change convergence and baseline length between cameras in the rig. Assume that the baseline length is determined by the 1/30th rule [6].
(2) Calibrate the camera using the camera calibration system in [1]
(3) Camerawork examination: Perform realtime 3D matchmoving by the combination of range data from the stereo rig and iterative closest point (ICP) algorithm [7].
(4) Repeat (1) – (3) for disparity examination by trial and error

3.3 Stereo Camera Tracking

In the proposed system, the stereo rig is used as a capture device and a vision-based range sensor. 3D positions of feature points are given to the system and the stereo camera pose is estimated using ICP algorithm. Given stereo correspondences, range data is calculated by a well-known formula,

$$Z = \frac{fB}{d} \tag{1}$$

where, Z is the depth, f is the focal length, B is the baseline length, and d is the disparity given by block matching between left and right images. To accelerate this process, we propose to limit its search range ($d_{\min}$, $d_{\max}$) by stereo uncertainty and native pixel parallax (NPP) respectively, which is the maximum disparity in S3D to avoid generating stereo images harmful to the eyes (Eq. (2)).

$$\left(d_{\min}, d_{\max}\right) = \left(\sqrt{\frac{\partial d f B}{2 \partial Z}}, \left(\frac{W_{interocular}}{W_{screen}}\right) W_{px}\right) \tag{2}$$

Here, $W_{interocular}$ is the interocular distance (= 2.5 [inches]), W_{screen} is the screen size in inches, and W_{px} is the width of input image in pixel. In the proposed system, W_{screen} is set as default to 41.06 [inches] because S3D MR-PreViz utilizes JVC GD-463D10 (46 inches 3D display).

We calculate camera pose from the first frame to the current frame. First, Lucas-Kanade (LK) tracker [8] continuously tracks feature points tracked in the previous frame. Second, newly observed points are matched using template matching instead of computationally expensive feature point descriptors. These results are given to ICP algorithm to calculate current camera pose.

Position of a feature point is refined by the following procedure. If the sum of the number of tracked feature points and that of newly matched feature points is small, range data in the current frame is added to the map. Range data is also used for refining the stored range data on the assumption that the same feature points are observed repeatedly while running S3D MR-PreViz because the rehearsal path is roughly determined in advance (Eq. (3)).

$$\mathbf{p}_i' = \frac{n_{ref}\mathbf{p}_i^{\mathrm{map}} + \mathbf{p}_i}{n_{ref} + 1} \tag{3}$$

Here, n_{ref} is the number of reference, $\mathbf{p}_i$ is the range data in the current frame, and $\mathbf{p}_i^{\mathrm{map}}$ is the range data in the stored range data. Because the above processes have to be repeated for each point, they are assigned to multiple threads for parallel processing. Multi-core processing is implemented using OpenMP. Fig. 4 shows the results of tracking and 3D reconstruction.

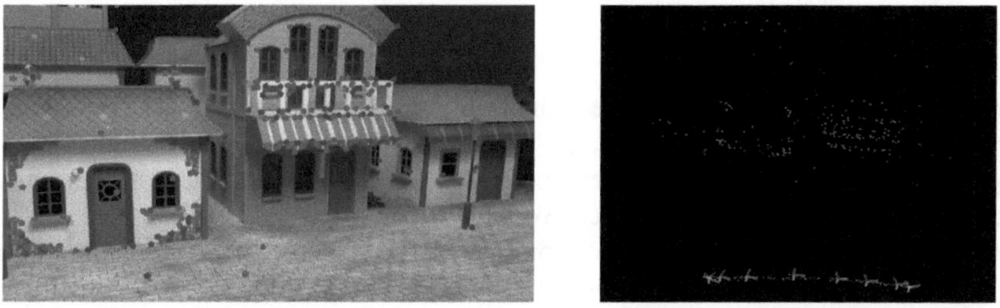

Fig. 4. Examples of tracking result. Left: Map reprojection. Three maps are reconstructed and each of them is colored just for visibility. Right: Bird's eye view of the 3D reconstruction and camera trajectory.

4 Results

Fig. 5 shows the results of the proposed system. An S3D MR-PreViz was shot interactively using the stereo rig. The stereo rig moved 900 [mm] from right to left and panned on a rail facing at the robot. Distance between the rig and the closest miniature house to the rig was 1,800 [mm]. Baseline length was set to 50 [mm] by 1/30th rule and stereo search range was limited to 7 – 40 [px] according to the baseline length. Number of images was 450 frames and image resolution was 720x405 [px]. Tracking worked in 14.9 [FPS] when average number of matched points was 122.4 points. In the proposed system, S3D MR-PreViz shooting and disparity examination are repeated quickly because there is no preparation except stereo camera calibration.

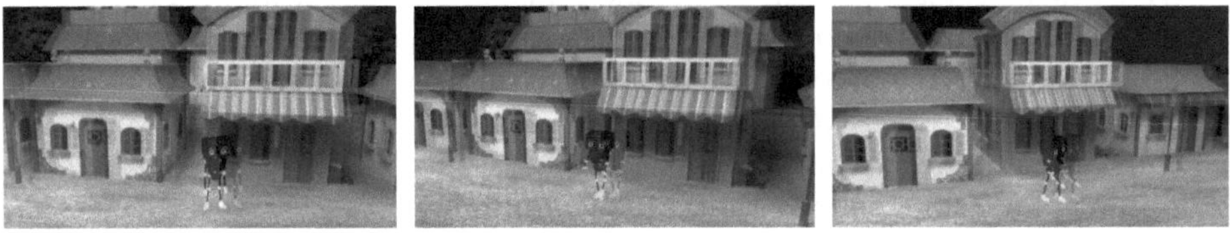

Fig. 5. Results of S3D MR-PreViz using the proposed system (Red-cyan color anaglyph)

5 Conclusion and Future Work

In this paper we presented a new MR-based PreViz shooting system for S3D films, which includes real-time 6-DOF stereo camera tracking using ICP algorithm. Our previous work required offline preparation but the process is accomplished in real-time using stereo vision in the proposed method. MR composite video was displayed in S3D properly. However, the proposed system suffered from tracking in a full-scale filming set due to short baseline setting for shooting scenes in S3D and convergence angle is not considered for simplifying stereo matching. Therefore, future work will include accuracy improvement of the tracking method and implementation of convergence examination.

References

1. Ichikari, R., et al.: Mixed reality pre-visualization for filmmaking: On-set camera-work authoring and action rehearsal. The Int. J. Virtual Reality 7(4), 25–32 (2008)
2. Mori, S., et al.: Enabling on-set stereoscopic MR-based previsualization for 3D filmmaking. In: SIGGRAPH ASIA 2011. Technical Sketch (2011)
3. Koppal, et al.: A view-centric editor for stereoscopic cinema. IEEE Trans. on Computer Graphics and Applications 31(1), 20–35 (2011)
4. Se, S., et al.: Local and global localization for mobile robots using visual landmarks. In: Proc. IEEE/RSJ Int. Conf. on Intelligent Robots and Systems, pp. 414–420 (2001)
5. Elinas, P., et al.: σSLAM: Stereo vision SLAM using the Rao-Blackwellised particle filter and a novel mixture proposal distribution. In: Proc. IEEE Int. Conf. on Robotics and Automation, pp. 1564–1570 (2006)
6. Mendiburu, B.: 3D movie making: Stereoscopic digital cinema from script to screen. Focal press (2009)
7. Besl, P., McKay, N.: A method for registration of 3-D shapes. IEEE Tran.s on Pattern Analysis and Machine Intelligence 14(2), 239–256 (1992)
8. Lucas, B., Kanade, T.: An iterative image registration technique with applications in stereo vision. In: Proc. DARPA Image Understanding Workshop, pp. 121–130 (1981)

Using Game Technology to Develop Snowboard Training Simulator

Changhoon Park and Junsuk Moon

Dept. of Game Engineering, Hoseo University,
165 Sechul-ri, Baebang-myun, Asan, Chungnam 336-795, Korea
chpark@hoseo.edu, mjs0806@imrlab.hoseo.edu

Abstract. The motion sensor, such as Kinect and Wii remote has attracted the attention especially for the development of virtual reality games. Most of games using motion sensor provides entertainment. These games have a limitation that if players want to learn and exercise practical sports skill. To overcome this, we aim to provide a sport-training program that is effective and applicable to real life sports. This paper will present a virtual simulator for the beginners to train and learn snowboarding skill. Player can practice five basic exercises[1] in the simulator. To accomplish this, following three main functions will be implemented based on sport science and advanced game technology.

Keywords: snowboard, simulator, virtual coach, feedback, presence.

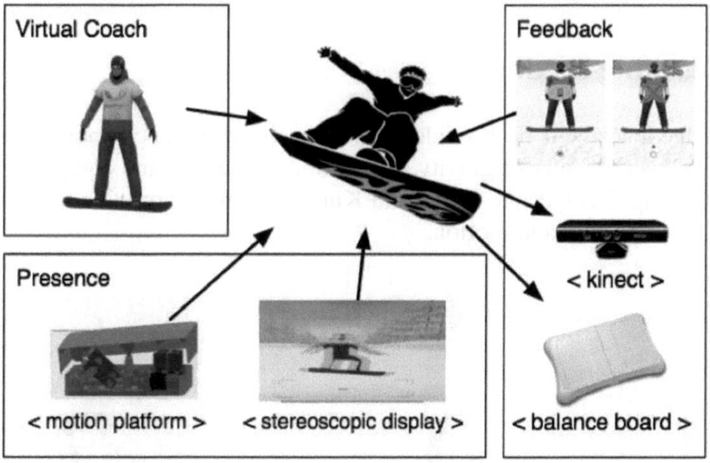

Fig. 1. Overview of a snowboard training simulator

[1] Five basic exercises include basic board position, heel-side slipping, toe-side slipping, heel-side pendulum and toe-side pendulum.

C. Stephanidis (Ed.): Posters, Part II, HCII 2013, CCIS 374, pp. 723–726, 2013.

1 Virtual Coach

Virtual coach is provided to allow the player to imitate the expert's behavior as shown in the below figure. Human-like 3d character is modeled for virtual coach. And, eleven character animation clips are created from a snowboarding video of an expert. These animation clips is composed for the training of five basic snowboard training. In addition to 3d character, expert's center of gravity is also presented. Training the center of gravity is important because it provides balance and control of turning. Then, the player can imitate movement and center of gravity at the same time.

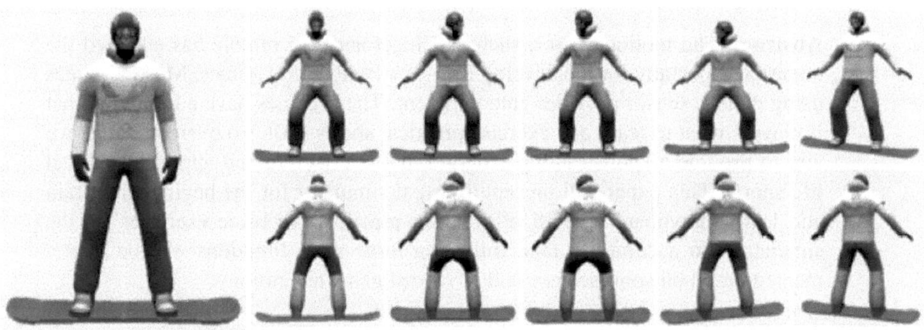

Fig. 2. 11 character animation clips for virtual coach

2 Coaching Feedback

Coaching feedback will be provided immediately to enhance sport learning. In the simulator, player's center of gravity and motion are sensed and compared with that of the expert using Wii balance board and Kinect. Then, we provide a proper feedback about center of gravity and motion.

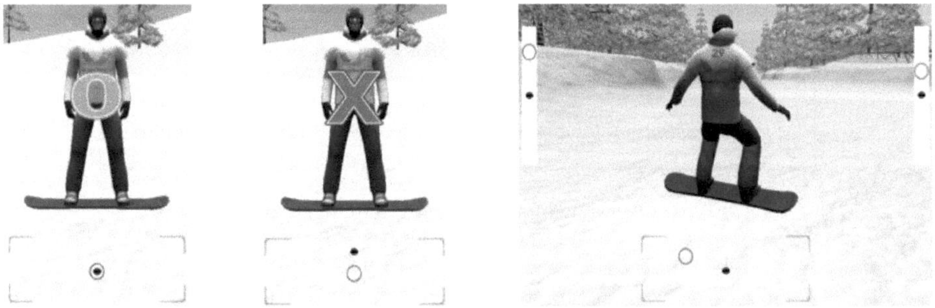

Fig. 3. Coaching feedback for success, failure and pendulum with the center of gravity

3 Presence

We will create the full illusion of movement on the slope by introducing stereoscopic display and motion platform. It is important to provide the feeling of presence for the effective training. Motion platform simulator allows to create the same loads as on the snowboard slope. Stereoscopic 3D display provides the illusion of depth in an image by means of stereopsis for binocular vision.

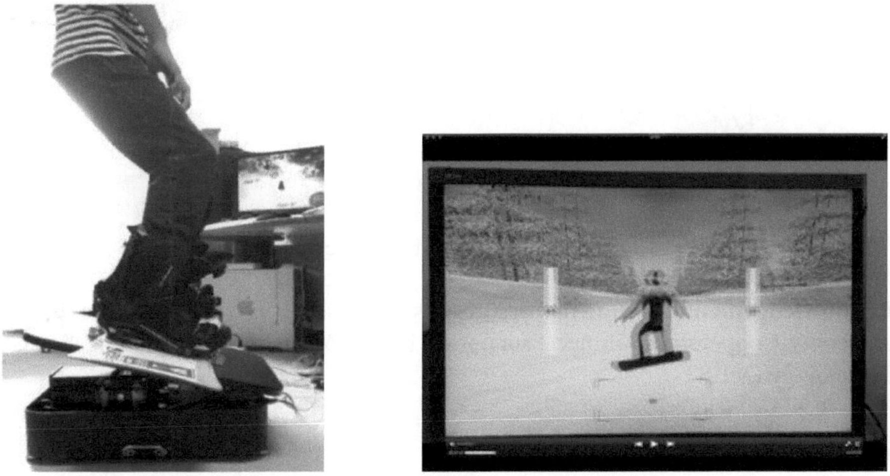

Fig. 4. Playing the game on motion platform with stereoscopic image

4 Conclusion

In the future, we will use multiple interfaces complexly to figure out player's motion finely for the advanced sport training. This paper presented a virtual simulator for substantive snowboard training. It could be effective training that various interface used in combination. In the future, we make the best use of Kinect so it will be improved training system, which can effective and realistic training. After all, the player can learn to snowboard in a safe environment without need to go to a slope.

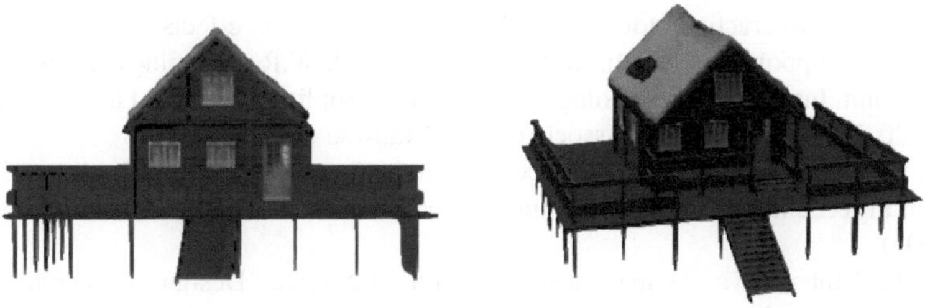

Fig. 5. Playing the game on motion platform with stereoscopic image

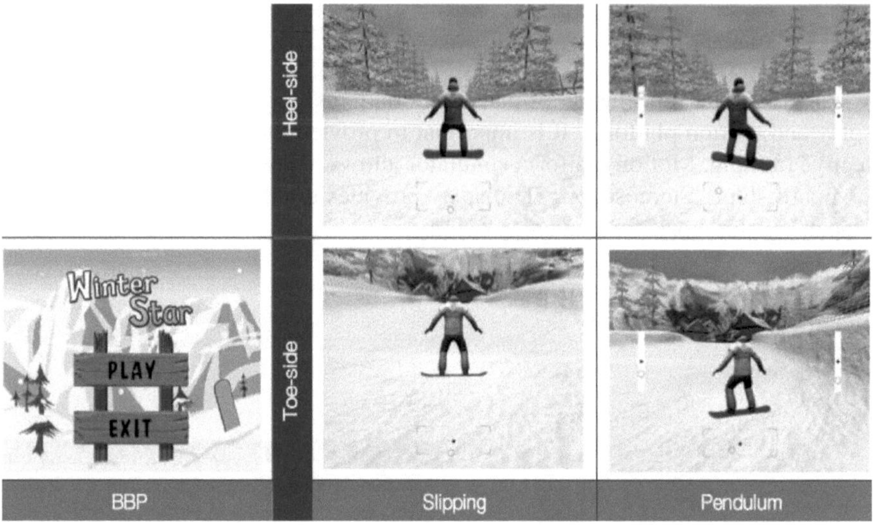

Fig. 6. Screenshots of game contents

Acknowledgements. Following are results of a study on the "Leaders Industry-university Cooperation" Project, supported by the Ministry of Education, Science 7 Technology (MEST).

References

1. Mokka, S., Vaatanen, A., Heinila, J., Valkkynen, P.: Fitness computer game with a bodily user interface. In: Proc. of the 2th Intl. Conference on Entertainment Computing, vol. 38 (2003)
2. Van Dan, N., Kameyama, M.: Bayesian-networks-based motion estimation for a highly-safe intelligent vehicle. In: SICE-ICASE International Joint Conference, pp. 6023–6026 (2006)
3. Park, C., Ko, H., Kim, T.: NAVER: Design and Implementation of VR Framework for Gyeongju VR Theater. Computer and Graphics 27(2), 223–236 (2003)
4. Ahn, S.H., Kang, K.B., Kim, E.J., Kim, S.-J., Lee, J.-W., Song, C.G.: Interactive 3D Golf Simulator. In: ICHIT-AMTA, November 10-11, International Convention Center, Jeju (2006)
5. Annesi, J.J., Mazas, J.: Effects of virtual reality-enhanced exercise equipment on adherence and exercise-induced feeling states. Percept. Mot. Skills 85, 835–844 (2006)
6. Lieberman, D.A.: Interactive video games for health promotion: effects on knowledge, self-efficacy, social support, and health. In: Street, R.L., Gold, W.R., Mannings, T. (eds.) Health Promotion and Interactive Technology: Theoretical Applications and Future Directions, pp. 103–120. Lawrence Erlbaum Associates Inc., Mahwah (1997)
7. Zhao, P., van de Panne, M.: User interfaces for interactive control of physics-based 3D characters. In: Proceedings of the 2005 Symposium on Interactive 3D Graphics and Games, I3D 2005 (2005)
8. Kim, H.-L.: Interactive Game-centric tangible Interface Design Research (2004), http://www.designdb.com/

Collision Avoidance Affected by Walker's Head Direction in a Virtual Environment

Shunya Ueda[1] and Michiteru Kitazaki[2]

[1] Graduate School of Engineering, Toyohashi University of Technology,
1-1 Hibarigaoka, Tempakucho, Toyohashi, Aichi, 441-8580, Japan
ueda@real.cs.tut.ac.jp
[2] Department of Computer Science and Engineering,
Toyohashi University of Technology,
1-1 Hibarigaoka, Tempakucho, Toyohashi, Aichi, 441-8580, Japan
mich@cs.tut.ac.jp

Abstract. We investigated participants' active response to avoid collision with an approaching walker in a virtual environment. The walker was approaching and then changed his direction leftward or rightward at a random timing. The walker's head rotated (yaw) leftward or rightward, or remained straight at 533ms before direction change of walking. Ten participants were asked to avoid collision by moving a mouse laterally to move own viewpoint. We found that participants' collision avoidance behavior was affected by head directions. They moved in the opposite direction to the other walker's head direction when the walker rotated his head. These results suggest that we utilize other people's head direction to avoid collision in active situation as well as static perceptual situation.

Keywords: Perception and action, Collision avoidance.

1 Introduction

We can perceive other people's walking direction very quickly and accurately. Its accuracy depends on spatial and temporal information such as presentation duration and body surface [1]. Ten to twenty point lights attached to body joints elicit biological motion perception such as walking and dancing [2]. The accuracy of direction perception of a point-light walker is lower than the gray-shaded computer graphics walker, but high enough [1][3]. Since human walker's gaze and head direction reflect the intended direction of walking [4], human observers utilize other people's eye direction [5] and head direction [3][6] to perceive the other's walking direction. These studies employed cognitive inferences [2] and perceptual judgments [3][6] of static participants, who were observing a walker approaching to the participant in a virtual environment. However, participants' active or behavioral response for approaching walkers has not been investigated. Active responses (actions) and passive perception (judgments) are differently induced by visual stimulation. Actions and manual control decreases visual illusions [7][8] and facilitates some aspects of visual perception [9]. Thus, illusory effects of head direction might be diminished by active responses.

C. Stephanidis (Ed.): Posters, Part II, HCII 2013, CCIS 374, pp. 727–731, 2013.

2 Methods

Ten naive observers with uncorrected or corrected normal vision participated in the experiment after written informed consent. The experiment was approved by the Committee for the Human-subject Studies at Toyohashi University of Technology. The stimulus was created and controlled by a computer (DELL, Precision workstation T1600, Intel Core i3-2120 3.30GHz, NVIDIA Quadro FX3700), and projected on a rear-screen (248 wide x 186 high cm) by a 3CRT projector (Barco, Cine7/II, 1024 x 768 pixel, 60 Hz, 0.0077 - 9.404 cd/m^2). The experiment was performed in a darkroom.

In a virtual environment of a corridor (10m width floor and ceiling with 2.5m height left and right walls that were filled with random dots: 10 dots/m^2), a walker (170 cm tall, Male) approached (2 steps/s, 2.94 km/h) to participants (Figure 1). The participants also moved ahead at the same speed. The other walker changed his direction randomly leftward or rightward (6.7 deg) at a random timing (1.67-2.67 s) after starting walking. The direction change took 300 ms. The walker's head rotated (yaw) leftward or rightward (20 deg), or remained straight at 533ms before direction change of walking. The head turn took 167 ms. These stimuli were presented on the rear-projection screen (63.60 x 49.88 deg in visual angle) and participants observed them at 200 cm viewing distance. All combinations of experimental conditions were repeated 20 times in random orders (Figure 2). Participants were asked to avoid collision by moving a mouse laterally to move their own viewpoint.

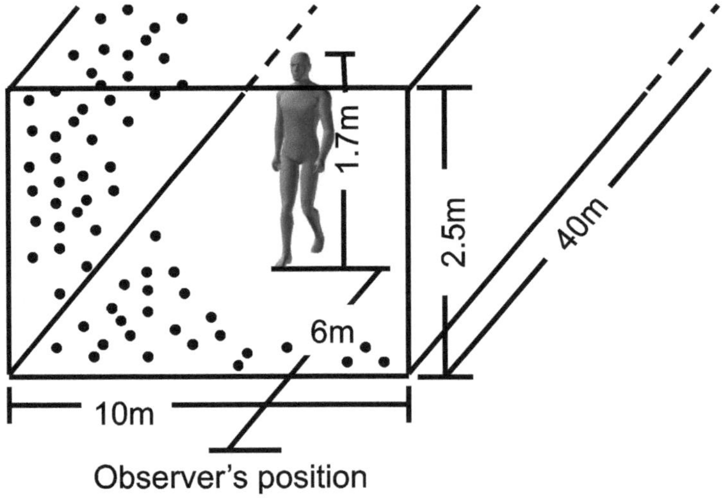

Fig. 1. Schematic of virtual environment. The corridor was made with four walls filled with random dots. Gray-shaded walker approached to the observer/participant.

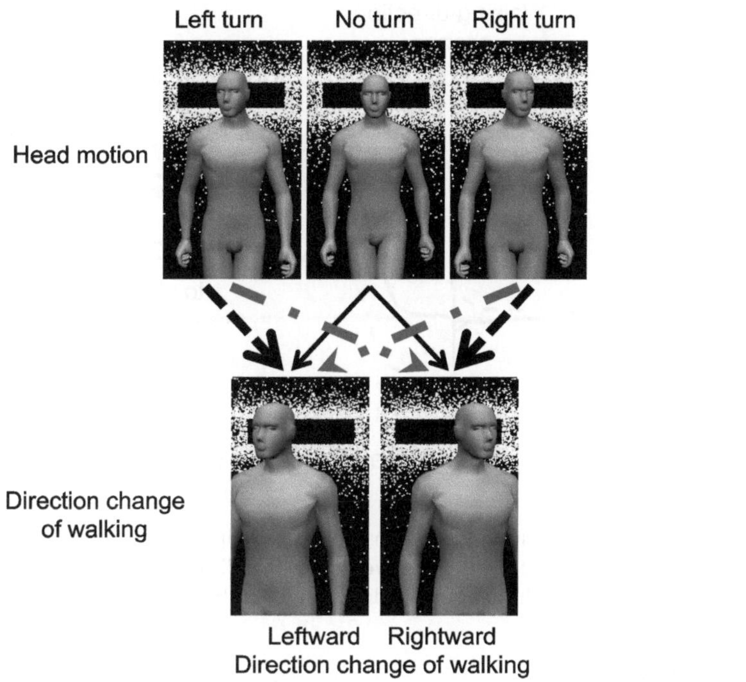

Fig. 2. Experimental conditions. The rotation directions of head and the following direction changes of walker were combined for setting 6 conditions. The combination of the left (right) head turn and the left (right) walking direction change is the consistent condition of head and walking, while the combination of the left (right) head turn and the right (left) walking direction change is the inconsistent condition.

3 Results

We found that participants' collision avoidance behavior was affected by head directions (Figure 3). They moved in the opposite direction to the other walker's head direction when the walker rotated his head. In the conditions that the head yaw was consistent with the walking direction change, collision avoidance began in the correct direction (opposite direction to the walker) approximately 500 ms before collision avoidance action in the conditions without head rotation. In the conditions that the head yaw was inconsistent with the walking direction change, collision avoidance began in the wrong direction (same direction as the walker) approximately 500 ms before the no-head-rotation conditions, then was being returned to the correct direction after 500 ms of the first action.

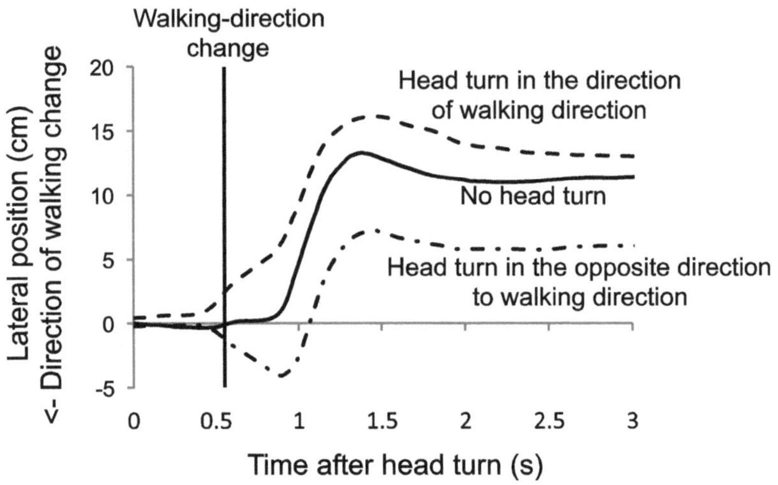

Fig. 3. Experimental results. Lateral position of participant's viewpoint was plotted against time after head turn. Positive value of the vertical axis indicated the opposite direction to walking-direction change, thus the appropriate direction for collision avoidance.

4 Discussion

These results suggest that we utilize other people's head direction to avoid collision in active situation as well as static perceptual situation. Thus, the effect of head rotation on walker's perception is not a visual illusory effect, but rather it supports the notion that our perception of and action to other walkers are related to our social cognition or social perception. Directions of eye and head often reflect walker's intention of walking and path finding. Thus, human observers utilize others' gaze and head direction to perceive and infer others' behavior. This kind of perception and inference seems to be a rudimentary social communication and important for human as social mobile observers. The fact that human perceptual accuracy of other's gaze is very high also supports this notion [10]. Perceptions of other walkers' motion and gaze shift elicit brain activities at the regions relating to social cognition [11][12]. These findings also support the importance of other walker's perception to investigate our social cognition.

Our findings can contribute to design robot' walking motions that facilitate human perception or inference of robot's heading change naturally and automatically. We should put appropriate motions of robot's head and eyes at an appropriate timing before heading change.

Acknowledgments. This research was partly supported by Grant-in-Aid for Scientific Research (B) #22300076 and Grant-in-Aid for Challenging Exploratory Research #23650060 from MEXT Japan.

References

1. Sato, T., Inoue, Y., Tani, Y., Matsuzaki, N., Kawamura, K., Kitazaki, M.: Perceiving the direction of walking. In: ECVP (European Conference on Visual Perception), Utrecht, Netherlands (2008); Perception 37(suppl.), 27 (2008)
2. Johansson, G.: Visual perception of biological motion and model for its analysis. Perception & Psychophysics 14(2), 201–211 (1973)
3. Kitazaki, M., Ono, K., Tsukada, Y., Murofushi, Y., Itakura, S.: Perception of walker: Human, robot, and point-lights, Workshop on Human-Robot Symbiosis: Synergistic Creation of Human-Robot Relationships. In: 11th IEEE-RAS International Conference on Humanoid Robots, Bled, Slovenia, October 26 (2011)
4. Hollands, M.A., Patla, A.E., Vickers, J.N.: Look where you're going!: Gaze behaviour associated with maintaining and changing the direction of locomotion. Experimental Brain Research 143, 221–230 (2002)
5. Nummenmaa, L., Hyönä, J., Hietanen, J.K.: I'll walk this way: Eyes reveal the direction of locomotion and make passersby look and go the other way. Psychological Science 20(12), 1454–1458 (2009)
6. Murofushi, Y., Ono, K., Sato, T., Kitazaki, M.: Perceived direction of human, robot and point-light walkers modulated by head direction. In: VSS (Vision Sciences Society Meeting), Naples, Florida, USA, May 13 (2012); Journal of Vision 12(9), 464 (2012), doi:10.1167/12.9.464
7. Goodale, M.A., Milner, A.D., Jakobson, L.S., Carey, D.P.: A neurological dissociation between perceiving objects and grasping them. Nature 349, 154–156 (1991)
8. Harman, K.L., Humphrey, G.K., Goodale, M.A.: Active manual control of object views facilitates visual recognition. Current Biology 9, 1315–1318 (1999)
9. Ichikawa, M., Masakura, Y.: Manual control of the visual stimulus reduces the flash-lag effect. Vision Research 46, 2192–2203 (2006)
10. Gamer, M., Hecht, H.: Are you looking at me? Measuring the cone of gaze. Journal of Experimental Psychology: Human Perception and Performance 33(3), 705 (2007)
11. Pelphrey, K.A., Viola, R.J., McCarthy, G.: When strangers pass: Processing of mutual and averted social gaze in the superior temporal sulcus. Psychological Science 15(9), 598–603 (2004)
12. Morris, J.P., Pelphrey, K.A., Mccarthy, G.: Regional brain activation evoked when approaching a virtual human on a virtual walk. Journal of Cognitive Neuroscience 17(11), 1744–1752 (2005)

Part XII
Security and Privacy

The Problem of Implicature in "Do Not Track" Choice Design

Lisa Harper, Deborah Kohl, and Kathryn Summers

University of Baltimore
Baltimore MD, 21201
{lisa.harper,dkohl,ksummers}@ubalt.edu

Abstract. In an observational study using an eye-tracker, subjects were presented with a modeless cookie choice dialog preceding a short survey on Internet privacy. Subjects were later asked whether they believed ad trackers were present on the site or not. 41% believed there either were or were not ad trackers on the site based on *n*ot clicking "allow" or "block", respectively. These results suggest that a pragmatic implicature is in play – information is suggested though not explicitly stated.

1 Introduction

The W3C Tracking Protection Working Group (TPWG) has been working toward a "Do Not Track" (DNT) policy intended to allow users to signal their intent with regard to browser-based tracking. DNT is not designed as a general purpose tool for communicating privacy practices. It is intended to simply communicate a user's preference not to be tracked.

The current Tracking Preference Expression draft specifies three possible states: DNT:1 (do not track), DNT:0 (allow tracking) and unset. In this third case, tracking preference is not enabled. The TPWG draft posits a number of reasons for why a user agent may not have tracking preference enabled:

1. The browser user agent does not implement DNT;
2. The user has not yet expressed a specific preference; or,
3. The user has not chosen to transmit a preference.

User preference mechanisms specified by the TPWG represent an earnest attempt to place some burden of policy implementation on browser developers rather than publishers: instead of forcing the user to make a choice for every website, the idea is that a user specifies choice in browser preferences and sets exceptions as desired. Nonetheless, it is conceivable that any given website may still offer a tracking preference choice.

2 Privacy Choice Design Problem

Though the TPWG intent is to provide a machine readable preference expression mechanism and not a user interface (UI) specification, the three options above map to common UI pattern: **modeless dialog control**.

C. Stephanidis (Ed.): Posters, Part II, HCII 2013, CCIS 374, pp. 735–739, 2013.

The research described in this paper raises the question: if a user is presented with a dialog control presenting a choice between opt-in, opt-out and dismiss, what does the user believe is the consequence of choosing to dismiss? One way to consider this problem is as a choice design problem (fig 1):

1. If I click "allow", I choose "allow" cookies
2. If I click "block", I choose "block" cookies
3. I can do neither ("dismiss")

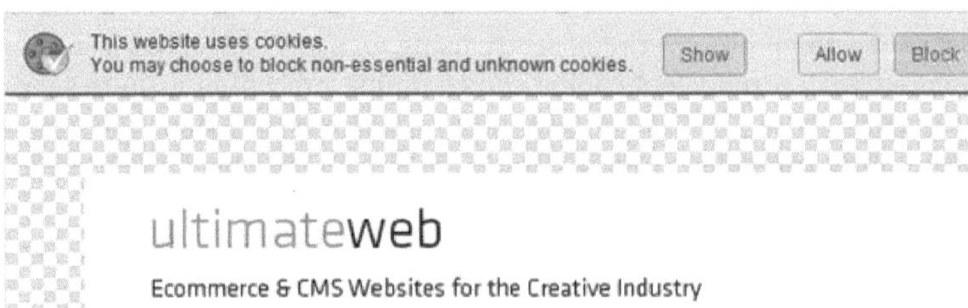

Fig. 1. Cookie dialog control from cookieguard.eu

Fair and unbiased choice design is a tricky problem. Default choices have a dramatic impact on user action [1]. Heuristic and bias reasoning theories account for a number of different situations leading to systematic bias. Biases including loss aversion (e.g., change from status quo), framing, and evaluation of options in relation to reference points (e.g., expectation and social comparison) have been well-described by Tversky and Kahneman [2,3].

Whether intentional or not, designers – both standards architects and web designers – have tremendous potential to influence choice [4].

3 Implicature

Previous work of decision-making in privacy research has focused on the effectiveness of communicating privacy risks to consumers [5], and confusability in user interface design [6]. This study concerns whether users confronted with a non-forced choice dialog box understand the meaning of their choices in the context of interaction.

Pragmatics is concerned with reasoning processes that go beyond conventional meaning. It is founded on the notion of language as action with communicative goals [7,8,9]. A common pragmatic phenomenon in linguistic understanding is implicature. An implicature represents a gap between what is expressed and what is communicated. Importantly, whether an implicature is true or not, does not affect the meaning of the message itself. For example,

1. Harry and Sally are married.

2. Tell a friend or colleague.
3. If you mow the lawn, I'll give you five dollars.

In (1) the implication is that Harry and Sally are married to each other. But, if they were not, and both married to someone else, this statement is still true. (2) exemplifies implicature derived by considering "or" as inclusive or exclusive. (3) is an *invited inference* [10] or *conditional promise* [11]. In (3), hearers understand the conditional relation between getting five dollars and mowing. But they may also infer "not to mow" means they will "not get five dollars." Fillenbaum [12] showed that the obverse of a conditional promise (in the example above, "I won't give you five dollars, if you don't mow the lawn") was an accepted inference for 85% of subjects tested.

In this study, we are concerned with whether a non-forced choice dialog has the potential to generate an implicature in user understanding. One way to view the choice problem above is as a discourse reasoning task where more than one conditional is given for interpretation in a single turn. In the cookie dialog choice decision described in this paper, not only must subjects interpret the meaning of each conditional independently, but they must do so in the context of choice between an additional explicit conditional and graphical third choice ("dismiss"). The particular question addressed here is what a user believes his choice to mean when he neither selects "allow" nor "block" – does he believe there are cookies present on the website? Why or why not?

4 Purpose and Procedure

The purpose of this study was to assess the feasibility of conducting a larger, online pilot. Specific questions addressed by this study addressed (1) whether the dialog was placed in such a way that subjects would likely read it; and, (2) whether subjects would consider the dialog as independent of the experiment. We needed to be confident that users were not influenced by the experiment to select a particular choice. To this end, we posed this study as a survey.

Subjects were recruited at the University of Baltimore from university business offices. Employees and students were invited to participate in a "10 minute survey" in the Information Arts and Technologies usability lab in exchange for a $5 dollar gift card. All were native English speakers who were comfortable using the Internet.

Using a Tobii T60 eye-tracker, subjects were presented with a choice banner ("This website uses cookies") preceding a short survey on Internet privacy. The choice banner was modified from the CookGuard plugin[1] designed to help website owners comply with European Union directives. A modification was made to include an "x" so that a third option – "if I click the x, I dismiss the control" – was explicit.

This banner was placed prominently on the start page of the Internet survey (fig 2). Generally, such banners are placed at the very top of a website, but we

[1] `http://cookieguard.eu`

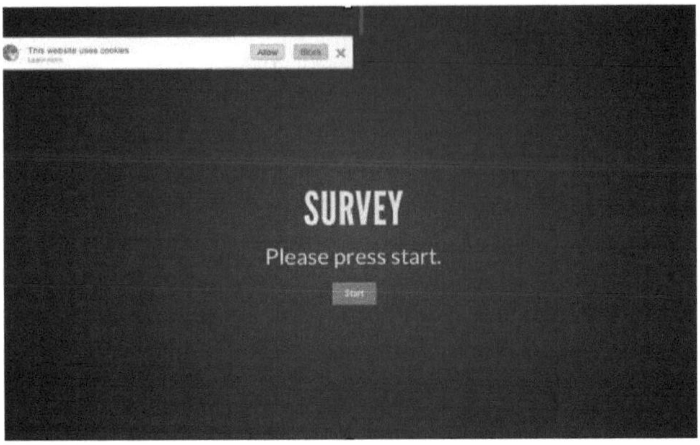

Fig. 2. User display

were concerned that subjects might not notice it there, so we positioned it in such a way to make it more visually distinct.

5 Results and Discussion

Of 17 subjects, 5 did not know what browser cookies were for, 14 reported that privacy was very important to them, and 15 reported that they would turn off tracking if it were easy. Notably, only 1 subject selected any option other than "dismiss" on the cookie banner.[2] He selected "block" cookies because "he didn't like cookies." No one clicked the provided link "learn more".

For the first goal of assessing likelihood that a subject would read the banner, we learned that, despite a sparsity of information on the start page, the first 9 subjects did not see the banner. For the remaining, subjects were verbally cued that there would be a cookie banner on the start page and that they could "choose however they wanted." Indeed, all but one did then see and read the banner.

For the second goal, we were were more successful. When presented the banner, subjects did not suspect that the cookie banner had anything to do with the following survey.

After presentation of the cookie banner and a number of demographic questions, subjects were asked whether they believed ad trackers were present on the site or not. 8 subjects believed that ad trackers were present while 9 did not. Of those that believed ad trackers were present, 1 subject believed that this was the case since he did not "block" cookies. Of the 9 that did not believe ad trackers were present, 6 believed this because they did not "allow" cookies. Accordingly, 7 of 17 (41%) believed there either were or were not ad trackers on the site based on *not* clicking "allow" or "block" cookies, respectively. These results suggest

[2] Note also that many subjects who selected to dismiss the cookie banner later indicated that privacy was very important to them.

that a pragmatic implicature was in play – information was suggested via the cookie banner though not explicitly stated.

6 Limitations

Results in this study were derived primarily to assess the feasibility of a larger pilot. Though results suggest that implicature is of concern for the design of modeless cookie dialogs, we cannot conclude that all such dialogs will invoke implicature. Issues that apply include the effect of dialog as conditional promise [13], distinguishing between assertions and implications in memory [14], attitude or belief about privacy, and the mixed use of linguistic and graphical information.

7 Conclusions

The definition of a technical specification and mechanism intended to represent user preference is undoubtably a difficult endeavor. Though results of a follow-up pilot are not yet available, this study emphasizes the need for the TPWG and designers to consider the unintended consequence of implicature in user choice design. Despite the rather limited nature of this study, we believe implicature may be inherent to the design of modeless dialogs. A solution may be to offer visual feedback conveying the consequence of a user choice decision.

References

1. Johnson, E.J., Bellman, S., Lohse, G.L.: Defaults, framing and privacy: Why opting in-opting out. Marketing Letters 13, 5–15 (2002)
2. Tversky, A., Kahneman, D.: The framing of decisions and the psychology of choice. Science 211, 453–458 (1981)
3. Kahneman, D., Tversky, A.: Choices, values, and frames. American Psychologist 39, 341 (1984)
4. Thaler, R., Sunstein, C., Balz, J.: Choice architecture. Available at SSRN 1583509 (2010)
5. McDonald, A.M., Cranor, L.F.: An empirical study of how people perceive online behavioral advertising (cmu-cylab-09-015) (2009)
6. Leon, P.G., Ur, B., Shay, R., Wang, Y., Balebako, R., Cranor, L.: Why Johnny can't opt out: A usability evaluation of tools to limit online behavioral advertising. Technical Report CMU-CyLab-11-017 (2012)
7. Grice, H.P.: Logic and conversation. In: Cole (ed.) Syntax and Semantics: Speech Acts, vol. 3, pp. 41–58. Elsevier (1975)
8. Levinson, S.C.: Pragmatics. Cambridge University Press (1983)
9. Clark, H.: Using Language. Cambridge University Press (1996)
10. Geis, M.L., Zwicky, A.M.: On invited inferences. Linguistic Inquiry (1971)
11. Searle, J.R.: What is a speech act. The Philosophy of Language 3, 1965–1996 (1971)
12. Fillenbaum, S.: IF: Some uses. Psychological Research (1975)
13. Horn, L.R.: From if to iff: Conditional perfection as pragmatic strengthening. Journal of Pragmatics 32, 289–326 (2000)
14. Brewer, W.F.: Memory for the pragmatic implications of sentences. Memory & Cognition 5, 673–678 (1977)

SpeechProtector: A Speech Protection System for Preventing Reporting Bias

Kazutaka Kurihara[1] and Koji Tsukada[2]

[1] National Institute of Advanced Industrial Science and Technology, Chuo Dai 2, 1-1-1 Umezono, Tsukuba, Ibaraki, Japan
k-kurihara@aist.go.jp
[2] JST PRESTO, 2-1-1 Otsuka Bunkyo-ku, Tokyo, Japan

Abstract. Freedom of expression is welcomed in democratic nations, but there is no end of cases in which recorded video is processed to report information not intended by the person in the video. For this article, we have developed a prototype system for preventing this sort of bias in reporting. The system is a smartphone application that allows users, who are the subject of news-gathering, to also record the material themselves, post it to a video sharing site, and to display a QR code containing a link to the video. The system enables a link to a video reproducing the original statements to be forcefully embedded in the report video, which should inhibit bias in the reporting as it is presented later.

Keywords: Reporting bias, QR code, smartphone, Youtube.

1 Introduction

Journalism is a type of expression that uses the media. Journalism and the right to knowledge are based on the right to freedom of expression. On the other hand, journalism must also maintain the principle of objective reporting. In spite of this, in actual reporting, the facts are very often not discussed as-is, but are reconstructed, incorporating the subjective biases of the reporting organization. For recordings of people making statements, the content is often split up or rearranged, contrary to the intentions of the speaker, and this can cause controversy.

The remedy to this is generally said to be that the receiver of the information must acquire media literacy and cultivate the ability to discern the truth of information they receive.

The goal of this research has been to reduce bias in journalistic reports that use statements made by people in presentations, speeches, press conferences or street interviews, even if the statements have been manipulated. This is done through technology that enables receivers of the information to access the speaker's statements as originally intended. This protects the credibility of the speaker in society, and can be expected to tighten global monitoring of bias in reporting.

C. Stephanidis (Ed.): Posters, Part II, HCII 2013, CCIS 374, pp. 740–744, 2013.

Fig. 1. Being filmed while using SpeechProtector. Note that this QR code is actually readable.

As the first step in this article, we describe development of the smartphone-based SpeechProtector prototype system for preserving reported statements (Figure 1). The system applies particularly to reports involving photographs and video. The user, who is the subject of the report, also records the entire session, posts it to a video sharing site, and forcefully inserts a link in the material used for reporting by displaying a QR code with a time-stamped link to this video during the whole session. The system provides a simple interface for accomplishing this.

Then, in whatever way the gathered video data and statements are modified, the receiver can easily access the original content using a mobile terminal such as an ordinary mobile phone, as long as the QR code remains in the report. If the user is not satisfied with the report, he/she can appeal to society using this link, through Social Networking Services or other personal publishing avenues.

2 Related Work

This research can be considered as an application of a type of electronic watermarking. Technologies like [1] , from Mitsubishi Electric, are the latest technologies able to embed and detect copyright information in Hi-Vision video. They are mainly useful when copyright holders want to control distribution of information. In this research, however, the person being recorded does not have the right to edit the material collected, so a way to force insertion of watermark information into the report is needed.

We next describe how this additional data can be embedded visually in the real world. QR codes [2] are a 2D-barcode technology developed by Denso Inc.

(currently Denso Wave Corp.) to overcome some shortcomings of conventional barcodes, with an explicit statement that patent rights will not be exercised. Today, many mobile devices include a function able to read them, and they have spread to the extent that almost everyone with a mobile phone can read them. They are widely used, such as in paper and various urban advertising media, and on packaging to indicate product qualities. A major way in which they are used is to apply a code to physical objects or content, linking to more detailed information. The particular visual characteristics of QR codes make them easily recognizable, which is another characteristic.

3 Design and Implementation of SpeechProtector

3.1 Problem Analysis and System Design

Behind the problem that reporting can be done contrary to the intentions of the person subject to reporting are facts that it is difficult to refuse information gathering, and there is no control over how the material gathered will eventually be edited and reported. Thus, we introduce a mechanism that allows the person to force his/her intentions to be reflected in the information gathered, and allows the viewer of the report to notice and access this information. The mechanism involves designing three aspects: (1) how can the person force his/her intentions to be reflected in the report, (2) how can the viewer's attention be drawn to them, and (3) how can they be expressed to the viewer?

For (1), sudden requests for news gathering can be accommodated using a system that operates on a smartphone, which can be expected to be carried at all times. The person being photographed can force the 2D barcode to be included in the image of his/her face by holding up an image of the barcode, (Figure 1). This action falls under his/her freedom of expression, and cannot be forbidden by anyone else. As long as the resolution is high-enough, this code will still be valid even if sections of the captured video are edited. Similarly, the code should still be valid when images are posted as still photos on the Net or in paper media.

For (2), QR codes can be used for the 2D barcodes in (1). QR codes have a particular visual form and are used widely in the public, so viewers recognize them easily. They can also be read easily using any mobile device in their possession, conveying the original intentions of the person being photographed.

Finally, (3) can be implemented by configuring the destination of a link in the QR code to a video of the original content, captured by the person themselves. This is because the originally stated content is the most effective and impartial way to critique bias in reporting. Further, adding Social Networking Services and other functions that enable third parties to discuss the critique with the associated video creates a mechanism that will promote interest in reporting bias within society.

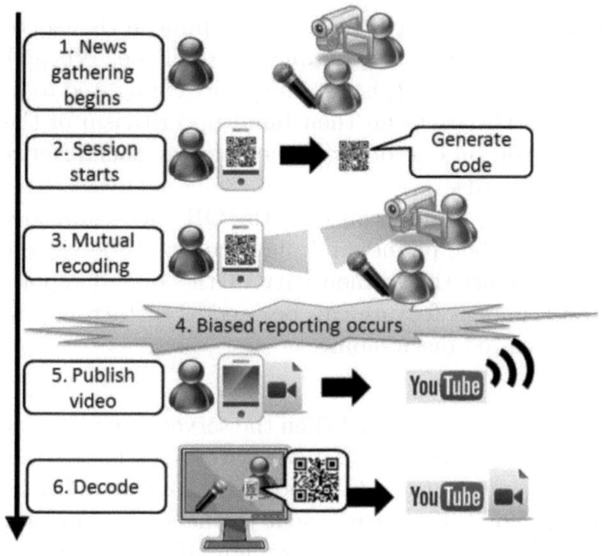

Fig. 2. Scenario using SpeechProtector

3.2 Implementation

We implemented the prototype SpeechProtector system for inhibiting bias in reporting using a client-server system. The server uses ASP.NET, and the client is implemented as a Windows Phone (smartphone) application. We used YouTube as the base for video hosting and Social Networking Service functions.

Usage Scenario. We outline the operation sequence with a hypothetical scenario (Figure 2) below.

(1)The user is conducting his everyday activities, carrying a smartphone, when confronted by a reporter.

(2)The user starts SpeechProtector on the smartphone, initiating a new session. This generates a QR code for the session.

(3)The reporter begins gathering material (filming). The user holds the smartphone near his/her own face while also recording video with SpeechProtector. While recording, the QR code created in (2) is displayed prominently on the smartphone, and the reporter cannot avoid photographing it when filming the user's face.

(4)Later, if the interview is reported according to the user's intentions, there is nothing to do. In such a case, a message indicating that "no corresponding video has been published" is displayed when the QR code is decoded. If not reported according to the user's intentions, he/she has the following means of opposing it.

(5)Simple operations in SpeechProtector will publish the video taken with the smartphone while the reporter was filming on YouTube. When this is done, the destination of the QR code in (2) is automatically configured to link to the video shared on YouTube. The user can then build up criticism of the biased report using comments on YouTube or other venues such as Social Networking Services or Internet bulletin boards.

(6)Later, any ordinary viewer can read the QR code embedded in the biased report using his/her mobile phone, and play the YouTube video of the recorded original statements. Thus the authenticity of the biased report is ascertained and the YouTube comment feature can be used as a starting point for criticism or participation in related discussion.

Client-Server Communication. When the server receives notification to start a session from the client, as in 3.2 (2), it generates a session URL, which is unique for each session. It then returns a QR code to the client indicating this URL.

The URL for the YouTube video is sent to the server after the video is published on YouTube in 3.2 (5), and it is configured as the forwarding address of the session URL.

4 Conclusion

In this article, we have proposed and prototyped the SpeechProtector system to control information bias in reporting, by helping the person being reported on to make his/her own recording of the news gathering, to post it on a video sharing site, and to force a link to this video into the news material being gathered, in the form of a QR code.

Acknowledgments. A part of this research was instigated by the Japan Science and Technology Agency and received support from a Grant-in-aid for Scientific Research (KAKENHI 23700155).

References

1. http://www.mitsubishielectric.co.jp/news/2011/pdf/1027-a.pdf
2. http://www.qrcode.com/en/index.html

Secure and Usable PIN-Entry Method with Shoulder-Surfing Resistance

Mun-Kyu Lee and Hyeonjin Nam

School of Computer and Information Engineering,
Inha University, Incheon 402-751, Korea
mklee@inha.ac.kr, jin0639@hanmail.net

Abstract. We propose a new PIN-entry method which prevents shoulder surfing attacks effectively. The proposed method uses a random mapping between the PIN digits and alphabets given as challenges to the users. The user's task is to recognize this mapping and to enter the mapped alphabet sequence instead of directly entering the PIN digits. The intuitive nature and easy interface of the proposed scheme enables the users to learn it easily, and the experimental results in the pilot test show that the new method guarantees fast and reliable authentication. To be precise, the average authentication time was 5.8 to 6.8 seconds, and the average error rate was 3.3 to 6.7%.

Keywords: user authentication, personal identification number, shoulder surfing attack.

1 Introduction

The personal identification number (PIN) is a well-known user authentication method used in many devices such as a smartphone, ATM, and an electronic doorlock. However, the regular PIN-entry method is quite vulnerable to the shoulder surfing attack (SSA) because its layout is fixed and the user always inputs the same information based on the PIN. To solve this problem, there have been various proposals for countermeasures involving random challenges and user's appropriate responses calculated from the secret PIN digits [1-7]. Those countermeasures require users either to perform complicated mental tasks or to use secondary channels to recognize audio and tactile information. Obviously, those proposals increase the authentication time and raise the rate of erroneous input, significantly degrading the usability of PIN-entry scheme.

We propose a new PIN-entry method without any secondary channel. We performed a pilot test with various settings. According to the experimental results, the authentication time is only twice the regular PIN-entry method and significantly faster than those of the existing SSA-resistant methods. In addition, the error rate is much lower than those of the existing methods.

C. Stephanidis (Ed.): Posters, Part II, HCII 2013, CCIS 374, pp. 745–748, 2013.

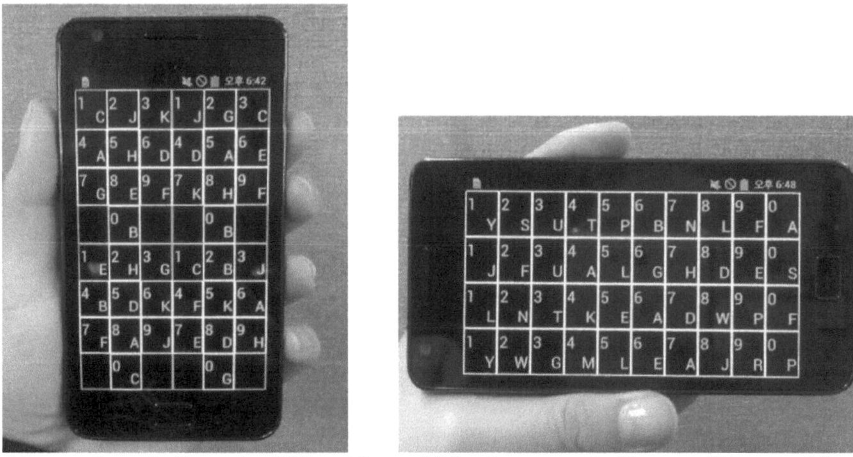

(a) portrait mode (4 regular PIN pads) (b) landscape mode (4 rows of linear pads)

Fig. 1. The challenge stage where random mappings between PIN digits and characters are given

2 Proposed PIN-Entry Method

The proposed method is composed of two stages; the challenge stage and the response stage. In the first stage, the user is given a challenge screen which provides a random mapping between the user's PIN digits and alphabet characters. In the example of Fig. 1(a), the user may find 4 regular PIN pads where each digit is associated with a character. Each of the 4 PIN pads are for each PIN digit. To be precise, the top left PIN pad is for the first PIN digit and the top right for the second. The bottom left PIN pad is for the third PIN digit and the bottom right for the final PIN digit. The required task of the user in this stage is to recognize this mapping and memorize the characters associated with his/her PIN digits. For example, let us assume that the PIN is 3146. Then, the matching character sequence is KJBA. For security reasons, this association between PIN digits and characters should be randomized for each authentication session.

The alphabets given as challenges may be selected from either the whole alphabet set (26-character mode) or the set of only 10 characters, A, B, C, D, E, F, G, H, J, and K (10-character mode). We do not consider the character 'I', because it may confuse the user with the digit, '1.' The example in Fig. 1(a) shows the 10-character mode.

We also may use a completely different layout such as Fig. 1(b). In this layout, the digits are not arranged as those of a PIN pad, but they are arranged in a row. To provide a complete mapping for a 4-digit PIN, the challenge screen is composed of 4 rows. In this example, if the user's PIN is 3146, the matching sequence will be UJKE. We name the layouts in Fig. 1(a) and Fig. 1(b) as a portrait mode and a landscape mode, respectively. In total, there are 4 combinations of modes (portrait vs. landscape as well as 26 vs. 10) which can be pre-configured according to the user's preference.

When the user touches any region in the screen in the first stage, the second stage begins. In this stage, the user inputs the 4 characters through a keypad (Fig.2).

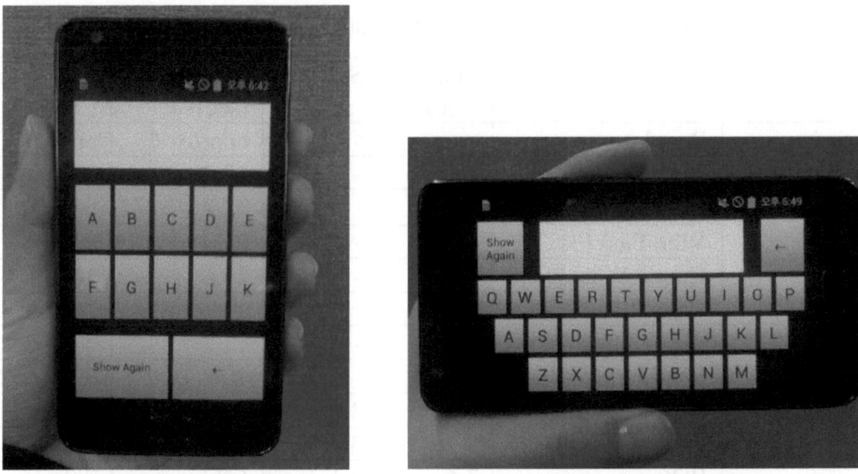

(a) 10-character mode (b) 26-character mode

Fig. 2. The response stage: One of (a) and (b) is performed according to the alphabet set given as the challenge in the previous stage

3 Performance Analysis

We performed a pilot test with various settings. According to the experimental results given in Table 1, the authentication time is 5.8 to 6.8 seconds, which is significantly faster than those of the existing SSA-resistant methods. The error rate is 3.3 to 6.7%, which is much smaller than those of the existing methods. What is more encouraging is that the data in Table 1 were measured from participants who were not sufficiently trained for the new method. We may expect that the time and error rate should be improved if the users become accustomed to the new method.

According to Table 1, the first and second stages seem to consume almost the same amount of time. Therefore, we cannot point out a specific bottleneck in our method which could have been a target for optimization. However, the data in Table 1 shows us non-negligible correlation between the performance and the configuration modes. Therefore, in our future research, we will find the optimal combination though extensive experiments involving a wide range of users. In addition, other factors that may affect the performance should be analyzed precisely. These factors include the font of digits and characters which decides the recognition speed of the user, and the size and arrangements of touch buttons which decide the amount of movement of fingers.

Regarding the security against shoulder surfing, the proposed method is significantly more secure than the regular PIN pad, because an ordinary human attacker cannot completely memorize the instant mapping shown in the challenge stage which lasts for only about 3 seconds. However, it would be desirable that this claim should be verified by experiments involving real human attackers, especially educated ones, which will be included in our future research. We also remark that the proposed method does not prevent recording attacks.

Table 1. Performance Comparison (Authentication Time and Error Rate)

Method		Stage 1 (sec)	Stage 2 (sec)	Total time (sec)	Error rate (%)
Existing	Regular	-	-	approx. 3	approx. 0
	Binary [1]	-	-	23.2	9.0
	Undercover [2]	-	-	32-45	> 31.5
	VibraPass [3]	-	-	8.2	> 14.8
	Haptic Wheel [4]	-	-	23.0	16.4
	ColorPIN [5]	-	-	13.3-13.9	N.A.
	Phone Lock [6]*	-	-	12.2	4.8(+6.9)
	SpinLock [7]*	-	-	10.8-16.9	3.3(+64.0)
Proposed**	L/26	3.8	3.0	6.8	6.7
	L/10	3.2	3.2	6.4	3.3
	P/26	3.6	3.1	6.7	3.3
	P/10	2.9	2.9	5.8	6.7

* Among the audio and tactile versions, we only consider the audio versions, which are more practical ones. ** L vs. P: landscape vs. portrait modes, 26 vs. 10: 26 vs. 10-character modes.

Acknowledgments. This research was supported by the MSIP, Korea, under the ITRC support program (NIPA-2013-H0301-13-1003) supervised by the NIPA and the IT R&D program of MOTIE/KEIT (10039180).

References

1. Roth, V., Richter, K., Freidinger, R.: A PIN-entry method resilient against shoulder surfing. In: Proceedings of the 11th ACM Conference on Computer and Communications Security, pp. 236–245 (October 2004)
2. Sasamoto, H., Christin, N., Hayshi, E.: Undercover: Authentication Usable in Front of Prying Eyes. In: CHI 2008, pp. 183–192 (April 2008)
3. Luca, A.D., Zezschwitz, E.V., Hußmann, H.: VibraPass-Secure Authentication Based on Shared Lies. In: CHI 2009, pp. 913–916 (April 2009)
4. Bianchi, A., Oakley, I., Lee, J.K., Kwon, D.S.: The Haptic Wheel: Design & Evalua-tion of a Tactile Password System. In: CHI 2010, pp. 3625–3630 (April 2010)
5. Luca, A.D., Hertzschuch, K., Hussmann, H.: ColorPIN – securing PIN entry through indirect input. In: CHI 2010, pp. 1103–1106 (April 2010)
6. Bianchi, A., Oakley, I., Kostakos, V., Kwon, D.S.: The Phone Lock: Audio and Haptic Shoulder-Surfing Resistant PIN Entry Methods for Mobile Devices. In: TEI 2011, pp. 197–200 (January 2011)
7. Bianchi, A., Oakley, I., Kwon, D.S.: Spinlock: A single-cue haptic and au-dio pin input technique for authentication. In: Cooper, E.W., Kryssanov, V.V., Ogawa, H., Brewster, S. (eds.) HAID 2011. LNCS, vol. 6851, pp. 81–90. Springer, Heidelberg (2011)

Optimized Anonymity for Intergenerational Communication Based on the Concept of Crowdsourcing

Yuki Nagai[1], Atsushi Hiyama[1], Takahiro Miura[1], Masaru Miyazaki[2], and Michitaka Hirose[1]

[1] Department of Mechano-Informatics, Graduate School of Information Science and Technology, The University of Tokyo, 7-3-1 Hongo, Bunkyo-ku, Tokyo Japan
{ynagai,atsushi,miu,hirose}@cyber.t.u-tokyo.ac.jp
[2] Science & Technology Research Laboratories, Japan Broadcasting Corporation (NHK), 1-10-11 Kinuta, Setagaya-ku, Tokyo Japan
miyazaki.m-fk@nhk.or.jp

Abstract. The grandparent-grandchild (GP-GC) relationship is considered important especially in hyper-aged societies with low birth rates. With the popular trend in information and communication technology (ICT) towards SNS-like crowdsourcing, our aim is to create GP-GC-like relationships among users of online social networks. As a first step, we conducted an experiment in which we connected seniors and young people on an SNS. Our results indicate that seniors are interested in young people's life-logs, but most of their comments in the experiment were in the form of overbearing or meaningless advice. On the basis of these results, in this paper, we also discuss the design of a system that facilitates an augmented GP-GC relationship.

Keywords: anonymity, seniors, crowdsourcing, SNS.

1 Introduction

The grandparent-grandchild (GP-GC) relationship is considered important [1] especially in hyper-aged societies with low birth rates. For grandchildren, grandparents seem to provide them with communication-based emotional support [2] similar to that provided by mentors. Grandparents also view the GP-GC relationship positively, because they feel joyful and proud when they communicate with their grandchildren [3]. However, these days, almost three-quarters of the population of older people in developed regions are living independently and the predominance of such people is likely to increase [4]. Many attempts have been made to connect grandparents and grandchildren using information and communication technology (ICT) as a bridge [5–7]. In the research studies conducted, the online GP-GC relationship was accepted and viewed favorably.

C. Stephanidis (Ed.): Posters, Part II, HCII 2013, CCIS 374, pp. 749–753, 2013.

With the facilitation provided by ICT, new forms of online communication, such as social networking services (SNSs), have become pervasive. Despite the digital divide that predominantly impacts seniors, some of them are still able to recount historical stories or give advice to young people on SNS platforms such as Twitter[1]. Furthermore, recent crowdsourcing platforms have become more SNS-like, in that they are no longer as mechanical as they were before. For example, Socialgift[2] and bemool[3] are systems for task sharing but have some features for online communication.

With the popular trend in ICT towards SNS-like crowdsourcing, our aim is to create GP-GC-like relationships among users of online social networks.

Our aim is to use SNS-like crowdsourcing to create GP-GC-like relationships among users of online social networks. As a first step, we connected seniors on an SNS called "Kashiwa Social" [8], an SNS for seniors, and young people on Twitter. In this paper, we report on how seniors reacted and interacted on the SNS and discuss the design of an augmented GP-GC relationship.

2 Methodology

SNS for Seniors

"Kashiwa Social" is an SNS used by seniors in Kashiwa [8]. The service is optimized for seniors (Fig. 1) and is based on Teleda, made by Japan Broadcasting Corporation (NHK). The service has 85 users, 70 seniors and 15 facilitators. The facilitators in the system promote communication among the seniors. The seniors range in age from 60 to 78 years, with the average age being 67.0 years. The facilitators range in age from 30 to 49, with the average being 37.7 years. Kashiwa Social consists of community groups, with each community centered around a discussion theme. We used the "Talk with young people" community in our experiment. In each community, topics are posted and commented on by users.

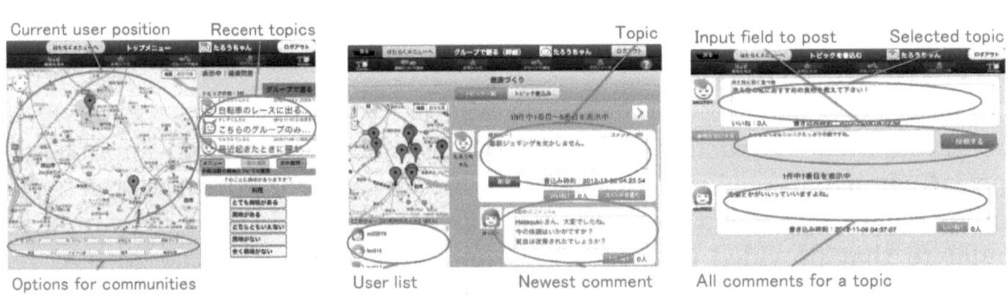

(a) Top page (b) Topic page (c) Comment page

Fig. 1. Kashiwa Social

[1] `https://twitter.com/aoikesi` (in Japanese)
[2] `http://www.socialgift.com/`
[3] `https://bemool.com/` (in Japanese)

Connect with Young Users on Twitter
We constructed a mediator system to connect Kashiwa Social, used by seniors, with young people on Twitter. The young participants comprised five male university students ranging in age from 22 to 24 years. The mediator system caught their tweets via the Twitter Streaming API[4]. If the tweet was not a reply to a specific topic, the system posted the message on Kashiwa Social as a comment on the user's topic. The system tweeted posts by seniors on Kashiwa Social using the system's Twitter account as replies to the young users. A system account was used to post seniors' posts so that young people could not determine exactly who posted the reply. When the young people replied to the tweet, the system replaced their Twitter screen names with names allocated to them on Kashiwa Social. In this way, seniors were able to determine whom the young people's replies were for. We used topics to introduce the young people's profiles, and gave more information gradually (Table 1), in order to determine the influence of anonymity (of the young people) on the actions of the seniors.

Table 1. Sample topics

Day	Title	Text
1	Nice to meet you.	I am a university student.
8	Thank you for your continued support.	I am researching the use of social media for intergenerational communication. I will work for a start-up company. I am interested in girls, wine, and ICT.
15	I have some questions I would like to ask you.	1. What kind of literature are you interested in? 2. What do you want to do on the Internet? 3. What are some important things to take into consideration when choosing a company to work for?

3 Results

Of the 70 seniors, 38 visited the community during the experiment. From time to time, the mediator system became inoperational due to network error. The system was inoperational over the period spanning the 22nd to the 33rd day, (Fig. 2(a)), and the number of views from the seniors in the community fell (Fig. 2(b)). This statistic indicates that the absence of new tweets from the young people resulted in seniors staying away. From this point on, we focus the results obtained up to the 21st day. From the viewpoint of anonymity, changes in the topics introduced did not seem to affect the number of views in this experiment (Fig. 2(b)). Over the three-week period, the number of views from the community was 143 and that of posts was 16 (Fig. 3). The number of posts was small; however, the results show that seniors are interested in young people's life-logs compared to other communities. The following are examples of the posts submitted by seniors:

[4] Twitter API: `https://dev.twitter.com`

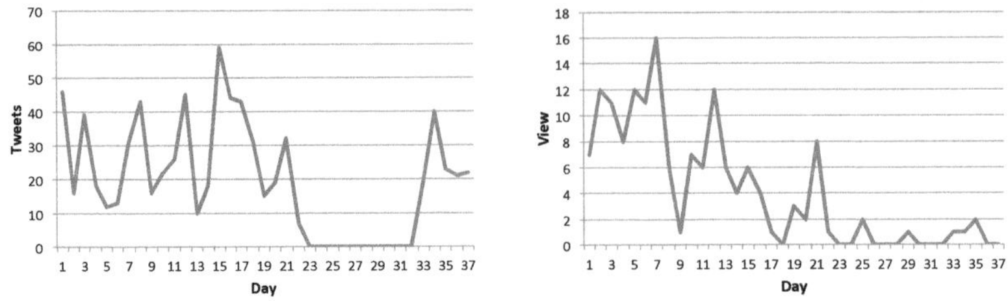

(a) Tweets from young people (b) Views of seniors

Fig. 2. Daily transition

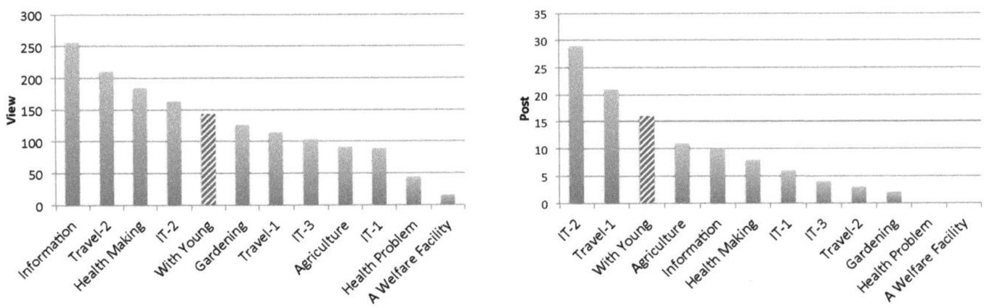

(a) Views (b) Posts

Fig. 3. Comparison of communities

- I want you to relax the tension and do your best.
- Rockefeller said, "The most important thing for a young man is to establish credit–reputation and character." Do your best.
- You said your English is poor, but you should study much harder before you say so.
- What do you think about the teaching of history topics such as Myths in the university?
- First, answer your question by yourself.

4 Discussion

The senior participants were more interested in our community on Kashiwa Social than they were in other communities, However, most of their comments were not the answers we expected to the questions posed by the young people. They sometimes gave us supportive comments, but some were overbearing or meaningless monologues. They complained in the interview, after the experiment on the SNS user interface, that the tweets from the young people were too difficult and complicated to understand. Further, we use tweets for selected contexts of the young people's lives, but they wanted to get more details about the young people, such as face, hobby, relationship status (single, in a relationship, or married). For the young people, we need to present the personalities of the seniors in abstract by making them into a crowd, but we also need to clearly identify the young people for the seniors.

5 Conclusion

In this paper, we reported on our first attempt at creating an augmented GP-GC relationship in which an SNS used by seniors was connected to young people on Twitter. Our results indicate that seniors are interested in this type of communication with young people than with other types of communities in the SNS. On the other hand, the replies from the seniors were found to be overbearing or meaningless. We used tweets from young people as a means of familiarizing the seniors with the young people's lives, but they wanted more details.

Acknowledgement. This research was partially supported by the Japan Science and Technology Agency, JST, under the Strategic Promotion of Innovative Research and Development Program.

References

1. Friedman, D., Hechter, M., Kreager, D.: A theory of the value of grandchildren. Rationality and Society 20(1), 31–63 (2008)
2. Mansson, D.H., Myers, S.A., Turner, L.H.: Relational maintenance behaviors in the grandchild–grandparent relationship. Communication Research Reports 27(1), 68–79 (2010)
3. Kemp, C.L.: Dimensions of grandparent-adult grandchild relationships: From family ties to intergenerational friendships. Canadian Journal on Aging/La Revue Canadienne Du Vieillissement 24, 161–177 (2005)
4. United Nations: Population Ageing and Department 2012. United Nations. Department of Economic and Social Affairs, Population Division (2012)
5. Neustaedter, C., Judge, T.K., Harrison, S., Sellen, A., Cao, X., Kirk, D., Kaye, J.: Connecting families: new technologies, family communication, and the impact on domestic space. In: Proceedings of the 16th ACM International Conference on Supporting Group Work, GROUP 2010, pp. 363–366. ACM, New York (2010)
6. Bentley, F., Basapur, S., Chowdhury, S.K.: Promoting intergenerational communication through location-based asynchronous video communication. In: Proc UbiComp, vol. 11 (2011)
7. Moffatt, K., David, J., Baecker, R.M.: Connecting grandparents and grandchildren. In: Neustaedter, C., Harrison, S., Sellen, A. (eds.) Connecting Families, pp. 173–193. Springer, London (2013)
8. Miyazaki, M., Sano, M., Mitsuya, S., Sumiyoshi, H., Naemura, M., Fujii, A.: Development and field trial of a social tv system for elderly people. In: HCI International (2013)

Laptop Security and Data Protection with Intel® Anti-Theft Service

Sasanka Prabhala and Jiphun C. Satapathy

Intel Corporation, 2111 NE 25th Avenue, Hillsboro, OR 97124, U.S.A.
{sasanka.v.prabhala,jiphun.c.satapathy}@intel.com

Abstract. With technology advancements and widespread adoption of connectivity, more and more users are using a wide range of devices to access information whenever and wherever they want. With increase in laptop usage, there is also an increase in laptop theft. This paper describes how Intel® Anti-Theft Service (IATS) powered by Intel® Anti-Theft Technology (Intel AT) helps protect both the asset (device) and data by locking down the device if lost or stolen. In this paper, we outline the working of Intel AT, operation of IATS, design and development of IATS from user experience viewpoint, and conclude with shared quantitative and qualitative metrics for implementation of Intel AT with customers and partners.

Keywords: Intel Anti-Theft Technology, Intel Anti-Theft Service, Anti-Theft Service, User Experience, Qualitative and quantitative metrics.

1 Introduction

With technology advancements and widespread adoption of connectivity, more and more users are using a wide range of devices to access information whenever and wherever they want. With increase in laptop usage, there is also an increase in laptop theft. For example, more than 12,000 laptops are lost or stolen in U.S. airports [1]. A laptop theft not only means theft of the physical device but also theft of valuable information that is stored on the device. Laptop theft also means data breach which is very significant to business and individuals.

To tackle the issue of laptop theft, Intel Corporation developed a technology solution known as Intel Anti-Theft Technology (Intel AT). Intel Anti-Theft service (IATS), powered by Intel AT, helps (a) asset protection – device lockdown if lost or stolen and (b) data protection - secure data files. Unlike other security solutions, Intel AT is hardware based solution and hence protects asset and data if the device is lost or stolen or when the device hard drive is swapped. In addition, IATS provides a mechanism to reactivate the recovered stolen device.

Services such as IATS should be designed to be simple and easy to use and at the same time provide peace of mind to end-users by protecting their asset and data. The paper is divided into four sections. The first section briefly outlines the different components that make up AT and their working. The second section describes the

C. Stephanidis (Ed.): Posters, Part II, HCII 2013, CCIS 374, pp. 754–758, 2013.

operation of IATS as related to asset and data protection. The third section overviews design and re-design of IATS from user experience viewpoint. The fourth and final section offers conclusive quantitative and qualitative metrics based on user experience testing for implementation of Intel AT with customers and partners.

2 Intel Anti-Theft Service Working

IATS is an end to end service based on Intel AT, a feature in most Intel Architecture (IA) platforms. It uses chipset firmware (FW) also known as Management Engine (ME) to store required information to achieve security and persistence. Figure 1 shows the high level block diagram for IATS. There are primarily two components for this service – (a) client side components and (b) server side components.

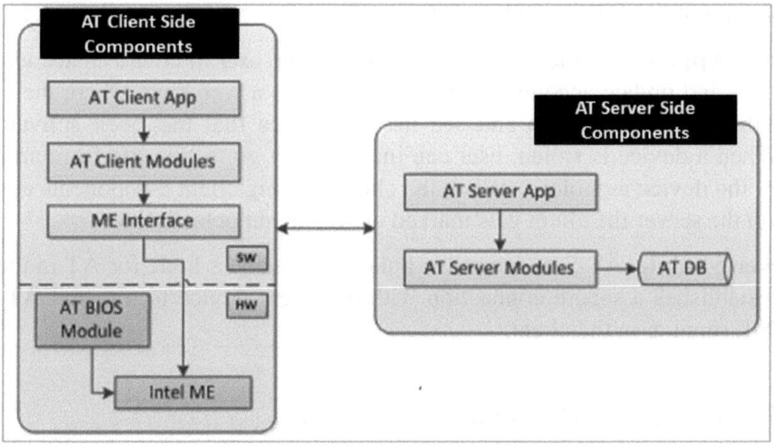

Fig. 1. High level block diagram for IATS

2.1 Client Side Components

Client side components are the required modules that run on the mobile devices and are made up of the following:

Anti-Theft (AT) Client App. This is the client console the user uses to configure or manage the device with IATS. For example the user can click on IATS tray icon and access the server. The user can also check the last time the client completed the sync with the server.

AT Client Modules. AT client modules are middleware run-time libraries which enable the AT Client App to communicate with ME. AT Client Modules expose various interfaces which the AT Client App uses to execute an action.

ME Interface. This is the driver running in the operating system (OS) which abstracts the interface for ME. This provides a tunnel to send and receive a message to ME.

AT BIOS Module. This is a module which runs in the BIOS and provides a mechanism to the user so that the user can unlock the device. When the user boots a stolen device, this BIOS authentication module comes up and requires a password from the user to unlock the device. This module prevents a thief from accessing or using the device when the device is marked as stolen.

Intel ME. This is the FW module which runs in chipset. Intel ME works as the secured engine for AT and performs all the crypto related activities. ME stores all the information in regards to timer and keys which provide persistence of data regardless OS components are compromised or not.

2.2 Server Side Components

Server side components are required to run on the server where the user can control the device remotely and are made up of the following:

AT Server App. This is the front-end console for the user to create an account, manage devices and update account information. This is a web page where the user can login with proper credentials and see list of devices that has been activated with IATS. When a device is stolen, user can immediately go to this site from any device and mark the device as stolen. When the client running client components communicates with the server the client gets marked as stolen and gets disabled.

AT Server Module. AT Server module builds the business logic for AT in the server side. It establishes a secure connection with the client device to transmit AT related data to ME running in the client.

3 Intel Anti-Theft Service Operation

3.1 Asset Protection (Device Lockdown)

Asset protection is the primary feature of IATS. IATS disables the device when it is stolen. If the device is stolen and the owner of that device updates the state of that device to be stolen in IATS server then IATS server sends a secured disable message to the client when the client does sync with the server. If for some reason the device does not interact with the server for a preconfigured period then the ME running in the client disables the client. Once the device is marked as stolen and disabled by ME the only way it can be reused is if the user of the device enters a correct password at the BIOS authentication module. Otherwise the device will power up, display the BIOS authentication module screen and shutdowns. User's asset is protected by device lockdown and making it useless to thieves.

3.2 Data Protection (Secure Data Vault)

IATS provides data protection for user's confidential data. Client application uses a symmetric key to encrypt user data and store it locally on the device. The key is encrypted with a user given password and is stored in the ME. This way if a device is marked as stolen, the key which protects the encrypted data cannot be read in the OS and the data stays secured.

4 Intel Anti-Theft Service User Experience Design

The authors have joined the team at which time version 1.0 of IATS was already launched. The authors were tasked with improving the overall user experience of version 1.0 service. Specifically, understand users' interest and reaction to the activation and enrollment process. To evaluate the user experience, user experience assessment (UXA) study was conducted. UXA measures users' experience (likes, dislikes, thoughts, perceptions, expectations, desirability, and value) based on their interaction with the service [2]. Typically, UXA study is conducted by screening and recruiting real users from targeted consumer segmentation (12 participants were recruited); interacting with the service or usage performing a variety of tasks (performed activation/enrollment, lock/unlock PC, suspend/unsubscribe, and secure data vault tasks); in a focus group or one-on-one setting (one-on-one method was employed); assessing consumer experiences. UXA study allowed us to do critical direction setting to provide the experience that users wanted and cared such as:

- Re-designed the service website to improve ease of use (figure 2)
- Included "step" roadmap during installation process to guide users
- Consolidated activation and enrollment steps into one continuous installation process to remove ambiguity
- Removed user input decision points during installation process to improve efficiency
- Consolidated asset protection functions into one page to simplify management and access to the functions
- Tightly coupled asset and data protection functions to enable easy access (figure 3)

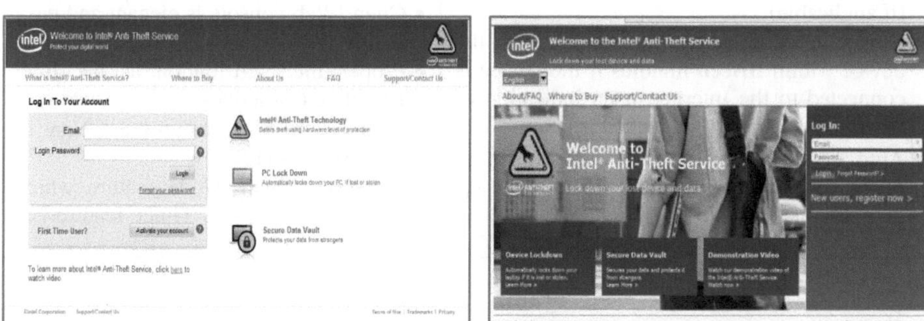

Fig. 2. Homepage of version 1.0 (left image) and of current version (right image)

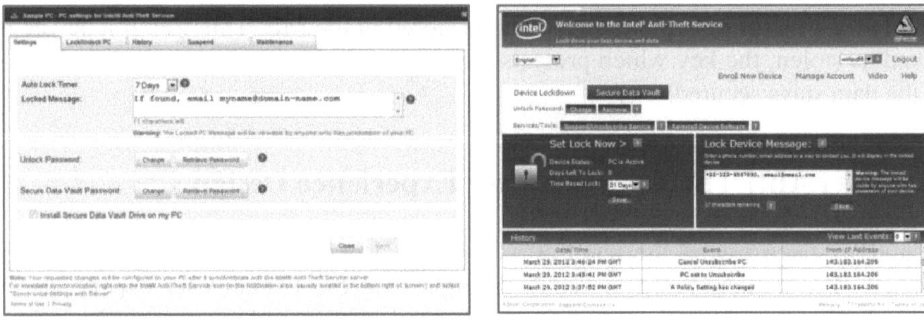

Fig. 3. Device lockdown and secure data vault function of version 1.0 (left image) and of current version (right image)

5 Conclusions

UXA study and heuristic evaluations confirmed that the re-designed IATS provided users with the user experience they wanted and valued. In addition to enhancing the user experience of IATS, quantitative and qualitative metrics (table 1) were identified and shared with industry partners integrating Intel AT into their product offerings. Future work includes integrating new usage models into IATS and Intel AT Services.

Table 1. Quantitative and qualitative metrics

Quantitative	Qualitative
• Device boot time impact of Intel AT Service should be **zero** • First time Intel AT Service activation and settings configuration should not take more than **five** steps • Intel AT Service software download/ installation should not be more than **one** click (if applicable) • Device Lockdown feature should lock the device within **fifteen** minutes if the device is connected to the Internet or an indication of when the device will be locked is given • Auto Lock Timer feature should default to **seven** days with provision for user to set between one and thirty days	• Simple and succinct description about Intel AT Service • Clear indication of Intel AT Service type and duration (free or subscription) • Automatic re-login into the user account immediately after account creation • Client/Web console is elegant and easy to use • Proper Intel Attribution as per Intel Branding Guidelines • Intel AT Service features are easy to understand and follow • Supports Repair Mode feature which disables Auto Lock Timer feature but protects files

References

1. Ponemon Institute: Airport insecurity: The case of missing and lost laptops (2008)
2. Beauregard, R., Younkin, A., Corriveau, P., Doherty, R., Salskov, E.: Assessing the quality of user experience. Intel. Technology Journal 11(1), 77–88 (2007)
3. Nielsen, J.: Usability Engineering, pp. 115–148. Academic Press, San Diego (1994)

Cyber Trust and Suspicion: A Human-Centric Approach

Hongbin Wang

School of Biomedical Informatics, University of Texas Health Science Center at Houston
Hongbin.Wang@uth.tmc.edu

Abstract. Conventional wisdom has regarded cyberspace security as a pure technology issue – sophisticated information techniques, tools, and policies are a must in order to detect and defeat threats. At a more foundational level, however, it is now clear that cyberspace security is also, if not more, a human-social phenomenon - how human operators, be they everyday internet users or national intelligence analysts, perceive and make sense of cyber events "closes the loop" and is therefore essential for the ultimate success (or failure) of cyberspace security. In this position paper we argue for the need of studying cyber trust and suspicion from a human-centric approach. Based on a principled abduction-based framework, the results will answer a full range of fundamental questions regarding cyber trust and suspicion.

Keywords: Cybersecurity, Trust and Suspicion, Human Belief Revision, Psychology, Computational Modeling.

1 Introduction

> *"... it's now clear this cyber threat is one of the most serious economic and national security challenges we face as a nation. It's also clear that we're not as prepared as we should be, as a government or as a country...."*
> *--- President Obama, 2009, on Securing Our Nation's Cyber Infrastructure*

With the rapid advances of information technology, cyberspace, a space of 0's and 1's, has become as real as our physical space. At the same time, cyberspace security is increasingly becoming a serious challenge [1]. Cyber attacks, such as identity theft, cooperate espionage, password sniffing, DDoS (Distributed Denial of Service), stuxnet, and email spamming, to name a few, have presented grave threats to human everyday life as well as national security. Conventional wisdom has regarded cyberspace security as a pure technology issue – sophisticated information techniques, tools, and policies are a must in order to detect and defeat threats (for defense) and develop and deliver attacks (for offense). At a more foundational level, however, it is now clear that cyberspace security is also, if not more, a human-social phenomenon - how human operators, be they everyday internet users or national intelligence analysts, perceive and make sense of cyber events "closes the loop" and is therefore essential for the ultimate success (or failure) of cyberspace security. Unfortunately, the significant role of the human operations in cyber security cycles has largely been ignored or less

C. Stephanidis (Ed.): Posters, Part II, HCII 2013, CCIS 374, pp. 759–763, 2013.

understood thus far. This is particularly true with regard to cyber trust and suspicion, two fundamental concepts in cyberspace security. Is the email just received trustworthy? Is the network activity pattern normal? The bottom line is that a cyber attack (e.g., worm or sabotage) is more damaging and harmful if it is stealthy and with disguise, and disasters occur when a non-trustworthy source is trusted. One central question in cyberspace security is therefore to understand how cyber trust and suspicion are represented, measured, monitored and managed. Any security-oriented algorithms and systems have to have some form of trust and suspicion management built-in, though often implicitly [2,3]. It is critical to realize that trust and suspicion are fundamentally psychological constructs and human traits. Automated trust and suspicion management systems through sophisticated computer algorithms are certainly desirable and have been quite successful [4]. We have to accept, however, that it is humans (but not machines) that trust and suspect, and that the computer algorithms have to be based on sound theorization of human trust and suspicion intuition in order to be useful. Such a theorization has the potential to make automated solutions even more powerful, robust, and realistic by inserting key human factors such as motivation, intention, attention, perception, belief, and emotion into the picture. In addition, in cases when computer algorithms are inconclusive, it is human operators' trust and suspicion insights and intuitions that often *connect the dots and close the loop*.

1.1 Cyber Trust and Suspicion

Trust and suspicion are fundamental concepts in many fields including philosophy, literature, law, and psychology [5,6]. They are often used to describe a person's relationship to another person, to a thing, to a factor/belief, or to nature. In ancient Greece, skepticism philosophers argued to assert nothing and suspend judgment. With the development of modernity and technology the concepts of trust and suspicion become even more relevant (rather than obsolete) [7]. In reality, for a piece of information, people can choose to trust, to distrust, or, very often, to be anywhere between. Being uncertain is simply a basic fact of human conditions.

Trust and suspicion are naturally loaded concepts. Dictionary definitions of "trust" link the term to "confidence", "reliability", "credibility", "predictability", and "benevolence". Trust is distinguished from "distrust" in that distrust is not equal to lack of trust, which is more related to the concept of "suspicion". Suspicion is a cognition or disposition of doubt, which often results from co-existence of conflicting beliefs or lack of evidence, and may lead to more vigilance and information seeking [8].

In a classic review of the concepts of trust and suspicion [9,10], Deutsch defines "trust" as follows: "An individual may be said to have trust in the occurrence of an event if he expects its occurrence and his expectation leads to behavior which he perceives to have greater negative motivational consequences if the expectation is not confirmed than positive motivational consequences if it is confirmed" [10]. And he defines "suspicion" as follows: "An individual may be said to be suspicious of the occurrence of an event if the disconfirmation of the expectation of the event's occurrence is preferred to its confirmation and if the expectation of its occurrence leads to behavior which is intended to reduce its negative motivational consequences" [10].

It is clear from these definitions that trust and suspicion are closely linked to motivations and subsequent decision making. A trust-minded person, compared to a suspicious person, is more willing to take risks in an uncertain environment and therefore is more likely to be caught off-guard if something goes wrong. It is in this sense trust and suspicion are relevant and important factors in cyberspace security [e.g., 3,11,12]. Cyberspace fundamentally alters the dynamics of inter-personal and human-machine relationships. Internet and social media allow never-met-before people to know each other and become "friends." Communications become so fast and cheap that everybody is exploded with information. In these situations, what do "trust" and "suspicion" mean? When we say we trust an email message, do we trust the message itself or trust the person who sends the message, or trust something else? We can use sophisticated machine learning techniques to mine past data and develop algorithms to tell us the precise likelihood and consequence of such trust in the past, however we may still be uncertain about the intention/implication of the message and the sender, and the action we should take. Needless to say, all these factors are interwoven and together they form the landscape of today's cyberspace security. A foundational understanding of the underlying dynamics of cyber trust and suspicion is clearly needed for achieving better cyber security. It can only be acquired when we close the loop between information systems and human operators and study their interactions.

1.2 Psychometrics of Cyber Trust and Suspicion

Not much work has been done in understanding how trust and suspicion work in cyberspace domains with humans in the loop. Relevant work often focuses on answering questions such as: What are they? How to measure them? What affects them? Can they be exploited [2,3,11-15]? Findings in these efforts are essential in our effort to develop a comprehensive computational model of cyber trust and suspicion that can capture the dynamics between human operators and systems. One major thrust is to find a credible way to measure trust or develop a cybertrust indicator [e.g., 13]. Jian *et al.* [3] explored the possibility of establishing an empirically tested (rather than theoretically driven) scale for measuring trust (human-human trust, human-machine trust, and trust in general) in computerized systems. Their results show that trust and distrust are better treated as the opposite ends of a single continuum. Barelka and colleagues [14] examined the relationship of trust and suspicion in IT domains. Using sophisticated statistical techniques, they found that trust in automation was best characterized by two orthogonal dimensions (trust and distrust) and trust and distrust were independent from IT suspicion. Interestingly, these results seem to be at odds with a recent functional brain imaging study, which shows that trust and distrust have distinct neural correlates in the brain [15]. More specifically, the study, using fMRI technology, shows that trust is associated with the brain's reward, prediction, and uncertainty areas (e.g., caudate, anterior paracingulate cortex, and the orbitofrontal cortex), while distrust is associated with the brain's intense emotions and fear of loss areas (e.g., the insular cortex and amygdala). The results support a 2-dimention view of trust-distrust relation and suggest that the brain uses distinct regions to represent trust (credibility and benevolence) and distrust (discredibility and malevolence).

Overall, the study provides insightful supporting evidence for the claim that trust and distrust are qualitatively distinct phenomena and distrust is not just the absence of trust.

2 Abductive Approach to Cyber Trust and Suspicion

The benevolence-malevolence dimension underlying trust indicates that a person who trusts is willing to be vulnerable to another person who is being trusted based on the belief that whatever the trustee does will not harm the trustor. Such a motivational or intentional inference is possible because of a critical human mental function called theory of mind (ToM), which refers to a person' ability to perceive and reason about others' mental states such as beliefs, desires, intentions, and feelings [16].

Inference for motivation or intention is therefore critical for cyber trust and suspicion. In an earlier effort we explored how such an inference can help a cyber attacker to deliver completely covert attacks [17]. Consider the following scenario: It is 12am and that John, an analyst, is working on a sensitive document on his computer and you have delivered a virus to his computer in order to take a peek. Ideally, you would like your operation is completely invisible to John, but unfortunately, one inevitable side effect of your virus is that John's computer becomes slow, which *John eventually notices and starts to become* ***suspicious***. Then John receives an alerting pop-out message informing him that the antivirus software on his computer has started scanning as scheduled and that so far no virus has been found. John now understands why his computer becomes slow, is relieved, and continues to work on his document, without realizing your peeking eyes.

Though hypothetical, this example highlights an important aspect of cyber trust and suspicion, which has to do with an understanding of how a human operator reasons and explains unexpected observations and if and when the operator becomes suspicious. We call this an abductive approach since it is based on a powerful inference type called abduction [18]. The general form of abduction is shown below,

A fact C is observed,
H can explain C;
Hence, H may be true.

Charniak and McDermott [19] characterize abduction as modus ponens turned backward. Modern researchers often regard abduction as a complex process of finding a best explanation for a set of observations [20,21]. Since "explaining" is an inevitable aspect of human everyday activities, abductive reasoning is almost ubiquitous. In battlefields, commanders have to infer the enemy's motivations based on observations and intelligence and then take proper actions. In cyberspace security, operators may have to infer if an attack has occurred given observations. We therefore argue that an abduction-based framework provides a psychologically plausible and computationally tractable solution for understanding and modeling cyber trust and suspicion.

Acknowledgments. This work is supported by an AFOSR grant (FA9550-12-1-0457, 26-0302-50-65) and an ONR grant (N00014-08-1-0042).

References

1. Andress, J., Winterfeld, S.: Cyber warfare: techniques, tactics and tools for security practitioners. Syngress, Waltham (2011)
2. Dzindolet, M.T., Peterson, S.A., Pomranky, R.A., Pierce, L.G., Beck, H.P.: The role of trust in automation reliance. Int. J. Hum.-Comput. Stud. 58, 697–718 (2003)
3. Jian, J., Bisantz, A.M., Drury, C.G.: Foundations for an Empirically Determined Scale of Trust in Automated Systems. International Journal of Cognitive Ergonomics 4, 53–71 (2000)
4. Liu, L., Chen, S., Yan, G., Zhang, Z.: BotTracer: Execution-based Bot-like Malware Detection. In: Proceedings of the 11th Information Security Conference, Taipei, China (2008)
5. Barber, B.: The logic and limits of trust. Rutgers University Press (1983)
6. Misztal, B.A.: Trust in Modern Societies: The Search for the Bases of Social Order. Polity Press, Cambridge (1996)
7. Sztompka, P.: Trust: Cultural Concerns. International Encyclopedia of the Social & Behavioral Sciences, 15913–15917 (2002)
8. Sinaceur, M.: Suspending judgment to createvalue: Suspicion and trust in negotiation. Journal of Experimental Social Psychology 46, 543–550 (2010)
9. Deutsch, M.: The effect of motivational orientation upon trust and suspicion. Human Relations 13, 123–139 (1960)
10. Deutsch, M.: Trust and suspicion. J. of Conflict Resolution 2, 265–279 (1958)
11. Bagherir, E., Ghorbani, A.A.: Exploiting trust and suspicion for real-time attack recognition in recommender applications. In: Etalle, S., Marsh, S. (eds.) Trust Management. IFIP, vol. 238, pp. 239–254. Springer, Heidelberg (2007)
12. Lee, J.D., See, K.A.: Trust in automation: designing for appropriate reliance. Hum Factors 46, 50–80 (2004)
13. Leon, P.G., Cranor, L., McDonald, A.M., McGuire, R.: Token Attempt: The Misrepresentation of Website Privacy Policies through the Misuse of P3P Compact Policy Tokens. CMU-CyLab-10-014, CMU (2010)
14. Lyons, J.B., Stokes, C.K., Eschleman, K.J., Alarcon, G.M., Barelka, A.J.: Trustworthiness and IT suspicion: an evaluation of the nomological network. Hum Factors 53, 219–229 (2011)
15. Dimoka, A.: What does the brain tell us about trust and distrust? evidence from a functional neuroimaging study. MIS Quarterly 34, 373–396 (2010)
16. Baron-Cohen, S.: Mindblindness: An essay on autism and theory of mind. MIT Press, Cambridge (1995)
17. Wang, H., Sun, Y.: An Abductive Approach to Covert Interventions. In: Proceedings of the 34th Annual Conf. of the Cognitive Science Society, Cognitive Science Society (2012)
18. Fann, K.T.: Peirce's theory of abduction. Martinus Nijhoff, The Hague (1970)
19. Charniak, E., McDermott, D.: Introduction to artificial intelligence. Addison-Wesley Publishing Company, Reading (1985)
20. Thagard, P.: Conceptual revolutions. Princeton University Press, Princeton (1992)
21. Josephson, J.R., Josephson, S.G.: Abductive inference: Computation, Philosophy, Technology. Cambridge University Press, Cambridge (1994)

Author Index

MIX
Papier aus verantwortungsvollen Quellen
Paper from responsible sources
FSC® C105338

If you have any concerns about our products,
you can contact us on
ProductSafety@springernature.com

In case Publisher is established outside the EU,
the EU authorized representative is:
Springer Nature Customer Service Center GmbH
Europaplatz 3, 69115 Heidelberg, Germany

Printed by Libri Plureos GmbH
in Hamburg, Germany